Tim Priest

Immune and Glial Regulation of Pain

Mission Statement of IASP Press®

IASP brings together scientists, clinicians, health care providers, and policy makers to stimulate and support the study of pain and to translate that knowledge into improved pain relief worldwide. IASP Press publishes timely, high-quality, and reasonably priced books relating to pain research and treatment.

Immune and Glial Regulation of Pain

Editors

Joyce A. DeLeo, PhD

Departments of Anesthesiology and Pharmacology,
Dartmouth-Hitchcock Medical Center, Lebanon,
New Hampshire, USA

Linda S. Sorkin, PhD

Department of Anesthesiology, University of California,
San Diego, California, USA

Linda R. Watkins, PhD

Department of Psychology, University of Colorado at Boulder,
Boulder, Colorado, USA

IASP PRESS® • SEATTLE

Library of Congress Cataloging-in-Publication Data

Immune and glial regulation of pain / editors, Joyce A. De Leo, Linda S. Sorkin, Linda R. Watkins.
Includes bibliographical references and index.
ISBN 978-0-931092-67-1 (softcover : alk. paper)
1. Pain--Pathophysiology. 2. Neuroimmunology. 3. Inflammation--Mediators. 4. Neuroglia. I. De Leo, Joyce A., 1960- II. Sorkin, Linda S., 1953- III. Watkins, Linda R., 1954- IV. International Association for the Study of Pain.
[DNLM: 1. Pain--metabolism. 2. Analgesics--therapeutic use. 3. Chronic Disease--drug therapy. 4. Glial Cell Line-Derived Neurotrophic Factors--physiology. 5. Pain--drug therapy. 6. Peripheral Nerves--metabolism. WL 704 I33 2007]

RB127.I46 2007
616'.0472--dc22

2007013915

Published by:

IASP Press
International Association for the Study of Pain
111 Queen Anne Ave N, Suite 501
Seattle, WA 98109-4955, USA
Fax: 206-283-9403
www.iasp-pain.org

Printed in the United States of America

Contents

Contributing Authors

Eric C. Beattie, PhD *Department of Neurosciences, California Pacific Medical Center Research Institute, San Francisco, California, USA*

Simon Beggs, PhD *University of Toronto Centre for the Study of Pain; Faculty of Dentistry, University of Toronto; Program in Neurosciences and Mental Health, Hospital for Sick Children, Toronto, Ontario, Canada*

Etty N. Benveniste, PhD *Department of Cell Biology, The University of Alabama at Birmingham, Birmingham, Alabama, USA*

David Busha, BS *Department of Psychology and Center for Neuroscience, University of Colorado at Boulder, Boulder, Colorado, USA*

W. Marie Campana, PhD *Department of Anesthesiology, University of California, San Diego, La Jolla, California, USA*

Earl Carstens, PhD *Section of Neurobiology, Physiology and Behavior, University of California, Davis, California, USA*

Jason M. Cuellar, PhD *Department of Anesthesia, Stanford University Medical Center, Stanford, California, USA*

Fernando Q. Cunha, MS, PhD *Department of Pharmacology, School of Medicine, Ribeirao Preto University, Sao Paulo, Brazil*

Thiago M. Cunha, MS *Department of Pharmacology, School of Medicine, Ribeirao Preto University, Sao Paulo, Brazil*

Joyce A. DeLeo, PhD *Department of Pharmacology and Toxicology, Dartmouth College, Hanover, New Hampshire, USA; Departments of Anesthesiology and Pharmacology, Dartmouth-Hitchcock Medical Center, Lebanon, New Hampshire, USA*

Biljana Djukic, PhD *Department of Pharmacology, University of North Carolina at Chapel Hill, Chapel Hill, North Carolina, USA*

Sérgio H. Ferreira, PhD *Department of Pharmacology, School of Medicine, Ribeirao Preto University, Sao Paulo, Brazil*

Todd A. Fiacco, PhD *Department of Pharmacology, University of North Carolina at Chapel Hill, Chapel Hill, North Carolina, USA*

Robert W. Gereau IV, PhD *Washington University Pain Center, Department of Anesthesiology, and Department of Anatomy and Neurobiology, Washington University School of Medicine, St. Louis, Missouri, USA*

Elisabeth Hansson, MD *Institute of Neuroscience and Physiology, Department of Clinical Neuroscience and Rehabilitation, The Sahlgrenska Academy at Göteborg University, Göteborg, Sweden*

Leif Hertz, MD, MSc *Department of Clinical Pharmacology, China Medical University, Shenyang, P.R. China*

Ping Hu, MB, MMed *Prince of Wales Medical Research Institute, Randwick, New South Wales, Australia*

Ru-Rong Ji, PhD *Pain Research Center, Department of Anesthesiology, Brigham and Women's Hospital and Harvard Medical School, Boston, Massachusetts, USA*

Ian N. Johnston, PhD *School of Psychology, University of Sydney, Sydney, New South Wales, Australia*

Jaro Karppinen, MD, MSc, PhD *Department of Musculoskeletal Disorders, Finnish Institute of Occupational Health, Oulu, Finland*

Michael L. LaCroix-Fralish, PhD *Department of Pharmacology and Toxicology, Dartmouth College, Hanover, New Hampshire, USA*

Robert H. LaMotte, PhD *Department of Anesthesiology, Yale University School of Medicine, New Haven, Connecticut, USA*

Annemarie Ledeboer, PhD *Department of Psychology and Center for Neuroscience, University of Colorado at Boulder, Boulder, Colorado, USA*

Halina Machelska, PhD *Clinic for Anesthesiology and Intensive Care, Charité University Medicine, Campus Benjamin Franklin, Berlin, Germany*

Steven F. Maier, PhD *Department of Psychology and Center for Neuroscience, University of Colorado at Boulder, Boulder, Colorado, USA*

Donald C. Manning, MD, PhD *Neurosciences Clinical Research and Development, Celgene Corporation, Summit, New Jersey, USA; Department of Anesthesiology and Pain Management, University of Virginia, Health Sciences Center, Charlottesville, Virginia, USA*

Ken D. McCarthy, PhD *Department of Pharmacology, University of North Carolina at Chapel Hill, Chapel Hill, North Carolina, USA*

Elspeth M. McLachlan, PhD, DSc, FAA *Prince of Wales Medical Research Institute, Randwick, New South Wales, Australia*

Erin D. Milligan, PhD *Department of Psychology and Center for Neuroscience, University of Colorado at Boulder, Boulder, Colorado, USA*

Patrick E. Monahan, BS *Department of Cell Biology, Neurobiology and Anatomy, Loyola University, Chicago, Maywood, Illinois, USA*

Maria Elena P. Morales, BS *Washington University Pain Center, Department of Anesthesiology, and Department of Anatomy and Neurobiology, Washington University School of Medicine, St. Louis, Missouri, USA*

Carlos A. Parada, MS, PhD *Department of Pharmacology, School of Medicine, Ribeirao Preto University, Sao Paulo, Brazil*

Stephen Poole, PhD *Division of Immunology and Endocrinology, National Institute for Biological Standards and Control, Potters Bar, Hertfordshire, United Kingdom*

Michael W. Salter, MD, PhD *University of Toronto Centre for the Study of Pain; Faculty of Dentistry, University of Toronto; Program in Neurosciences & Mental Health, Hospital for Sick Children, Toronto, Ontario, Canada*

Maria Schäfers, MD *Department of Neurology, University of Duisberg-Essen, Essen, Germany*

Yehuda Shavit, PhD *Department of Psychology, The Hebrew University of Jerusalem, Mount Scopus, Jerusalem, Israel*

Evan M. Sloane, BS *Department of Psychology and Center for Neuroscience, University of Colorado at Boulder, Boulder, Colorado, USA*

Claudia Sommer, MD *Department of Neurology, University of Würzburg, Würzburg, Germany*

Linda S. Sorkin, PhD *Department of Anesthesiology, University of California, San Diego, La Jolla, California, USA*

Christoph Stein, MD *Department of Anesthesiology, Free University of Berlin, Berlin, Germany*

David Stellwagen, PhD *Department of Psychiatry, Stanford Medical School, Palo Alto, California, USA*

Camilla I. Svensson, PhD *Department of Anesthesiology, University of California, San Diego, La Jolla, California, USA*

Vivianne L. Tawfik, PhD *Department of Pharmacology, Dartmouth Medical School, Hanover, New Hampshire, USA*

Tuan Trang, PhD *Program in Neurosciences & Mental Health, Hospital for Sick Children, Toronto, Ontario, Canada*

Nurcan Üçeyler, MD *Department of Neurology, University of Würzburg, Würzburg, Germany*

Waldiceu A. Verri, Jr., MS, PhD *Department of Pharmacology, School of Medicine, Ribeirao Preto University, Sao Paulo, Brazil*

Linda R. Watkins, PhD *Department of Psychology and Center for Neuroscience, University of Colorado at Boulder, Boulder, Colorado, USA*

R. Frederick Westbrook, PhD *School of Psychology, University of New South Wales, Sydney, New South Wales, Australia*

Fletcher A. White, PhD *Department of Cell Biology, Neurobiology and Anatomy, Loyola University, Chicago, Maywood, Illinois, USA; Department of Anesthesiology, Loyola University Health System, Maywood, Illinois, USA*

Gilly Wolf, MA *Department of Psychology, The Hebrew University of Jerusalem, Mount Scopus, Jerusalem, Israel*

Tony L. Yaksh, PhD *Department of Anesthesiology, University of California, San Diego, La Jolla, California, USA*

Raz Yirmiya, PhD *Department of Psychology, The Hebrew University of Jerusalem, Mount Scopus, Jerusalem, Israel*

Preface

We were very excited when the IASP Press asked us to consider editing a book on immune and glial regulation of pain. This once heretical view has now matured into an accepted subject in the pain field. This is evident by the exponential growth of publications over the last 15 years or so, directed at both basic science and clinical research. Conceivably, glial-immune cell interactions may be targeted to prevent or decrease neuronal sensitization, and hopefully reduce the clinical manifestations of persistent pain. This concept has been explored in developing strategies for the treatment of many neurodegenerative diseases. The pain field would also benefit from this approach as we understand more about the complexity of the synapse in both normal and pathological conditions.

In considering the layout of this book and potential contributors, we wanted to carefully balance providing an overview of glial and immune biology with representing high-quality research from many of the laboratories actively working in this field. The book is divided into seven distinct sections ranging from a broad overview of glial biology to the implications for clinical pain control. Part I provides an overview of immune and glial cells with contributions from two internationally renowned classical glial biologists, Lief Hertz (Chapter 2) and Etty Benveniste (Chapter 3). Linda Sorkin and Maria Schäfers (Chapter 1) set the stage for these chapters by describing peripheral immune cell function in the context of pain states.

Part II is devoted to immune-pain interactions at the periphery. Pain facilitation by proinflammatory cytokines at peripheral nerve terminals is described by Fernando Cunha, Sergio Ferreira, and colleagues (Chapter 4) and via retrograde signaling by Maria Schäfers, Claudia Sommer, and Linda Sorkin (Chapter 5). This section would not be complete without a chapter on the enhancement of opioid analgesia by peripheral immune activation from the laboratory of Halina Machelska and Christoph Stein (Chapter 6).

Part III is focused on the dorsal root ganglia (DRG) with contributions by Fletcher White and colleagues on chemokines as pain sensitizers (Chapter 7), electrophysiological evidence of increased nociceptive transmission in response to nerve root damage by Jason Cuellar and Earl Carstens (Chapter 8), and DRG signaling and erythropoietin as a protective agent by W. Marie Campana (Chapter 9). As discussed by Elspeth McLachlan and her colleague (Chapter 10), the recognition that DRG satellite cells and trafficking leukocytes into the DRG may directly affect primary afferent signaling enhances the complexity of glial-immune interactions and also provides an additional anatomical target for drug development.

Numerous studies have shown that astrocytes and microglia intimately participate in neuronal sensitization, not only via indirect mechanisms (release of cytokines and various neuroligands), but also more directly via release of glutamate and/or by evoking changes in synaptic ion homeostasis. The concept that the functional unit, which includes an astrocyte, a microglial cell, and pre- and postsynaptic neuronal terminals, is a critical contributor to the generation and maintenance of the end-product of excessive excitatory transmission in the synapse is the focus of Part IV. Maria Elena Morales and Robert Gereau (Chapter 11), Eric Beattie and David Stellwagen (Chapter 12), and Ken McCarthy and colleagues (Chapter 13) each address different aspects of glial regulation of neuronal functions relevant to pain.

In Part V, we move to the spinal cord and brain with an emphasis on intra-cellular signaling: steroid hormone regulation of astrocyte function by Michael LaCroix-Fralish and Joyce DeLeo (Chapter 14); ERK/MAPK described by Ru-Rong Ji (Chapter 15); ATP and microglia by Michael Salter and colleagues (Chapter 16); p38 MAP kinase by Camilla Svensson and colleagues (Chapter 17); and the use of an anti-inflammatory cytokine, IL-10, given intrathecally to control neuropathic pain behaviors by Erin Milligan, Linda Watkins, and colleagues (Chapter 18). An exciting explosion in the glial-immune field is the finding that similar players and interactions that have been demonstrated in chronic pain states also occur in morphine tolerance and opioid hyperalgesia. Part VI highlights these data with comprehensive chapters by Vivianne Tawfik and Joyce DeLeo (Chapter 19) and Yehuda Shavit and colleagues (Chapter 20). Finally, we end with the implications of these data for pain control in patients in Part VII. This connection has often met with some frustration in the ability to measure peripheral versus cerebrospinal fluid cytokine levels or in treatment variability in patients with chronic pain syndromes. Jaro Karppinen (Chapter 21), Donald Manning (Chapter 22), and Nurcan Üçeyler and Claudia Sommer (Chapter 23) each have summarized their findings in human populations that will lead the reader into contemplating future directions in this area.

Finally, we would like to thank IASP Press for choosing this subject as one of their timely books for the pain community. Their decision to publish a volume on this subject reflects the devotion of IASP to understanding the mechanisms of pain with the eventual realization of improved care of patients through the development of novel therapies, perhaps targeted to immune and glial cells.

We sincerely hope that both basic scientists and clinicians find this compilation of expertise informative as well as inspiring to generate new directions in this field.

JOYCE A. DELEO, PHD
LINDA S. SORKIN, PHD
LINDA R. WATKINS, PHD

Part I

Overview of Immune Cells and Glial Cells

Immune and Glial Regulation of Pain, edited by Joyce A. DeLeo, Linda S. Sorkin, and Linda R. Watkins, IASP Press, Seattle, © 2007.

1

Immune Cells in Peripheral Nerve

Linda S. Sorkin[a] and Maria Schäfers[b]

[a]Department of Anesthesiology University of California, San Diego, USA;
[b]Department of Neurology, University of Duisberg-Essen, Essen, Germany

Activation of cells within the innate immune system and the subsequent release of immunoactive agents in both the spinal cord and peripheral nervous system contribute to nociception and pain. The concept that neuroinflammation in the periphery, in the absence of overt nerve injury or axonal degeneration, is sufficient to induce pain took hold in the literature after Maves et al. (1993) showed a dose-response relationship between the amount of chromic gut suture used to create a focal nerve injury in the chronic constriction injury model and the degree of nociceptive behavior induced. Indeed, merely placing short lengths of chromic gut suture next to the exposed nerve, in the absence of overt nerve damage, was sufficient to induce hyperalgesia. Other more direct models of localized induced immune responses utilizing local administration of tumor necrosis factor α (TNF-α) (Wagner and Myers 1996a; Sorkin and Doom 2000), carrageenan, complete Freund's adjuvant (Eliav et al. 1999), or zymosan (Chacur et al. 2001) to the sciatic nerve trunk uniformly produce mechanical allodynia referred to the paw, with the only disagreement being the involvement of thermal hyperalgesia. In these models, a marked infiltration of immune cells to the nerve (Clatworthy and Grose 1999; Eliav et al. 1999; Gazda et al. 2001) occurred within several days of the initial insult. Combining an inflammatory substance with physical nerve injury enhances pain behavior (Clatworthy et al. 1995; Clatworthy and Grose 1999; Eliav et al. 1999). Concurrent suppression of the immune response with the corticosteroid dexamethasone (Clatworthy et al. 1995) or the immunosuppressant cyclosporine A (Bennett 1999) dose-dependently reduced both immune cell infiltration and nerve-injury-induced hyperalgesia.

Generation of a more global autoimmune neuritis that mimics Guillain-Barré syndrome—experimental autoimmune neuropathy (EAN)—involves focal infiltration of lymphocytes and macrophages into peripheral nerves, demyelination of axons, and release of several proinflammatory cytokines and immune cell chemotactic agents (Gold et al. 2000). A recent study found both mechanical allodynia and thermal hyperalgesia in animals with EAN (Moalem-Taylor et al. 2007). These behaviors both develop and dissipate in parallel to the motor deficits seen in EAN. Most of the anti-inflammatory therapies that are effective in EAN are also beneficial in neuropathic pain models (Zettl et al. 1994). Contributions of T cells and of the adaptive immune system are better understood in EAN than in the "classic" pain models (Jung et al. 1992; Zettl et al. 1994; Mäurer et al. 2002a,b). Thus, previous experiments performed on EAN animals may provide clues for further work in various pain models to help identify potential therapeutic targets.

Following sciatic nerve axotomy, encasing the injury site (nerve stump) in tubing to reduce contact with infiltrating immune cells and their products is sufficient to reduce axotomy-induced pain-like behavior (autotomy) for weeks while simultaneously reducing the number of mast cells, macrophages, and lymphocytes intercalated among the nerve fibers (Okuda et al. 2006). Cui et al. (2000) demonstrated a strong correlation between the presence of mechanical allodynia in three different nerve injury models and the degree of local macrophage/monocyte infiltration as well as the number of cells containing TNF-α and interleukin (IL)-6, but found no correlation with the number of IL-1-containing cells. Thus, there is strong circumstantial evidence to link the inflammatory milieu (immune cells and their secreted mediators) with continued immune cell infiltration, enhanced activity in nociceptive pathways, and pain behavior. These interactions can occur at all levels of the nerve from the peripheral terminals to the spinal nerve. Local tissue inflammation accompanied by increased numbers of activated immune cells and release of their contents is associated with excitation of peripheral nociceptive terminals and nociceptors en passant along the axons and with subsequently generated pain.

In the periphery, immune-competent cells include not only the infiltrating phagocytes (neutrophils and macrophages) and natural killer cells, but also mast cells, supportive Schwann cells along the axons, satellite cells in the dorsal root ganglia (DRG), fibroblasts, and epithelial cells. All of these cell types can secrete the mediators classically associated with immune cell activation (McMahon et al. 2005). While interruption or activation of several of these cell types is able to block or initiate pain behavior, respectively, it must be remembered that these cells form a functional cascade with multiple positive feedback loops. Alteration of any element will modulate the activity in most of the others. Some of these cells and their mediators are depicted schematically in Fig. 1. The adaptive immune system can also play a substantial role in activating nociceptive systems. However, due to the complexity of these pathways, this discussion will concentrate on cells of the innate immune system.

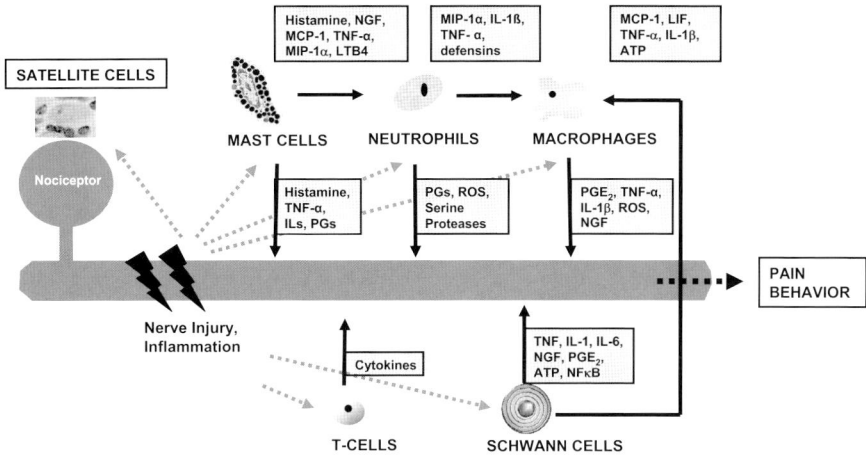

Fig. 1. Schematic of several peripheral immune cells and agents released by them. Arrows indicate actions on nerves or in attracting/activating other immune cells. Feedback loops are not indicated. Abbreviations: IL = interleukin, LIF = leukemia inhibitory factor, LTB4 = leukotriene B4, MCP-1 = monocyte chemoattractant protein-1, MIP-1α = macrophage inflammatory protein-1-α, NFκB = nuclear factor κB, NGF = nerve growth factor, PGs = prostaglandins, ROS = reactive oxygen species, TNF-α = tumor necrosis factor-α.

MAST CELLS

Mast cells are generated in the bone marrow and circulate in the blood in an immature form, maturing once they enter the tissue. They are activated by bacteria, viruses, neuropeptides such as substance P, endothelin-1, TNF-α, IL-1β, phospholipase A2 (PLA2), and prostaglandin E_2 (see Galli et al. 2005 for a comprehensive list). Resident mast cells are found along the axons in normal nerves (Zuo et al. 2003), and importantly, they are juxtaposed to "free nerve endings" in peripheral tissues (Kruger et al. 1985; Heppelmann et al. 1995), usually in the immediate vicinity of small blood vessels. Heppleman and colleagues (1995) proposed a functional relationship among these three elements, with releasable mast cell contents directly activating or sensitizing nociceptor terminals. Indeed, with the exception of bradykinin, mast cells release all of the components of the traditional inflammatory soup—such as histamine, serotonin (in rodents only), and prostaglandins—that is frequently used experimentally to sensitize nociceptor populations (Kessler et al. 1992; Davis et al. 1993; Galli et al. 2005). In addition, depending on the stimulus and environmental factors, mast cells can release a wide variety of proinflammatory cytokines including TNF-α, interleukins (IL-6 and IL-1β), tryptase and other serine proteases, nerve growth factor (NGF) (Bonini et al. 2003), free radicals, and arachadonic acid metabolites, generated by both cyclooxygenase (COX) and lipoxygenase

(Reynier-Rebuffel et al. 1992; Galli et al. 2005; Groneberg et al. 2005). These agents directly stimulate receptors on nociceptive terminals, axons, or cell bodies and may result in neuronal activation and/or sensitization. Administration of many of these factors intradermally (Cunha et al. 1992; Bennett et al. 1998; Evans et al. 2000; Kawabata et al. 2001), epineurially (Sorkin and Doom 2000), or endoneurially (Wagner and Myers 1996a; Ruiz et al. 2004; Zelenka et al. 2005) results in pain behavior. Some released factors, including leukotriene B4 (LTB4), NGF, and the chemokines monocyte chemoattractant protein-1 (MCP-1/CCL2) and macrophage inflammatory protein-1α (MIP-1α/CCL3), serve as chemoattractants and activators for other immune cells from the vasculature, most notably neutrophils and leukocytes (see Moalem and Tracey 2006 for review). Histamine can also aid in chemoattraction of leukocytes; it is also known to excite subtypes of nociceptive and chemosensitive itch afferent fibers.

Many of the agents released from mast cells cause vasodilation and increased vascular permeability, either directly or via neurogenic inflammation (Gamse et al. 1987; Raud 1989; Junger and Sorkin 2000). For instance, bradykinin, serotonin, and other algesic agents from the circulation also contribute to the inflammatory environment. Bradykinin degranulates mast cells and elicits further release of histamine (Reissmann et al. 2000). ATP-gated $P2X_7$ receptors are found on most peripheral immune cells, including mast cells, macrophages, and T-lymphocytes, as well as on activated Schwann cells (Kim et al. 2001; Chessell et al. 2005). While $P2X_7$ receptors apparently have little influence on measures of acute pain, their loss prevents the development of thermal and mechanical hyperalgesia following nerve injury and inhibits thermal hyperalgesia elicited by peripheral inflammation (Chessell et al. 2005). Mast cells that have been stimulated by tumor necrosis factor can express major histocompatibility complex (MHC) II molecules and may serve as antigen-presenting cells under certain conditions (Henz et al. 2001; Galli et al. 2005), although this is probably a minor determinant of subsequent adaptive responses.

Intraneural injection of compound 48/80 degranulates mast cells and markedly increases endoneurial fluid pressure and edema secondary to increased vascular permeability and migration of leukocytes into the endoneurial space (Powell et al. 1999). Similar findings, most notably mast cell degranulation, are seen in nerves of animals with EAN (Powell et al. 1983) and in the galactose intoxication model of diabetic neuropathy (Powell et al. 1981). Mast cells degranulate in response to partial ligation or crushing of the nerve, at and distal to the lesion (Olsson 1967). Degranulation of resident cells can begin within minutes, and degranulated mast cells are found in the nerve for weeks to months (Zuo et al. 2003). The total number of mast cells does not change at the site of sciatic nerve transection within the first 2 days (but see Zuo et al. 2003). However, 1–4 weeks after injury, mast cell density is greatly increased at the neuroma, and a steady increase has been reported over the first 6 months (Nennesmo and Reinholt 1986; Zochodne et al. 1994; Okuda et al. 2006). Many of these new mast cells are associated with the vascular plexus surrounding the neuroma. Mild mechanical trauma of the neuroma is sufficient to degranulate localized mast cells. Release of mast cell contents has been postulated to contribute to neuroma pain (Nennesmo and Reinholt 1986). Stabilization with cromoglycate reduces mast cell degranulation in partially ligated nerves and coincidently decreases injury-induced recruitment of neutrophils and macrophages as well as induction of hyperalgesia (Zuo et al. 2003). However, mast cells also might contribute to hyperalgesia via synthesis and release of eiconanoids, cytokines, and chemokines in the absence of overt degranulation (Moalem and Tracey 2006).

NEUTROPHILS

Neutrophils (polymorphonuclear leukocytes) are mature white blood cells that normally constitute approximately 60% of the circulating leukocytes. They are typically among the first circulating immune cells recruited to sites of inflammation or injury and thus form one of the earliest defense mechanisms of the innate immune system to microbial invasion. Indeed, neutrophil infiltration is frequently used as an index of acute dermal or muscle inflammation (Daemen et al. 1998; Sorkin et al. 2003). Neutrophils are attracted to inflammatory sites by various chemotactic factors: the early wave of influx during the first hour is probably mediated by both mast-cell- and endothelial-cell-derived platelet-activating factor (Gaboury et al. 1995), and other chemoattractants including proinflammatory cytokines (TNF-α), chemokines, and LTB4 become involved shortly thereafter. Several chemokines, including IL-8 and growth-related gene product α, are also released by activated neutrophils. Thus, once started, a positive feedback cycle with increasing neutrophil recruitment continues until anti-inflammatory mechanisms are triggered (Scapini et al. 2000).

Open wounds, carrageenan, zymosan, N-formyl peptides, delayed type hypersensitivity reactions, NGF, complement factor C5a and lipoxygenase products induce neutrophil infiltration into the skin (Bennett et al. 1998; Daemen et al. 1998 Dhabhar 2002; Sorkin et al. 2003). While some neutrophil attractants work independently in parallel, others apparently work in series. Interleukin-1 and histamine chemoattractant effects on neutrophils are independent of NGF, whereas NGF effects are upstream of LTB4 (Bennett et al. 1998). Interestingly, acute stress enhances neutrophil migration into tissue. In contrast, at least in some cases, chronic exposure to stress (perhaps including pain) inhibits neutrophil infiltration (Dhabhar 2002). The prevailing opinion is that the critical aspect of nerve injury leading to neutrophil infiltration and perhaps hyperalgesia is local neuroinflammation (Moalem and Tracey 2006) rather than retrograde transport or neurogenic inflammation as previously proposed.

Partial ligation of the sciatic nerve induces massive neutrophil infiltration at the injury site and immediately proximal and distal to the ligation within 8 hours; migration peaks at 12–24 hours and then dissipates over the following few days (Perkins and Tracey 2000; Zuo et al. 2003). More distally, neutrophil content of the nerve in the knee peaks 3 days after injury; no change in neutrophil number was seen in the plantar paw skin in this preparation (Perkins and Tracey 2000). However, earlier studies involving complete transection of the sciatic nerve (Levine et al. 1990) and chronic constriction injury of the nerve (Daemen et al. 1998) demonstrated neutrophil accumulation in the dorsal skin and muscle of the denervated hindpaw. Pretreatment with dexamethasone reduces neutrophil infiltration and thermal hyperalgesia (Clatworthy et al. 1995). Depletion of neutrophils prior to the surgery reduces the injury-induced thermal hyperalgesia and may delay induction of inflammation. However, neutrophil depletion does not diminish hyperalgesia after other mononuclear cells further down the cascade have been activated (Perkins and Tracey 2000).

Neutrophil activation has two components: (1) oxidative metabolism, the respiratory burst, which starts with assembly of nicotinamide adenine dinucleotide phosphate (NADPH) oxidase, followed by its activation in the plasma membrane, and (2) release of the preformed neutrophil granule contents (Witko-Sarsat et al. 2000). Activation of NADPH generates reactive oxygen species. Interleukins 1 and 6 and TNF-α prime pathways that also contribute to NADPH oxidase activation, and myeloperoxidase adds to the process by acting on H_2O_2 to produce reactive intermediaries including nitric oxide. This process is more pronounced in murine than in human neutrophils (Witko-Sarsat et al. 2000). Extracellular release of serine proteases found in neutrophil granules (see Pham 2006 for review) have a myriad of functions that could affect nociception, including cleavage of pro-IL-1 to its active form in the absence of specific converting enzymes and shedding of membrane-bound TNF-α to soluble TNF-α (Robache-Gallea et al. 1995; Coeshott et al. 1999), as well as catalysis of some protein-activated (PARs-2) receptors (Uehara et al. 2003; Sambrano et al. 2000) and activation of toll-like receptor 4 (Pham 2006).Defensins, antimicrobial peptides released by infiltrating neutrophils, are mitogenic for epithelial cells and fibroblasts (Murphy et al. 1993; Witko-Sarsat et al. 2000); other types of neutrophil granules contain PLA2 (Murphy et al. 1993). Neutrophils also synthesize a variety of pro- and anti-inflammatory cytokines, chemokines, and growth factors including TNF-α, IL-1α, IL-1β, IL-8, MIP-1α, MIP-1β, IL-1 receptor antagonist, and Fas ligand (see Cassatella 1999 for a more complete list). Chemokine production depends on the recent history of the neutrophil as well as on the specific nature of the stimulus. Many of the chemokines released are chemoattractants for a variety of immune cells including macrophages and Th1 lymphocytes. Thus, neutrophils have a central role in orchestrating the inflammatory response (Cassatella 1999). There is a strong correlation between neutrophil accumulation in the tissue and hyperalgesia following injection of proinflammatory mediators (Bennett et al. 1998; Fecho and Valtschanoff 2006). This association between peripheral neutrophil content and pain behavior can be seen in the differences between inbred Fisher and Lewis rats. Fisher rats exhibit higher basal levels of dermal neutrophils, as well as greater neutrophil influx, compared to Lewis rats after equivalent carrageenan injections (Fecho and Valtschanoff 2006). The Fisher rats also develop more intense carrageenan-induced mechanical and thermal hyperalgesia and paw swelling. While this pattern continues for thermal hyperalgesia in a nerve injury model, the converse is true for mechanical stimulation. Lewis, but not Fischer, rats develop nerve-injury-induced mechanical allodynia and hyperalgesia (Fecho and Valtschanoff 2006).

Neutrophil accumulation in the tissue by itself is not sufficient to elicit pain behavior because neither attraction of neutrophils with glycogen nor injection of supernatant from nonactivated neutrophils is sufficient to induce hyperalgesia. However, injection of the lipid soluble fraction of supernatant from activated neutrophils causes a marked sensitivity to mechanical stimulation (Levine et al. 1985). Hyperalgesia produced by this pathway is cyclooxygenase independent.

Intradermal injection of NGF, LTB4, and other neutrophil attractants and activators including complement factor C5a induces mechanical and thermal hyperalgesia (Levine et al. 1984, 1985; Bennett et al. 1998; Schuligoi 1998). NGF-induced hyperalgesia is dependent on LTB4, given that pretreatment with a 5-lipoxygenase inhibitor prevents the pain behavior (Amann et al. 1996). The time course of the sensitization/accumulation is rapid, with onset of C5a -induced hyperalgesia as early as 10 minutes after injection (Levine et al. 1985). Sensitization is at the level of the peripheral terminal; the vast majority of C nociceptors are profoundly sensitized by LTB4, and there is a strong correlation between LTB4 and capsaicin sensitivity (Martin et al. 1988; Martin 1990). Systemic depletion of neutrophils (Levine et al. 1985; Bennett et al. 1998) or prevention of neutrophil accumulation with colchicine (Schuligoi 1998) blocks LTB4-, C5a-, and NGF-induced hyperalgesia.

MACROPHAGES

Macrophages (from the Greek *macros* and *phagein,* meaning "big eaters") are phagocytic leukocytes that participate in both innate and acquired immune systems. In peripheral nerves, resident macrophages are supplemented by infiltrating activated hematogenous macrophages (Bendszus and Stoll 2003) via the endoneurial vasculature after a variety of insults, ranging from neuroinflammation in the absence of Wallerian degeneration triggered by local application of Freund's adjuvant to the nerve trunk (Eliav et al. 1999) to all examined nerve injuries involving axotomy and injured Schwann cells. Seven days after axotomy, 85% of the macrophages found in the nerve are activated and contain axonal debris and phagocytosed myelin (Perrin et al. 2005). When degeneration is ongoing, macrophages are frequently found between openings in the basal laminae and cytoplasm of Schwann cells, in close proximity to the axons (Frisen et al. 1993).

Neutrophils release several substances that recruit macrophages to an injury or site of neuroinflammation. These substances include MIP-1α and IL-1β (Witko-Sarsat et al. 2000). Endoneurial administration of antibodies against MIP-1α and IL-1β suppresses myelin clearance and reduces both the total number of macrophages and the number of phagocytic macrophages found in an injured nerve (Perrin et al. 2005). The number of infiltrated macrophages and the degree of nerve degeneration both peak at the time of maximal hyperalgesia (Myers et al. 1996). Activated Schwann cells produce and release MCP-1 (Rutkowski et al. 1999) and leukemia inhibitory factor (LIF) (Tofaris et al. 2002). Blockade of either of these two factors substantially reduces macrophage infiltration (Tofaris et al. 2002; Perrin et al. 2005), and intraplantar injection of MCP-1 induces mechanical allodynia (Abbadie et al. 2003). Mice lacking chemotactic cytokine receptor 2 (CCR2), the receptor for MCP-1, do not develop mechanical allodynia following partial sciatic nerve ligation and have reduced inflammation-induced mechanical allodynia. Inflammation-induced thermal hyperalgesia is normal in these mice, as are acute measures of thermal sensitivity (Abbadie et al. 2003).

Depletion of circulating monocytes decreases thermal hyperalgesia following partial sciatic nerve ligation (Liu et al. 2000). However, Rutkowski et al. (2000), employing an L5 spinal nerve transection model and using mechanical hyperalgesia as their outcome measure, have disputed this observation. Chronic constriction injury in mice with delayed macrophage recruitment and Wallerian degeneration (C57BL/WLD) results in a greatly reduced thermal hyperalgesia temporally associated with reduced numbers of phagocytic cells in the injured nerve (Myers et al. 1996; Sommer and Schäfers 1998). The duration of mechanical allodynia was significantly prolonged in C57BL/WLD mice in accordance with the delay in regeneration of sensory nerve fibers in these mice (Sommer and Schäfers 1998). Although these studies seem to indicate that infiltrating macrophages contribute to thermal, but not mechanical, postinjury pain states, the complete answer is not as clear. Ramer et al. (1997) reported reductions of both thermal hyperalgesia and mechanical allodynia using the same procedure on the C57BL/WLD mice, and Cui et al. (2000) have shown a strong correlation between the number of macrophages in a nerve and withdrawal threshold to mechanical stimulation in both the chronic constriction injury and partial sciatic ligation models of neuropathic pain.

Macrophages produce many algogenic substances that can directly activate or sensitize nociceptors, including prostaglandins, lipoxygenases, TNF-α, IL-1β, and reactive oxygen species (Nathan 1987; Shamash et al. 2002). Released ATP binds to $P2X_7$ receptors and activates a cryopyrin (also known as NALP3)-containing inflammasome which, in turn, activates caspase-1 (Martinon et al. 2002). Caspase-1 cleaves pro-IL-1β to form biologically active IL-1β (Hogquist et al. 1991), which results in downstream increases in expression of COX-2 and nitric oxide. Cropyrin and activated inflammasomes are also necessary intermediaries for toll-like receptor activation-induced release of IL-1β and IL-18, but are not required for nuclear factor (NF)-κB signaling (Mariathasan et al. 2006). After injury, TNF-α colocalizes in macrophages with the matrix metalloproteinase MMP-9 and TNF-α-converting enzyme (TACE) (Shubayev and Myers 2002). Macrophages also synthesize components of the complement cascade and mitogens for Schwann cells (Baichwal et al. 1988) and induce synthesis of NGF in other non-neuronal cell types as well as creating NGF themselves (Heumann et al. 1987). In vitro, these actions are increased by substance P, which induces oxidative bursts in macrophages with enhanced release of oxygen free radicals and cytokines (Hartung and Toyka 1983). Interestingly, macrophages in injured nerves begin to express $α_{2A}$-adrenergic receptors, and their activation results in long-lasting amelioration of mechanical hyperalgesia following partial sciatic nerve ligation (Lavand'homme et al. 2002), indicating that the activated macrophage is a potential target for local clonidine treatment.

SCHWANN CELLS

Schwann cells in the peripheral nervous system are traditionally regarded as support cells that release trophic factors and provide electrical insulation to the axons that they envelop. Injury to a myelinated axon initiated by disease or physical trauma results in activation of these cells and their increased expression and release of a wide range of proinflammatory substances and growth factors and can initiate changes in receptor expression and in ion channels. TNF-α is likely to be a major player in the process of Schwann cell activation after injury (Myers et al. 2006), possibly via receptor-mediated activation of NFκB, via c-jun, and via increased expression of the p75 NGF receptor (Bonetti et al. 2000). Increased signal for NFκB is found in Schwann cell nuclei of patients with chronic inflammatory demyelinating polyradiculoneuritis (Bonetti et al. 2000). Nerve injury induces a modest increase in Na^+ channels in Schwann cells (Devor et al. 1993). The receptor GPR7 is expressed on Schwann cells in humans and rats; expression increases in patients with either immune-mediated or inflammatory neuropathies, many of which are painful, as well as in rats with either physical injuries to the nerve or EAN (Zaratin et al. 2005). Endogenous agonists to this receptor (NPB, NPW) are postulated to have a role in pain signaling. In vitro, Schwann cells release ATP in response to extracellular glutamate. This release appears to be AMPA-receptor mediated (Liu and Bennett 2003). However, in vivo, Schwann cells are reported to have low levels of NMDA and kainate receptors, but not of AMPA receptors (Kinkelin et al. 2000). Thus, the physiological relevance of this mechanism is unknown.

Any injury that results in some degree of Wallerian generation results in increased expression and release of the cytokines TNF-α, IL-1, IL-6, and IL-8 in Schwann cells (Bergsteinsdottir et al. 1991; Bolin et al. 1995; Wagner and Myers 1996b; Rutkowski et al. 1999; Shubayev and Myers 2000; Shamash et al. 2002; Tofaris et al. 2002). Expression of TNF-α converting enzyme, TACE, increases as well; as its name implies, TACE aids in the conversion of inactive, membrane-bound TNF-α to mature, soluble TNF-α (Shubayev and Myers 2002). IL-6 induces increased expression of LIF, while IL-1 and LIF induce Schwann cells to synthesize the monocyte chemoattractant MCP-1 (Tofaris et al. 2002). IL-1 via LIF increases NK-1-receptor mRNA in sympathetic ganglia explants (Ludlam et al. 1995) as well as inducible nitric oxide synthase (Levy et al. 1999). Physical trauma also results in the release of prostaglandin E_2 and NGF (Obata et al. 2002).

Schwann cell release of chemokines and cytokines is blocked by treatment with anti-inflammatory drugs, including dexamethasone (Rutkowski et al. 1999). Injury-induced increases of TNF-α in the nerve and hyperalgesia are both blocked by pretreatment with the hematopoietic cytokine erythropoietin (EPO) through its action on EPO receptors (Campana et al. 2006), which are localized to neurons and Schwann cells (Li et al. 2005). Following nerve injury, Schwann cell EPO receptors increase, while those in the axoplasm decrease (Campana and Myers 2001). Physical trauma also activates extracellular signal-related kinase (ERK1/2) in Schwann cells with a significantly slower onset and longer time course than is seen in the neurons. Following compression of the dorsal root ganglia, phospho-ERK increases starting at 1 hour after injury and remains elevated for the 24 hours of observation (Doya et al. 2005). Nerve-injury-induced increases in Schwann cell phospho-ERK are blocked by antagonizing the Janus kinase (JAK)-2 pathway (Li et al. 2005).

Schwann cells do not constitutively express MHC II either under normal cell culture conditions or in vivo. However, if Schwann cells are co-cultured with activated T cells, induction of MHC II will occur in most cells; quiescent T cells are not sufficient (Kingston et al. 1989). In vivo, local injection of bacterial antigens or nerve crush is sufficient to induce MHC II expression in a subpopulation of Schwann cells (Bergsteinsdottir et al. 1992).

SATELLITE CELLS

Satellite cells are glia in the DRG that envelop the soma of the sensory neurons. As these are small cells, it takes several satellite cells to cover each neuron. This set of glia is postulated to form a functional unit that supports and controls the environment for its neuronal cell body (Hanani 2005). Many (about 1 in 5) satellite cells are functionally coupled via gap junctions (Hanani et al. 2002). After axotomy, the number of gap junctions increases, and satellite cells surrounding different neurons become coupled to each other (Hanani et al. 2002). Similar to astrocytes in the CNS, satellite cells are thought to locally buffer changes in the extracellular milieu by taking up excess ions and neurotransmitters. While research has been minimal, it is known that satellite cells possess at least two types of K^+ channels (Cherkas et al. 2004) as well as both glutamate and γ-aminobutyric acid (GABA) transporters (Berger and Hediger 2000). They also express a diverse population of receptors under basal conditions, including those for P2Y (Weick et al. 2003), IL-1 (Copray et al. 2001), acetylcholine (muscarinic receptors) (Bernardini et al. 1999), and endothelin B (Pomonis et al. 2001). Endothelin B receptors are located on satellite cells and nonmyelinating Schwann cells and are not found on DRG neurons (Pomonis et al. 2001). Loss of functional endothelin B receptors using either a specific antagonist or knockout mice prevents inflammatory pain and significantly reduces neutrophil infiltration (Griswold et al. 1999).

After injury to the nerve, satellite cells proliferate, undergo hypertrophy, and increase their expression of glial markers (Woodham et al. 1989; Ohtori et al. 2004), TNF-α (Ohtori et al. 2004; Takahashi et al. 2006), TNF receptor 1 (Ohtori et al. 2004), NGF and NT3 (Zhou et al. 1999), transforming growth factor-α (Xian and Zhou 1999), and several cell adhesion molecules (Zhang et al. 2000). Upregulation of TNF-α in satellite cells is also seen after injury to the ventral root, indicating that neuroinflammation rather that physical damage to the axons is sufficient (Xu et al. 2006). Interestingly, several substances, including TNF-α, are increased in satellite cells contralateral to the injury. Binding and internalization of NGF by satellite cells has been postulated to decrease extracellular NGF levels and thus to control dendritic growth and to create an "NGF depository" for future release (Hanani 2005). Increases in NGF elicit increases in phospho-ERK in satellite cells (Averill et al. 2001), as does topical application of TNF-α to the nerve root (Takahashi et al. 2006).

CONCLUSIONS

The innate immune system is an integral player in the generation of pain in the periphery. Various cell types participate in carefully choreographed roles culminating in release of cytokines, other inflammatory mediators, and neuroactive agents. This process results in some degree of neuroinflammation and leads to pain perception. Understanding the multiple steps of this interplay will result in the development of new therapies and better treatments for chronic pain.

ACKNOWLEDGMENTS

We would like to thank Dr. Gary Firestein for reading an early version of this manuscript.

REFERENCES

Abbadie C, Lindia JA, Cumiskey AM, et al. Impaired neuropathic pain responses in mice lacking the chemokine receptor CCR2. *Proc Natl Acad Sci USA* 2003; 100:7947–7952.

Amann R, Schuligoi R, Lanz I, Peskar BA. Effect of a 5-lipoxygenase inhibitor on nerve growth factor-induced thermal hyperalgesia in the rat. *Eur J Pharmacol* 1996; 306:89–91.

Averill S, Delcroix JD, Michael GJ, et al. Nerve growth factor modulates the activation status and fast axonal transport of ERK 1/2 in adult nociceptive neurones. *Mol Cell Neurosci* 2001; 18:183–196.

Baichwal RR, Bigbee JW, DeVries GH. Macrophage-mediated myelin-related mitogenic factor for cultured Schwann cells. *Proc Natl Acad Sci USA* 1988; 85:1701–1705.

Bendszus M, Stoll G. Caught in the act: in vivo mapping of macrophage infiltration in nerve injury by magnetic resonance imaging. *J Neurosci* 2003; 23:10892–10896.

Bennett GJ. Does a neuroimmune interaction contribute to the genesis of painful peripheral neuropathies? *Proc Natl Acad Sci USA* 1999; 96:7737–7738.

Bennett G, al-Rashed S, Hoult JR, Brain SD. Nerve growth factor induced hyperalgesia in the rat hind paw is dependent on circulating neutrophils. *Pain* 1998; 77:315–322.

Berger UV, Hediger MA. Distribution of the glutamate transporters GLAST and GLT-1 in rat circumventricular organs, meninges, and dorsal root ganglia. *J Comp Neurol* 2000; 421:385–399.

Bergsteinsdottir K, Kingston A, Mirsky R, Jessen KR. Rat Schwann cells produce interleukin-1. *J Neuroimmunol* 1991; 34:15–23.

Bergsteinsdottir K, Kingston A, Jessen KR. Rat Schwann cells can be induced to express major histocompatibility complex class II molecules in vivo. *J Neurocytol* 1992; 21:382–390.

Bernardini N, Levey AI, Augusti-Tocco G. Rat dorsal root ganglia express m1-m4 muscarinic receptor proteins. *J Peripher Nerv Syst* 1999; 4:222–232.

Bolin LM, Verity AN, Silver JE, Shooter EM, Abrams JS. Interleukin-6 production by Schwann cells and induction in sciatic nerve injury. *J Neurochem* 1995; 64:850–858.

Bonetti B, Valdo P, Stegagno C, et al. Tumor necrosis factor alpha and human Schwann cells: signalling and phenotype modulation without cell death. *J Neuropathol Exp Neurol* 2000; 59:74–84.

Bonini S, Rasi G, Bracci-Laudiero ML, Procoli A, Aloe L. Nerve growth factor: neurotrophin or cytokine? *Int Arch Allergy Immunol* 2003; 131:80–84.

Campana WM, Myers RR. Erythropoietin and erythropoietin receptors in the peripheral nervous system: changes after nerve injury. *FASEB J* 2001; 15:1804–1806.

Campana WM, Li X, Shubayev VI, et al. Erythropoietin reduces Schwann cell TNF-alpha, Wallerian degeneration and pain-related behaviors after peripheral nerve injury. *Eur J Neurosci* 2006; 23:617–626.

Cassatella MA. Neutrophil-derived proteins: selling cytokines by the pound. *Adv Immunol* 1999; 73:369–509.

Chacur M, Milligan ED, Gazda LS, et al. A new model of sciatic inflammatory neuritis (SIN): induction of unilateral and bilateral mechanical allodynia following acute unilateral peri-sciatic immune activation in rats. *Pain* 2001; 94:231–244.

Cherkas PS, Huang TY, Pannicke T, et al. The effects of axotomy on neurons and satellite glial cells in mouse trigeminal ganglion. *Pain* 2004; 110:290–298.

Chessell IP, Hatcher JP, Bountra C, et al. Disruption of the P2X7 purinoceptor gene abolishes chronic inflammatory and neuropathic pain. *Pain* 2005; 114:386–396.

Clatworthy AL, Grose E. Immune-mediated alterations in nociceptive sensory function in *Aplysia californica*. *J Exp Biol* 1999; 202:623–630.

Clatworthy AL, Illich PA, Castro GA, Walters ET. Role of peri-axonal inflammation in the development of thermal hyperalgesia and guarding behavior in a rat model of neuropathic pain. *Neurosci Lett* 1995; 184:5–8.

Coeshott C, Ohnemus C, Pilyavskaya A, et al. Converting enzyme-independent release of tumor necrosis factor alpha and IL-1beta from a stimulated human monocytic cell line in the presence of activated neutrophils or purified proteinase 3. *Proc Natl Acad Sci USA* 1999; 96:6261–6266.

Copray JC, Mantingh I, Brouwer N, et al. Expression of interleukin-1 beta in rat dorsal root ganglia. *J Neuroimmunol* 2001; 118:203–211.

Cui J-G, Holmin S, Mathiesen T, Meyerson B, Linderoth B. Possible role of inflammatory mediators in tactile hypersensitivity in rat models of mononeuropathy. *Pain* 2000; 88:239–248.

Cunha FQ, Poole S, Lorenzetti BB, Ferreira SH. The pivotal role of tumour necrosis factor alpha in the development of inflammatory hyperalgesia. *Br J Pharmacol* 1992; 107:660–664.

Daemen MA, Kurvers HA, Kitslaar PJ, et al. Neurogenic inflammation in an animal model of neuropathic pain. *Neurol Res* 1998; 20:41–45.

Davis K, Meyer R, Campbell J. Chemosensitivity and sensitization of nociceptive afferents that innervate the hairy skin of monkey. *J Neurophysiol* 1993; 69:1071–1081.

Devor M, Govrin-Lippmann R, Angelides K. Na+ channel immunolocalization in peripheral mammalian axons and changes following nerve injury and neuroma formation. *J Neurosci* 1993; 13:1976–1992.

Dhabhar FS. Stress-induced augmentation of immune function—the role of stress hormones, leukocyte trafficking, and cytokines. *Brain Behav Immun* 2002; 16:785–798.

Doya H, Ohtori S, Takahashi K, et al. Extracellular signal-regulated kinase mitogen-activated protein kinase activation in the dorsal root ganglion (DRG) and spinal cord after DRG injury in rats. *Spine* 2005; 30:2252–2256.

Eliav E, Herzberg U, Ruda MA, Bennett GJ. Neuropathic pain from an experimental neuritis of the rat sciatic nerve. *Pain* 1999; 83:169–182.

Evans AR, Junger H, Southall MD, et al. Isoprostanes, novel eicosanoids that produce nociception and sensitize rat sensory neurons. *J Pharmacol Exp Ther* 2000; 293:912–920.

Fecho K, Valtschanoff JG. Acute inflammatory and neuropathic pain in lewis and Fischer rats. *J Neuroendocrinol* 2006; 18:504–513.

Frisen J, Risling M, Fried K. Distribution and axonal relations of macrophages in a neuroma. *Neuroscience* 1993; 55:1003–1013.

Gaboury JP, Johnston B, Niu XF, Kubes P. Mechanisms underlying acute mast cell-induced leukocyte rolling and adhesion in vivo. *J Immunol* 1995; 154:804–813.

Galli SJ, Nakae S, Tsai M. Mast cells in the development of adaptive immune responses. *Nat Immunol* 2005; 6:135–142.

Gamse R, Posch M, Saria A, Jancso G. Several mediators appear to interact in neurogenic inflammation. *Acta Physiol Hung* 1987; 69:343–354.

Gazda LS, Milligan ED, Hansen MK, et al. Sciatic inflammatory neuritis (SIN): behavioral allodynia is paralleled by peri-sciatic proinflammatory cytokine and superoxide production. *J Peripher Nerv Syst* 2001; 6:111–129.

Gold R, Hartung HP, Toyka KV. Animal models for autoimmune demyelinating disorders of the nervous system. *Mol Med Today* 2000; 6:88–91.

Griswold DE, Douglas SA, Martin LD, et al. Endothelin B receptor modulates inflammatory pain and cutaneous inflammation. *Mol Pharmacol* 1999; 56:807–812.

Groneberg DA, Serowka F, Peckenschneider N, et al. Gene expression and regulation of nerve growth factor in atopic dermatitis mast cells and the human mast cell line-1. *J Neuroimmunol* 2005; 161:87–92.

Hanani M. Satellite glial cells in sensory ganglia: from form to function. *Brain Res Brain Res Rev* 2005; 48:457–476.

Hanani M, Huang TY, Cherkas PS, Ledda M, Pannese E. Glial cell plasticity in sensory ganglia induced by nerve damage. *Neuroscience* 2002; 114:279–283.

Hartung HP, Toyka KV. Activation of macrophages by substance P: induction of oxidative burst and thromboxane release. *Eur J Pharmacol* 1983; 89:301–305.

Henz BM, Maurer M, Lippert U, Worm M, Babina M. Mast cells as initiators of immunity and host defense. *Exp Dermatol* 2001; 10:1–10.

Heppelmann B, Messlinger K, Neiss WF, Schmidt RF. Fine sensory innervation of the knee joint capsule by group II and group IV nerve fibers in the cat. *J Comp Neurol* 1995; 51:415-428.

Heumann R, Lindholm D, Bandtlow C, et al. Differential regulation of mRNA encoding nerve growth factor and its receptor in rat sciatic nerve during development, degeneration, and regeneration: role of macrophages. *Proc Natl Acad Sci USA* 1987; 84:8735–8739.

Hogquist KA, Nett MA, Unanue ER, Chaplin DD. Interleukin 1 is processed and released during apoptosis. *Proc Natl Acad Sci USA* 1991; 88:8485–8489.

Jung S, Kramer S, Schluesener HJ, et al. Prevention and therapy of experimental autoimmune neuritis by an antibody against T cell receptors-alpha/beta. *J Immunol* 1992; 148:3768–3775.

Junger H, Sorkin LS. Nociceptive and inflammatory effects of subcutaneous TNF. *Pain* 2000; 85:145–151.

Kawabata A, Kawao N, Kuroda R, et al. Peripheral PAR-2 triggers thermal hyperalgesia and nociceptive responses in rats. *Neuroreport* 2001; 12:715–719.

Kessler W, Kirchhoff C, Reeh PW, Handwerker HO. Excitation of cutaneous afferent nerve endings in vitro by a combination of inflammatory mediators and conditioning effect of substance P. *Exp Brain Res* 1992; 91:467–476.

Kim M, Spelta V, Sim J, North RA, Surprenant A. Differential assembly of rat purinergic P2X7 receptor in immune cells of the brain and periphery. *J Biol Chem* 2001; 276:23262–23267.

Kingston AE, Bergsteinsdottir K, Jessen KR, et al. Schwann cells co-cultured with stimulated T cells and antigen express major histocompatibility complex (MHC) class II determinants without interferon-gamma pretreatment: synergistic effects of interferon-gamma and tumor necrosis factor on MHC class II induction. *Eur J Immunol* 1989; 9:177–183.

Kinkelin I, Brocker EB, Koltzenburg M, Carlton SM. Localization of ionotropic glutamate receptors in peripheral axons of human skin. *Neurosci Lett* 2000; 283:149–152.

Kruger L, Sampogna SL, Rodin BE, et al. Thin-fiber cutaneous innervation and its intraepidermal contribution studied by labeling methods and neurotoxin treatment in rats. *Somatosens Res* 1985; 2:335–356.

Lavand'homme PM, Ma W, De Kock M, Eisenach JC. Perineural alpha$_{2A}$-adrenoceptor activation inhibits spinal cord neuroplasticity and tactile allodynia after nerve injury. *Anesthesiology* 2002; 97:972–980.

Levine JD, Lau W, Kwait G, Goetzl EJ. Leukotriene B4 produces hyperalgesia that is dependent on polymorphinuclear leukocytes. *Science* 1984; 225:743–745.

Levine JD, Gooding J, Donatoni P, Borden L, Goetzl EJ. The role of the polymorphonuclear leukocyte in hyperalgesia. *J Neurosci* 1985; 5:3025–3029.

Levine JD, Coderre TJ, Covinsky K, Basbaum AI. Neural influences on synovial mast cell density in rat. *J Neurosci Res* 1990; 26:301–307.

Levy D, Hoke A, Zochodne DW. Local expression of inducible nitric oxide synthase in an animal model of neuropathic pain. *Neurosci Lett* 1999; 260:207–209.

Li X, Gonias SL, Campana WM. Schwann cells express erythropoietin receptor and represent a major target for Epo in peripheral nerve injury. *Glia* 2005; 51:254–265.

Liu GJ, Bennett MR. ATP secretion from nerve trunks and Schwann cells mediated by glutamate. *Neuroreport* 2003; 14:2079–2083.

Liu T, van Rooijen N, Tracey DJ. Depletion of macrophages reduces axonal degeneration and hyperalgesia following nerve injury. *Pain* 2000; 86:25–32.

Ludlam WH, Chandross KJ, Kessler JA. LIF-and IL-1 beta-mediated increases in substance P receptor mRNA in axotomized, explanted or dissociated sympathetic ganglia. *Brain Res* 1995; 685:12–20.

Mariathasan S, Weiss DS, Newton K, et al. Cryopyrin activates the inflammasome in response to toxins and ATP. *Nature* 2006; 440:228–232.

Martin HA. Leukotriene B4 induced decrease in mechanical and thermal thresholds of C-fiber mechanoreceptors in rat hairy skin. *Brain Res* 1990; 509:273–279.

Martin HA, Basbaum AI, Goetzl EJ, Levine JD. Leukotriene B4 decreases the mechanical and thermal thresholds of C-fiber nociceptors in the hairy skin of the rat. *J Neurophysiol* 1988; 60:438–445.

Martinon F, Burns K, Tschopp J. The inflammasome: a molecular platform triggering activation of inflammatory caspases and processing of proIL-beta. *Mol Cell* 2002; 10:417–426.

Mäurer M, Toyka KV, Gold R. Immune mechanisms in acquired demyelinating neuropathies: lessons from animal models. *Neuromuscul Disord* 2002a; 12:405–414.

Mäurer M, Toyka KV, Gold R. Cellular immunity in inflammatory autoimmune neuropathies. *Rev Neurol (Paris)* 2002b; 158:S7–15.

Maves TJ, Pechman PS, Gebhart GF, Meller ST. Possible chemical contribution from chronic-gut sutures produces disorders of pain sensation like those seen in man. *Pain* 1993; 54:57–69.

McMahon SB, Cafferty WB, Marchand F. Immune and glial cell factors as pain mediators and modulators. *Exp Neurol* 2005; 192:444–462.

Moalem G, Tracey DJ. Immune and inflammatory mechanisms in neuropathic pain. *Brain Res Brain Res Rev* 2006; 51:240–264.

Moalem-Taylor G, Allbutt HN, Iordanova MD, Tracey DJ. Pain hypersensitivity in rats with experimental autoimmune neuritis, an animal model of human inflammatory demyelinating neuropathy. *Brain Behav Immunol* 2007; in press.

Murphy CJ, Foster BA, Mannis MJ, Selsted ME, Reid TW. Defensins are mitogenic for epithelial cells and fibroblasts. *J Cell Physiol* 1993; 155:408–413.

Myers RR, Heckman HM, Rodriguez M. Reduced hyperalgesia in nerve-injured WLD mice: relationship to nerve fiber phagocytosis, axonal degeneration and regeneration in normal mice. *Exp Neurol* 1996; 141:94–101.

Myers RR, Campana WM, Shubayev VI. The role of neuroinflammation in neuropathic pain: mechanisms and therapeutic targets. *Drug Discov Today* 2006; 11:8–20.

Nathan CF. Secretory products of macrophages. *J Clin Invest* 79:319–326.

Nennesmo I, Reinholt F. Mast cells in nerve end neuromas of mice. *Neurosci Lett* 1986; 69:296–301.

Obata K, Tsujino H, Yamanaka H, et al. Expression of neurotrophic factors in the dorsal root ganglion in a rat model of lumbar disc herniation. *Pain* 2002; 99:121–132.

Ohtori S, Takahashi K, Moriya H, Myers RR. TNF-alpha and TNF-alpha receptor type 1 upregulation in glia and neurons after peripheral nerve injury: studies in murine DRG and spinal cord. *Spine* 2004; 29:1082–1088.

Okuda T, Ishida O, Fujimoto Y, et al. The autotomy relief effect of a silicone tube covering the proximal nerve stump. *J Orthop Res* 2006; 24:1427–1437.

Olsson Y. Degranulation of mast cells in peripheral nerve injuries. *Acta Neurol Scand* 1967; 43:365–374.

Perkins NM, Tracey DJ. Hyperalgesia due to nerve injury: role of neutrophils. *Neuroscience* 2000; 101:745–757.

Perrin FE, Lacroix S, Aviles-Trigueros M, David S. Involvement of monocyte chemoattractant protein-1, macrophage inflammatory protein-1alpha and interleukin-1beta in Wallerian degeneration. *Brain* 2005; 128:854–866.

Pham CT. Neutrophil serine proteases: specific regulators of inflammation. *Nat Rev Immunol* 2006; 6:541–550.

Pomonis JD, Rogers SD, Peters CM, Ghilardi JR, Mantyh PW. Expression and localization of endothelin receptors: implications for the involvement of peripheral glia in nociception. *J Neurosci* 2001; 21:999–1006.

Powell HC, Costello ML, Myers RR. Galactose neuropathy. Permeability studies, mechanism of edema, and mast cell abnormalities. *Acta Neuropathol (Berl)* 1981; 55:89–95.

Powell HC, Braheny SL, Myers RR, Rodriguez M, Lampert PW. Early changes in experimental allergic neuritis. *Lab Invest* 1983; 48:332–338.

Powell HC, Garrett RS, Brett FM, et al. Response of glia, mast cells and the blood brain barrier, in transgenic mice expressing interleukin-3 in astrocytes, an experimental model for CNS demyelination. *Brain Pathol* 1999; 9:219–235.

Ramer MS, French GD, Bisby MA. Wallerian degeneration is required for both neuropathic pain and sympathetic sprouting into the DRG. *Pain* 1997; 72:71–78.

Raud J. Intravital microscopic studies on acute mast cell-dependent inflammation. *Acta Physiol Scand Suppl* 1989; 578:1–58.

Reissmann S, Pineda F, Vietinghoff G, et al. Structure activity relationships for bradykinin antagonists on the inhibition of cytokine release and the release of histamine. *Peptides* 2000; 21:527–533.

Reynier-Rebuffel AM, Callebert J, Dimitriadou V, et al. Carbachol induces granular cell exocytosis and serotonin release in rabbit cerebral arteries. *Am J Physiol* 1992; 262:R105–111.

Robache-Gallea S, Morand V, Bruneau JM, et al. In vitro processing of human tumor necrosis factor-alpha. *J Biol Chem* 1995; 270:23688–23692.

Ruiz G, Ceballos D, Banos JE. Behavioral and histological effects of endoneurial administration of nerve growth factor: possible implications in neuropathic pain. *Brain Res* 2004; 1011:1–6.

Rutkowski JL, Tuite GF, Lincoln PM, et al. Signals for proinflammatory cytokine secretion by human Schwann cells. *J Neuroimmunol* 1999; 101:47–60.

Sambrano GR, Huang W, Faruqi T, et al. Cathepsin G activates protease-activated receptor-4 in human platelets. *J Biol Chem* 2000; 275:6819–6823.

Scapini P, Lapinet-Vera JA, Gasperini S, et al. The neutrophil as a cellular source of chemokines. *Immunol Rev* 2000; 177:195–203.

Schuligoi R. Effect of colchicine on nerve growth factor-induced leukocyte accumulation and thermal hyperalgesia in the rat. *Naunyn Schmiedebergs Arch Pharmacol* 1998; 358:264–269.

Shamash S, Reichert F, Rotshenker S. The cytokine network of Wallerian degeneration: tumor necrosis factor-alpha, interleukin-1alpha, and interleukin-1beta. *J Neurosci* 2002; 22:3052–3060.

Shubayev VI, Myers RR. Upregulation and interaction of TNFalpha and gelatinases A and B in painful peripheral nerve injury. *Brain Res* 2000; 855:83–89.

Shubayev VI, Myers RR. Endoneurial remodeling by TNFalpha and TNFalpha-releasing proteases. A spatial and temporal co-localization study in painful neuropathy. *J Peripher Nerv Syst* 2002; 7:28–36.

Sommer C, Schäfers M. Painful mononeuropathy in C57BL/Wld mice with delayed wallerian degeneration: differential effects of cytokine production and nerve regeneration on thermal and mechanical hypersensitivity. *Brain Res* 1998; 784:154–162.

Sorkin L, Doom C. Epineurial application of TNF elecits an acute mechanical hyperalgesia in the awake rat. *J Peripher Nerv Syst* 2000; 5:96–1000.

Sorkin LS, Moore J, Boyle DL, Yang L, Firestein GS. Regulation of peripheral inflammation by spinal adenosine: role of somatic afferent fibers. *Exp Neurol* 2003; 184:162–168.

Takahashi N, Kikuchi S, Shubayev VI, Campana WM, Myers RR. TNF-alpha and phosphorylation of ERK in DRG and spinal cord: insights into mechanisms of sciatica. *Spine* 2006; 31:523–529.

Tofaris GK, Patterson PH, Jessen KR, Mirsky R. Denervated Schwann cells attract macrophages by secretion of leukemia inhibitory factor (LIF) and monocyte chemoattractant protein-1 in a process regulated by interleukin-6 and LIF. *J Neurosci* 2002; 22:6696–6703.

Uehara A, Muramoto K, Takada H, Sugawara S. Neutrophil serine proteinases activate human nonepithelial cells to produce inflammatory cytokines through protease-activated receptor 2. *J Immunol* 2003; 170:5690–5696.

Wagner R, Myers RR. Endoneurial injection of TNF-alpha produces neuropathic pain behaviors. *Neuroreport* 1996a; 7:2897–2901.

Wagner R, Myers RR. Schwann cells produce tumor necrosis factor alpha: expression in injured and non-injured nerves. *Neurosci* 1996b; 73:625–629.

Weick M, Cherkas PS, Hartig W, et al. P2 receptors in satellite glial cells in trigeminal ganglia of mice. *Neuroscience* 2003; 120:969–977.

Witko-Sarsat V, Rieu P, Descamps-Latscha B, Lesavre P, Halbwachs-Mecarelli L. Neutrophils: molecules, functions and pathophysiological aspects. *Lab Invest* 2000; 80:617–653.

Woodham P, Anderson PN, Nadim W, Turmaine M. Satellite cells surrounding axotomised rat dorsal root ganglion cells increase expression of a GFAP-like protein. *Neurosci Lett* 1989; 98:8–12.

Xian CJ, Zhou XF. Neuronal-glial differential expression of TGF-alpha and its receptor in the dorsal root ganglia in response to sciatic nerve lesion. *Exp Neurol* 1999; 157:317–326.

Xu JT, Xin WJ, Zang Y, Wu CY, Liu XG. The role of tumor necrosis factor-alpha in the neuropathic pain induced by Lumbar 5 ventral root transection in rat. *Pain* 2006; 123:306–321.

Zaratin PF, Quattrini A, Previtali SC, et al. Schwann cell overexpression of the GPR7 receptor in inflammatory and painful neuropathies. *Mol Cell Neurosci* 2005; 28:55–63.

Zelenka M, Schafers M, Sommer C. Intraneural injection of interleukin-1beta and tumor necrosis factor-alpha into rat sciatic nerve at physiological doses induces signs of neuropathic pain. *Pain* 2005; 116:257–263.

Zettl UK, Gold R, Hartung HP, Toyka KV. Apoptotic cell death of T-lymphocytes in experimental autoimmune neuritis of the Lewis rat. *Neurosci Lett* 1994; 176:75–79.

Zhang Y, Roslan R, Lang D, et al. Expression of CHL1 and L1 by neurons and glia following sciatic nerve and dorsal root injury. *Mol Cell Neurosci* 2000; 16:71–86.

Zhou XF, Deng YS, Chie E, et al. Satellite-cell-derived nerve growth factor and neurotrophin-3 are involved in noradrenergic sprouting in the dorsal root ganglia following peripheral nerve injury in the rat. *Eur J Neurosci* 1999; 11:1711–1722.

Zochodne DW, Nguyen C, Sharkey KA. Accumulation and degranulation of mast cells in experimental neuromas. *Neurosci Lett* 1994; 182:3–6.

Zuo Y, Perkins NM, Tracey DJ, Geczy CL. Inflammation and hyperalgesia induced by nerve injury in the rat: a key role of mast cells. *Pain* 2003; 105:467–479.

Correspondence to: Linda S. Sorkin, PhD, Anesthesiology Research Laboratory 0818, University of California, San Diego, 9500 Gilman Drive, La Jolla, CA 92093-0818, USA. Tel: 1-619-543-3498; fax: 1-619-543-6070; email: lsorkin@ucsd.edu.

Immune and Glial Regulation of Pain, edited by Joyce
A. DeLeo, Linda S. Sorkin, and Linda R. Watkins,
IASP Press, Seattle, © 2007.

2

Roles of Astrocytes and Microglia in Pain Memory

Leif Hertz[a] and Elisabeth Hansson[b]

[a]Department of Clinical Pharmacology, China Medical University, Shenyang, P.R. China; [b]Institute of Neuroscience and Physiology, Department of Clinical Neuroscience and Rehabilitation, The Sahlgrenska Academy at Göteborg University, Göteborg, Sweden

Astrocytes and microglia are two very different types of glial cells, both of which are attracting wide interest in the pain field on account of their roles in the development, spread, and maintenance of persistent neuropathic pain secondary to peripheral nerve damage, inflammatory neuritis, or intrathecally induced glial activation (Garrison et al. 1991; Meller et al. 1994; Colburn et al. 1997; Milligan et al. 2000; Chacur et al. 2001; Tanga et al. 2004; DeLeo et al. 2006). Transmitters released in pain-conducting pathways, such as calcitonin gene-related peptide (CGRP), substance P, and glutamate, together with serotonin (5-HT) released by descending fibers, activate microglia and astrocytes. Generally, microglial activation is transient and precedes astrocytic activation, which is much longer-lasting; however, activation of either of the two cell types promotes pain (Tanga et al. 2004).

Besides microglial activation in the spinal cord, a similar, transient activation occurs along afferent nociceptive pathways ascending to the thalamus and parietal and frontal cortex (Hansson and Zügner 2005; Hansson 2006; Huber et al. 2006). Also, permeability of the blood-brain barrier is increased (Huber et al. 2001) by an effect on capillary endothelial cells (Abbott et al. 2006), which may be important for the invasion of peripheral monocytes/macrophages.

ANATOMY AND ULTRASTRUCTURE OF ASTROCYTES AND MICROGLIA

Astrocytes and microglia are both glial cells. There are many more glial cells than neurons in the mammalian brain, but since the glial cells are smaller, they account for no more that one-third of the volume of the brain cortex (Williams et al. 1980; Wolff and Chao 2004; Kimelberg 2005). Astrocytes are the most numerous glial cells in the cortex, whereas microglia account for only about 10% of all glial cells (Wolff and Chao 2004).

Like neurons, astrocytes are derived from the neuroectoderm, whereas microglial cells are derived from mesoderm. During early development, microglial cells invade brain parenchyma as individual cells via intracerebral blood vessels (Morest and Silver 2003). They retain their migratory potential in the adult brain and can be chemotactically guided toward damaged areas. There are approximately 5,000 microglial cells/mm^3 of tissue volume with little regional variability, and the individual cells have little, if any, contact with each other (Wolff and Chao 2004). Astrocytic cell density is 5–10 times as high, with considerable regional differences, and neighboring astrocytes interdigitate to some extent. Moreover, they form a syncytial network, coupled by gap junctions, that allows passage of a multitude of substances, including potassium ions (K^+), calcium ions (Ca^{2+}), cyclic adenosine monophosphate (cAMP), inositol trisphosphate (IP_3), glucose, lactate, and glutamate (Scemes and Spray 2004). Gap junctions are plentiful in spinal astrocytes (Li and Nagy 2000; Scemes et al. 2000). There are different subtypes of astrocytes (Hansson 1988; Walz 2000b; Matthias et al. 2003; Kimelberg 2004), but the importance of these differences for persistent pain is unknown. However, injury to sensory afferents causes the formation of "reactive astrocytes," characterized by an increased expression of glial fibrillary protein (GFAP) (Raghavendra and DeLeo 2004).

Astrocytes virtually enclose the synaptic cleft, giving rise to the expression "the tripartite synapse" (Araque et al. 1999). They ensheathe the larger part of many dendrites, such as those of Purkinje cells (Peters et al. 1991), and they cover the circumference of many neuronal somata (Hirrlinger et al. 2004). Most of the surface of brain capillaries is invested by astrocytic processes, and astrocytes surround pre- and postcapillary vessels with astrocytic endfeet (Wolff and Chao 2004), which may play a major role in the regulation of blood flow (Anderson and Nedergaard 2003; Zonta et al. 2003; Mulligan and McVicar 2004; Metea and Newman 2006). Minute surface extensions (threadlike filopodia about 3 μm long and 0.2 μm wide, and equally thin, sheetlike lamellipodia), also called peripheral astrocyte processes, account for 40% of the volume and 80% of the surface area of a typical astrocyte (Derouiche 2004; Wolff and Chao 2004). Lamellipodia are able to glide along neuronal surfaces, and filopodia are continuously extended and withdrawn (Hirrlinger et al. 2004), altering the topographical relationship with other astrocytes, neuronal constituents, and the extracellular space.

Microglia are related to monocytes and dendritic cells, but at the same time they are bona fide brain cells. In the "resting" state their cell bodies and primary branches are almost immobile, whereas the higher-order branches of the ramified processes undergo rapid extension and retraction, lasting seconds to minutes, occurring at a speed of 1–1.5 µm/minute, and extending for several micrometers (Davalos et al. 2005; Nimmerjahn et al. 2005). Following a small laser ablation or mechanical injury, cells within 50–100 µm respond within a minute with enlargement of the processes closest to the site of the injury and retraction of the processes in the opposite direction. Within 30 minutes their processes have reached the damaged site and fused together, forming a spherical containment around the site of injury.

MICROGLIAL FUNCTION

Physiological signals for process motility. The rapid movement of microglial processes toward a damaged site can be mimicked by local, atraumatic administration of adenosine triphosphate (ATP), adenosine diphosphate (ADP), and uridine triphosphate (UTP), which are potent agonists at purinergic P2X ligand-gated ion channels and P2Y G-protein-coupled receptors. Antagonist studies suggest that it is the activation of P2Y receptors that is necessary for the response to injury (Davalos et al. 2005).

Microglial-neuronal interactions. Given that activation of microglia without astrocytic activation is capable of producing allodynia, direct signaling from microglia to neurons is likely to take place. One potential mechanism for this process has been described by Coull et al. (2005). According to their studies, cultures of microglia respond to ATP with release of brain-derived neurotropic factor (BDNF), a neurotrophin known to be expressed by activated microglia (Nakajima et al. 2002) and recognized as an endogenous modulator of pain hypersensitivity (Mannion et al. 1999; Thompson et al. 1999). Microinjection of ATP-stimulated microglia into the spinal cord in vivo causes allodynia, which is due to a depolarizing shift in the anion reversal potential in spinal lamina 1 neurons in response to the effect of released BDNF on TrkB (tropomyosin-related kinase B) receptors. This shift reflects a collapse of the transmembrane anion gradient with an increase in intracellular chloride ion (Cl^-) concentration. Thus, the Cl^- channel opening in response to stimulation by γ-aminobutyric acid (GABA) does not result in the usual inactivating hyperpolarization, but rather in a depolarization that may even cause neuronal excitation (Coull et al. 2003, 2005). There is also an effect of neurons on microglia, given that microglia express receptors for glutamate (Noda et al. 2000), GABA (Charles et al. 2003; Kuhn et al. 2004), norepinephrine (Mori et al. 2002; Dello Russo et al. 2004), dopamine (Farber et al. 2005), and serotonin (Mahe et al. 2005), all of which can modulate release of cytokines or nitric oxide production.

Microglia-astrocyte interaction. Neuronal injury induces interleukin-1 (IL-1) expression, primarily in microglia, which subsequently release IL-1, interleukin-6 (IL-6), and tumor necrosis factor-α (TNF-α) (Griffin and Stanley 1993; Kyrkanides et al. 1999; John et al. 2003; Andersson et al. 2005). IL-1 has two isoforms, IL-1α and IL-1β, which are almost identical and act on the same receptors. IL-1 release from microglia stimulates astrocytic production of TNF-α, of IL-1β itself, and of IL-6 (Fiebich et al. 1999; Hu and van Eldik 1999; Sutton et al. 1999; John et al. 2003), although microglia appear to be the principal source of these cytokines, both in disease conditions and in culture systems (Aloisi 2001; Persson et al. 2005; Andersson et al. 2005). It is consistent with a special, initial role of IL-1 in microglia in response to noxious conditions that the first cells to produce cytokines after an excitotoxic lesion of the immature rat brain are a microglial population expressing IL-1β and TNF-α (Acarin et al. 2000), and that intracerebral injections of IL-1-receptor antagonist can reduce the expression of TNF-α, measured 18 hours after initiation of seizures (De Simoni et al. 2000). Also, while irradiation of cultured rat astrocytes has little effect on the phenotype of the cells, irradiation of a mixed population of microglia/astrocytes changes astrocyte phenotype into cells with more processes (Hwang et al. 2006).

In the normal brain, few, if any, astrocytes express IL receptors, but after local injury reactive astrocytes show IL-1 binding (Ban 1994; Friedman 2001). Astrocytes in primary cultures have repeatedly been found to express IL-1 receptor mRNA (Rubio 1994; Tomozawa et al. 1995). IL-1 induces the expression of inducible nitric oxide synthase (iNOS or NOS2) in astrocytes via a mechanism dependent on nuclear factor (NF)-κB (Chao et al. 1997; Pahan et al. 1997), and it induces the expression of a plethora of other genes (John et al. 2005). Reports of potential effects of IL-1 on glutamate uptake are inconsistent (Piani et al. 1993; Hu et al. 2000; Okada et al. 2005), whereas cytokine-mediated enhancement of purinergic receptor expression and/or increase of Ca^{2+} wave propagation, despite decreased gap junction permeability (Meme et al. 2004, 2006), have been observed repeatedly (John et al. 1999; Narcisse et al. 2005).

IL-6 expression is low in the normal brain, but is elevated after injury and during inflammation (Van Wagoner and Benveniste 1999). Activated astrocytes may be a major source of IL-6, which is among the cytokines released from primary cultures of astrocytes and from astrocytoma cell lines by stimulation with IL-1, lipopolysaccharide (LPS), or IL-6 itself (Benveniste et al. 1990; Blom et al. 1997; Forloni et al. 1997; van Wagoner et al. 1999).

Astrocytes also express receptors for TNF-α (Aranguez et al. 1995). Excitotoxic lesions in young rats induced by *N*-methyl-D-aspartate (NMDA) leads initially to production of TNF-α and TNF-β in a subpopulation of microglial cells, located in the surviving tissue, and later to expression of TNF-α in reactive astrocytes (Acarin et al. 2000). Many of the effects by IL-1 on astrocytes can also be evoked by TNF-α, and the combined effect of the two cytokines may exceed that of either one alone. A decrease in glutamate uptake in astrocytes by TNF-α has consistently been reported (Fine et al. 1996; Ye and Sontheimer 1996; Hu et al. 2000; Korn et al. 2005). In mouse cerebellar astrocytes, stimulation of NOS activity requires the joint presence of IL-1α and TNF-α (Chao et al. 1995; Da Silva et al. 1997). TNF-α also has effects that are not shared with either IL-1β or IL-6. Thus, it depolarizes cultured cortical astrocytes by reducing their selectively high K^+ conductance, a response that neither of the two other cytokines evokes (Koller et al. 1996, 1998). TNF-α stimulates the astrocytic exchange of intracellular H^+ with extracellular Na^+ (Benos et al. 1994), and the resulting intracellular alkalinization may affect other parameters (Kovacs et al. 2004). Also, the normally observed increase in free cytosolic calcium ion concentration ($[Ca^{2+}]_i$) during exposure of cultured astrocytes to glutamate is reduced by preincubation with TNF-α but not by preincubation with IL-1β or IL-6 (Koller et al. 2001). Again, the interactions appear to be bidirectional, because it has been shown in mixed astrocyte-microglia cultures that astrocyte-derived ATP induces release of IL-1β from microglia through $P2X_7$-receptor channels (Morigiwa et al. 2000; Bianco et al. 2005).

Although microglial involvement is generally considered to occur under pathological conditions only, Ziv et al. (2006) identified T lymphocytes and microglia as important for the maintenance of spatial learning abilities and hippocampal neurogenesis in adulthood.

ASTROCYTE FUNCTION

Glutamatergic activity. Astrocytes are intimately involved in glutamatergic activity. They are necessary for production of transmitter glutamate from glucose, due to the astrocytic but not neuronal expression of the enzyme pyruvate carboxylase (Fig. 1) (Hertz and Zielke 2004). They provide the major mechanism for inactivation of released transmitter glutamate by cellular uptake (Danbolt 2001). Astrocytes convert part—normally about two-thirds (Hertz et al. 2007)—of the accumulated glutamate to glutamine, an astrocyte-specific process (Norenberg and Martinez-Hernandez 1977), and they release glutamine for uptake and resynthesis of transmitter glutamate in neurons via the glutamate-glutamine (Glu-Gln) cycle (Fig. 1). They oxidize the remaining part of the accumulated glutamate, thereby necessitating continuous production of transmitter glutamate from glucose (Fig. 1). They express receptors for glutamate—mainly metabotropic glutamate receptors and ionotropic glutamate receptors of the AMPA (α-amino-3-hydroxy-5-methyl-4-isoxazole propionic

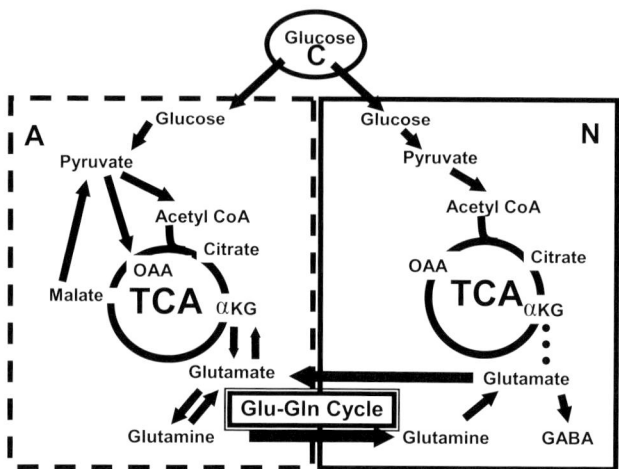

Fig. 1. Net synthesis of glutamate and glutamine from glucose and their net degradation occurs in astrocytes but not in neurons. Glucose enters both neurons (N) and astrocytes (A) from capillaries (C), and in both cell types it is converted via pyruvate to acetyl coenzyme A (acetyl CoA). During energy metabolism, acetyl CoA condenses with preformed oxaloacetate (OAA) in the tricarboxylic acid (TCA) cycle to form citrate, and OAA is regenerated in the TCA cycle ready to combine with another molecule of acetyl CoA. Thus, there is no net synthesis of any TCA cycle intermediate, but a considerable production of energy (ATP) during each turn of the cycle. In addition astrocytes, but not neurons, can form OAA from pyruvate by pyruvate carboxylation, catalyzed by the astrocyte-specific pyruvate carboxylase. This OAA can condense with acetyl CoA to form a "new" molecule of citrate, from which α-ketoglutarate (α-KG), an immediate precursor of glutamate, is formed. Newly synthesized glutamate is carried as glutamine in the glutamate-glutamine (Glu-Gln) cycle to neurons and is used for synthesis of transmitter glutamate (and GABA). In addition the Glu-Gln cycle transports previously released transmitter glutamate back to neurons (as glutamine) after its preferential astrocytic accumulation. Astrocytes, but not neurons, are also able to degrade glutamate and glutamine oxidatively. After conversion to α-KG, another TCA cycle intermediate, malate, is formed, exits the TCA cycle, and is converted by another astrocyte-specific enzyme, cytosolic malic enzyme, to pyruvate, which is then oxidized. The dotted line between α-KG and glutamate indicates that in spite of the absence of net formation of glutamate from α-KG in neurons there is a rapid bidirectional exchange between α-KG and glutamate that leads to accumulation of label in glutamate after administration of ^{13}C-labeled glucose or pyruvate.

acid) subtype—and react to neuronally released glutamate with an increase in IP$_3$ and in $[Ca^{2+}]_i$. By releasing glutamate locally in response to the increased astrocytic $[Ca^{2+}]_i$, astrocytes enhance synaptic activity, and by releasing glutamate at different locations in response to Ca^{2+} waves traveling through the astrocytic syncytium, they activate previously resting neurons. These interactions will be described in more detail in the section on Ca^{2+} homeostasis.

Given that astrocytic glutamate uptake is reduced by TNF-α, the extracellular glutamate concentration in the spinal cord may be increased during chronic pain. Glutamate transport is also regulated by many other factors, including

α_1-adrenergic stimulation (Hansson and Rönnbäck 1992; Alexander et al. 1997), intracellular pH (Judd et al. 1996), redox potential (Trotti et al. 1997), and BDNF, which causes an upregulation of the glutamate transporter GLT-1 (Rodriguez-Kern et al. 2003). An initial upregulation of the two astrocytic glutamate transporters GLAST and GLT-1 during the first 4 days of neuropathic pain, followed by a downregulation, has been reported by Sung et al. (2003). An increased extracellular glutamate concentration has been reported in the spinal cord during chronic pain (Skyba et al. 2005), which may play a role in stimulation of nociceptive pathways (Watkins et al. 1997; Sung et al. 2003; Hansson and Rönnbäck 2004; Raghavendra and DeLeo 2004).

Pyruvate carboxylase mediates effective synthesis of new molecules of constituents of the tricarboxylic acid (TCA) cycle that are precursors for glutamate synthesis from glucose, which requires formation of both acetyl coenzyme A (acetyl CoA) and the TCA cycle intermediate oxaloacetate, formed by pyruvate carboxylation (Fig. 1). Both astrocytes and neurons can synthesize acetyl CoA, which is an intermediate during energy production from glucose, but due to their lack of pyruvate carboxylase, neurons cannot perform net synthesis of oxaloacetate (Yu et al. 1983; Shank et al. 1985; Kaufman and Driscoll 1992). In the brain in vivo there is a constant synthesis of glutamate from glucose, which is balanced by a similar glutamate oxidation after its conversion to malate in the TCA cycle and decarboxylation of malate to pyruvate by malic enzyme, mainly in astrocytes; continuous synthesis and ensuing oxidation of glutamate accounts for 20% of total glucose metabolism in the normal resting brain cortex of both rats and humans (Hertz et al. 2007).

Astrocytic formation of glutamate from glucose and oxidative degradation of glutamate can be temporally dissociated, so that enhanced formation and net accumulation of glutamate from glucose occur during brain activation. Studies by LaNoue have indicated a 30% increase in pyruvate carboxylation during an increase in glutamatergic activity in the retina (K.F. LaNoue, personal communication). Also, an increase of both glutamate and glutamine pool sizes has been demonstrated in day-old chicks during memory formation (Hertz et al. 2003; Gibbs et al. 2007), and nuclear magnetic resonance (NMR) spectroscopy has shown an increase of glutamine content in the hippocampus of amygdaloid-kindled rats (Shirayama et al. 2005). An increase in glutamate contents of the dorsal spinal cord has also been demonstrated during chronic pain (Kawamata and Omote 1996).

Ca^{2+} homeostasis. The concentration of $[Ca^{2+}]_i$ serves as an essential intracellular messenger in virtually any type of cell. This concentration is regulated by Ca^{2+} entering or leaving across the cell membrane and by $[Ca^{2+}]_i$ release and/or binding to intracellular structures, resulting in an average $[Ca^{2+}]_i$ in mammalian cells of about 1×10^{-4} mM (100 nM). The steep Ca^{2+} gradient from an extracellular Ca^{2+} concentration of ~1 mM is maintained by control of channel-mediated Ca^{2+} entry into the cell (through transmitter-operated or voltage-dependent channels or in exchange with other ions), by Ca^{2+} outflow from the cell mediated by Ca^{2+}-ATPase or Ca^{2+}/Na^+ exchange (Ketelaars et al. 2004), and by controlled sequestration of Ca^{2+} in the cell interior by binding to or release from intracellular organelles (Scapagnini et al. 2004). Exposure to glutamate induces increases in $[Ca^{2+}]_i$ in cultured or microdissected astrocytes and in astrocytes in brain slices (Enkvist et al. 1989; Cornell-Bell et al. 1990, 2004; Thorlin et al. 1998), including spinal cord astrocytes (Ahmed et al. 1990). These increases are often oscillating (Zur Nieden and Deitmer 2006), with the frequency dependent on the strength of the stimulus (Pasti et al. 1997) and on previous stimulation (Pasti et al. 1995).

Local cross-talk at a glutamatergic synapse between neurons and astrocytes in the "tripartite synapse" can maintain transmission in the stimulated synapse long after cessation of the original stimulus by neuronal release of glutamate. The glutamate-mediated increase in $[Ca^{2+}]_i$ in astrocytes, in turn, leads to release of glutamate from astrocytes and neuronal excitation (Nadkarni and Jung 2004). This phenomenon may be important for maintaining the pain sensation, constituting a form of "pain memory" (DeLeo et al. 2004; Hansson and Zügner 2005; Hansson 2006). Also, stimulation of astrocytic AMPA receptors causes release of D-serine (Miller 2004), a cofactor during NMDA-receptor activation.

Several other transmitters also cause increases in $[Ca^{2+}]_i$ in astrocytes in primary cultures. Thus, astrocytes express $5\text{-}HT_{2A}$ and $5\text{-}HT_{2B}$ receptors, stimulation of which increases $[Ca^{2+}]_i$ (Hagberg et al. 1998; Sandén et al. 2000; Kong et al. 2002). Coculture of astrocytes with endothelial cells, which furthers astrocyte differentiation (Abbot et al. 2006), changes the response from a single peak (Fig. 2A) to Ca^{2+} oscillations (Fig. 2B), and the oscillations become much more pronounced in cells that have been pre-incubated with CGRP and substance P for 60 minutes (Fig. 2D). Beta-endorphin, an antinociceptive transmitter, suppressed the magnitude of the amplitude of 5-HT-induced intracellular Ca^{2+} release and reduced the number of oscillations in astrocytes that had been cocultured with endothelial cells (Fig. 2C), and it abolished the effect of preincubation with CGRP and substance P (Fig. 2E) by both reducing the amplitude of the $[Ca^{2+}]_i$ increase and preventing the oscillations.

Astrocytic increases in $[Ca^{2+}]_i$ can spread slowly (0.5–1 mm/minute) from the stimulated center as waves in the astrocytic syncytium (Cornell-Bell et al. 1990, 2004; Blomstrand et al. 1999; Haas et al. 2006; Wang et al. 2006) and eventually modify the activity of distant neurons by releasing glutamate (causing neuronal excitation) or ATP, which is hydrolyzed extracellularly to adenosine (causing neuronal inhibition) (Haydon 2001; Newman 2003a, 2006; Fiacco and McCarthy 2004). Many different factors, including neuronal activity, modify Ca^{2+} wave propagation (Rouach et al. 2004), and astrocytes are capable of spontaneous increases in $[Ca^{2+}]_i$ (Nilsson et al. 1991; Parri and Crunelli 2003). Wave propagation from cell to cell is triggered by IP_3 transfer from cell to cell through gap junctions and by subsequent IP_3-induced release of Ca^{2+}, and/or by stimulation of purinergic P2Y receptors by ATP released from the cells through $P2X_7$-receptor channels (Suadicani et al. 2006). The astrocytic $[Ca^{2+}]_i$ waves can excite the neurons they encounter by vesicular release of glutamate (Parpura and Haydon 2000; Newman 2003b; Fellin et al. 2004; Montana et al. 2004; Zhang et al. 2004; Anlauf and Derouiche 2005). Such neuronal-astrocytic interactions could be upregulated in chronic pain and may contribute both to an expansion of the region of local pain and to distribution of pain to the contralateral part of the body.

Potassium ion (K^+) homeostasis. In the cerebral cortex the extracellular K^+ concentration ($[K^+]_e$) is close to 3 mM under resting conditions. During normal neuronal excitation, it rises by at most 1 or 2 mM, but during intense stimulation or seizures, $[K^+]_e$ may reach 12 mM, and during ischemia and spreading depression it rises to much higher levels (Walz and Hertz 1983). It is of crucial importance for central nervous system (CNS) function and metabolism that increases of $[K^+]_e$—both during normal functioning and in pathophysiological conditions—are rapidly reversed, whereas correction of the corresponding intracellular loss of K^+ is less urgent.

In cerebral cortical tissue, it has been convincingly demonstrated that an energy-requiring, ouabain-inhibitable cellular uptake of K^+ restores the balance between intra- and extracellular concentrations of K^+ after neuronal excitation (Xiong and Stringer 2000; D'Ambrosio et al. 2002). The neuronal Na^+,K^+-ATPase is stimulated by the excitation-induced increase in the intracellular concentration of Na^+, but not by an above-normal concentration of $[K^+]_e$, because it has an affinity for K^+ that is so high that the enzyme is saturated at resting $[K^+]_e$. An observation that the kinetics of the decrease of $[K^+]_e$ are similar after an increase by neuronal excitation (with an increase in intraneuronal concentration of Na^+) and by iontophoretic administration of K^+ (with no increase in intraneuronal concentration of Na^+) (Walz 2000a, 2004) provides strong evidence that the major uptake mechanism for active clearance of raised $[K^+]_e$ is directly dependent upon the elevation of $[K^+]_e$. This conclusion means that uptake is mainly astrocytic, not neuronal, because astrocytic uptake of K^+ is stimulated by an increase in $[K^+]_e$.

An active K^+ uptake in astrocytes, mediated by the Na^+,K^+-ATPase, was suggested more than 40 years ago (Hertz 1965). It is now known that two K^+-stimulated mechanisms exist for uptake of K^+ in astrocytes. One is an Na^+,K^+-ATPase-mediated uptake of K^+ in exchange with Na^+, and the second a cotransporter-mediated uptake of Na^+, K^+, and 2 Cl^- (Fig. 3). The cotransporter

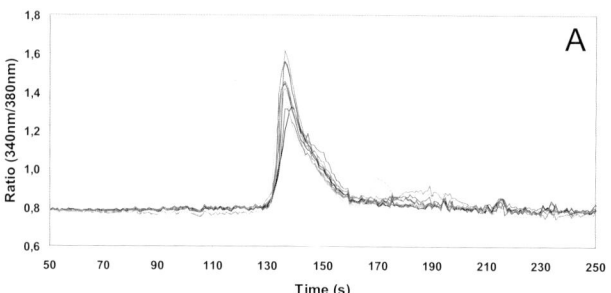

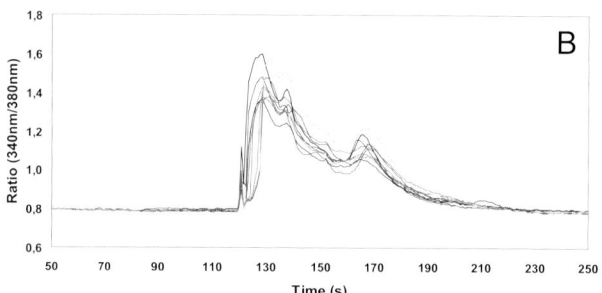

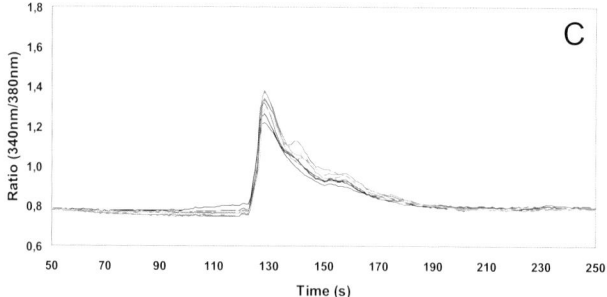

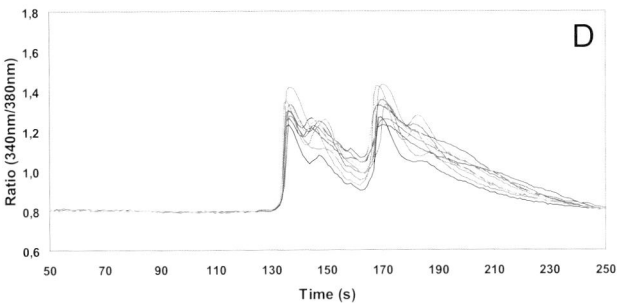

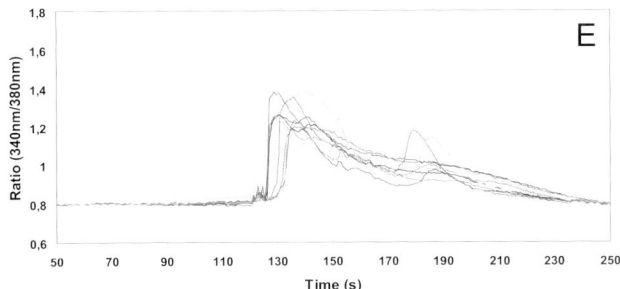

Fig. 2. Transients of free cytosolic calcium ion concentration ($[Ca^{2+}]_i$) in rat astrocyte cultures exposed to serotonin (5-HT) under different experimental conditions. (A) Astrocytes in primary cultures from cerebral cortex of newborn rats, grown in culture for 16 days, were exposed to 5-HT (10^{-5} M). Changes in $[Ca^{2+}]_i$ were monitored using the Ca^{2+}-sensitive fluorophore probe Fura-2/AM (loaded with 8 μM at 22°C for 30 minutes). Data are presented as the 340/380 nm ratio of fluorescence intensities, measured with an inverted epifluorescence microscope. Each line represents a separate sample. (B) Astrocytes in primary culture, which had been differentiated by coculturing with endothelial cells in primary culture for 9 days, responded to 5-HT (10^{-5} M) with Ca^{2+} oscillations. (C) Cultures grown as in panel B, which were exposed to 5-HT together with β-endorphin (10^{-6} M), responded with reduced Ca^{2+} amplitudes and oscillations. (D) Cultures grown as in panel B, which had been exposed to calcitonin gene-related peptide (CGRP) (10^{-7} M) and substance P (10^{-7} M) for 60 minutes before stimulation with 5-HT, responded with Ca^{2+} oscillations that were more pronounced than in panel B. (E) Cultures that had been treated with CGRP and substance P as in panel D responded to administration of β-endorphin together with 5-HT with a reduction in amplitude, and the oscillations had disappeared. (From previously unpublished experiments by Elisabeth Hansson.)

is not directly dependent upon energy metabolism or Na^+,K^+-ATPase activity (it is driven by the inwardly directed electrochemical gradient for Na^+). However, because the accumulated Na^+ subsequently is actively transported out of the cell by the Na^+,K^+-ATPase (maintaining a Na^+ gradient driving the cotransporter-mediated uptake), it is indirectly dependent on Na^+,K^+-ATPase activity. Both

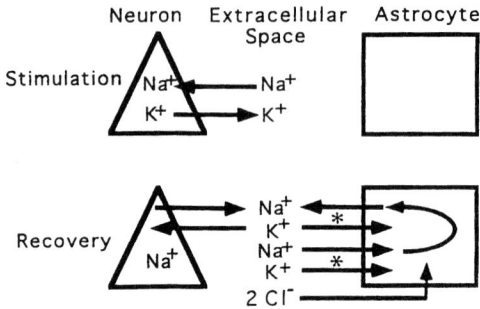

Fig. 3. Diagram of sodium (Na⁺), potassium (K⁺), and chloride (Cl⁻) ion fluxes in neurons and astrocytes during neuronal stimulation and subsequent recovery. During stimulation there is a passive Na⁺ uptake and K⁺ release in neurons, but there are no ion movements in astrocytes; during the subsequent recovery, two concentrative uptake mechanisms transport K⁺ into astrocytes: the Na⁺,K⁺-ATPase system, exchanging extracellular K⁺ with intracellular Na⁺, and a cotransport system, transporting in conjunction 1 Na⁺, 1 K⁺, and 2 Cl⁻ ions into the cell. Astrocytic Na⁺,K⁺-ATPase is stimulated at its extracellular K⁺-sensitive site by the increase in extracellular K⁺ concentration resulting from neuronal excitation (indicated by an asterisk); in neurons it is stimulated at its intracellular Na⁺-sensitive site by the stimulus-induced increase in intracellular Na⁺ concentration. Uptake of Na⁺, K⁺, and Cl⁻ into astrocytes by the cotransport system is energetically driven by the Na⁺ gradient, and is stimulated by entry of calcium ions (Ca²⁺) through voltage-sensitive Ca²⁺ channels by K⁺-mediated depolarization (indicated by an asterisk), followed by a Na⁺,K⁺-ATPase-dependent extrusion of Na⁺ by stimulation of the intracellular, Na⁺-sensitive site of the astrocytic Na⁺,K⁺-ATPase. The joint operation of the Na⁺,K⁺-ATPase and the cotransport system leads to a reaccumulation of K⁺, together with Cl⁻, but without any concomitant uptake of Na⁺. If intracellular Na⁺ is still elevated in neurons (as a result of Na⁺ entry during the previous stimulation) after completed clearance of excess K⁺ from the extracellular space, neuronal Na⁺,K⁺-ATPase activity will remain stimulated and will lead to an "undershoot" in the extracellular concentration of K⁺. From Hertz (2005).

the Na⁺,K⁺-ATPase and the cotransporter are stimulated by increases in $[K^+]_e$ of the magnitude occurring in the extracellular space during neuronal excitation; the astrocytic Na⁺,K⁺-ATPase is stimulated by a direct effect at its extracellular K⁺-sensitive site, which has a sufficiently low affinity to be stimulated by any above-normal K⁺ concentration (Grisar et al. 1979; Mercado and Hernandez 1992; Hajek et al. 1996), and the cotransporter is stimulated by a depolarization-mediated increase in $[Ca^{2+}]_i$ (Su et al. 2000). The importance of the cotransporter for clearance of excess $[K^+]_e$ after neuronal excitation in intact brain tissue is indicated by the finding that $[K^+]_e$ in slices of dentate gyrus reaches a higher level during induced epileptic activity when the cotransporter is inhibited by furosemide (Xiong and Stringer 2000) and by evidence that clearance of a stimulus-induced increase in extracellular K⁺ concentration in the spinal cord is delayed by furosemide (Hertz et al. 1996).

A different mechanism for regulation of $[K^+]_e$, involving redistribution of locally increased $[K^+]_e$ through astrocytes to different locations without any net uptake in the astrocytes, was suggested by Kuffler and coworkers (Orkand et al. 1966). This "spatial buffer" mechanism is based on (1) selective K^+ permeability of the glial cell membrane and (2) electrical coupling of glial cells into a functional syncytium. During exposure to a *local* increase in extracellular K^+, evoked by neuronal firing, the K^+ equilibrium potential at this location becomes lower (less negative) than the membrane potential, and K^+ enters passively. An initially higher membrane potential in the remainder of the glial cell and the glial syncytium creates electrical currents moving toward the depolarized region, primarily carried by a flow of K^+ in the opposite direction. As a result, the K^+ equilibrium potential at these locations becomes higher (more negative) than the membrane potential, and K^+ leaves the cell. The whole process is capable of redistributing a raised local $[K^+]_e$, *across relatively short distances* (Walz 2000a, 2004), but it does *not* involve any measurable cellular *uptake* of K^+, and it ceases once $[K^+]_e$ has re-equilibrated. The spatial buffer plays a major role in clearing excess $[K^+]_e$ after neuronal excitation in the retina (Kofuji et al. 2002; Kofuji and Newman 2004). However, although it is still commonly believed that the spatial buffer has a similar role in the brain, this is probably not the case (Xiong and Stringer 2000), although it may modulate the subsequent undershoot in $[K^+]_e$ (D'Ambrosio et al. 2002; Neusch et al. 2006). In reactive astrocytes an increased Cl^- conductance facilitates a channel-mediated uptake of K^+ together with Cl^- (Walz, 2004). Potassium channel phosphorylation suppresses channel conductance and accelerates channel deactivation, and in chronic pain astrocytic KIR (K^+ inward rectifier) channels are phosphorylated (Ippolito et al. 2005).

CONCLUDING REMARKS

Astrocytes interact functionally with neurons in many different ways, all of which have profound effects on neuronal excitability, which can be influenced via glutamatergic signaling, Ca^{2+} signaling, and K^+ signaling. Pain transduction can influence astrocytic functions, both directly and via initial effects on microglia. It is often assumed that astrocytic dysfunction is the reason why astrocytes are able to sustain persistent pain. However, astrocytic dysfunction is more likely to reduce CNS activity than to enhance it. For example, astrocytes are responsible not only for termination of glutamatergic neurotransmitter activity by uptake of extracellular glutamate, but also for production of neurotransmitter glutamate from glucose and for the return of accumulated neurotransmitter glutamate to neurons. Glutamate content increases in the brain during learning and in the dorsal horn during chronic pain. Moreover, astrocytes express glutamate receptors, and a glutamate-mediated increase in astrocytic $[Ca^{2+}]_i$ can reinforce and strengthen ongoing synaptic activity and even excite previously resting neurons. Neurotransmitters involved in pain transduction increase Ca^{2+} transients, which may enhance astrocytic-neuronal interactions in excitatory activity. KIR channel function is reduced in chronic pain, but the functional importance of the reduction is difficult to evaluate because spatial buffering does not contribute significantly to removal of the increased $[K^+]_e$ following neuronal stimulation, although it modulates the undershoot. However, a channel-mediated uptake of K^+ together with Cl^- can occur in reactive astrocytes, and reduction of this uptake may, again, increase neuronal excitability. Thus, chronic pain may not reflect a dysfunction of one or a few functions in astrocytes, but rather indicate a concerted effort by astrocytes and microglia to respond to increased nociceptive transmission – perhaps in an effort to register and remember neuronal activation. This response may maintain pain sensation even after the original injury or inflammation has healed, converting it to chronic pain by altering neuronal excitability in the spinal cord or brain.

REFERENCES

Abbott NJ, Rönnbäck L, Hansson E. Astrocyte-endothelial interactions at the blood-brain barrier. *Nat Rev Neurosci* 2006; 7:41–53.

Acarin L, Gonzalez B, Castellano B. Neuronal, astroglial and microglial cytokine expression after an excitotoxic lesion in the immature rat brain. *Eur J Neurosci* 2000; 12:3505–3520.

Ahmed Z, Lewis CA, Faber DS. Glutamate stimulates release of Ca^{2+} from internal stores in astroglia. *Brain Res* 1990; 516:165–169.

Alexander GM, Grothusen JR, Gordon SW, Schwartzman RJ. Intracerebral microdialysis study of glutamate reuptake in awake, behaving rats. *Brain Res* 1997; 766:1–10.

Aloisi F. Immune function of microglia. *Glia* 2001; 36:165–179.

Anderson CM, Nedergaard M. Astrocyte-mediated control of cerebral microcirculation. *Trends Neurosci* 2003; 26:340–344.

Andersson AK, Rönnbäck L, Hansson E. Lactate induces tumour necrosis factor-α, interleukin-6 and interleukin-1β release in microglial- and astroglial-enriched primary cultures. *J Neurochem* 2005; 93:1327–1333.

Anlauf E, Derouiche A. Astrocytic exocytosis vesicles and glutamate: a high-resolution immunofluorescence study. *Glia* 2005; 49:96–106.

Aranguez I, Torres C, Rubio N. The receptor for tumor necrosis factor on murine astrocytes: characterization, intracellular degradation, and regulation by cytokines and Theiler's murine encephalomyelitis virus. *Glia* 1995; 13:185–194.

Araque A, Parpura V, Sanzgiri RP, Haydon PG. Tripartite synapses: glia, the unacknowledged partner. *Trends Neurosci* 1999; 22:208–215.

Ban EM. Interleukin-1 receptors in the brain: characterization by quantitative in situ autoradiography. *Immunomethods* 1994; 5:31–40.

Benos DJ, McPherson S, Hahn BH, Chaikin MA, Benveniste EN. Cytokines and HIV envelope glycoprotein gp120 stimulate Na+/H+ exchange in astrocytes. *J Biol Chem* 1994; 269:13811–13816.

Benveniste EN, Sparacio SM, Norris JG, Grenett HE, Fuller GM. Induction and regulation of interleukin-6 gene expression in rat astrocytes. *J Neuroimmunol* 1990; 30:201–212.

Bianco F, Pravettoni E, Colombo A, et al. Astrocyte-derived ATP induces vesicle shedding and IL-1 beta release from microglia. *J Immunol* 2005; 174:7268–7277.

Blom MA, van Twillert MG, de Vries SC, et al. NSAIDS inhibit the IL-1 beta-induced IL-6 release from human post-mortem astrocytes: the involvement of prostaglandin E2. *Brain Res* 1997; 777:210–218.

Blomstrand F, Khatibi S, Muyderman H, et al. 5-Hydroxytryptamine and glutamate modulate velocity and extent of intercellular calcium signalling in hippocampal astroglial cells in primary cultures. *Neuroscience* 1999; 88:1241–1253.

Chacur M, Milligan ED, Gazda LS, et al. A new model of sciatic inflammatory neuritis (SIN): induction of unilateral and bilateral mechanical allodynia following acute unilateral peri-sciatic immune activation in rats. *Pain* 2001; 94:231–244.

Chao CC, Hu S, Ehrlich L, Peterson PK. Interleukin-1 and tumor necrosis factor-alpha synergistically mediate neurotoxicity: involvement of nitric oxide and of N-methyl-D-aspartate receptors. *Brain Behav Immun* 1995; 9:355–365.

Chao CC, Lokensgard JR, Sheng WS, Hu S, Peterson PK. IL-1-induced iNOS expression in human astrocytes via NF-kappa B. *Neuroreport* 1997; 8:3163–3166.

Charles KJ, Deuchars J, Davies CH, Pangalos MN. GABA-B receptor subunit expression in glia. *Mol Cell Neurosci* 2003; 24:214–223.

Colburn RW, DeLeo JA, Rickman AJ, et al. Dissociation of microglial activation and neuropathic pain behaviors following peripheral nerve injury in the rat. *J Neuroimmunol* 1997; 79:163–175.

Cornell-Bell AH, Finkbeiner SM, Cooper MS, Smith SJ. Glutamate induces calcium waves in cultured astrocytes: long-range glial signaling. *Science* 1990; 247:470–473.

Cornell-Bell AH, Jung P, Trinkaus-Randall V. Decoding calcium wave signaling. In: Hertz L (Ed). *Non-Neuronal Cells of the Nervous System: Function and Dysfunction.* Amsterdam: Elsevier, 2004, pp 661–687.

Coull JA, Boudreau D, Bachand K, et al. Trans-synaptic shift in anion gradient in spinal lamina I neurons as a mechanism of neuropathic pain. *Nature* 2003; 424:938–942.

Coull JA, Beggs S, Boudreau D, et al. BDNF from microglia causes the shift in neuronal anion gradient underlying neuropathic pain. *Nature* 2005; 438:1017–1021.

D'Ambrosio R, Gordon DS, Winn HR. Differential role of KIR channel and Na$^+$/K$^+$-pump in the regulation of extracellular K$^+$ in rat hippocampus. *J Neurophysiol* 2002; 87:87–102.

Danbolt N. Glutamate uptake. *Prog Neurobiol* 2001; 65:1–105.

Da Silva J, Pierrat B, Mary JL, Lesslauer W. Blockade of p38 mitogen-activated protein kinase pathway inhibits inducible nitric-oxide synthase expression in mouse astrocytes. *J Biol Chem* 1997; 272:28373–28380.

Davalos D, Grutzendler J, Yang G, et al. ATP mediates rapid microglial response to local brain injury in vivo. *Nat Neurosci* 2005; 8:752–758.

DeLeo JA, Tanga FY, Tawfik VL. Neuroimmune activation and neuroinflammation in chronic pain and opioid tolerance/hyperalgesia. *Neuroscientist* 2004; 10:40–52.

DeLeo JA, Tawfik VL, LaCroix-Fralish ML. The tetrapartite synapse: path to CNS sensitization and chronic pain. *Pain* 2006; 122:17–21.

Dello Russo C, Boullerne AI, Gavrilyuk V, Feinstein DL. Inhibition of microglial inflammatory responses by norepinephrine: effects on nitric oxide and interleukin-1beta production. *J Neuroinflammation* 2004; 1:1–9.

Derouiche A. The perisynaptic astrocyte process as a glial compartment: immunolabeling for glutamine synthetase and other glial markers. In: Hertz L (Ed). *Non-Neuronal Cells of the Nervous System: Function and Dysfunction.* Amsterdam: Elsevier, 2004, pp 147–163.

Enkvist MO, Holopainen I, Åkerman KE. Glutamate receptor-linked changes in membrane potential and intracellular Ca^{2+} in primary rat astrocytes. *Glia* 1989; 2:397–402.

Farber K, Pannasch U, Kettenmann H. Dopamine and noradrenaline control distinct functions in rodent microglial cells. *Mol Cell Neurosci* 2005; 29:128–138.

Fellin T, Pascual O, Gobbo S, et al. Neuronal synchrony mediated by astrocytic glutamate through activation of extrasynaptic NMDA receptors. *Neuron* 2004; 43:729–743.

Fiacco TA, McCarthy KD. Intracellular astrocyte calcium waves in situ increase the frequency of spontaneous AMPA receptor currents in CA1 pyramidal neurons. *J Neurosci* 2004; 24:722–732.

Fiebich BL, Hofer TJ, Lieb K, et al. The non-steroidal anti-inflammatory drug tepoxalin inhibits interleukin-6 and alpha1-anti-chymotrypsin synthesis in astrocytes by preventing degradation of I kappa B-alpha. *Neuropharmacology* 1999; 38:1325–1333.

Fine SM, Angel RA, Perry SW, et al. Tumor necrosis factor alpha inhibits glutamate uptake by primary human astrocytes. Implications for pathogenesis of HIV-1 dementia. *J Biol Chem* 1996; 271:15303–15306.

Forloni G, Mangiarotti F, Angeretti N, Lucca E, De Simoni MG. Beta-amyloid fragment potentiates IL-6 and TNF-alpha secretion by LPS in astrocytes but not in microglia. *Cytokine* 1997; 9:759–762.

Friedman WJ. Cytokines regulate expression of the type 1 interleukin-1 receptor in rat hippocampal neurons and glia. *Exp Neurol* 2001; 168:23–31.

Garrison CJ, Dougherty PM, Kajander KC, Carlton SM. Staining of glial fibrillary acidic protein (GFAP) in lumbar spinal cord increases following a sciatic nerve constriction injury. *Brain Res* 1991; 565:1–7.

Gibbs ME, Lloyd HGE, Santa T, Hertz L. Glycogen is a preferred glutamate precursor during learning in day-old chick: biochemical and behavioral evidence. *J Neurosci Res* 2007; Epub April 23.

Griffin WST, Stanley L. Glial activation as a common denominator in neurodegenerative disease: a hypothesis in neuropathophysiology. In: Fedoroff S, Juurlink BHJ, Doucette R (Eds). *Biology and Pathology of Astrocyte-Neuron Interactions*. New York: Plenum Press, 1993, pp 359–381.

Grisar T, Frère JM, Franck G. Effect of K^+ ions on kinetic properties of the $(Na^+; K^+)$-ATPase (EC 3.6.1.3) of bulk isolated glial cells; perikarya and synaptosomes from rabbit brain cortex. *Brain Res* 1979; 165:87–103.

Haas B, Schipke CG, Peters O, et al. Activity-dependent ATP-waves in the mouse neocortex are independent from astrocytic calcium waves. *Cerebral Cortex* 2006; 16:237–246.

Hagberg G-B, Blomstrand F, Nilsson M, Tamir H, Hansson E. Stimulation of 5-HT$_{2A}$ receptors on astrocytes in primary culture opens voltage-independent Ca^{2+} channels. *Neurochem Int* 1998; 32:153–162.

Hajek I, Subbarao KV, Hertz L. Stimulation of Na^+,K^+-ATPase activity in astrocytes and neurons by K^+ and/or noradrenaline. *Neurochem Int* 1996; 28:335–342.

Hansson E. Astroglia from defined brain regions as studied with primary cultures. *Prog Neurobiol* 1988: 30:369–397.

Hansson E. Could chronic pain and spread of pain sensation be induced and maintained by glial activation? *Acta Physiol Scand* 2006; 187:321–327.

Hansson E, Rönnbäck L. Adrenergic receptor regulation of amino acid neurotransmitter uptake in astrocytes. *Brain Res Bull* 1992; 29:297–301.

Hansson E, Rönnbäck L. Altered neuronal-glial signaling in glutamatergic transmission as a unifying mechanism in chronic pain and mental fatigue. *Neurochem Res* 2004; 29:989–996.

Hansson E, Zügner R. Can chronic pain and spreading of pain be induced via glial mechanisms? New hypotheses on the generation and maintenance of protracted pain conditions. *Lakartidningen* 2005; 102:3552–3558.

Haydon PG. GLIA: listening and talking to the synapse. *Nat Rev Neurosci* 2001; 2:185–193.

Hertz L. Possible role of neuroglia: a potassium-mediated neuronal-neuroglial- neuronal impulse transmission system. *Nature* 1965; 206:1091–1094.

Hertz L. The neuronal-glial brain: fine structure, ion homeostasis and glucose metabolism. In: Coleman RM (Ed). *Focus on Neurochemistry Research*. Hauppauge, NY: Nova Science, 2005, pp 1–60.

Hertz L, Zielke HR. Astrocytic control of glutamatergic activity: astrocytes as the stars of the show. *Trends Neurosci* 2004: 27:735–743.

Hertz L, Gibbs ME, O'Dowd BS, et al. Astrocyte-neuron interaction during one-trial aversive learning in the neonate chick. *Neurosci Biobehav Rev* 1996; 20:537–551.

Hertz L, O'Dowd BS, Ng KT, Gibbs ME. Reciprocal changes in forebrain contents of glycogen and of glutamate/glutamine during early memory consolidation in the day-old chick. *Brain Res* 2003; 994:226–233.

Hertz L, Peng L, Dienel GA. Energy metabolism in astrocytes: high rate of oxidative metabolism and spatiotemporal dependence on glycolysis/glycogenolysis. *J Cereb Blood Flow Metab* 2007; 27:219–249.

Hirrlinger J, Hulsmann S, Kirchhoff F. Astroglial processes show spontaneous motility at active synaptic terminals *in situ*. *Eur J Neurosci* 2004; 20:2235–2239.

Hu J, Van Eldik LJ. Glial-derived proteins activate cultured astrocytes and enhance beta amyloid-induced glial activation. *Brain Res* 1999; 842:46–54.

Hu S, Sheng WS, Ehrlich LC, Peterson PK, Chao CC. Cytokine effects on glutamate uptake by human astrocytes. *Neuroimmunomodulation* 2000; 7:153–159.

Huber JD, Witt KA, Hom S, et al. Inflammatory pain alters blood-brain barrier permeability and tight junctional protein expression. *Am J Physiol Heart Circ Physiol* 2001; 280:H1241–H1248.

Huber JD, Campos CR, Mark KS, Davis TP. Alterations in blood-brain barrier ICAM-1 expression and brain microglial activation after lambda-carrageenan-induced inflammatory pain. *Am J Physiol Heart Circ Physiol* 2006; 290:H732–740.

Hwang SY, Jung JS, Kim TH, et al. Ionizing radiation induces astrocyte gliosis through microglia activation. *Neurobiol Dis* 2006; 21:457–467.

Ippolito DL, Xu M, Bruchas MR, Wickman K, Chavkin C. Tyrosine phosphorylation of $K_{ir}3.1$ in spinal cord is induced by acute inflammation, chronic neuropathic pain, and behavioral stress. *J Biol Chem* 2005; 280:41683–41693.

John GR, Scemes E, Suadicani SO, et al. IL-1beta differentially regulates calcium wave propagation between primary human fetal astrocytes via pathways involving P2 receptors and gap junction channels. *Proc Natl Acad Sci USA* 1999; 96:11613–11618.

John GR, Lee SC, Brosnan CF. Cytokines: powerful regulators of glial cell activation. *Neuroscientist* 2003; 9:10–22.

John GR, Lee SC, Song X, Rivieccio M, Brosnan CF. IL-1-regulated responses in astrocytes: relevance to injury and recovery. *Glia* 2005; 49:161–176.

Judd, M.G. Nagaraja TN, Brookes N. Potassium-induced stimulation of glutamate uptake in mouse cerebral astrocytes: the role of intracellular pH. *J Neurochem* 1996; 66:169–176.

Kaufman EE, Driscoll BF. Carbon dioxide fixation in neuronal and astroglial cells in culture. *J Neurochem* 1992; 58:258–262.

Kawamata M, Omote K. Involvement of increased excitatory amino acids and intracellular Ca^{2+} concentration in the spinal dorsal horn in an animal model of neuropathic pain. *Pain* 1996; 68:85–96.

Ketelaars SO, Gorter JA, Aronica E, Wadman WJ. Calcium extrusion protein expression in the hippocampal formation of chronic epileptic rats after kainate-induced status epilepticus. *Epilepsia* 2004; 45:1189–1201.

Kimelberg HK. The problem of astrocyte identity. *Neurochem Int* 2004; 45:191–202.

Kimelberg HK. Astrocytic swelling in cerebral ischemia as a possible cause of injury and target for therapy. *Glia* 2005; 50:389–397.

Kofuji P, Newman EA. Potassium buffering in the central nervous system. *Neuroscience* 2004;129:1045–1056.

Kofuji P, Biedermann B, Siddharthan V, et al. Kir potassium channel subunit expression in retinal glial cells: implications for spatial potassium buffering. *Glia* 2002; 39:292–303.

Koller H, Thiem K, Siebler M. Tumour necrosis factor-alpha increases intracellular Ca^{2+} and induces a depolarization in cultured astroglial cells. *Brain* 1996; 119:2021–2027.

Koller H, Allert N, Oel D, Stoll G, Siebler M. TNF alpha induces a protein kinase C-dependent reduction in astroglial K^+ conductance. *Neuroreport* 1998; 9:1375–1378.

Koller H, Trimborn M, von Giesen H, Schroeter M, Arendt G. TNF-alpha reduces glutamate induced intracellular Ca^{2+} increase in cultured cortical astrocytes. *Brain Res* 2001; 893:237–243.

Kong EK, Peng L, Chen Y, Yu ACH, Hertz L. Up-regulation of 5-HT$_{2B}$ receptor density and receptor-mediated glycogenolysis in mouse astrocytes by long-term fluoxetine administration. *Neurochem Res* 2002; 27:113–120.

Korn T, Magnus T, Jung S. Autoantigen specific T cells inhibit glutamate uptake in astrocytes by decreasing expression of astrocytic glutamate transporter GLAST: a mechanism mediated by tumor necrosis factor-alpha. *FASEB J* 2005; 19:1878–1880.

Kovacs EZ, Bush BA, Benos DJ. Glycoprotein gp120-mediated astrocytic dysfunction. In: Hertz L (Ed). *Non-Neuronal Cells of the Nervous System: Function and Dysfunction.* Amsterdam: Elsevier, 2004, pp 921–949.

Kuhn SA, van Landeghem FK, Zacharias R, et al. Microglia express GABA$_B$ receptors to modulate interleukin release. *Mol Cell Neurosci* 2004; 25:312–322.

Kyrkanides S, Olschowka JA, Williams JP, Hansen JT, O'Banion MK. TNF alpha and IL-1beta mediate intercellular adhesion molecule-1 induction via microglia-astrocyte interaction in CNS radiation injury. *J Neuroimmunol* 1999; 95:95–106.

Li WE, Nagy JI. Activation of fibres in rat sciatic nerve alters phosphorylation state of connexin-43 at astrocytic gap junctions in spinal cord: evidence for junction regulation by neuronal-glial interactions. *Neuroscience* 2000; 97:113–923.

Mahe C, Loetscher E, Dev KK, et al. Serotonin 5-HT7 receptors coupled to induction of interleukin-6 in human microglial MC-3 cells. *Neuropharmacology* 2005; 49:40–47.

Mannion RJ, Costigan M, Decosterd I, et al. Neurotrophins: peripherally and centrally acting modulators of tactile stimulus-induced inflammatory pain hypersensitivity. *Proc Natl Acad Sci USA* 1999; 96:9385–9390.

Matthias K, Kirchhoff F, Seifert G, et al. Segregated expression of AMPA-type glutamate receptors and glutamate transporters defines distinct astrocyte populations in the mouse hippocampus. *J Neurosci* 2003; 23:1750–1758.

Meller ST, Dykstra C, Grzybycki D, Murphy S, Gebhart GF. The possible role of glia in nociceptive processing and hyperalgesia in the spinal cord of the rat. *Neuropharmacology* 1994; 33:1471–1478.

Meme W, Ezan P, Venance L, Glowinski J, Giaume C. ATP-induced inhibition of gap junctional communication is enhanced by interleukin-1 beta treatment in cultured astrocytes. *Neuroscience* 2004; 126:95–104.

Meme W, Calvo CF, Froger N, et al. Proinflammatory cytokines released from microglia inhibit gap junctions in astrocytes: potentiation by beta-amyloid. *FASEB J* 2006; 20:494–496.

Mercado R, Hernandez J. Regulatory role of a neurotransmitter (5-HT) on glial Na^+,K^+-ATPase in the rat brain. *Neurochem Int* 1992; 21:119–127.

Metea MR, Newman EA. Glial cells dilate and constrict blood vessels: a mechanism of neurovascular coupling. *J Neurosci* 2006; 26:2862–2870.

Miller RF. D-Serine as a glial modulator of nerve cells. *Glia* 2004; 47:275–283.

Milligan ED, Mehmert KK, Hinde JL, et al. Thermal hyperalgesia and mechanical allodynia produced by intrathecal administration of the human immunodeficiency virus-1 (HIV-1) envelope glycoprotein, gp120. *Brain Res* 2000; 861:105–116.

Montana V, Ni Y, Sunjara V, Hua X, Parpura V. Vesicular glutamate transporter-dependent glutamate release from astrocytes. *J Neurosci* 2004; 24:2633–2642.

Morest DK, Silver J. Precursors of neurons, neuroglia, and ependymal cells in the CNS: What are they? Where are they? How do they get where they are going? *Glia* 2003; 43:6–18.

Mori K, Ozaki E, Zhang B, et al. Effects of norepinephrine on rat cultured microglial cells that express alpha1, alpha2, beta1 and beta2 adrenergic receptors. *Neuropharmacology* 2002; 43:1026–1034.

Morigiwa K, Quan M, Murakami M, Yamashita M, Fukuda Y. P2 purinoceptor expression and functional changes of hypoxia-activated cultured rat retinal microglia. *Neurosci Lett* 2000; 282:153–156.

Mulligan SJ, MacVicar BA. Calcium transients in astrocyte endfeet cause cerebrovascular constrictions. *Nature* 2004; 431:195–199.

Nadkarni S, Jung P. Dressed neurons: modeling neural-glial interactions. *Phys Biol* 2004; 1:35–41.

Nakajima K, Tohyama Y, Kohsaka S, Kurihara T. Ceramide activates microglia to enhance the production/secretion of brain-derived neurotrophic factor (BDNF) without induction of deleterious factors in vitro. *J Neurochem* 2002; 80:697–705.

Narcisse L, Scemes E, Zhao Y, Lee SC, Brosnan CF. The cytokine IL-1beta transiently enhances P2X7 receptor expression and function in human astrocytes. *Glia* 2005; 49:245–258.

Neusch C, Papadopoulos N, Müller M, et al. Lack of the KIR4.1 channel subunit abolishes K^+ buffering properties of astrocytes in the ventral respiratory group: impact on extracellular K^+ regulation. *J Neurophysiol* 2006; 95:1843-1852.

Newman EA. Glial cell inhibition of neurons by release of ATP. *J Neurosci* 2003a; 23:1659–1666.

Newman EA. New roles for astrocytes: regulation of synaptic transmission. *Trends Neurosci* 2003b; 26:536–542.

Newman EA. A purinergic dialogue between glia and neurons in the retina. *Novartis Found Symp* 2006; 276:193–202.

Nilsson M, Hansson E, Rönnbäck L. Heterogeneity among astroglial cells with respect to 5HT-evoked cytosolic Ca^{2+} responses. A microspectrofluorimetric study on single cells in primary culture. *Life Sci* 1991; 49:1339–1350.

Nimmerjahn A, Kirchhoff F, Helmchen F. Resting microglial cells are highly dynamic surveillants of brain parenchyma in vivo. *Science* 2005; 308:1314–1318.

Noda M, Nakanishi H, Nabekura J, Akaike N. AMPA-kainate subtypes of glutamate receptor in rat cerebral microglia. *J Neurosci* 2000; 20:251–258.

Norenberg MD, Martinez-Hernandez A. Fine structural localization of glutamine synthetase in astrocytes of rat brain. *Brain Res* 1977; 161:303–310.

Okada K, Yamashita U, Tsuji S. Modulation of Na^+-dependent glutamate transporter of murine astrocytes by inflammatory mediators. *J UOEH* 2005; 27:161–170.

Orkand RK, Nicholls JG, Kuffler SW. Effect of nerve impulses on the membrane potential of glial cells in the central nervous system of amphibia. *J Neurophysiol* 1966; 29:788–806.

Pahan K, Sheikh FG, Namboodiri AM, Singh I. Lovastatin and phenylacetate inhibit the induction of nitric oxide synthase and cytokines in rat primary astrocytes, microglia, and macrophages. *J Clin Invest* 1997; 100:2671–2679.

Parpura V, Haydon PG. Physiological astrocytic calcium levels stimulate glutamate release to modulate adjacent neurons. *Proc Natl Acad Sci USA* 2000; 97:8629–8634.

Parri HR, Crunelli V. The role of Ca^{2+} in the generation of spontaneous astrocytic Ca^{2+} oscillations. *Neuroscience* 2003; 120:979–992.

Pasti L, Pozzan T, Carmignoto G. Long-lasting changes of calcium oscillations in astrocytes. A new form of glutamate-mediated plasticity. *J Biol Chem* 1995; 270:15203–15210.

Pasti L, Volterra A, Pozzan T, Carmignoto G. Intracellular calcium oscillations in astrocytes: a highly plastic, bidirectional form of communication between neurons and astrocytes in situ. *J Neurosci* 1997; 17:7817–7830.

Persson M, Brantefjord M, Hansson E, Rönnbäck L. Lipopolysaccharide increases microglial GLT-1 expression and glutamate uptake capacity in vitro by a mechanism dependent on TNF-α. *Glia* 2005; 51:111–120.

Peters A, Palay SL, Webster H de F. *The Fine Structure of the Nervous System. Neurons and their Supporting Cells,* 3rd ed. Oxford: Oxford University Press, 1991.

Piani D, Frei K, Pfister HW, Fontana A. Glutamate uptake by astrocytes is inhibited by reactive oxygen intermediates but not by other macrophage-derived molecules including cytokines, leukotrienes or platelet-activating factor. *J Neuroimmunol* 1993; 48:99–104.

Raghavendra V, DeLeo JA. The role of astrocytes and microglia in persistent pain. In: Hertz L (Ed). *Non-Neuronal Cells of the Nervous System: Function and Dysfunction.* Amsterdam: Elsevier, 2004, pp 951–966.

Rodriguez-Kern A, Gegelashvili M, Schousboe A, et al. Beta-amyloid and brain-derived neurotrophic factor, BDNF, up-regulate the expression of glutamate transporter GLT-1/EAAT2 via different signaling pathways utilizing transcription factor NF-kappa-B. *Neurochem Int* 2003; 43:363–370.

Rouach N, Koulakoff A, Giaume C. Neurons set the tone of gap junctional communication in astrocytic networks. *Neurochem Int* 2004; 45:265–272.

Rubio N. Demonstration of the presence of an interleukin-1 receptor on the surface of murine astrocytes and its regulation by cytokines and Theiler's virus. *Immunology* 1994; 82:178–183.

Sandén N, Thorlin T, Blomstrand F, Persson PAI, Hansson E. 5-Hydroxytryptamine$_{2B}$ receptors stimulate Ca^{2+} increases in cultured astrocytes from three different brain regions. *Neurochem Int* 2000; 36:427–434.

Scapagnini G, Nelson TJ, Alkon DL. 2004. Regulation of Ca^{2+} stores in glial cells. In: Hertz L (Ed). *Non-Neuronal Cells of the Nervous System: Function and Dysfunction.* Amsterdam: Elsevier, 2004, pp 635–660.

Scemes E, Spray, DC. 2004. The astrocytic syncytium. In: Hertz L (Ed). *Non-Neuronal Cells of the Nervous System: Function and Dysfunction.* Amsterdam: Elsevier, 2004, pp 165–179.

Scemes E, Suadicani SO, Spray DC. Intercellular communication in spinal cord astrocytes: fine tuning between gap junctions and P2 nucleotide receptors in calcium wave propagation. *J Neurosci* 2000; 20:1435–1445.

Shank RP, Bennett GS, Freytag SO, Campbell GL. Pyruvate carboxylase: an astrocyte-specific enzyme implicated in the replenishment of amino acid neurotransmitter pools. *Brain Res* 1985; 329:364–367.

Shirayama Y, Takahashi S, Minabe Y, Ogino T. In vitro ^1H NMR spectroscopy shows an increase in N-acetylaspartylglutamate and glutamine content in the hippocampus of amygdaloid-kindled rats. *J Neurochem* 2005; 92:1317–1326.

Skyba DA, Lisi TL, Sluka KA. Excitatory amino acid concentrations increase in the spinal cord dorsal horn after repeated intramuscular injection of acidic saline. *Pain* 2005; 119:142–149.

Su G, Haworth RA, Dempsey RJ, Sun D. Regulation of Na^+-K^+-Cl cotransporter in primary astrocytes by dibutyryl cAMP and high $[K^+]_o$. *Am J Physiol Cell Physiol* 2000; 279:1710–1721.

Suadicani SO, Brosnan CF, Scemes E. P2X7 receptors mediate ATP release and amplification of astrocytic intercellular Ca^{2+} signaling. *J Neurosci* 2006; 26:1378–1385.

Sung B, Lim G, Mao J. Altered expression and uptake activity of spinal glutamate transporters after nerve injury contribute to the pathogenesis of neuropathic pain in rats. *J Neurosci* 2003; 23:2899–2910.

Sutton ET, Thomas T, Bryant MW, et al. Amyloid-beta peptide induced inflammatory reaction is mediated by the cytokines tumor necrosis factor and interleukin-1. *J Submicrosc Cytol Pathol* 1999; 31:313–323.

Tanga FY, Raghavendra V, DeLeo JA. Quantitative real-time RT-PCR assessment of spinal microglial and astrocytic activation markers in a rat model of neuropathic pain. *Neurochem Int* 2004; 45:397–407.

Thompson SW, Bennett DL, Kerr BJ, Bradbury EJ, McMahon SB. Brain-derived neurotrophic factor is an endogenous modulator of nociceptive responses in the spinal cord. *Proc Natl Acad Sci USA* 1999; 96:7714–7718.

Thorlin T, Eriksson PS, Rönnbäck L, Hansson E. Receptor-activated Ca^{2+} increases in vibrodissociated cortical astrocytes: a nonenzymatic method for acute isolation of astrocytes. *J Neurosci Res* 1998; 54:390–401.

Tomozawa Y, Inoue T, Satoh M. Expression of type I interleukin-1 receptor mRNA and its regulation in cultured astrocytes. *Neurosci Lett* 1995; 195:57–60.

Trotti D, Nussberger S, Volterra A, Hediger MA. Differential modulation of the uptake currents by redox interconversion of cysteine residues in the human neuronal glutamate transporter EAAC1. *Eur J Neurosci* 1997; 9:2207–2212.

Van Wagoner NJ, Benveniste EN. Interleukin-6 expression and regulation in astrocytes. *J Neuroimmunol* 1999; 100:124–139.

Van Wagoner NJ, Oh JW, Repovic P, Benveniste EN. Interleukin-6 (IL-6) production by astrocytes: autocrine regulation by IL-6 and the soluble IL-6 receptor. *J Neurosci* 1999; 19:5236–5244.

Vezzani A, Moneta D, Conti M, et al. Powerful anticonvulsant action of IL-1 receptor antagonist on intracerebral injection and astrocytic overexpression in mice. *Proc Natl Acad Sci USA* 2000; 97:11534–11539.

Walz W. Role of astrocytes in the clearance of excess extracellular potassium. *Neurochem Int* 2000a; 36:291–300.

Walz W. Controversy surrounding the existence of discrete functional classes of astrocytes in adult gray matter. *Glia* 2000b; 31:95–103.

Walz W. Potassium homeostasis in the brain at the organ and cell level. In: Hertz L (Ed). *Non-Neuronal Cells of the Nervous System: Function and Dysfunction.* Amsterdam: Elsevier, 2004, pp 595–609.

Walz W, Hertz L. Functional interactions between neurons and astrocytes II. Potassium homeostasis at the cellular level. *Prog Neurobiol* 1983; 20:133–183.

Wang X, Lou N, Xu Q, et al. Astrocytic Ca^{2+} signaling evoked by sensory stimulation in vivo. *Nat Neurosci* 2006; 9:816–823.

Watkins LR, Martin D, Ulrich P, Tracey KJ, Maier SF. Evidence for the involvement of spinal cord glia in subcutaneous formalin induced hyperalgesia in the rat. *Pain* 1997; 71:225–235.

Williams V, Grossman RG, Edmunds SM. Volume and surface area estimates of astrocytes in the sensorimotor cortex of the cat. *Neuroscience* 1980; 5:1151–1159.

Wolff J, Chao TI. Cytoarchitectonics of non-neuronal cells in the central nervous system. In: Hertz L (Ed). *Non-Neuronal Cells of the Nervous System: Function and Dysfunction.* Amsterdam: Elsevier, 2004, pp 1–52.

Xiong ZQ, Stringer JL. Sodium pump activity, not glial spatial buffering, clears potassium after epileptiform activity induced in the dentate gyrus. *J Neurophysiol* 2000; 83:1443–1451.

Ye ZC, Sontheimer H. Cytokine modulation of glial glutamate uptake: a possible involvement of nitric oxide. *Neuroreport* 1996; 7:2181–2185.

Yu ACH, Drejer J, Hertz L, Schousboe A. Pyruvate carboxylase activity in primary cultures of astrocytes and neurons. *J Neurochem* 1983; 41:1484–1487.

Zhang Q, Fukuda M, Van Bockstaele E, Pascual O, Haydon PG. Synaptotagmin IV regulates glial glutamate release. *Proc Natl Acad Sci USA* 2004; 101:9441–9446.

Ziv Y, Ron N, Butovsky O, et al. Immune cells contribute to the maintenance of neurogenesis and spatial learning abilities in adulthood. *Nat Neurosci* 2006; 9:268-275.

Zonta M, Angulo MC, Gobbo S, et al. Neuron-to-astrocyte signaling is central to the dynamic control of brain microcirculation. *Nat Neurosci* 2003; 6:43–50.

Zur Nieden R, Deitmer JW. The role of metabotropic glutamate receptors for the generation of calcium oscillations in rat hippocampal astrocytes in situ. *Cereb Cortex* 2006; 16:676–687.

Correspondence to: Leif Hertz, MD, DSc, RR 2, Box 245 (738 Dickey Lake Road), Gilmour, Ontario, Canada K0L 1W0. Email: lhertz@northcom.net.

Immune and Glial Regulation of Pain, edited by Joyce
A. DeLeo, Linda S. Sorkin, and Linda R. Watkins,
IASP Press, Seattle, © 2007.

3

Intracellular Signaling Cascades in Glia

Etty N. Benveniste

*Department of Cell Biology, The University of Alabama at Birmingham,
Birmingham, Alabama, USA*

Cytokines, chemokines, and growth factors influence the survival, growth, differentiation, and gene expression pattern in all cell types, including glial cells. These secreted proteins initiate communication with cells through cell surface receptors or receptor complexes that trigger intracellular signaling pathways that determine the timing, nature, and duration of the cellular response. The ultimate response of cells to external stimuli requires the coordinated activity of a large network of intracellular signaling cascades, which ultimately depend on a small number of molecular mechanisms (Natarajan et al. 2006).

A myriad of intracellular signaling pathways are activated upon receptor engagement. These pathways include Janus kinases (JAK)/signal transducers and activators of transcription (STAT), nuclear factor (NF)-κB, mitogen-activated protein kinase (MAPK), and phosphoinositide-3 kinase (PI3K) cascades. In this chapter, we will provide an overview of the JAK/STAT and NF-κB signaling pathways and describe how these pathways are activated in glia and regulate glial cell functions.

THE JAK/STAT PATHWAY

Most cytokines and interferons utilize the JAK/STAT pathway as the predominant means of signal transduction (Shuai and Liu 2003; Campbell 2005; Platanias 2005). JAKs are receptor-associated tyrosine kinases, and STATs are the specific transcription factors that they activate. There are four members of the JAK family (JAK1, JAK2, JAK3, and tyrosine kinase-2 [TYK2]) and seven members of the STAT family (STATs 1, 2, 3, 4, 5A, 5B, and 6). Cytokine and interferon receptors, upon stimulation with their corresponding ligand, induce oligomerization of receptor subunits, activating JAKs that are bound to membrane proximal regions of the receptor subunits. JAKs then sequentially phosphorylate critical tyrosine residues on each other, as well as in the cyto-plasmic domain of the receptors. These receptor phosphotyrosine residues serve to recruit specific members of the STAT family to the receptor complex, where the STATs are phosphorylated by JAKs on specific tyrosine residues. Activated STATs then dimerize and translocate to the nucleus to induce gene transcription. Binding of activated STATs to response elements results in the rapid, but transient, induction of ligand-specific programs of gene expression.

Cytokines and interferons implicated in central nervous system (CNS) responses, particularly with respect to neuroinflammatory responses, include interferon (IFN)-γ, IFN-β, and interleukin (IL)-6 family members. Examples describing the specific JAK/STAT pathways used by these stimuli are as follows. The IFN-γ receptor (IFNGR) consists of two subunits, IFNGR1 and IFNGR2, that are constitutively associated with JAKs: IFNGR1 with JAK1 and IFNGR2 with JAK2. Binding of IFN-γ to the IFN-γ receptor leads to trans-phosphorylation and reciprocal activation of the JAKs. The activated JAKs then phosphorylate IFNGR1, creating a recruitment site for latent STAT-1α. Tyrosine phosphorylation of STAT-1α by JAKs results in its dissociation from the receptor complex, in the formation of STAT-1α homodimers, and in the translocation of STAT-1α into the nucleus, where it binds to IFN-γ activated sequence (GAS) elements in the promoters of IFN-γ-inducible genes, leading to activation of transcription (Shuai and Liu 2003) (Fig. 1A). Serine phosphorylation at residue 727 increases the transactivation potential of STAT-1α (Decker and Kovarik 2000). IFN-β binds to its receptor, which is composed of two subunits, IFNARI and IFNAR2, which are associated with TYK2 and JAK1, respectively. IFN-β stimulation leads to the tyrosine phosphorylation of STAT-2 and STAT-1, which then associate with the interferon regulatory factor (IRF)-9 transcription factor. This complex, known as IFN stimulated gene factor 3 (ISGF3), translocates to the nucleus and binds to IFN-stimulated response elements (ISREs) to initiate transcription (Fig. 1B). Less frequently, a STAT-1α homodimer is formed in response to IFN-β, which binds to GAS elements (Fig. 1B). Interleukin-6 is the prototypic member of the IL-6 family of cytokines, which includes IL-6, IL-11, oncostatin M (OSM), leukemia inhibitory factor (LIF), and ciliary neurotrophic factor (CNTF) (Van Wagoner and Benveniste 1999b; Naka et al. 2002). These cytokines exert their biological effects by the formation of receptor complexes that include the shared 130-kDa receptor subunit, gp130. IL-6 requires a ligand-specific receptor, which is found in both membrane-associated and soluble forms. Interestingly, the IL-6 soluble receptor (sIL-6R) functions as an agonist of IL-6 (Rose-John et al. 1995), and makes cells expressing gp130 (but not the membrane-bound IL-6R) responsive to IL-6 upon addition of the sIL-6R. IL-6 signals through a receptor complex composed of IL-6, either membrane-bound IL-6R or the sIL-6R, and gp130, which results in the

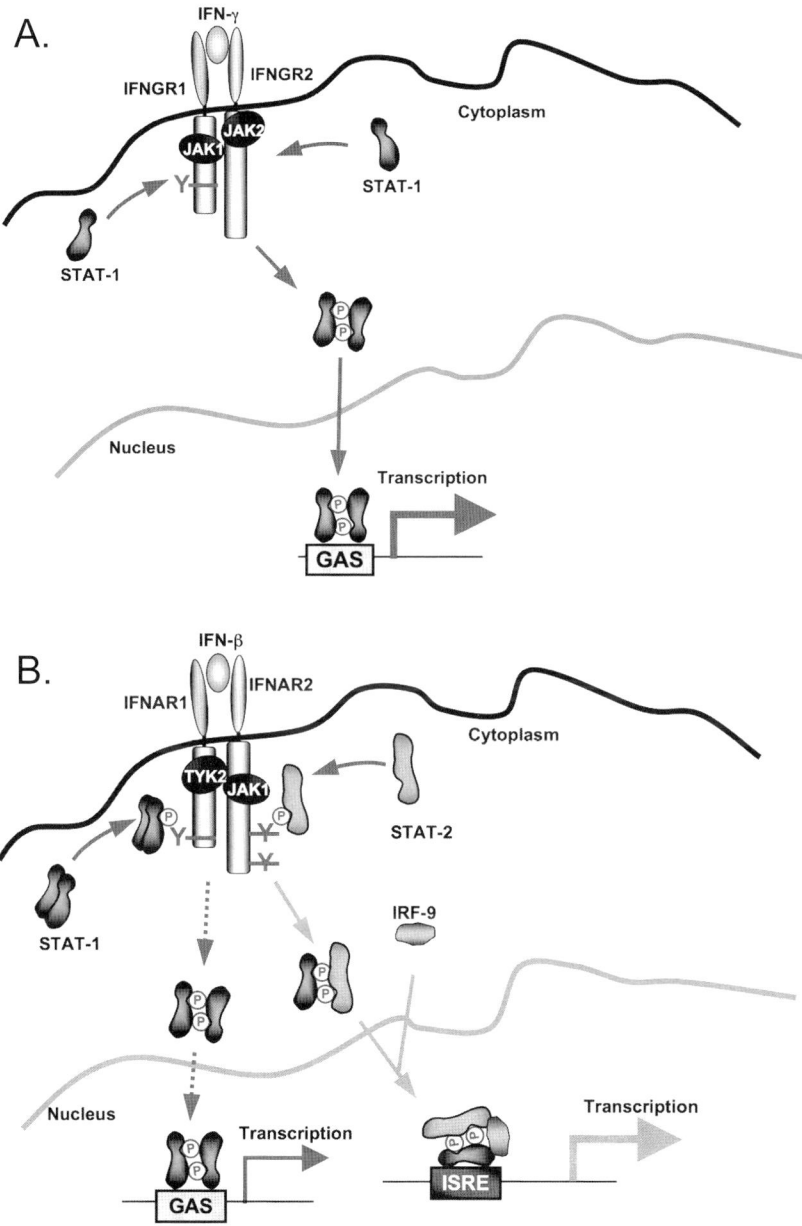

Fig. 1. A schematic representation of the Janus kinase (JAK)-signal transducer and activator of transcription (STAT) pathway. The activation of JAKs after interferon (IFN)-γ (A) and IFN-β (B) stimulation results in the phosphorylation of STATs, which then dimerize and translocate to the nucleus to activate gene transcription. GAS = interferon-gamma-activated sequence, IRF-9 = interferon regulatory factor-9, ISRE = interferon-stimulated response elements, TYK2 = tyrosine kinase 2. Adapted from Schindler (2006).

activation of JAK1 and JAK2 (Rodig et al. 1998). The cytoplasmic domain of gp130 becomes phosphorylated by the JAKs, allowing for the interaction of STAT proteins, predominantly STAT-3. Upon phosphorylation, STAT-3 dimers translocate to the nucleus and activate transcription from IL-6 target gene promoters that contain a GAS-like element known as the sis-inducible element (SIE). IL-6 signaling also leads to activation of the mitogen-activated protein kinase (MAPK) pathway (Fig. 2).

ACTIVATION OF THE JAK/STAT PATHWAY IN GLIA BY INTERFERONS

Astrocytes, microglia, and oligodendrocytes comprise the glial cell elements of the CNS and have important physiological properties in both the healthy and damaged CNS. Astrocytes, the most numerous of the glial cells,

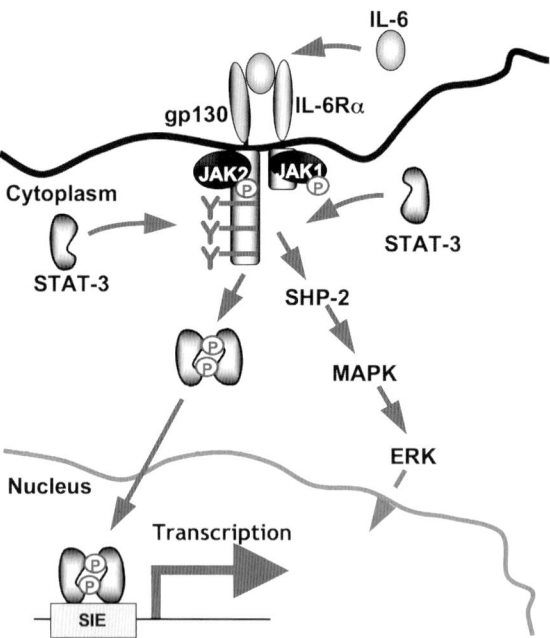

Fig. 2. The interleukin-6 (IL-6) signaling pathway. IL-6 stimulates cells through a receptor complex composed of the IL-6R or the sIL-6R and gp130. This process leads to activation of gp130-associated Janus kinases (JAKs), which phosphorylate gp130 to provide docking and activation sites for STAT-3, which then activates IL-6-responsive genes. IL-6 signal transduction also occurs through activation of the mitogen-activated protein kinase (MAPK)/extracellular regulated kinase (ERK) signaling pathway. SHP-2 = Src homology phosphatase 2, SIE = sis-inducible element. Adapted from Schindler (2006).

affect neuronal function by the release of neurotrophic factors, guide neuronal development, contribute to the metabolism of neurotransmitters, and regulate extracellular concentrations of ions and metabolites (Volterra and Meldolesi 2005). Furthermore, recent evidence implicates astrocytes in synaptogenesis and synaptic transmission (Allen and Barres 2005; Stellwagen and Malenka 2006). Astrocytes also have important roles in contributing to both the structural and functional integrity of the blood-brain barrier. Accordingly, when astrocyte function is perturbed, these cells contribute to the pathogenesis of numerous CNS diseases such as multiple sclerosis (MS), HIV-1 associated dementia, Alzheimer's disease, spinal cord injury (SCI), and amyotrophic lateral sclerosis, just to name a few (Dong and Benveniste 2001; John et al. 2003; Benveniste and Benos 2005; Volterra and Meldolesi 2005). Astrocyte involvement in such diseases stems in part from their ability to promote immunological and inflammatory events in the CNS (Dong and Benveniste 2001; John et al. 2003; Benveniste and Benos 2005).

Astrocytes can be induced to secrete a number of immunoregulatory cytokines and chemokines such as interleukin (IL)-1, IL-6, IL-8, and IL-27, tumor necrosis factor-α (TNF-α), transforming growth factor-β (TGF-β), monocyte chemoattractant protein-1 (MCP-1, also known as CCL2), IFN-γ inducible protein-10 KDa (IP-10, also known as CXCL10), and stromal derived factor-1 (SDF-1, also known as CXCL12). The induction of many of these genes is provoked by IFN-γ or IFN-β activation of the JAK/STAT pathway, specifically the formation of STAT-1α homodimers upon IFN-γ stimulation, and by formation of the ISGF3 complex upon IFN-β treatment (Oh et al. 1999; Satoh and Kuroda 2001; Hua et al. 2002; Okada et al. 2005). In general, IFN-γ promotes the expression of proinflammatory gene products, while IFN-β regulates expression of anti-inflammatory genes. In this regard, IFN-γ treatment induces expression of the transcription factor IRF-1 (a STAT-1α-dependent gene) in astrocytes, which in turn induces expression of proinflammatory proteins (Dong et al. 2001; Satoh and Kuroda 2001), whereas IFN-β treatment preferentially induces the IRF-7 transcription factor, which is mediated by the ISGF3 complex (Satoh and Kuroda 2001). IRF-7 can then amplify IFN-β production, resulting in a positive feedback loop. Both IFN-γ and IFN-β responses involve the STAT-1α transcription factor, and in astrocytes, both IFNs are capable of enhancing STAT-1α gene expression (Lee and Benveniste 1996; Satoh and Kuroda 2001). Other effects of IFN-β on astrocytes are complex and appear to be gene-dependent. IFN-β inhibits astrocyte production of IL-1/IFN-γ-induced TNF-α, IL-6, and inducible nitric oxide synthase (iNOS), in part by inhibiting IFN-γ-induced STAT-1α binding activity (Hua et al. 2002). In contrast, IFN-β synergizes with IL-1 to induce regulated upon activation, normal T-cell-expressed and secreted (RANTES/CCL5) expression in astrocytes, and it augments RANTES expression induced by both IL-1 and IFN-γ (Kim et al. 2004), providing an example of a case in which IFN-β does not antagonize the effect of IFN-γ. IFN-β also has the ability to inhibit responses in astrocytes through the JAK/STAT pathway. IFN-β inhibits the expression of phorbol-12-myristate-13-acetate (PMA)-induced matrix metalloproteinase-9 (MMP-9) and IL-8 in astrocytes, and this inhibitory effect is dependent on the STAT-1α transcription factor (Ma et al. 2001; Nozell et al. 2006). These genes do not have GAS elements or ISREs in their promoters, so the inhibitory effect is probably due to STAT-1α or ISGF3 sequestration of important transcriptional activators of MMP-9 and IL-8 gene expression such as CREB-binding protein.

Microglia are the resident brain macrophages, and have functions similar to those of other tissue macrophages including phagocytosis, antigen presentation, and production of cytokines, chemokines, eicosanoids, complement components, MMPs, oxidative radicals, and nitric oxide (Carson 2002; Hanisch 2002; Town et al. 2005). Activated macrophages and microglia have a well documented pathogenic role in MS, Alzheimer's disease, and HIV-1 associated dementia (Hanisch 2002; John et al. 2003). IFN-γ is a potent activator of microglia, particularly with respect to its ability to induce class II transactivator (CIITA) and subsequent class II major histocompatibility complex (MHC) expression, and expression of co-stimulatory molecules such as cluster of differentiation (CD) molecules CD40, CD80, and CD86 (O'Keefe et al. 2002). Expression of these genes is critical for the microglial cell to function as an antigen-presenting cell in the CNS, and contributes to promotion of immune reactivity during disease states. The promoters for CIITA, CD40, CD80, and CD86 all have GAS elements, which are critical for IFN-γ induction of these genes. Furthermore, using STAT-1α-deficient microglia, we have shown that STAT-1α is required for IFN-γ induction of CIITA and CD40 (Nguyen and Benveniste 2000; O'Keefe et al. 2002). In human microglia, IFN-β induces expression of the chemokines RANTES (CCL5) and macrophage inflammatory protein (MIP-1α) (CCL3), but IFN-γ has no such effect (Hua and Lee 2000; McManus et al. 2000). It was further demonstrated that IFN-β activation of numerous signaling cascades, including JAK/STAT, was responsible for chemokine expression in these cells (Kim et al. 2002).

Oligodendrocytes are responsible for the synthesis and maintenance of myelin in the CNS, and therefore are critical for function in health and disease (Popko and Baerwald 1999). Damage to myelin and/or to the oligodendrocyte is a common feature in numerous neurological disorders; one example is MS, which is the most common human demyelinating disease of the CNS. IFN-γ is thought to have a deleterious role in immune-mediated demyelinating diseases, in part through direct effects on oligodendrocytes and their progenitor cells. IFN-γ has been shown to induce death of both developing and mature oligodendrocytes (Vartanian et al. 1995; Baerwald and Popko 1998; Chew et al. 2005). This effect may be mediated directly by IFN-γ or by the upregulation of the death receptor Fas on these cells (Pouly et al. 2000). The effect of IFN-γ depends in large part on the developmental stage of the oligodendrocyte lineage. More recent studies have examined the molecular basis by which IFN-γ damages oligodendrocytes, and two major signaling pathways appear to be involved. Horiuchi et al. (2006) demonstrated that simultaneous activation of the STAT pathway by IFN-γ and of the extracellular regulated kinase (ERK) pathway by stimuli such as platelet-derived growth factor and fibroblast growth factor-2 contributed to IFN-γ-induced cytotoxicity of oligodendrocyte precursors. Transgenic expression of IFN-γ in the CNS results in oligodendrocyte loss and hypomyelination, which involves activation of STAT-1α in oligodendrocytes (Balabanov et al. 2006). Thus, these results indicate that IFN-γ can utilize several signaling cascades (ERK and STAT) to adversely affect oligodendrocytes and the process of myelination.

ACTIVATION OF THE JAK/STAT PATHWAY
IN GLIA BY IL-6 CYTOKINES

Cytokines of the IL-6 family exert their diverse biological effects by engagement of receptor complexes that are characterized by the presence of the shared 130-kDa receptor subunit, gp130 (Fig. 2). Gp130 is ubiquitously expressed and has been detected on astrocytes, microglia, and oligodendrocytes (Blass-Kampmann et al. 1997; Marmur et al. 1998; Nakashima et al. 1999; Yanagisawa et al. 2000). Members of the IL-6 cytokine family (IL-6, IL-11, OSM, LIF, CNTF) play pivotal roles in immune, hematopoietic, nervous, and endocrine systems, and also function in inflammation and acute phase responses, and many of these responses are mediated through the STAT-3 transcription factor (Hirano et al. 2000).

Astrocytes do not express the membrane-bound form of the IL-6R; rather, they respond to IL-6 only in the presence of the sIL-6R (Van Wagoner and Benveniste 1999b). IL-6/sIL-6R is a potent activator of STAT-3 in astrocytes, and leads to the expression of IL-6 (Van Wagoner et al. 1999a) and α_1-antichymotrypsin (Kordula et al. 1998). Furthermore, OSM is a strong activator of STAT-3 in astroglial cells, and leads to expression of vascular endothelial growth factor (VEGF) in these cells (Repovic et al. 2003). The process of astrogliosis is associated with the rapid, but transient, activation of the STAT-3 pathway by IL-6 cytokines (Sriram et al. 2004). Activation of the STAT-3 signaling pathway in reactive astrocytes has been well documented (Xia et al. 2002; Okada et al. 2005). In vivo studies demonstrate that reactive astrocytes have an important role in the healing process after SCI, and that this function of reactive astrocytes is largely dependent on STAT-3 activation (Okada et al. 2006).

Oligodendrocyte survival and myelination is in large part mediated by members of the IL-6 family of cytokines, notably IL-6, LIF and CNTF. Signaling of CNTF, IL-6/sIL-6R, and LIF through gp130 increases the proliferation of oligodendrocyte precursors (Barres 1991; Valerio et al. 2002) and enhances myelination (Stankoff et al. 2002). In addition, IL-6 and the sIL-6R prevent oligodendrocyte degeneration and demyelination induced by NMDA through activation of both STAT-1 and STAT-3 (Pizzi et al. 2004). LIF and CNTF promote the survival of oligodendrocytes in vivo, especially in the context of neuroinflammation (Butzkueven et al. 2002, 2006; Linker et al. 2002; Kuhlmann et al. 2006). The protective effect of LIF was shown to be mediated directly through signaling within oligodendrocytes, and through activation of STAT-3 in these cells (Emery et al. 2006). Thus, there is strong interest in using IL-6 family members to treat neurodegenerative and demyelinating diseases because of their protective effects on oligodendrocytes. In addition, a recent study has shown that LIF promotes neural stem cell self-renewal, leading to an expansion of this pool of cells (Bauer and Patterson 2006). The authors speculated that this may be important for promoting regeneration in the CNS.

IL-6 also has destructive properties in the CNS, especially when chronically expressed at high levels (Campbell et al. 1993). Transgenic mice in which IL-6 is expressed under the control of the astrocyte-specific glial fibrillary acidic protein (GFAP) promoter display neurodegeneration, breakdown of the blood-brain-barrier, CNS inflammation and angiogenesis, and increased expression of complement proteins (Campbell et al. 1993; Barnum et al. 1996). The brains of these mice also display strong activation of STAT-3, as assessed by tyrosine phosphorylation (Campbell 2005). Another important consequence of IL-6 over-expression in the CNS is the induction of cytokines such as IL-1 and TNF-α (Di Santo et al. 1996, 1997), which in general have proinflammatory properties, and are also overexpressed in the brain in MS and HIV-1 associated dementia.

NEGATIVE REGULATION OF THE JAK/STAT PATHWAY: SOCS PROTEINS

Precise regulation of the magnitude and duration of JAK activity and of STAT activation is essential for the orchestration of numerous biological processes, and dysregulation of the JAK/STAT pathway has pathological implications (Shuai and Liu 2003). A number of mechanisms have evolved that negatively regulate the JAK/STAT pathway, thereby attenuating biological responses. Control via a negative feedback loop, which is accomplished by suppressors of cytokine signaling (SOCS), is one of the major mechanisms for the inhibition of signal transduction through the JAK/STAT pathway (Kubo et al. 2003; Alexander and Hilton 2004; Campbell 2005). There are eight members of the SOCS protein family: cytokine-inducible Src homology 2 (SH2)-domain-containing protein (CIS) and SOCS-1 through SOCS-7. Each has a central SH2 domain, an N-terminal domain of variable length, and a C-terminal 40-amino-acid module called the SOCS box (Fig. 3A). SOCS proteins attenuate

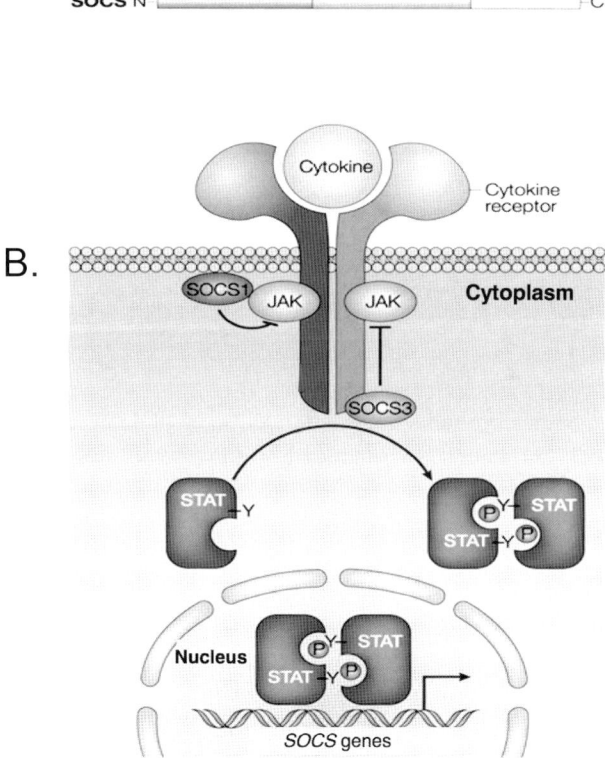

Fig. 3. The SOCS (suppressors of cytokine signaling) family of proteins. (A) Domain struc-ture of SOCS proteins. The SOCS family of proteins has eight members: cytokine-inducible SH2-domain-containing protein (CIS) and SOCS-1–SOCS-7. SOCS proteins contain an Src homology 2 (SH2) domain that is flanked by a variable amino-terminal domain and a carboxy-terminal SOCS box. The SOCS box can bind to elongins B and C, which are known compo-nents of a ubiquitin E3 ligase complex. (B) Inhibition of the JAK-STAT-signaling pathway by SOCS proteins has distinct mechanisms. SOCS-1 binds directly to tyrosine-phosphorylated JAKs through the SH2 domain, resulting in the inhibition of kinase activity. SOCS-3 inhibits JAKs by binding to the receptor. Adapted from Kubo et al. (2003).

JAK/STAT signaling by binding to phosphorylated tyrosine residues on receptor chains and on JAKs through their SH2 domain. For example, SOCS-1 interacts with a tyrosine residue in the activation loop of JAKs, thereby inhibiting kinase activity, while SOCS-3 binds to JAK-proximal sites on cytokine receptors and inhibits JAK activity (Fig. 3B). The SOCS box has been shown to couple the substrate-specific interactions of the SH2 domain to the ubiquitin ligation machinery, leading to subsequent degradation in the proteosome. Therefore, SOCS proteins combine specific inhibition of JAK activity with a generic mechanism of targeting interacting proteins for proteosomal degradation.

The SOCS-1 protein is a key regulator of IFN-γ signaling via STAT-1α in vivo. SOCS-1-deficient mice display a lethal perinatal syndrome that includes fatty degeneration, necrosis of the liver, and damage to the pancreas, heart, and skin due to infiltrating T cells, macrophages, and eosinophils (Naka et al. 1998; Starr et al. 1998). The disease is eliminated upon treatment with antibodies to IFN-γ, and it does not affect mice deficient in IFN-γ in addition to SOCS-1 (Alexander et al. 1999). Thus, the actions of SOCS-1 are necessary to attenuate the duration of IFN-γ signaling through STAT-1α, allowing for the beneficial immunological effects of IFN-γ, but preventing the pathological consequences of uncontrolled IFN-γ responses.

Given that SOCS-3 deficiency is lethal to the embryo, conditional gene targeting has been used to elucidate the function of this protein. The SOCS-3 protein is critical for regulating signaling by IL-6 cytokine family members, which utilize the STAT-3 protein. Targeted deletion of SOCS-3 in macrophages results in markedly enhanced IL-6-induced STAT-3 activation, demonstrating that SOCS-3 targets gp130-dependent signal transduction pathways. In vivo studies suggest that SOCS-3 is a negative regulator of inflammatory diseases.

SOCS EXPRESSION AND FUNCTION
IN THE CENTRAL NERVOUS SYSTEM

SOCS-1 and SOCS-3 have been implicated in regulating responses in glial cells, so the focus of this section will be on these two SOCS proteins. SOCS-1 and SOCS-3 mRNA and protein are present at very low levels in unstimulated cells, perhaps because of active repression (Jegalian and Wu 2002; Mostecki et al. 2005). SOCS-1 and SOCS-3 gene transcription is rapidly induced in glial cells upon stimulation with numerous stimuli (Table I). In primary astrocytes and human astroglioma cell lines, SOCS-1 and SOCS-3 expression is induced by the cytokines IFN-γ, IFN-β, and OSM, and by peroxisome proliferator-activated receptor (PPAR)-γ agonists such as 15d-PGJ$_2$ and rosiglitazone (Park et al. 2003; Stark et al. 2004; B. Baker and E.N. Benveniste, 2007, unpublished observations). PPAR-γ agonists are recognized as having anti-inflammatory

Table I
SOCS-1 and SOCS-3 gene induction in glial cells

SOCS-1		SOCS-3	
Cell Type	Inducer(s)	Cell Type	Inducer(s)
Primary astrocytes	15d-PGJ$_2$, RSG, IFN-γ, IFN-β, OSM	Primary astrocytes	15d-PGJ$_2$, RSG, IFN-γ, IFN-β, OSM
BV-2 microglial cells	15d-PGJ$_2$, RSG	Primary microglia	IFN-γ, IFN-β, LPS
Primary microglia	IFN-γ, IFN-β, LPS, IL-4	RAW264.7 (macrophage)	Lovastatin, IFN-γ, IFN-β, LPS
RAW264.7 (macrophage)	IFN-γ, IFN-β, LPS, IL-10, IL-4	Primary oligodendrocytes	LIF
Primary oligodendrocytes	IFN-γ		

Abbreviations: IFN = interferon; IL = interleukin; LIF = leukemia inhibitory factor; LPS = lipopolysaccharide; OSM = oncostatin M; PGJ$_2$ = prostaglandin J$_2$; RSG = rosiglitazone; SOCS = suppressor of cytokine signaling.

effects by suppressing cytokine actions, and they also showed beneficial effects in experimental allergic encephalomyelitis (EAE)— an animal model of MS—by inhibiting cytokine and chemokine induction (Diab et al. 2002; Feinstein et al. 2002; Feinstein 2003). In primary microglia, microglial cell lines, and macrophage cell lines, SOCS-1 and SOCS-3 are induced by cytokines such as IFN-γ, IFN-β, IL-10, and IL-4, by lipopolysaccharide (LPS) signaling through Toll-like receptor 4 (TLR4), and by the PPAR-γ agonists 15d-PGJ$_2$ and rosiglitazone (Table I); (Park et al. 2003; Qin et al. 2006a,b). The ability of IL-10 and LPS to induce SOCS-3 is dependent upon STAT-3 activation, because a STAT-3 dominant-negative mutant prevents this response (Qin et al. 2006b). Interestingly, lovastatin has recently been shown to induce SOCS-3 expression in RAW264.7 macrophage cells (Huang et al. 2003). Statins are relevant to CNS inflammatory diseases because they have beneficial effects in ameliorating the clinical course of EAE, and more importantly, they have proven efficacious in two clinical trials of relapsing-remitting MS (Greenwood et al. 2006). Statins have also been shown to reduce the risk of Alzheimer's disease in persons less than 80 years old (Rockwood et al. 2002). Oligodendrocytes have recently been shown to express SOCS-1 upon stimulation with IFN-γ (Balabanov et al. 2006; Emery et al. 2006a), and they express SOCS-3 upon exposure to LIF (Emery et al. 2006a,b).

Studies on the expression or function of SOCS family members in the CNS are limited. In the brain of transgenic mice with chronic astrocyte production of IL-12 (GF-IL-12), which exhibit a spontaneous neuroimmune disease, presymptomatic mice had low constitutive expression of SOCS-1 and SOCS-3.

However, in symptomatic GF-IL-12 mice, there was a marked increase in SOCS-1 and SOCS-3 mRNA expression in infiltrating CD3-positive cells and lesion-associated macrophages and microglia (Maier et al. 2002). In the EAE model, SOCS-1 and SOCS-3 mRNA transcripts increased significantly in the cerebellum and spinal cord at the height of the disease and then declined (Maier et al. 2002). Stark and Cross (2005) analyzed SOCS-1 and SOCS-3 expression in two models of EAE—SJL mice with relapsing-recruiting EAE, and B6 mice with a more chronic course without complete remissions. SOCS-1 and SOCS-3 mRNA was elevated throughout active disease in both strains, although B6 mice expressed less SOCS-3 than SJL mice at the peak of disease, suggesting a more proinflammatory CNS environment in B6 mice. The authors speculate that the failure of B6 mice to completely recover after acute EAE may be due to inadequate production of SOCS-3.

A beneficial effect of SOCS-1 in EAE has recently been shown. Using a mimetic of SOCS-1 (TKip), Mujtaba et al. (2005) demonstrated TKip inhibition of STAT-1α activation, as well as a protective effect of TKip in EAE. The protective effect correlated with lower myelin basic protein (MBP) antibody titers, suppression of MBP-induced splenocyte proliferation, and inhibition of TNF-α activity. Furthermore, targeted expression of SOCS-1 in oligodendrocytes protects against the injurious effects of IFN-γ (Balabanov et al. 2006), demonstrating another beneficial effect of the SOCS-1 protein in the CNS. However, the role of SOCS proteins is complex, as illustrated by three recent studies. SOCS-3 has been suggested to have neuroprotective effects, as antisense knockdown of SOCS-3 expression increases the severity of stroke symptoms (Carmichael 2003). Emery et al. (2006b) have shown that SOCS-3 expression in oligodendrocytes limits LIF-induced protection against demyelination. SOCS-3 is detrimental to axonal growth through the inhibition of STAT-3 activation (Miao et al. 2006). Thus, the effects of SOCS-1 and SOCS-3 in cells of the CNS are complex. These proteins have important roles in mitigating the pathogenic effects of inflammatory cytokines during neuroinflammatory diseases, but they also adversely affect the growth of oligodendrocytes and neurons.

THE NUCLEAR FACTOR-KAPPA-B PATHWAY

The NF-κB family of transcription factors consists of five structurally similar members that each contain a Rel homology domain (RHD) (Fig. 4A) (Greten et al. 2004; Hayden and Ghosh 2004; Monks et al. 2004; Viatour et al. 2005). These proteins are classified into two groups. The first group, consisting of p65 (RelA), RelB, and c-Rel, are synthesized in their mature forms and contain a C-terminal transactivation domain (TAD). The second group, consisting of

NF-κB1 (p105/p50) and NF-κB2 (p100/p52), lack a TAD and are first synthesized as large precursors (p105 and p100), which are later processed to result in the mature form (p50 and p52). Through their RHDs, NF-κB members are able to form numerous homo- and heterodimers that are competent to bind DNA. However, only the NF-κB dimers that contain p65, RelB, or c-Rel, and thus a TAD, are able to positively regulate gene expression. In many cell types, the most common NF-κB dimer is composed of p65 and p50, and this dimer is specifically referred to as NF-κB.

In unstimulated cells, NF-κB is inactive and sequestered in the cytosol through interactions with inhibitor of NF-κB (IκB) proteins, which bind to the RHD of NF-κB and mask the nuclear localization signal (Fig. 4B) (Greten et

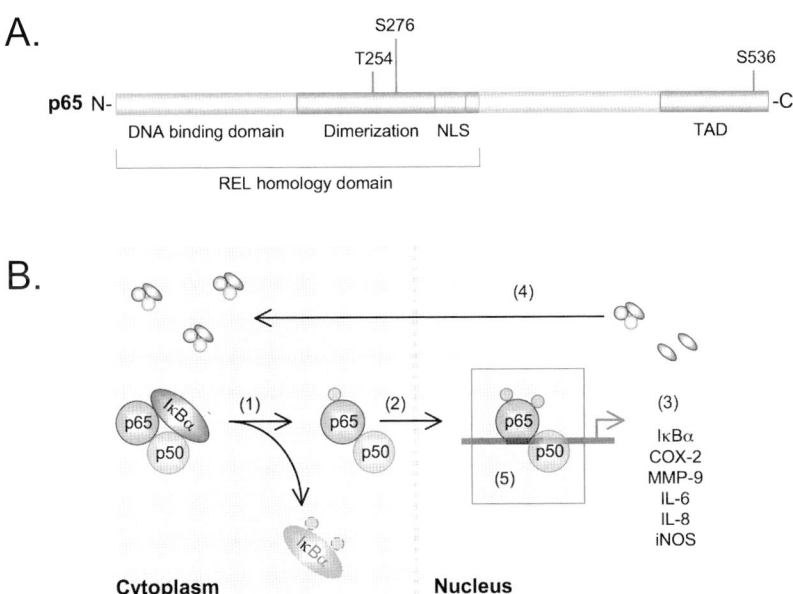

Fig. 4. The nuclear factor (NF)-κB pathway. A. NF-κB p65 contains an N-terminal DNA-binding domain known as the Rel homology domain (RHD), a C-terminal transactivation domain, a dimerization domain, and a nuclear localization signal (NLS). Phosphorylation of p65 at threonine 254 (T254), serine 276 (S276), and S536 enhances DNA binding and transactivation. (B) The prototypic NF-κB dimer contains p65 and p50 and is maintained in the inactive state by interactions with an inhibitor of NF-κB (IκBα). In response to stimuli, IκBα is phosphorylated and rapidly degraded (1). Once released, NF-κB may be post-translationally modified and migrate into the nucleus (2). In the nucleus, NF-κB binds to κB response elements and activates the expression of numerous genes, including the genes for IκBα, cyclooxygenase-2 (COX-2), matrix metalloproteinase-9 (MMP-9), interleukin (IL)-6, IL-8, and inducible nitric oxide synthase (iNOS) (3). NF-κB signaling is partially terminated when newly synthesized IκBα escorts NF-κB molecules into the cytoplasm (4). While at the promoters of target genes, little is known about NF-κB regulation (5).

al. 2004; Hayden and Ghosh 2004; Monks et al. 2004; Moynagh 2005; Viatour et al. 2005). In response to proinflammatory cytokines such as TNF-α or IL-1β, the IκB kinase (IKK) complex is activated and phosphorylates IκB proteins, causing their ubiquitin-dependent degradation. This process allows the newly liberated NF-κB dimers to translocate into the nucleus, bind κB elements present in the promoters of target genes, and activate gene expression. Given the repertoire of genes that it activates, NF-κB is a critical regulator of the inflammatory response; of cell proliferation, invasion, migration, and adhesion; and of the processes of apoptosis and angiogenesis.

ACTIVATION OF THE NUCLEAR FACTOR-KAPPA-B PATHWAY IN GLIA

Astrocytes are activated by a wide array of stimuli that lead to NF-κB activation and downstream gene expression (Kaltschmidt et al. 2005; Memet 2006). Some of these stimuli include TNF-α, IL-1β, PMA, β-amyloid, LPS, and ethanol (Sparacio et al. 1992; Moynagh et al. 1993; Friedman et al. 1996; Akama et al. 1998; Lee et al. 1998; Kemler and Fontana 1999; Srinivasan et al. 2004; Blanco et al. 2005; Griffin and Moynagh 2006; Nozell et al. 2006). NF-κB-driven genes that are induced in astrocytes include intercellular adhesion molecule-1 (ICAM-1), vascular cell adhesion molecule-1 (VCAM-1), IL-8, iNOS, TNF-α, IL-6, nerve growth factor (NGF), and MMP-9 (Memet 2006); it is notable that many of these gene products are associated with inflammation. In general, activation of the NF-κB pathway in astrocytes is thought to contribute to inflammatory responses within the CNS.

Microglia also respond to a variety of stimuli that activate NF-κB; these include TNF-α, IL-12, β-amyloid, ATP, LPS, IFN-β, brain-derived neurotropic factor (BDNF) and neurotrophin (NT-3) (Pahan et al. 2001; Kim et al. 2002; Chen et al. 2005; Kaltschmidt et al. 2005; Qin et al. 2005). Again, many genes associated with inflammation are induced by these stimuli, which include iNOS, IL-12, CD40, IP-10, IL-8, TNF-α, IL-1β, IL-6, RANTES, MCP-1, MIP-1α, ICAM-1, B7-1 and B7-2 (Pahan et al. 2001; Olson and Miller 2004; Si et al. 2004; Jack et al. 2005; Qin et al. 2005). Furthermore, NF-κB signaling in microglia induced by β-amyloid is critical for neuronal death, which may contribute to β-amyloid-dependent neurodegeneration (Chen et al. 2005). Thus, NF-κB activation and downstream responses in microglia may contribute to both neuroinflammation and neurodegeneration.

Activation of NF-κB in oligodendrocytes has not been studied as intensely, although there are reports that NGF and H_2O_2 activate NF-κB in these cells (Kaltschmidt et al. 2005). H_2O_2-mediated apoptotic cell death of oligodendrocytes is dependent on NF-κB activation (Vollgraf et al. 1999). Schwann cells are responsible for myelination in the peripheral nervous system. Activation of NF-κB in Schwann cells is essential for formation of peripheral myelin (Nickols et al. 2003), so it is possible that NF-κB may influence myelin formation by oligodendrocytes in the CNS.

A number of recent in vivo studies have implicated astrocytic NF-κB in contributing to disease induction and severity in both SCI and EAE. Selective inhibition of astrocytic NF-κB by expression of a dominant-negative form of IκB-α resulted in significant improvement in functional recovery after contusive SCI (Brambilla et al. 2005). This improvement was correlated with reduced lesion volume, increased white matter preservation, and reduced expression of the chemokines IP-10 (CXCL10) and MCP-1 (CCL2). These findings indicate that NF-κB-dependent events initiated in astrocytes are responsible for damage after SCI, in contrast to STAT-3 signaling in astrocytes, which was shown to be important for repair after SCI (Okada et al. 2006). These findings suggest that activation of STAT-3 and NF-κB in astrocytes leads to distinct responses that either promote or inhibit recovery from SCI, respectively. Van Loo et al. (2006) blocked the catalytic subunit IKK2 or the regulatory NEMO subunit in astrocytes, leading to inactivation of NF-κB in these cells, and found that this strategy ameliorated disease in an EAE model. The inhibition of NF-κB prevented the expression of proinflammatory cytokines such as IFN-γ, IL-1β, and TNF-α and chemokines such as MIP-1α (CCL3), IP-10 (CXCL10), and RANTES (CCL5), and also inhibited VCAM-1 expression by astrocytes. These results imply that NF-κB activation in astrocytes contributes to the pathogenesis of CNS inflammation.

CONCLUSIONS

This chapter has provided an overview of the JAK/STAT and NF-κB pathways, describing their involvement in glial cell function. This overview is by no means complete or comprehensive since other signaling pathways such as MAPK, PI3K, cyclic adenosine monophosphate/protein kinase A, protein kinase C, and small mothers against decapentaplegic (SMAD) signaling are also critical for regulating the function of glial cells (Kielian 2004; Rivest 2003; Wesemann and Benveniste 2004; Shankar et al. 2006; Ubogu et al. 2006). Critical for the ability of glial cells to respond to multiple stimuli is the expression of specific receptors that transmit signals from interferons and numerous cytokines. A key feature that dictates the magnitude of intracellular signaling is the level of expression of receptors at the cell surface. In addition, it has recently been suggested that receptors and associated adapters can accumulate within the nucleus and exert novel functions within this subcellular compartment (Massie and Mills 2006). This possibility adds to the level of complexity in signaling cascades that alter gene expression and cellular functions.

In the context of the CNS, glial cell responses to interferons and cytokines can be both neuroprotective and neurodestructive, depending on which glial cell responds and on the timing, magnitude, and duration of the signal. A current challenge in the field of signal transduction is to understand how multiple intracellular signals are integrated within cells and elucidate the molecular mechanisms that dictate cellular responses to such signals (Natarajan et al. 2006). Specifically for the CNS, a deeper understanding of glial cell signal transduction cascades will provide important information for therapeutic interventions to diminish inflammation, promote myelination or remyelination, and enhance neuroprotective effects.

ACKNOWLEDGMENTS

This work was supported by grants from the National Institutes of Health (NS54158, CA97247, NS45290, NS50665) and the National Multiple Sclerosis Society (RG3661-A-10, RG3892-A-12). I thank Cheryl Lyles for outstanding secretarial assistance.

REFERENCES

Akama KT, Albanese C, Pestell RG, et al. Amyloid β-peptide stimulates nitric oxide production in astrocytes through an NFκB-dependent mechanism. *Proc Natl Acad Sci USA* 1998; 95:5795–5800.

Alexander WS, Hilton DJ. The role of suppressors of cytokine signaling (SOCS) proteins in regulation of the immune response. *Annu Rev Immunol* 2004; 22:503–529.

Alexander WS, Starr R, Fenner JE, et al. SOCS1 is a critical inhibitor of interferon γ signaling and prevents the potentially fatal neonatal actions of this cytokine. *Cell* 1999; 98:597–608.

Allen NJ, Barres BA. Signaling between glia and neurons: focus on synaptic plasticity. *Curr Opin Neurobiol* 2005; 15:542–548.

Baerwald KD, Popko B. Developing and mature oligodendrocytes respond differently to the immune cytokine interferon-gamma. *J Neurosci Res* 1998; 52:230–239.

Balabanov R, Strand K, Kemper A, et al. Suppressor of cytokine signaling 1 expression protects oligodendrocytes from the deleterious effects of interferon-gamma. *J Neurosci* 2006; 26:5143–5152.

Barnum SR, Jones JL, Müller-Ladner U, et al. Chronic complement C3 gene expression in the CNS of transgenic mice with astrocyte-targeted interleukin-6 expression. *Glia* 1996; 18:107–117.

Barres BA. New roles for glia. *J Neurosci* 1991; 11:3685–3694.

Bauer S, Patterson PH. Leukemia inhibitory factor promotes neural stem cell self-renewal in the adult brain. *J Neurosci* 2006; 26:12089–12099.

Benveniste EN, Benos DJ. Astrocyte immunobiology. In: Gendelman HE, Grant I, Everall IP, Lipton SA, Swindells S (Eds). *The Neurology of AIDS.* New York: Oxford University Press, 2005, pp 211–223.

Blanco AM, Valles SL, Pascual M, et al. Involvement of TLR4/Type I IL-1 receptor signaling in the induction of inflammatory mediators and cell death induced by ethanol in cultured astrocytes. *J Immunol* 2005; 175:6893–6899.

Blass-Kampmann S, Kindler-Rohrborn A, Deissler H, et al. In vitro differentiation of neural progenitor cells from prenatal rat brain: common cell surface glycoprotein on three glial cell subsets. *J Neurosci Res* 1997; 48:95–111.

Brambilla R, Bracchi-Ricard V, Hu WH. et al. Inhibition of astroglial nuclear factor κB reduces inflammation and improves functional recovery after spinal cord injury. *J Exp Med* 2005; 202:145–156.

Butzkueven H, Zhang J-G, Soilu-Hanninen M, et al. LIF receptor signaling limits immune-mediated demyelination by enhancing oligodendrocyte survival. *Nat Med* 2002; 8:613–619.

Butzkueven H, Emery B, Cipriani T, et al. Endogenous leukemia inhibitory factor production limits autoimmune demyelination and oligodendrocyte loss. *Glia* 2006; 53:696–703.

Campbell IL. Cytokine-mediated inflammation, tumorigenesis, and disease-associated JAK/STAT/SOCS signaling circuits in the CNS. *Brain Res Rev* 2005; 48:166–177.

Campbell IL, Abraham CR, Masliah E, et al. Neurologic disease induced in transgenic mice by cerebral overexpression of interleukin 6. *Proc Natl Acad Sci USA* 1993; 90:10061–10065.

Carmichael ST. Gene expression changes after focal stroke, traumatic brain and spinal cord injuries. *Curr Opin Neurol* 2003; 16:699–704.

Carson MJ. Microglia as liaisons between the immune and central nervous systems: functional implications for multiple sclerosis. *Glia* 2002; 40:218–231.

Chen J, Zhou Y, Mueller-Steiner S, et al. SIRT1 protects against microglia-dependent amyloid-β toxicity through inhibiting NF-κB signaling. *J Biol Chem* 2005; 280:40364–40374.

Chew LJ, King WC, Kennedy A, et al. Interferon-gamma inhibits cell cycle exit in differentiating oligodendrocyte progenitor cells. *Glia* 2005; 52:127–143.

Decker T, Kovarik P. Serine phosphorylation of STATs. *Oncogene* 2000; 19:2628–2637.

Di Santo E, Alonzi T, Fattori E, et al. Overexpression of interleukin-6 in the central nervous system of transgenic mice increases central but not systemic proinflammatory cytokine production. *Brain Res* 1996; 740:239–244.

Di Santo E, Alonzi T, Poli V, et al. Differential effects of IL-6 on systemic and central production of TNF: a study with IL-6-deficient mice. *Cytokine* 1997; 9:300–306.

Diab A, Deng C, Smith JD, et al. Peroxisome proliferator-activated receptor-γ agonist 15-deoxy-$\Delta^{12,14}$-prostaglandin J$_2$ ameliorates experimental autoimmune encephalomyelitis. *J Immunol* 2002; 168:2508–2515.

Dong Y, Benveniste EN. Immune function of astrocytes. *Glia* 2001; 36:180–190.

Dong Y, Tang L, Letterio JJ, et al. The Smad3 protein is involved in TGF-β inhibition of class II transactivator and class II MHC expression. *J Immunol* 2001; 167:311–319.

Emery B, Butzkueven H, Snell C, et al. Oligodendrocytes exhibit selective expression of suppressor of cytokine signaling genes and signal transducer and activator of transcription 1 independent inhibition of interferon-γ-induced toxicity in response to leukemia inhibitory factor. *Neuroscience* 2006a; 137:463–472.

Emery B, Cate HS, Marriott M, et al. Suppressor of cytokine signaling 3 limits protection of leukemia inhibitory factor receptor signaling against central demyelination. *Proc Natl Acad Sci USA* 2006b; 103:7859–7864.

Feinstein DL. Therapeutic potential of peroxisome proliferator-activated receptor agonists for neurological disease. *Diabetes Technol Ther* 2003; 5:67–73.

Feinstein DL, Galea E, Gavrilyuk V, et al. Peroxisome proliferator-activated receptor-gamma agonists prevent experimental autoimmune encephalomyelitis. *Ann Neurol* 2002; 51:694–702.

Friedman WJ, Thakur S, Seidman L, et al. Regulation of nerve growth factor mRNA by interleukin-1 in rat hippocampal astrocytes is mediated by NF-κB. *J Biol Chem* 1996; 271:31115–31120.

Greenwood J, Steinman L, Zamvil SS. Statin therapy and autoimmune disease: from protein prenylation to immunomodulation. *Nat Rev Immunol* 2006; 6:358–370.

Greten FR, Eckmann L, Greten TF, et al. IKKβ links inflammation and tumorigenesis in a mouse model of colitis-associated cancer. *Cell* 2004; 118:285–296.

Griffin BD, Moynagh PN. Persistent interleukin-1β signaling causes long term activation of NFκB in a promoter-specific manner in human glial cells. *J Biol Chem* 2006; 281:10316–10326.

Hanisch U-K. Microglia as a source and target of cytokines. *Glia* 2002; 40:140–155.

Hayden MS, Ghosh S. Signaling to NF-kappaB. *Genes Dev* 2004; 18:2195–2224.

Hirano T, Ishihara K, Hibi M. Roles of STAT3 in mediating the cell growth, differentiation and survival signals relayed through the IL-6 family of cytokine receptors. *Oncogene* 2000; 19:2548–2556.

Horiuchi M, Itoh A, Pleasure D, et al. MEK-ERK signaling is involved in interferon-γ-induced death of oligodendroglial progenitor cells. *J Biol Chem* 2006; 281:20095–20106.

Hua LL, Lee SC. Distinct patterns of stimulus-inducible chemokine mRNA accumulation in human fetal astrocytes and microglia. *Glia* 2000; 30:74–81.

Hua LL, Kim MO, Brosnan CF, et al. Modulation of astrocyte inducible nitric oxide synthase and cytokine expression by interferon γ is associated with induction and inhibition of interferon γ-activated sequence binding activity. *J Neurochem* 2002; 83:1120–1128.

Huang KC, Chen CW, Chen JC, et al. Statins induce suppressor of cytokine signaling-3 in macrophages. *FEBS Lett* 2003; 555:385–389.

Jack CS, Arbour N, Manusow J, et al. TLR signaling tailors innate immune responses in human microglia and astrocytes. *J Immunol* 2005; 175:4320–4330.

Jegalian AG, Wu H. Regulation of Socs gene expression by the proto-oncoprotein GFI-1B: two routes for STAT5 target gene induction by erythropoietin. *J Biol Chem* 2002; 277:2345–2352.

John GR, Lee SC, Brosnan CF. Cytokines: powerful regulators of glial cell activation. *Neuroscientist* 2003; 9:10–22.

Kaltschmidt B, Widera D, Kaltschmidt C. Signaling via NF-kappaB in the nervous system. *Biochim Biophys Acta* 2005; 1745:287–299.

Kemler I, Fontana A. Role of IκBα and IκBβ in the biphasic nuclear translocation of NF-κB in TNF-α-stimulated astrocytes and in neuroblastoma cells. *Glia* 1999; 26:212–220.

Kielian T. Microglia and chemokines in infectious diseases of the nervous system: views and reviews. *Front Biosci* 2004; 9:732–750.

Kim MO, Si Q, Zhou JN, et al. Interferon-β activates multiple signaling cascades in primary human microglia. *J Neurochem* 2002; 81:1361–1371.

Kim MO, Suh HS, Brosnan CF, et al. Regulation of RANTES/CCL5 expression in human astrocytes by interleukin-1 and interferon-γ. *J Neurochem* 2004; 90:297–308.

Kordula T, Rydel RE, Brigham EF, et al. Oncostatin M and the interleukin-6 and soluble interleukin-6 receptor complex regulate $α_1$-antichymotrypsin expression in human cortical astrocytes. *J Biol Chem* 1998; 273:4112–4118.

Kubo M, Hanada T, Yoshimura A. Suppressors of cytokine signaling and immunity. *Nat Immunol* 2003; 4:1169–1176.

Kuhlmann T, Remington L, Cognet I, et al. Continued administration of ciliary neurotrophic factor protects mice from inflammatory pathology in experimental autoimmune encephalomyelitis. *Am J Pathol* 2006; 169:584–598.

Lee SJ, Hou J, Benveniste EN. Transcriptional regulation of intercellular adhesion molecule-1 in astrocytes involves NF-κB and C/EBP isoforms. *J Neuroimmunol* 1998; 92:196–207.

Lee YJ, Benveniste EN. STAT-1α expression is involved in IFN-γ induction of the class II transactivator and class II MHC genes. *J Immunol* 1996; 157:1559–1568.

Linker RA, Mäurer M, Gaupp S, et al. CNTF is a major protective factor in demyelinating CNS disease: A neurotrophic cytokine as modulator in neuroinflammation. *Nat Med* 2002; 8:620–624.

Ma Z, Qin H, Benveniste EN. Transcriptional suppression of matrix metalloproteinase-9 gene expression by IFN-γ and IFN-β: critical role of STAT-1α. *J Immunol* 2001; 167:5150–5159.

Maier J, Kincaid C, Pagenstecher A, et al. Regulation of signal transducer and activator of transcription and suppressor of cytokine-signaling gene expression in the brain of mice with astrocyte-targeted production of interleukin-12 or experimental autoimmune encephalomyelitis. *Am J Pathol* 2002; 160:271–288.

Marmur R, Kessler JA, Zhu G, et al. Differentiation of oligodendroglial progenitors derived from cortical multipotent cells requires extrinsic signals including activation of gp130/LIFbeta receptors. *J Neurosci* 1998; 18:9800–9811.

Massie C, Mills IG. The developing role of receptors and adaptors. *Nat Rev Cancer* 2006; 6:403–409.

McManus CM, Liu JSH, Hahn MT, et al. Differential induction of chemokines in human microglia by type I and II interferons. *Glia* 2000; 29:273–280.

Memet S. NF-κB functions in the nervous system: from development to disease. *Biochem Pharmacol* 2006; 72:1180–1195.

Miao T, Wu D, Zhang Y, et al. Suppressor of cytokine signaling-3 suppresses the ability of activated signal transducer and activator of transcription-3 to stimulate neurite growth in rat primary sensory neurons. *J Neurosci* 2006; 26:9512–9519.

Monks NR, Biswas DK, Pardee AB. Blocking anti-apoptosis as a strategy for cancer chemotherapy: NF-κB as a target. *J Cell Biochem* 2004; 92:646–650.

Mostecki J, Showalter BM, Rothman PB. Early growth response-1 regulates lipopolysaccharide-induced suppressor of cytokine signaling-1 transcription. *J Biol Chem* 2005; 280:2596–2605.

Moynagh PN. The NF-κB pathway. *J Cell Sci* 2005; 118:4589–4592.

Moynagh PN, Williams DC, O'Neill LAJ. Interleukin-1 activates transcription factor NF-κB in glial cells. *Biochem J* 1993; 294:343–347.

Mujtaba MG, Flowers LO, Patel CB, et al. Treatment of mice with the suppressor of cytokine signaling-1 mimetic peptide, tyrosine kinase inhibitor peptide, prevents development of the acute form of experimental allergic encephalomyelitis and induces stable remission in the chronic relapsing/remitting form. *J Immunol* 2005; 175:5077–5086.

Naka T, Matsumoto T, Narazaki M, et al. Accelerated apoptosis of lymphocytes by augmented induction of Bax in SSI-1 (STAT-induced STAT inhibitor-1) deficient mice. *Proc Natl Acad Sci USA* 1998; 95:15577–15582.

Naka T, Nishimoto N, Kishimoto T. The paradigm of IL-6: from basic science to medicine. *Arthritis Res* 2002; 4(Suppl 3):S233–S242.

Nakashima K, Wiese S, Yanagisawa M, et al. Developmental requirement of gp130 signaling in neuronal survival and astrocyte differentiation. *J Neurosci* 1999; 19:5429–5434.

Natarajan M, Lin KM, Hsueh RC, et al. A global analysis of cross-talk in a mammalian cellular signalling network. *Nat Cell Biol* 2006; 8:571–580.

Nguyen VT, Benveniste EN. Involvement of STAT-1α and ETS family members in interferon-γ induction of CD40 transcription in macrophages/microglia. *J Biol Chem* 2000; 271:23674–23684.

Nickols JC, Valentine W, Kanwal S, et al. Activation of the transcription factor NF-κB in Schwann cells is required for peripheral myelin formation. *Nat Neurosci* 2003; 6:161–167.

Nozell S, Laver T, Patel K, et al. Mechanism of IFN-beta-mediated inhibition of IL-8 gene expression in astroglioma cells. *J Immunol* 2006; 177:822–830.

O'Keefe GM, Nguyen VT, Benveniste EN. Regulation and function of class II major histocompatibility complex, CD40, and B7 expression in macrophages and microglia: implications in neurological diseases. *J Neurovirol* 2002; 8:496–512.

Oh J-W, Schwiebert LM, Benveniste EN. Expression of CC and CXC chemokine by human astrocytes. *J Neurovirol* 1999; 5:82–94.

Okada K, Kuroda E, Yoshida Y, et al. Effects of interferon-γ on the cytokine production of astrocytes. *J Neuroimmunol* 2005; 159:48–54.

Okada S, Nakamura M, Katoh H, et al. Conditional ablation of Stat3 or Socs3 discloses a dual role for reactive astrocytes after spinal cord injury. *Nat Med* 2006; 12:829–834.

Olson JK, Miller SD. Microglia initiate central nervous system innate and adaptive immune responses through multiple TLRs. *J Immunol* 2004; 173:3916–3924.

Pahan K, Sheikh FG, Liu X, et al. Induction of nitric-oxide synthase and activation of NF-κB by interleukin-12 p40 in microglial cells. *J Biol Chem* 2001; 276:7899–7905.

Park EJ, Park SY, Joe EH, et al. 15d-PGJ2 and rosiglitazone suppress Janus kinase-STAT inflammatory signaling through induction of suppressor of cytokine signaling 1 (SOCS1) and SOCS3 in glia. *J Biol Chem* 2003; 278:14747–14752.

Pizzi M, Sarnico I, Boroni F, et al. Prevention of neuron and oligodendrocyte degeneration by interleukin-6 (IL-6) and IL-6 receptor/IL-6 fusion protein in organotypic hippocampal slices. *Mol Cell Neurosci* 2004; 25:301–311.

Platanias LC. Mechanisms of type-I- and type-II-interferon-mediated signalling. *Nat Rev Immunol* 2005; 5:375–386.

Popko B, Baerwald KD. Oligodendroglial response to the immune cytokine interferon gamma. *Neurochem Res* 1999; 24:331–338.

Pouly S, Becher B, Blain M. et al. Interferon-γ modulates human oligodendrocyte susceptibility to fas-mediated apoptosis. *J Neuropathol Exp Neurol* 2000; 59:280–286.

Qin H, Wilson CA, Lee SJ, et al. LPS induces CD40 gene expression through the activation of NF-κB and STAT-1α in macrophages and microglia. *Blood* 2005; 106:3114–3122.

Qin H, Wilson C, Lee SJ, et al. IFN-β induced SOCS-1 negatively regulates CD40 gene expression in macrophages and microglia. *FASEB J* 2006a; 20:985–987.

Qin H, Wilson C, Roberts K, et al. IL-10 inhibits lipopolysaccharide-induced CD40 gene expression through induction of suppressor of cytokine signaling-3. *J Immunol* 2006b; 177:7761–7771.

Repovic P, Fears CY, Gladson CL, et al. Oncostatin-M induction of vascular endothelial growth factor expression in astroglioma cells. *Oncogene* 2003; 22:8117–8124.

Rivest S. Molecular insights on the cerebral innate immune system. *Brain Behav Immun* 2003; 17:13–19.

Rockwood K, Kirkland S, Hogan DB, et al. Use of lipid-lowering agents, indication bias, and the risk of dementia in community-dwelling elderly people. *Arch Neurol* 2002; 59:223–227.

Rodig SJ, Meraz MA, White JM, et al. Disruption of the JAK1 gene demonstrates obligatory and nonredundant roles of the JAKs in cytokine-induced biologic responses. *Cell* 1998; 93:373–383.

Rose-John S, Ehlers M, Grötzinger J, et al. The soluble interleukin-6 receptor. *Ann NY Acad Sci* 1995; 762:207–220.

Satoh J, Kuroda Y. Differing effects of IFNβ vs IFNγ in MS: gene expression in cultured astrocytes. *Neurology* 2001; 57:681–6855.

Schindler C. Cytokine receptors and Jak-STAT signaling. *Sci STKE* 2006; tr7. Available at: http://stke.sciencemag.org/cgi/content/full/sigtrans;2006/338/tr7.

Shankar SL, O'Guin K, Kim M, et al. Gas6/Axl signaling activates the phosphatidylinositol 3-kinase/Akt1 survival pathway to protect oligodendrocytes from tumor necrosis factor alpha-induced apoptosis. *J Neurosci* 2006; 26:5638–5648.

Shuai K, Liu B. Regulation of JAK-STAT signalling in the immune system. *Nat Rev Immunol* 2003; 3:900–911.

Si Q, Zhao ML, Morgan AC, et al. 15-deoxy-Delta12,14-prostaglandin J2 inhibits IFN-inducible protein 10/CXC chemokine ligand 10 expression in human microglia: mechanisms and implications. *J Immunol* 2004; 173:3504–3513.

Sparacio SM, Zhang Y, Vilcek J, et al. Cytokine regulation of interleukin-6 gene expression in astrocytes involves activation of an NF-kappa B-like nuclear protein. *J Neuroimmunol* 1992; 39:231–242.

Srinivasan D, Yen JH, Joseph DJ, et al. Cell type-specific interleukin-1beta signaling in the CNS. *J Neurosci* 2004; 24:6482–6488.

Sriram K, Benkovic SA, Hebert MA, et al. Induction of gp130-related cytokines and activation of JAK2/STAT3 pathway in astrocytes precedes upregulation of GFAP in the MPTP model of neurodegeneration: key signaling pathway for astrogliosis in vivo? *J Biol Chem* 2004; 279:19936–19947.

Stankoff B, Aigrot M-S, Noël F, et al. Ciliary neurotrophic factor (CNTF) enhances myelin formation: a novel role for CNTF and CNTF-related molecules. *J Neurosci* 2002; 22:9221–9227.

Stark JL, Cross AH. Differential expression of suppressors of cytokine signaling-1 and -3 and related cytokines in central nervous system during remitting versus non-remitting forms of experimental autoimmune encephalomyelitis. *Int Immunol* 2005; 18:347–353.

Stark JL, Lyons JA, Cross AH. Interferon-gamma produced by encephalitogenic cells induces suppressors of cytokine signaling in primary murine astrocytes. *J Neuroimmunol* 2004; 151:195–200.

Starr R, Metcalf D, Elefanty AG, et al. Liver degeneration and lymphoid deficiencies in mice lacking suppressor of cytokine signaling-1. *Proc Natl Acad Sci USA* 1998; 95:14395–14399.

Stellwagen D, Malenka RC. Synaptic scaling mediated by glial TNF-α. *Nature* 2006; 440:1054–1059.

Town T, Nikolic V, Tan J. The microglial "activation" continuum: from innate to adaptive responses. *J Neuroinflammation* 2005; 2:1–10.

Ubogu EE, Cossoy MB, Ransohoff RM. The expression and function of chemokines involved in CNS inflammation. *Trends Pharmacol Sci* 2006; 27:48–55.

Valerio A, Ferrario M, Dreano M, et al. Soluble interleukin-6 (IL-6) receptor/IL-6 fusion protein enhances in vitro differentiation of purified rat oligodendroglial lineage cells. *Mol Cell Neurosci* 2002; 21:602–615.

van Loo G, De Lorenzi R, Schmidt H, et al. Inhibition of transcription factor NF-κB in the central nervous system ameliorates autoimmune encephalomyelitis in mice. *Nat Immunol* 2006:1038–1046.

Van Wagoner NJ, Benveniste EN. Interleukin-6 expression and regulation in astrocytes. *J Neuroimmunol* 1999b; 100:124–139.

Van Wagoner N, Oh J-W, Repovic P, et al. IL-6 production by astrocytes: autocrine regulation by IL-6 and the soluble IL-6 receptor. *J Neurosci* 1999a; 19:5236–5244.

Vartanian T, Li Y, Zhao M, et al. Interferon-γ-induced oligodendrocyte cell death: implications for the pathogenesis of multiple sclerosis. *Mol Med* 1995; 1:732–743.

Viatour P, Merville MP, Bours V, et al. Phosphorylation of NF-κB and IκB proteins: implications in cancer and inflammation. *Trends Biochem Sci* 2005; 30:43–52.

Vollgraf U, Wegner M, Richter-Landsberg C. Activation of AP-1 and nuclear factor-κB transcription factors is involved in hydrogen peroxide-induced apoptotic cell death of oligodendrocytes. *J Neurochem* 1999; 73:2501–2509.

Volterra A, Meldolesi J. Astrocytes, from brain glue to communication elements: the revolution continues. *Nat Rev Neurosci* 2005; 6:626–640.

Wesemann D, Benveniste EN. Cytokine and chemokine receptors and signaling. In: Kettenmann H, Ransom BR (Eds). *Neuroglia.* Oxford: Oxford University Press, 2004, pp 147–162.

Xia XG, Hofmann HD, Deller T, et al. Induction of STAT3 signaling in activated astrocytes and sprouting septal neurons following entorhinal cortex lesion in adult rats. *Mol Cell Neurosci* 2002; 21:379–392.

Yanagisawa M, Nakashima K, Arakawa H, et al. Astrocyte differentiation of fetal neuroepithelial cells by interleukin-11 via activation of a common cytokine signal transducer, gp130, and a transcription factor, STAT3. *J Neurochem* 2000; 74:1498–1504.

Correspondence to: Etty (Tika) Benveniste, PhD, Department of Cell Biology, University of Alabama at Birmingham, 1530 3rd Avenue South, MCLM 395, Birmingham, AL 35294-0005, USA. Tel: 1-205-934-7667; fax: 1-205-975-6748; email: tika@uab.edu.

Part II

Immune-Pain Interactions: Peripheral Tissue and Nerves

Immune and Glial Regulation of Pain, edited by Joyce
A. DeLeo, Linda S. Sorkin, and Linda R. Watkins,
IASP Press, Seattle, © 2007.

4

Pain Facilitation by Proinflammatory Cytokine Actions at Peripheral Nerve Terminals

Thiago M. Cunha,[a] Waldiceu A. Verri, Jr.,[a]
Stephen Poole,[b] Carlos A. Parada,[a]
Fernando Q. Cunha,[a] and Sérgio H. Ferreira[a]

[a]*Department of Pharmacology, School of Medicine, Ribeirao Preto University,
Sao Paulo, Brazil;* [b]*Division of Immunology and Endocrinology, National
Institute for Biological Standards and Control, Hertfordshire, United Kingdom*

It is now broadly accepted that sensitization of primary sensory neurons is essential to inflammatory pain. Nonetheless, for a long time the sensitization of nociceptors was regarded as a result of the excitatory action of a "soup" of various inflammatory mediators released at the site of inflamed or damaged tissue (Lynn 1984). This hypothesis was challenged by the discovery of the mechanism of action of nonsteroidal anti-inflammatory drugs by Vane's group (1971) and by the demonstration, in humans (Ferreira 1972) and in animals (Ferreira 1972), that eicosanoids do not cause overt pain but sensitize nociceptors.

Other inflammatory mediators, including sympathetic amines (Nakamura and Ferreira 1987; Hannington-Kiff 1989), endothelin (Ferreira et al. 1989; Zhou et al. 2001), substance P (Henry 1976; Nakamura-Craig and Gill 1991; Xu et al. 1992), bradykinin (Staszewska-Barczak and Dusting 1977), and nerve growth factor (Lewin and Mendell 1993; Lewin et al. 1993), also possess the same nociceptor-sensitizing property. These mediators act directly on neuronal receptors, triggering molecular mechanisms that ultimately facilitate the electrical activity of the neuronal membrane. Although our understanding of the molecular mechanisms of nociceptor sensitization is incomplete, there is general agreement that stimulation of G-protein-coupled receptors by inflammatory mediators activates the enzyme adenylate cyclase to produce cyclic adenosine monophosphate (cAMP). This substance, in turn, triggers the activation of a group of protein kinases (PKA and PKC), which in turn leads to phosphorylation of ion channels in the membrane. The results are a facilitation of the inward sodium current via tetrodotoxin (TTX)-resistant Na^+ channels, a facilitation of inward Ca^{2+} currents, and an inhibition of outward K^+ currents. This sequence of events is probably the basic peripheral mechanism of hyperalgesia, a state in which a slight or normally non-noxious thermal, mechanical, or chemical stimulus becomes painful.

We refer to the mediators that act directly on the primary nociceptor as "final mediators," in contrast with "intermediate" mediators, released during inflammation by resident and migrating cells or by plasma, which stimulate the release of the final mediators. While the inflammatory signs and symptoms are similar, the resident and migrating cells and the intermediate and final mediators may vary, depending on the time frame, the type of tissue, and the type of inflammatory stimuli. In general, measurements of mediators in exudates or inflamed tissues at a single time point give a distorted picture of the evolution of the pathological process and suggest a disorganized "soup" of cells and mediators. In fact, sequential release of inflammatory mediators or cellular events observed after challenge by inflammatory stimuli can be observed only by performing a series of measurements. Most of the time, it is this temporal and pathophysiological hierarchy that allows the researcher to discover the site of action of existing drugs or to propose targets for new drug development. The cascade of hyperalgesic cytokines that we describe in this chapter is one of these pathophysiological hierarchical processes that our laboratory helped to discover during the last two decades (recently reviewed by Verri et al. 2006a). Cytokines in general act as intermediate mediators, releasing other cytokines as well as final mediators. In some instances, however, cytokines may act as final mediators and have been described as being involved in the development of neuronal damage, contributing to the symptom described in humans as allodynia.

One of the major problems created by the taxonomy adopted in 1982 by the International Association for the Study of Pain (IASP) was indiscriminate use of the term "allodynia" by animal researchers. The IASP defined allodynia based upon the painful characteristics of the stimulus: "Pain due to a stimulus which does not normally provoke pain." This simple definition induced scientists working in the area of analgesics and experimental nociception to use behavior assays such as the von Frey filament test as a measure of allodynia, with the assumption that they were quantifying neuropathic pain. The scientists and editors of scientific journals were unaware that this term was coined to be used for human symptoms. Bonica (1992) called attention to the fact that "allodynia involves a change in the *quality* of a sensation, whether tactile, thermal or of any other sort." Furthermore, an allodynic region, although painful to touch, is frequently insensitive to strong mechanical stimulation. Since the IASP definition was published in 1982, the term "allodynia" has been used more than 600 times for studies in rats (first in 1984) and 200 times for studies in mice (first in 1993) in research publications (based on the PubMed database). The IASP Task Force on Taxonomy has recently returned to a discussion of the concepts of allodynia and hyperalgesia (IASP pain terminology is available at www.iasp-pain.org). There is now a word of caution regarding use of the term allodynia: "It is important to recognize that allodynia involves a change in the quality of a sensation, whether tactile, thermal, or of any other sort. The original modality is normally nonpainful, but the response is painful. There is thus a loss of specificity of a sensory modality. By contrast, hyperalgesia (q.v.) represents an augmented response in a specific mode, viz., pain. With other cutaneous modalities, hyperesthesia is the term which corresponds to hyperalgesia, and as with hyperalgesia, the quality is not altered. In allodynia, the stimulus mode and the response mode differ, unlike the situation with hyperalgesia." Thus, no experimental tests in rats or mice are capable of differentiating allodynia from hyperalgesia. Most of the animal experiments were carried out with modifications of the von Frey filament test, which is a useful test for investigation of human allodynia (Chaplan et al. 1994). On the other hand, in the electronic von Frey test, applied to normal and damaged areas of rats or mice, there is a response to different intensities of pressure (Cunha et al. 2004). Thus, the von Frey filament test measures allodynia, whereas the electronic version measures hyperalgesia. In both situations there is no detection of "loss of specificity of a sensory modality," characteristic of allodynia. However, with both instruments it is possible to quantify an increase in the intensity of the nociceptive response, which we believe to be better described as "hypernociception." In this sense, if the injury causes a pathological lesion to a sensory neuron, the phenomenon may be classified as "neuropathic hypernociception." On the other hand, if the reaction is mainly tissue inflammation, with increased nociception, we may describe the event as "inflammatory hypernociception." Therefore, in this chapter we use the term "hypernociception" to describe any increase in the sensitivity of primary nociceptive neurons in animal models.

PERIPHERAL PROINFLAMMATORY CYTOKINES AND INFLAMMATORY PAIN

Cytokines are defined as proteins produced and released in a coordinated sequence by cells in response to a variety of inflammatory stimuli, such as viruses, parasites, or bacteria and their products, or in response to other cytokines (Aggarwal and Puri 1995; Vilcek 2003). In general, cytokines constitute a link between cellular injuries or immunological recognition of non-self and the local or systemic signs of inflammation (Dinarello 2000; Hopkins 2003; Conti et al. 2004; Verri et al. 2006b).

Although chemokines are considered cytokines, they belong to a particular group of cytokines with specific chemical and functional properties. These chemotactic cytokines are usually smaller than the other cytokines (8–10 kDa), and they direct the recruitment of leukocytes from the blood stream to the extravascular tissues by acting on receptors that are differentially expressed on leukocyte subsets. Today, besides their role in leukocyte recruitment during inflammation, chemokines are considered to have other functions such as angiogenesis and modulation of the immune response, including fever (Rossi and Zlotnik 2000).

In inflammation, resident cells such as dendritic cells, macrophages, mast cells, and lymphocytes recognize inflammatory stimuli and release cytokines. These cytokines play an essential role in the development of inflammatory pain as well as other inflammatory events such as leukocyte migration. The principal cytokines described as participating in the development of inflammatory pain are interleukin (IL)-1β, tumor necrosis factor (TNF)-α, IL-6, and the chemokines IL-8, chemokine-induced neutrophil chemoattractant (CINC)-1, and keratinocyte-derived chemokine (KC) (Ferreira et al. 1988; Cunha et al. 1991, 1992, 2005; Watkins et al. 1994; Safieh-Garabedian et al. 1995; Nicol. et al. 1997; Lorenzetti et al. 2002; for review see Verri et al. 2006a). Recently, it has been demonstrated that IL-15, IL-18, and IL-12 also induce inflammatory hypernociception (Verri et al. 2004, 2005, 2006b, 2007). The role of these cytokines and chemokines and the interaction between them are discussed below.

A CASCADE OF CYTOKINES MEDIATES INFLAMMATORY HYPERNOCICEPTION

After the discovery of cytokines, a great deal of effort was applied to characterizing their function. In the 1980s, researchers described the participation of cytokines in the induction of inflammatory signals such as the recruitment of white blood cells, fever, acute-phase protein release, and the increase in permeability of blood vessels (Dinarello 1984; Granstein et al. 1986). With the research community's new understanding of these findings, IL-1β, one of the first cytokines characterized, entered the inflammatory pain scene.

Different cell types including macrophages, monocytes, and glial cells produce IL-1β, which in turn induces the production of other inflammatory mediators (Dinarello 1998). Evidence that IL-1β stimulates the production of prostaglandins (Bernheim et al. 1980; Zucali et al. 1986) and that prostaglandins ultimately sensitize nociceptors (Handwerker 1976; Ferreira and Nakamura 1979) prompted us to investigate IL-1β as an inflammatory hypernociceptive mediator. We made the seminal finding that IL-1β is important in the genesis of inflammatory hypernociception in experimental animals (Ferreira et al. 1988). In fact, intraplantar injection of IL-1β produces severe mechanical hypernociception, which we knew to be dependent on prostanoid production because local pretreatment with indomethacin, a cyclooxygenase (COX) inhibitor, blocked its effects. Moreover, we observed that IL-1β, via prostaglandins, mediates inflammatory hypernociception induced by local administration of carrageenan or lipopolysaccharide into the rat paw (Ferreira et al. 1988). In fact, carrageenan- or lipopolysaccharide-induced mechanical hypernociception was inhibited by 50% by previous local treatment with antibodies against IL-1β (Cunha et al. 1992). This partial inhibition suggests that another hypernociceptive pathway besides that mediated by IL-1β/prostanoids is involved in the mechanical inflammatory hypernociception induced by carrageenan. As mentioned earlier, it seems that sympathetic amines account for the other component of inflammatory pain, at least in this experimental model.

Thereafter, we turned our attention to elucidating the sympathetic component of inflammatory hypernociception. While studying the role of chemokines in inflammatory hypernociception, we found that whereas IL-1β induces the release of prostanoids, the neutrophil chemoattractant chemokine IL-8/CXCL8 (in humans) or CINC-1/CXCL1 (in rats) mediates the participation of sympathetic components of inflammatory hypernociception. In fact, we demonstrated that mechanical hypernociception induced by IL-8/CXCL8 or CINC-1/CXCL1 is inhibited by β-adrenergic receptor antagonists, but not by COX inhibitors. Moreover, anti-IL-8/CXCL8 antiserum also partially inhibited carrageenan-induced hypernociception by 50% in rats (Cunha et al. 1991). The mechanism by which CXC chemokines induce hypernociception seems to depend on the tissue evaluated. For instance, in contrast with the hypernociception induced by the administration of IL-8 in cutaneous hindpaw tissue, in rat knee joints IL-8 induces mechanical hypernociception that is prevented by IL-1 receptor antagonist (IL-1ra) (Davis and Perkins 1994).

Following these observations, another proinflammatory cytokine, TNF-α, was considered to be a key molecule in the initiation of the inflammatory process. Generally, it is the first cytokine released in response to inflammatory stimuli such as a bacterial infection (Beutler and Cerami 1988; Tartaglia and Goeddel 1992; Ware 2005). Moreover, the finding that TNF-α could stimulate the release of IL-1β and CXC chemokines indicates its possible involvement in the initiation of inflammatory hypernociception.

Again, we were the first to demonstrate that TNF-α induces mechanical hypernociception in the hindpaw of rats. The TNF-α hypernociceptive effect was partially inhibited by indomethacin (a COX inhibitor) and atenolol (a β-adrenoreceptor antagonist) and was abolished by coadministration of these drugs, suggesting that TNF-α-induced hypernociception is mediated by prostanoids and sympathetic amines. Furthermore, treatment with anti-IL-1β or anti-IL-8/CINC-1 antiserum partially inhibited TNF-α-induced hypernociception, and the combination of both antisera completely abolished TNF-α effects, suggesting that IL-1β and IL-8/CINC-1 also mediate TNF-α-induced hypernociception. In addition, the mechanical hypernociceptive effects of IL-1β and IL-8/CINC-1 are inhibited by indomethacin and atenolol, respectively. These data suggest that TNF-α induces hypernociception in rats via two independent and parallel pathways:

1) TNF-α → IL-1β → prostanoids
2) TNF-α → CINC-1 → sympathetic amines

(Fig. 1). Moreover, carrageenan- or lipopolysaccharide-induced hypernociception is abolished by pretreatment with anti-TNF-α antiserum. Thus, TNF-α plays a pivotal role in carrageenan- and lipopolysaccharide-induced hypernociception in rats, acting via the two parallel pathways described above (Cunha et al. 1992; Poole et al. 1995).

In the same manner as TNF-α, IL-1β, and IL-8/CINC-1, IL-6 also produces mechanical hypernociception in rats, which is inhibited by indomethacin, anti-IL-1β antiserum, or IL-1ra. Regarding the cytokine cascade underlying IL-6-induced inflammatory hypernociception, we demonstrated that antiserum against IL-6 inhibits TNF-α-induced mechanical hypernociception in rats (Cunha et al. 1992). Thus, it seems that TNF-α, IL-6, and IL-1β sequentially precede the release of prostanoids to induce hypernociception in rats.

These experiments strongly support our above-mentioned hypothesis that in rats there is a cascade of cytokines that constitutes a link between injuries and the release of primary hypernociceptive mediators. This concept allows us to understand why the inhibition of one cytokine (IL-1β or TNF-α) or several (by glucocorticoids) inhibits the onset of hypernociception. The clinical success of anti-TNF-α in rheumatoid arthritis also exemplifies this concept (Rankin et al. 1995), which opposes the old idea that inflammatory hyperalgesia results from a "soup of inflammatory mediators."

Other groups also find a sequential role of cytokines in different hypernociceptive models in rats. For example, TNF-α triggers IL-1β-mediated thermal and mechanical hypernociception induced by intraplantar administration of complete Freund's adjuvant (CFA) (Woolf et al. 1997). In this model, IL-1β induces the release of nerve growth factor (NGF), rather than stimulating prostanoid production. In fact, antibodies against NGF inhibited the hypernociception induced by CFA and IL-1β. In addition, IL-1ra inhibited CFA- and IL-1β-induced, but not NGF-induced, mechanical and thermal hypernociception, suggesting the following sequential release of these mediators:

CFA → TNF-α → IL-1β → NGF → nociceptor sensitization

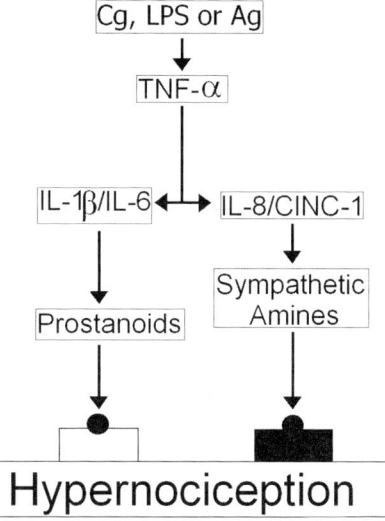

Fig. 1. Inflammatory stimulus-induced cytokine cascades mediate mechanical hypernociception in rats. The scheme represents the coordinated release of mediators triggered by the different inflammatory stimuli. Ag = antigen, Cg = carrageenan, CINC-1 = chemokine-induced neutrophil chemoattractant 1, IL = interleukin, LPS = lipopolysaccharide, TNF-α = tumor necrosis factor-α. (Based on Ferreira et al. 1988; Cunha et al. 1991, 1992; Lorenzetti et al. 2002; Cunha et al. 2003.)

(Safieh-Garabedian et al. 1995, Woolf et al. 1997). Moreover, in a different model of peripheral sensitization, the intraperitoneal administration of lithium chloride or lipopolysaccharide sensitized the rat to the tail-flick test. It has been hypothesized that this sensitization is mediated by sequential release of TNF-α and IL-1β, which activates the subdiaphragmatic vagal afferents (Watkins et al. 1994).

The relevance of a biological experimental concept depends on its confirmation in more than one model and animal species. In this regard, our hypothesis was further supported by recent findings that mechanical inflammatory hypernociception in mice is also mediated by a peripheral cascade of cytokines (Cunha et al. 2005). In mice, the carrageenan inflammatory stimulus induces the release of TNF-α and KC/CXCL1, which brings about the subsequent release of IL-1β followed by prostanoid production. KC/CXCL1 also stimulates the sympathetic component of inflammatory hypernociception (Fig. 2).

In support of the experimental models, clinical studies have also suggested a contribution of TNF-α to inflammatory pain. Evidence indicates that TNF-α may be associated with musculoskeletal pain syndromes and with pain states associated with nucleus pulposus herniation (Onda et al. 2003; Schafers et al. 2003). Furthermore, the pain associated with mandibular movement and tenderness (allodynia) on posterior palpation of the temporomandibular joint has been related to the level of TNF-α in the synovial fluid (Nordahl et al. 2000).

Thus, a great deal of data suggests a role of cytokines as intermediary hypernociceptive mediators, mostly in the peripheral tissues, supporting the likelihood that these molecules are a therapeutic target for controlling inflammatory pain states. Our group thus developed several peptides based on the amino acid sequence structure of IL-1β. Among them, the tripeptide KD(P)T consistently inhibited IL-1β and inflammatory mechanical hypernociception. Recently, a selective IL-1 receptor antagonist that differs from naturally occurring IL-1ra by the presence of a methionine group named anakinra was developed. Anakinra was tested in models of inflammatory diseases and is under clinical evaluation (Vila et al. 2005; den Broeder et al. 2006).

Besides IL-1β, TNF has also become a target for the treatment of inflammatory diseases such as arthritis. Drugs such as infliximab (a chimeric anti-TNF-α antibody), etanercept (a p75 TNF-α receptor/immunoglobulin G fusion protein), and recently, adalimumab (a fully humanized monoclonal anti-TNF-α antibody) are available. These anti-TNF-α therapies have shown efficacy in different diseases that are generally associated with pain, such as uveitis (Smith et al. 2005) and skin and joint manifestations of psoriasis (Tobin and Kirby 2005), but mainly in rheumatoid arthritis (Murray and Dahl 1997; Moreland et al. 1999; Weinblatt et al. 1999; Haraoui 2005).

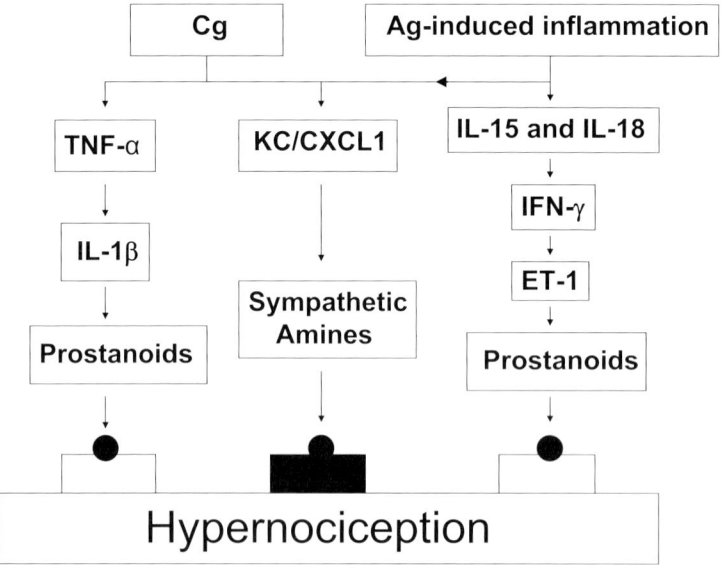

Fig. 2. Cascades of cytokines mediate mechanical hypernociception induced by inflammation from carrageenan (Cg) and antigen (Ag) in mice. ET-1 = endothelin-1, IFN-γ = interferon-gamma, KC/CXCL1 = keratinocyte-derived chemokine/CXC chemokine ligand 1; other abbreviations are as in Fig. 1. (Based on Cunha et al. 2005; Verri et al. 2006b, 2007, and submitted data.)

Despite the wealth of data concerning the nociceptive role of TNF-α and the beneficial effect of anti-TNF drugs on inflammatory diseases as mentioned above, there are few studies suggesting that these drugs inhibit the induction of hypernociception. Etanercept as well as anti-TNF antibodies reduced experimental inflammation and neuropathy-induced hypernociception (Sommer et al. 2001a,b; Inglis et al. 2005), and infliximab therapy significantly reduced pain scores in rheumatoid arthritis (Rankin et al. 1995; Maini et al. 1998). Long-term use of anti-TNF therapies may cause adverse effects, including in some cases heart failure, as well as immune suppression, which may lead to serious infections such as tuberculosis (Bickston et al. 1999; Cush 2004).

Although specific cytokine inhibitors such as anakinra, etanercept, and infliximab are available, the high cost of these therapies must be considered. Some established drugs have emerged as alternative cytokine inhibitors. We have investigated the potential of pentoxifylline and thalidomide for reducing inflammatory hypernociception (Ribeiro et al. 2000; Vale et al. 2004). In fact, both drugs reduced hypernociception associated with inflammation by a mechanism dependent on the inhibition of cytokine production, mainly at the peripheral site. Therefore, the cost-benefit profile of pentoxifylline and thalidomide favors the use of these drugs or others with similar mechanisms of action to control inflammatory pain.

CYTOKINES MEDIATE HYPERNOCICEPTION INDUCED BY THE IMMUNE INFLAMMATORY RESPONSE: THE ROLE OF IL-15 AND IL-18

Immune inflammatory responses mediated by T-helper type 1 (Th1) cells are involved in the development of different diseases including rheumatoid arthritis, myocarditis, encephalomyelitis, diabetes, and lupus (for reviews, see Fehniger and Caligiuri 2001; Brombacher et al. 2003; Strengell et al. 2003; Watford et al. 2004). Most of these inflammatory diseases are frequently accompanied by hyperalgesia, and the development of inflammatory nociception models that mimic these diseases is of great importance. Such models would facilitate rational studies of the pathophysiology of those conditions and could lead to better and more specific therapies. For example, antigen-induced inflammatory hypernociception in previously immunized animals serves as a model of the immune inflammation triggered by Th1 responses (Verri et al. 2006b).

An expanded nociceptive role for cytokines (TNF-α, IL-1β, IL-8/CINC-1, and IL-6) was revealed when it was demonstrated that they also play an important role in hypernociception induced by an immune challenge. In fact, specific anti-rat TNF-α, anti-rat IL-1β, and anti-human IL-8 antiserum or IL-1ra decreased antigen-induced hypernociception, and the levels of these cytokines were elevated in the paw after the administration of the antigen in immunized rats and mice (Cunha et al. 2003; T.M. Cunha, unpublished observation, 2006; Figs. 1 and 2). Additionally, besides the role of these well-known hyperalgesic cytokines as described above, other cytokines (IL-15, IL-18) seem important during hypernociception resulting from Th1-mediated immune inflammatory responses.

It has been demonstrated that IL-18 and IL-15 share a role in the development of rheumatoid arthritis (RA), in mediating Th1 responses, and in initiating the production of interferon-gamma (IFN-γ) (for reviews, see Fehniger and Caligiuri 2001; Nakanishi et al. 2001; Brombacher et al. 2003; Strengell et al. 2003). In fact, therapies targeting IL-15 and IL-18 ameliorate collagen-induced arthritis, a classical model of RA (Ruchatz et al. 1998; Gracie et al. 1999; Wei et al. 2001). Based on this experimental evidence, Baslund et al. (2005) performed a clinical trial to evaluate the therapeutic potential of an IL-15-targeting drug for treatment of RA. The study found that treatment with anti-IL-15 antibody had a beneficial effect in RA patients.

Taking this evidence into account, we have recently reported that IL-15 and IL-18 mediate Th1-like-induced inflammatory hypernociception via the sequential release of IFN-γ, endothelin-1 (ET-1), and prostaglandin E_2 (PGE_2). The hypernociception induced by IL-15 is independent from that induced by IL-18, suggesting that the molecules are acting synergistically (Verri et al. 2006b, 2007; Fig. 2). Therefore, therapies that target IL-15 and IL-18 might also be of importance for downregulating hypernociception induced by adaptive immune inflammation, and compared to anti-TNF therapies they probably would have a lower incidence of side effects such as propensity to infections (Bickston et al. 1999; Cush et al. 2004).

Besides IL-15 and IL-18, IL-12 is also an important cytokine for arthritis development (Leung et al. 2000; for review, see Brombacher et al. 2003). Its pronociceptive effect was demonstrated in rats. IL-12 injection induces mechanical hypernociception, which is mediated by ET-1's action on ET_B receptors and is not dependent on prostanoids, sympathetic amines, or leukotrienes (Verri et al. 2005). This effect is important because human volunteers have reported pain at the site of an IL-12 injection during clinical trials for cancer treatment or vaccine adjuvant (for discussion, see Verri et al. 2005).

CYTOKINES AND DIRECT SENSITIZATION OF NOCICEPTORS

Despite the evidence described above indicating that the hypernociceptive effects of cytokines are indirect, it has been reported that sensory neurons express cytokine receptors, which implies that these cytokines might also directly sensitize the nociceptor during inflammation. In effect, some research groups have demonstrated that cytokines such as TNF-α evoke action potentials in nociceptive neurons when applied topically to peripheral axons in vivo, thereby increasing neuronal sensitivity to mechanical and chemical stimuli (Nicol et al. 1997; Sorkin et al. 1997; Junger and Sorkin 2000). In an attempt to elucidate the mechanism by which TNF provokes this direct effect in neurons, Jin and Gereau (2006) investigated the effect of this cytokine on TTX-resistant Na^+ activity. It was demonstrated that TNF-α acting on TNFR1 enhances TTX-resistant Na^+ currents in primary afferent nociceptive neurons by activating the neuronal mitogen-activated protein (MAP) kinase (p38) pathway.

A direct effect of IL-1β, IL-6, and chemokines on nociceptors has also been demonstrated. For instance, IL-1β and IL-6, together with their soluble receptor (sIL-6R), are able to sensitize sensory neurons to heat (Obreja et al. 2002, 2005). The IL-6 effect was due to the activation of Janus tyrosine kinase and the PKC intracellular signaling pathway (Obreja et al. 2002, 2005). Moreover, macrophage inflammatory protein-1α (MIP-1α)/CCL3 sensitizes dorsal root ganglion neurons to capsaicin or anandamide by a mechanism dependent on G_i protein, phospholipase C, and PKC in vitro (Zhang et al. 2005).

Nevertheless, it is important to be careful in the interpretation of these results, and other possibilities should be considered. First, although the cytokines are acting directly on sensory neurons, they could produce secondary mediators, such as prostanoids, which might in fact be sensitizing the nociceptors. Nicol et al. (1997) demonstrated that TNF-α enhances the sensitivity of cultured neurons to capsaicin in a manner dependent on COX products. They also found that cytokines act on cells other than sensory neurons, such as dorsal root ganglion satellite cells, which in turn produce direct sensitizing mediators, and demonstrated the relevance of the direct effect of cytokines to the genesis of inflammatory hypernociception. In this context, Parada et al. (2003) showed that the effective attenuation of TNFR1 expression in peripheral sensory neurons by intrathecal treatment with antisense oligodeoxynucleotides to this receptor did not alter acute mechanical hypernociception induced when either TNF-α or carrageenan was injected into rat paws. Therefore, it seems that TNF-α acting on sensory neuron membrane TNFR1 is not necessary for the onset of peripheral acute inflammatory hypernociception. Thus, similar experiments must be performed with IL-6 and IL-1β to determine the importance of their direct effects on nociceptive neurons for the genesis of inflammatory hypernociception.

CHRONIC INFLAMMATORY PAIN MEDIATED BY CYTOKINES

The contribution of cytokines to the genesis of acute inflammatory pain has been extensively demonstrated, as mentioned above. However, the role of cytokines in chronic inflammatory pain states is still unclear. One problem is that there are few experimental models of chronic inflammatory pain. Although some acute inflammatory models, such as CFA-induced inflammation, could be maintained for longer periods, they would still represent unresolved acute inflammation. The clinically important chronic pain cases are those in which the lesion has already resolved but the pain persists.

In an attempt to study these cases, we developed an experimental model to elucidate the mechanism of chronic inflammatory pain. We induced a persistent hypernociceptive state with successive daily injections of PGE_2 or dopamine. After 14 daily injections of the stimulus, the sensitivity of the nociceptor did not return to its basal level but, instead, reached a plateau that persisted for more than 30 days (Ferreira et al. 1990). Other studies have reported that persistent hypernociception can also be triggered by maintaining the nociceptive stimuli (Covey et al. 2000).

In line with PGE_2- or dopamine-induced persistent hypernociception, repeated intraplantar injections of IL-1β, IL-8, or TNF-α also cause persistent mechanical hypernociception that is prevented by daily treatment with indomethacin and atenolol. In fact, daily treatment with indomethacin or atenolol inhibited 50% of the persistent hypernociception induced by TNF-α, and the combination of indomethacin and atenolol blocked the onset of the process (Sachs et al. 2002). These results suggest that, as in the case of acute hypernociception, the persistent hypernociception induced by IL-1β and IL-8 is due to the endogenous release of eicosanoids and sympathetic amines, respectively. Moreover, both mediators play a role in the development of the persistent hypernociception induced by TNF-α (Sachs et al. 2002).

In addition to the data generated using the model of persistent hypernociception described above, further support for the possible role of TNF-α in chronic pain came from results obtained using hypernociceptive priming. In this animal model, the injection of carrageenan induces an inflammatory hypernociception lasting hours to days, which produces a "primed" state lasting several weeks. During this time, injection of PGE_2 induces hypernociception that is markedly enhanced and prolonged compared to PGE_2-induced hypernociception in normal "unprimed" rats (Aley et al. 2000).

Studying the genesis of the priming state, Parada et al. (2003) showed that intrathecal administration of antisense oligodeoxynucleotide to TNFR1, which reduced TNFR1 mRNA in sensory neurons, but not in the peripheral tissue, attenuated either carrageenan- or TNF-α-induced priming without affecting acute hypernociception. The mechanism by which TNF-α induces chronic hypernociceptive priming is not completely clear, but it has been suggested that this cytokine induces an increase of PKC-ε levels in the nociceptor (Parada et al. 2005). Moreover, the modulation of TTX-resistant Na^+ currents via p38 activation could also be responsible for amplifying this effect of PGE_2 on this channel's activity during chronic priming.

CONCLUSIONS

This chapter reinforces the crucial role of cytokines and chemokines in mediating inflammatory pain in most of the experimental nociceptive models published so far. The central goal of this chapter was to demonstrate that cytokine/chemokine cascades link inflammatory stimuli with the release of the final mediators (prostaglandins and sympathetic amines) that ultimately are responsible for nociceptor sensitization. In addition, this chapter describes how cytokines and chemokines may also directly sensitize nociceptors. Thus, substances that block the synthesis or action of nociceptive cytokines and chemokines could be useful for treating inflammatory pain.

ACKNOWLEDGMENTS

The authors wish to express their appreciation to Ieda Regina dos Santos Schivo, Sérgio Roberto Rosa, and Giuliana Bertozi Francisco for excellent technical assistance. This work was supported by grants from FAPESP and CNPq. The authors apologize for references not discussed due to limited space.

REFERENCES

Aggarwal BB, Puri RK. Common and uncommon features of cytokines and cytokines receptors: an overview. In: Aggarwal BB, Puri RK (Eds). *Human Cytokines: Their Role in Disease and Therapy*, Vol. 1. Ann Arbor: Blackwell Science, 1995, pp 3–24.

Aley KO, Messing RO, Mochly-Rosen D, Levine JD. Chronic hypersensitivity for inflammatory nociceptor sensitization mediated by the epsilon isozyme of protein kinase C. *J Neurosci* 2000; 20:4680–4685.

Baslund B, Tvede N, Danneskiold-Samsoe B, et al. Targeting interleukin-15 in patients with rheumatoid arthritis: a proof-of-concept study. *Arthritis Rheum* 2005; 52:2686–2692.

Bernheim HA, Gilbert TM, Stitt JT. Prostaglandin E levels in third ventricular cerebrospinal fluid of rabbits during fever and changes in body temperature. *J Physiol* 1980; 301:69–78.

Beutler B, Cerami A. Tumor necrosis, cachexia, shock, and inflammation: a common mediator. *Annu Rev Biochem* 1988; 57:505–518.

Bickston SJ, Lichtenstein GR, Arseneau KO, Cohen RB, Cominelli F. The relationship between infliximab treatment and lymphoma in Crohn's disease. *Gastroenterology* 1999; 117:1433–1437.

Bonica JJ. Clinical importance of hyperalgesia. In: Willis WD Jr (Ed). *Hyperalgesia and Allodynia*, Vol. 1. New York: Raven Press, 1992, pp 17–43.

Brombacher F, Kastelein RA, Alber G. Novel IL-12 family members shed light on the orchestration of Th1 responses. *Trends Immunol* 2003; 24:207–212.

Chaplan SR, Bach FW, Pogrel JW, et al. Quantitative assessment of tactile allodynia in the rat paw. *J Neurosci Methods* 1994; 53:55–63.

Conti B, Tabarean I, Andrei C, Bartfai T. Cytokines and fever. *Front Biosci* 2004; 9:1433–1449.

Covey WC, Ignatowski TA, Knight PR, Spengler RN. Brain-derived TNF-alpha: involvement in neuroplastic changes implicated in the conscious perception of persistent pain. *Brain Res* 2000; 859:113–122.

Cunha FQ, Lorenzetti BB, Poole S, Ferreira SH. Interleukin-8 as a mediator of sympathetic pain. *Br J Pharmacol* 1991; 104:765–767.

Cunha FQ, Poole S, Lorenzetti BB, Ferreira SH. The pivotal role of tumour necrosis factor alpha in the development of inflammatory hyperalgesia. *Br J Pharmacol* 1992; 107:660–664.

Cunha JM, Sachs D, Canetti CA, et al. The critical role of leukotriene B4 in antigen-induced mechanical hyperalgesia in immunised rats. *Br J Pharmacol* 2003; 139:1135–1145.

Cunha TM, Verri WA Jr, Vivancos GG, et al. An electronic pressure-meter nociception paw test for mice. *Braz J Med Biol Res* 2004; 37:401–407.

Cunha TM, Verri WA Jr, Silva JS, et al. A cascade of cytokines mediates mechanical inflammatory hypernociception in mice. *Proc Natl Acad Sci USA* 2005; 102:1755–1760.

Cush JJ. Unusual toxicities with TNF inhibition: heart failure and drug-induced lupus. *Clin Exp Rheumatol* 2004; 22(5 Suppl 35):S141–147.

Davis AJ, Perkins MN. The involvement of bradykinin B1 and B2 receptor mechanisms in cytokine-induced mechanical hyperalgesia in the rat. *Br J Pharmacol* 1994; 113:63–68.

den Broeder AA, de Jong E, Franssen MJ, et al. Observational study on efficacy, safety, and drug survival of anakinra in rheumatoid arthritis patients in clinical practice. *Ann Rheum Dis* 2006; 65:760–762.

Dinarello CA. Interleukin 1 as mediator of the acute-phase response. *Surv Immunol Res* 1984; 3:29–33.

Dinarello CA. Interleukin-1, interleukin-1 receptors and interleukin-1 receptor antagonist. *Int Rev Immunol* 1998; 16:457–499.

Dinarello CA. Proinflammatory cytokines. *Chest* 2000; 118:503–508.

Ferreira SH. Prostaglandins, aspirin-like drugs and analgesia. *Nat New Biol* 1972; 240:200–203.

Fehniger TA, Caligiuri MA. Interleukin 15: biology and relevance to human disease. *Blood* 2001; 97:14–32.

Ferreira SH, Nakamura M. Prostaglandin hyperalgesia, a cAMP/Ca^{2+} dependent process. *Prostaglandins* 1979; 18:179–190.

Ferreira SH, Lorenzetti BB, Bristow AF, Poole S. Interleukin-1 beta as a potent hyperalgesic agent antagonized by a tripeptide analogue. *Nature* 1988; 334:698–700.

Ferreira SH, Romitelli M, de Nucci G. Endothelin-1 participation in overt and inflammatory pain. *J Cardiovasc Pharmacol* 1989; 13(Suppl 5):S220–222.

Ferreira SH, Lorenzetti BB, De Campos DI. Induction, blockade and restoration of a persistent hypersensitive state. *Pain* 1990; 42:365–371.

Gracie JA, Forsey RJ, Chan WL, et al. A proinflammatory role for IL-18 in rheumatoid arthritis. *J Clin Invest* 1999; 104:1393–1401.

Granstein RD, Margolis R, Mizel SB, Sauder DN. In vivo inflammatory activity of epidermal cell-derived thymocyte activating factor and recombinant interleukin 1 in the mouse. *J Clin Invest* 1986; 77:1020–1027.

Handwerker HO. Influences of algogenic substances and prostaglandins on the discharges of unmyelinated cutaneous nerve fibers identified as nociceptors. In: Bonica JJ, Albe-Fessard D (Eds). *Proceedings of the First World Congress on Pain*, Advances in Pain Research and Therapy, Vol. 1. New York: Raven Press, 1976, pp 41–45.

Hannington-Kiff FG. Antisympathetic drugs in limbs. In: Wall PD, Melzack R (Eds). *Textbook of Pain*, Vol. 1. Edinburgh: Churchill Livingstone, 1989, pp 754–766.

Haraoui B. The anti-tumor necrosis factor agents are a major advance in the treatment of rheumatoid arthritis. *J Rheumatol Suppl* 2005; 72:46–47.

Henry JL. Effects of substance P on functionally identified units in cat spinal cord. *Brain Res* 1976; 114:439–451.

Hopkins SJ. The pathophysiological role of cytokines. *Leg Med (Tokyo)* 2003; 5(Suppl 1): S45–57.

Inglis JJ, Nissim A, Lees DM, et al. The differential contribution of tumour necrosis factor to thermal and mechanical hyperalgesia during chronic inflammation. *Arthritis Res Ther* 2005; 7:R807–816.

Jin X, Gereau RWT. Acute p38-mediated modulation of tetrodotoxin-resistant sodium channels in mouse sensory neurons by tumor necrosis factor-alpha. *J Neurosci* 2006; 26:246–255.

Junger H, Sorkin LS. Nociceptive and inflammatory effects of subcutaneous TNF-alpha. *Pain* 2000; 85:145–151.

Leung BP, McInnes IB, Esfandiari E, Wei XQ, Liew FY. Combined effects of IL-12 and IL-18 on the induction of collagen-induced arthritis. *J Immunol* 2000; 164:6495–6502.

Lewin GR, Mendell LM. Nerve growth factor and nociception. *Trends Neurosci* 1993; 16:353–359.

Lewin GR, Ritter AM, Mendell LM. Nerve growth factor-induced hyperalgesia in the neonatal and adult rat. *J Neurosci* 1993; 13:2136–2148.

Lorenzetti BB, Veiga FH, Canetti CA, et al. Cytokine-induced neutrophil chemoattractant 1 (CINC-1) mediates the sympathetic component of inflammatory mechanical hypersensitivity in rats. *Eur Cytokine Netw* 2002; 13:456–461.

Lynn B. The detection of injury and tissue damage. In: Wall P, Melzack R (Eds). *Textbook of Pain*, Vol. 1. Edinburgh: Churchill Livingstone, 1984, pp 19–33.

Maini RN, Breedveld FC, Kalden JR, et al. Therapeutic efficacy of multiple intravenous infusions of anti-tumor necrosis factor alpha monoclonal antibody combined with low-dose weekly methotrexate in rheumatoid arthritis. *Arthritis Rheum* 1998; 41:1552–1563.

Moreland LW. The role of cytokines in rheumatoid arthritis: inhibition of cytokines in therapeutic trials. *Drugs Today (Barc)* 1999; 35:309–319.

Murray KM, Dahl SL. Recombinant human tumor necrosis factor receptor (p75) Fc fusion protein (TNFR:Fc) in rheumatoid arthritis. *Ann Pharmacother* 1997; 31:1335–1338.

Nakamura M, Ferreira SH. A peripheral sympathetic component in inflammatory hyperalgesia. *Eur J Pharmacol* 1987; 135:145–153.

Nakamura-Craig M, Gill BK. Effect of neurokinin A, substance P and calcitonin gene related peptide in peripheral hyperalgesia in the rat paw. *Neurosci Lett* 1991; 124:49–51.

Nakanishi K, Yoshimoto T, Tsutsui H, Okamura H. Interleukin-18 is a unique cytokine that stimulates both Th1 and Th2 responses depending on its cytokine milieu. *Cytokine Growth Factor Rev* 2001; 12:53–72.

Nicol GD, Lopshire JC, Pafford CM. Tumor necrosis factor enhances the capsaicin sensitivity of rat sensory neurons. *J Neurosci* 1997; 17:975–982.

Nordahl S, Alstergren P, Kopp S. Tumor necrosis factor-alpha in synovial fluid and plasma from patients with chronic connective tissue disease and its relation to temporomandibular joint pain. *J Oral Maxillofac Surg* 2000; 58:525–530.

Obreja O, Biasio W, Andratsch M, et al. Fast modulation of heat-activated ionic current by proinflammatory interleukin 6 in rat sensory neurons. *Brain* 2005; 128(Pt 7):1634–1641.

Obreja O, Rathee PK, Lips KS, Distler C, Kress M. IL-1 beta potentiates heat-activated currents in rat sensory neurons: involvement of IL-1RI, tyrosine kinase, and protein kinase C. *Faseb J* 2002; 16:1497–1503.

Onda A, Yabuki S, Kikuchi S. Effects of neutralizing antibodies to tumor necrosis factor-alpha on nucleus pulposus-induced abnormal nociresponses in rat dorsal horn neurons. *Spine* 2003; 28:967–972.

Parada CA, Reichling DB, Levine JD. Chronic hyperalgesic priming in the rat involves a novel interaction between cAMP and PKC-epsilon second messenger pathways. *Pain* 2005; 113:185–190.

Parada CA, Yeh JJ, Joseph EK, Levine JD. Tumor necrosis factor receptor type-1 in sensory neurons contributes to induction of chronic enhancement of inflammatory hyperalgesia in rat. *Eur J Neurosci* 2003; 17:1847–1852.

Poole S, Cunha FQ, Selkirk S, Lorenzetti BB, Ferreira SH. Cytokine-mediated inflammatory hyperalgesia limited by interleukin-10. *Br J Pharmacol* 1995; 115:684–688.

Rankin EC, Choy EH, Kassimos D, et al. The therapeutic effects of an engineered human anti-tumour necrosis factor alpha antibody (CDP571) in rheumatoid arthritis. *Br J Rheumatol* 1995; 34:334–342.

Ribeiro RA, Vale ML, Ferreira SH, Cunha FQ. Analgesic effect of thalidomide on inflammatory pain. *Eur J Pharmacol* 2000; 391:97–103.

Rossi D, Zlotnik A. The biology of chemokines and their receptors. *Annu Rev Immunol* 2000; 18:217–242.

Ruchatz H, Leung BP, Wei XQ, McInnes IB, Liew FY. Soluble IL-15 receptor alpha-chain administration prevents murine collagen-induced arthritis: a role for IL-15 in development of antigen-induced immunopathology. *J Immunol* 1998; 160:5654–5660.

Sachs D, Cunha FQ, Poole S, Ferreira SH. Tumour necrosis factor-alpha, interleukin-1beta and interleukin-8 induce persistent mechanical nociceptor hypersensitivity. *Pain* 2002; 96:89–97.

Safieh-Garabedian B, Poole S, Allchorne A, Winter J, Woolf CJ. Contribution of interleukin-1 beta to the inflammation-induced increase in nerve growth factor levels and inflammatory hyperalgesia. *Br J Pharmacol* 1995; 115:1265–1275.

Schafers M, Sorkin LS, Sommer C. Intramuscular injection of tumor necrosis factor-alpha induces muscle hyperalgesia in rats. *Pain* 2003; 104:579–588.

Smith JA, Thompson DJ, Whitcup SM, et al. A randomized, placebo-controlled, double-masked clinical trial of etanercept for the treatment of uveitis associated with juvenile idiopathic arthritis. *Arthritis Rheum* 2005; 53:18–23.

Sommer C, Lindenlaub T, Teuteberg P, et al. Anti-TNF-neutralizing antibodies reduce pain-related behavior in two different mouse models of painful mononeuropathy. *Brain Res* 2001a; 913:86–89.

Sommer C, Schafers M, Marziniak M, Toyka KV. Etanercept reduces hyperalgesia in experimental painful neuropathy. *J Peripher Nerv Syst* 2001b; 6:67–72.

Sorkin LS, Xiao WH, Wagner R, Myers RR. Tumour necrosis factor-alpha induces ectopic activity in nociceptive primary afferent fibres. *Neuroscience* 1997; 81:255–262.

Staszewska-Barczak J, Dusting GJ. Sympathetic cardiovascular reflex initiated by bradykinin-induced stimulation of cardiac pain receptors in the dog. *Clin Exp Pharmacol Physiol* 1977; 4:443–452.

Strengell M, Matikainen S, Siren J, et al. IL-21 in synergy with IL-15 or IL-18 enhances IFN-gamma production in human NK and T cells. *J Immunol* 2003; 170:5464–5469.

Tartaglia LA, Goeddel DV. Two TNF receptors. *Immunol Today* 1992; 13:151–153.

Tobin AM, Kirby B. TNF alpha inhibitors in the treatment of psoriasis and psoriatic arthritis. *BioDrugs* 2005; 19:47–57.

Vale ML, Benevides VM, Sachs D, et al. Antihyperalgesic effect of pentoxifylline on experimental inflammatory pain. *Br J Pharmacol* 2004; 143:833–844.

Vane JR. Inhibition of prostaglandin synthesis as a mechanism of action for aspirin-like drugs. *Nat New Biol* 1971; 231:232–235.

Verri WA Jr, Schivo IR, Cunha TM, et al. Interleukin-18 induces mechanical hypernociception in rats via endothelin acting on ETB receptors in a morphine-sensitive manner. *J Pharmacol Exp Ther* 2004; 310:710–717.

Verri WA Jr, Molina RO, Schivo IR, et al. Nociceptive effect of subcutaneously injected interleukin-12 is mediated by endothelin (ET) acting on ETB receptors in rats. *J Pharmacol Exp Ther* 2005; 315:609–615.

Verri WA Jr, Cunha TM, Parada CA, et al. Hypernociceptive role of cytokines and chemokines: targets for analgesic drug development? *Pharmacol Ther* 2006a; 112:116–138.

Verri WA Jr, Cunha TM, Parada CA, et al. IL-15 mediates immune inflammatory hypernociception by triggering a sequential release of IFN-gamma, endothelin, and prostaglandin. *Proc Natl Acad Sci US A* 2006b; 103:9721–9725.

Verri WA Jr, Cunha TM, Parada CA, et al. Antigen-induced inflammatory mechanical hypernociception in mice is mediated by IL-18. *Brain Behav Immun* 2007; 21:535–543.

Vila AT, Puig L, Fernandez-Figueras MT, et al. Adverse cutaneous reactions to anakinra in patients with rheumatoid arthritis: clinicopathological study of five patients. *Br J Dermatol* 2005; 153:417–423.

Vilcek J. The cytokines: an overview. In: Thomson AWS, Lotze MT (Eds). *The Cytokine Handbook*, Vol. 1. London: Academic Press, 2003, pp 3–18.

Ware CF. Network communications: lymphotoxins, LIGHT, and TNF. *Annu Rev Immunol* 2005; 23:787–819.

Watford WT, Hissong BD, Bream JH, et al. Signaling by IL-12 and IL-23 and the immunoregulatory roles of STAT4. *Immunol Rev* 2004; 202:139–156.

Watkins LR, Wiertelak EP, Goehler LE, et al. Characterization of cytokine-induced hyperalgesia. *Brain Res* 1994; 654:15–26.

Wei XQ, Leung BP, Arthur HM, McInnes IB, Liew FY. Reduced incidence and severity of collagen-induced arthritis in mice lacking IL-18. *J Immunol* 2001; 166:517–521.

Weinblatt ME, Kremer JM, Bankhurst AD, et al. A trial of etanercept, a recombinant tumor necrosis factor receptor: Fc fusion protein, in patients with rheumatoid arthritis receiving methotrexate. *N Engl J Med* 1999; 340:253–259.

Woolf CJ, Allchorne A, Safieh-Garabedian B, Poole S. Cytokines, nerve growth factor and inflammatory hyperalgesia: the contribution of tumour necrosis factor alpha. *Br J Pharmacol* 1997; 121:417–424.

Xu XJ, Dalsgaard CJ, Wiesenfeld-Hallin Z. Spinal substance P and *N*-methyl-D-aspartate receptors are coactivated in the induction of central sensitization of the nociceptive flexor reflex. *Neuroscience* 1992; 51:641–648.

Zhang N, Inan S, Cowan A, et al. A proinflammatory chemokine, CCL3, sensitizes the heat- and capsaicin-gated ion channel TRPV1. *Proc Natl Acad Sci USA* 2005; 102:4536–4541.

Zhou QL, Strichartz G, Davar G. Endothelin-1 activates ET(A) receptors to increase intracellular calcium in model sensory neurons. *Neuroreport* 2001; 12:3853–3857.

Zucali JR, Dinarello CA, Oblon DJ, et al. Interleukin 1 stimulates fibroblasts to produce granulocyte-macrophage colony-stimulating activity and prostaglandin E2. *J Clin Invest* 1986; 77:1857–1863.

Correspondence to: Sérgio Henrique Ferreira, PhD, Faculdade de Medicina de Ribeirão Preto, USP, Av. Bandeirantes, 3900, Ribeirão Preto, SP, Brazil 14049-900. Tel: 55-16-602-3222; fax: 55-16-633-0021; email: shferreir@fmrp.usp.br.

Immune and Glial Regulation of Pain, edited by Joyce A. DeLeo, Linda S. Sorkin, and Linda R. Watkins, IASP Press, Seattle, © 2007.

5

Proinflammatory Cytokines and Neuropathic Pain: Retrograde Signaling and Dorsal Root Ganglion Changes after Peripheral Nerve Injury

Maria Schäfers,[a] Claudia Sommer,[b] and Linda S. Sorkin[c]

aDepartment of Neurology, University of Duisberg-Essen, Essen, Germany;
bDepartment of Neurology, University of Würzburg, Würzburg, Germany;
cDepartment of Anesthesiology, University of California, San Diego, California, USA

CYTOKINES AND NEUROPATHIC PAIN

Cytokines are protein mediators of cell-to-cell communication that influence the behavior of other cells. Cytokines are called "pleiotropic," due to their broad range of redundant, frequently overlapping functions, and they can have autocrine, paracrine, or endocrine actions. Some cytokines are labeled proinflammatory, others anti-inflammatory, depending on their effects on immune cells, in particular on lymphocytes.

TUMOR NECROSIS FACTOR ALPHA

Tumor necrosis factor-α (TNF-α) is widely considered the prototypical proinflammatory cytokine due to its principal role in initiating the activation cascade of other cytokines and growth factors in the inflammatory response. Correlations between tissue levels of TNF-α and pain and hyperalgesia have been reported in a number of diseases, such as leprosy, painful neuropathies, postherpetic neuralgia, and sciatica (Barnes et al. 1992; Shafer et al. 1994; Tak et al. 1997; Lindenlaub and Sommer 2003).

Intraplantar or intramuscular administration of TNF-α in rats induces inflammatory hyperalgesia (Cunha et al. 1992; Perkins et al. 1995); it causes plasma extravasation as well as excitation and leads to a dose-dependent sensitization of peripheral C fibers (Junger and Sorkin 2000). Similar allodynia or hyperalgesia can be induced by endo- or epineurial administration of TNF-α (Wagner and Myers 1996b; Sorkin et al. 1997; Zelenka et al. 2005), and TNF-α-mediated neuronal excitation occurs when this cytokine is applied directly to the nerve trunk (Sorkin et al. 1997) or to dorsal root ganglia (DRG) (Liu et al. 2002; Zhang et al. 2002; Schäfers et al. 2003d; Ozaktay et al. 2006). Importantly, intraplantar TNF-α activates downstream pathways involving activation of other proinflammatory cytokines including interleukin (IL)-1β, IL-6, and IL-8 and initiates a positive feedback synthesis of itself. Nerve growth factor (NGF) and prostaglandins are also increased downstream of TNF-α activation (Cunha et al. 1992; Woolf et al. 1997).

There is considerable evidence for the involvement of TNF-α in neuropathic pain. Several studies have shown a correlation between the level of TNF-α expression and the development of allodynia or hyperalgesia in neuropathic pain models (Wagner and Myers 1996a; Sommer and Schäfers 1998; George et al. 1999, 2004; Cui et al. 2000; Okamoto et al. 2001; Kleinschnitz et al. 2004). Nerve injury initiates a potent immune response typified by the early release of TNF-α from infiltrating and resident macrophages (George et al. 1999) and Schwann cells (Wagner and Myers 1996a; Sommer and Schäfers 1998). Within 5 hours after nerve injury, TNF-α levels are elevated within resident Schwann cells, which owing to their close proximity can directly sensitize nearby neurons (Shamash et al. 2002). Mice that experience delayed Wallerian degeneration (OLA/WLD) have deficient TNF-α production and show reduced mechanical and thermal hypersensitivity after chronic constriction injury (Myers et al. 1996; Sommer and Schäfers 1998; Shamash et al. 2002). Liefner et al. used TNF-α knockout mice to demonstrate that the main contribution of TNF-α to Wallerian degeneration is induction of macrophage recruitment from the vasculature (Liefner et al. 2000).

Antagonism of TNF-α has the opposite effect. Thalidomide, which reduces the production of TNF-α by activated macrophages, attenuates thermal hyperalgesia following peripheral nerve injury (Sommer and Myers 1994; George et al. 2000). Despite its deleterious side effects (see Manning, this volume), thalidomide is still used in the clinic for the treatment of various painful TNF-α-mediated diseases (Apfel and Zochodne 2004). Etanercept is a recombinant human TNF-α receptor 2 (TNFR2)-Fc fusion protein that binds to the biologically active TNF-α protein before it encounters receptors on cell surfaces; it has been used experimentally to treat painful neuropathies (Sommer et al. 2001; Schäfers et al. 2003a,d). Interestingly, preemptive, but not delayed, treatment inhibited mechanical allodynia in neuropathic pain models, which suggests that TNF-α is particularly important in the initiation of neuropathic pain (Sommer et al. 1998, 2001; Schäfers et al. 2003a,d). Etanercept has been used in open trials and case reports to treat low back pain (Tobinick and Britschgi-Davoodifar 2003; Genevay et al. 2004). Infliximab is a chimeric monoclonal TNF-α antibody that has been studied in experimental spinal disk herniations (Olmarker et al. 2003). However, it was not effective in a randomized trial for pain in patients with disk-herniation-induced sciatica (Korhonen et al. 2005). Adalimumab is a complete human recombinant immunoglobulin G1 anti-TNF-α monoclonal antibody and is the newest TNF-α biological response modifier.

As in neuropathic animals, thalidomide reduces inflammatory hyperalgesia (Ribeiro et al. 2000). Knocking out TNF-α receptor 1 (TNFR1) diminishes, but does not abolish, carrageenan-induced hyperalgesia (Cunha et al. 2005), despite the fact that neutralizing antisera to TNF-α is effective (Cunha et al. 1992). This finding implies that TNF-α is exerting its effect via mechanisms other than activation of TNFR1 alone. Several studies have shown a correlation between the level of TNF-α expression and the development of allodynia or hyperalgesia in neuropathic pain models (Wagner and Myers 1996a; Sommer and Schäfers 1998; George et al. 1999, 2004; Cui et al. 2000; Okamoto et al. 2001; Kleinschnitz et al. 2004).

Hyperalgesia induced by intraplantar TNF-α is significantly reduced by systemic pentoxifylline, possibly by diminution of further TNF-α production from infiltrated macrophages, because pentoxifylline reduces TNF-α produced in inflamed joint exudates and in stimulated peritoneal macrophages (Vale et al. 2004).

INTERLEUKIN-1 BETA

Interleukin-1β (IL-1β) is a potent proinflammatory cytokine that seems to be involved in neuropathic pain (Sommer et al. 1999; Schäfers et al. 2001). IL-1β is produced and secreted under conditions that are associated with increased pain and hyperalgesia, such as neuropathies, tumor growth, or chronic inflammatory diseases including rheumatoid arthritis (Eastgate et al. 1988; Watkins et al. 1999). Under such conditions, IL-1β can be expressed in, and released from, many cell types such as mononuclear cells, fibroblasts, synoviocytes, Schwann cells, and endothelial cells. IL-1β is also involved in Wallerian degeneration; its production is upregulated in Schwann cells after peripheral nerve injury (Shamash et al. 2002). IL-1β gene expression in sciatic nerve is increased 7 days after nerve injury, at the time of peak thermal hyperalgesia (Okamoto et al. 2001). In addition, expression of IL-1 receptor type I mRNA was detected in DRG neurons, suggesting a possible autocrine or paracrine action of IL-1β on sensory processing (Copray et al. 2001).

Intraneural injection of IL-1β induces thermal hyperalgesia and mechanical allodynia (Zelenka et al. 2005). Epineurial administration of neutralizing antibodies to IL-1 receptor reduces both thermal hyperalgesia and mechanical allodynia associated with experimental neuropathy and attenuates the endoneurial increase of TNF-α immunoreactivity (Sommer et al. 1999). Whereas intrathecal IL-1β antagonists alone are seemingly without effect in nerve injury models, they act synergistically with TNF-α antagonists to cause a further reduction of allodynia (Sweitzer et al. 2001).

Deletion of IL-1 receptor type I and transgenic overexpression of the IL-1-receptor antagonist have recently been shown to delay the onset and reduce the severity of autotomy behavior after sciatic/saphenous nerve axotomy as well as to reduce spontaneous ectopic activity following spinal nerve injury (Wolf et al. 2006). Similarly, time to onset, duration, and magnitude of mechanical allodynia were reduced in two models of neuropathic pain—spinal nerve ligation (SNL) and chronic constriction injury (CCI)—in mice lacking both IL-1α and IL-1β genes (Honore et al. 2006).

However, the mechanism of IL-1β action in the periphery is unclear. Several studies indicate that IL-1β might be involved in a complex signaling cascade that leads to the production of pronociceptive compounds such as nitric oxide, NGF, and prostaglandins from immune cells or Schwann cells. For example, IL-1β induces transcription of NGF in Schwann cells (Lindholm et al. 1987), and IL-1β-induced hyperalgesia can be prevented by anti-NGF antibodies (Safieh-Garabedian et al. 1995), suggesting that IL-1β hyperalgesia is mediated via increased NGF in inflamed nerves. Prolonged exposure of primary afferent neurons to IL-1β induces substance P release via the cyclooxygenase (COX)-2 system (Inoue et al. 1999). Intraneural injection of IL-1β increases the expression of p38 mitogen-activated protein kinase (p38 MAPK) and nuclear factor (NF)-κB in DRG neurons, suggesting cytokine-dependent activation of primary afferent fibers (Zelenka et al. 2005). Some of these compounds can lead to changes in gene expression and neuronal excitability (including the development of spontaneous activity) in intact nociceptors.

IL-1β also directly excites nociceptive fibers (Fukuoka et al. 1994) and DRG neurons (Ozaktay et al. 2006). Nociceptive fibers are activated within 1 minute of IL-1β application (Fukuoka et al. 1994). In a skin-nerve in vitro preparation, brief exposure of the skin to IL-1β facilitated heat-evoked release of calcitonin gene-related peptide (CGRP) (Opree and Kress 2000). The short latency of this effect and the absence of the neuronal soma in that study suggest an effect independent of changes in gene expression or receptor upregulation. Brief applications of IL-1β to nociceptive neurons potentiate heat-activated inward currents and shift activation thresholds toward lower temperatures without altering intracellular calcium levels. This IL-1β-induced heat sensitization is mediated by activation of protein kinases. IL-1 receptor is expressed in DRG neurons, such that IL-1β can act directly on sensory neurons to increase their susceptibility to noxious heat (Obreja et al. 2002). Application of IL-1β to the DRG in vivo results in discharge of group II units and, at the highest dose range, causes increased mechanosensitivity of receptive fields (Ozaktay et al. 2006).

INTERLEUKIN-6

Another cytokine implicated in neuropathic pain is interleukin-6 (IL-6), which signals intracellularly via its unique membrane-bound receptor (IL-6R) and glycoprotein 130 (for review, see De Jongh et al. 2003). Increased IL-6 serum levels have been detected in patients with neuropathies, malignant tumors, musculoskeletal disorders, burn injuries, and autoimmune and chronic inflammatory conditions. The affected tissue in all these disorders commonly displays tenderness and hypersensitivity.

Most experimental studies report proinflammatory and pronociceptive roles for IL-6. Mechanical allodynia has been correlated with increasing levels of IL-6 immunoreactivity or mRNA in the sciatic nerve and DRG after CCI (Murphy et al. 1999). In the peripheral nerves, IL-6 is upregulated in invading macrophages in a prostaglandin E_2-dependent manner (Ma and Quirion 2006).

Intraplantar or intrathecal injection of IL-6 induces hyperalgesia or allodynia in rats (Vissers et al. 2005). Spinal administration of IL-6, in contrast, appears to reduce electrically evoked C-fiber activity (Flatters et al. 2003). IL-6 knockout mice show less thermal hyperalgesia and mechanical allodynia in the CCI model compared with wild-type mice. However, one group reported a decrease in mechanical allodynia, but not in thermal hyperalgesia, in IL-6 knockout mice, at least for the first 10 days after injury (Ramer et al. 1998, 1999). Intrathecal application of anti-IL-6 antibodies decreases tactile allodynia following SNL. Epineurial injection of antibodies to the IL-6 receptor attenuates thermal hyperalgesia and mechanical allodynia in the CCI model.

The mechanism of action of IL-6 is not well established, but it might be related to sympathetic sprouting in the DRG (Ramer et al. 1998). IL-6 induces the production of galanin in sensory neurons (Thompson et al. 1998). Changes in neurotransmitter expression may contribute to altered pain processing after nerve injury. However, acutely in inflammatory hyperalgesia, IL-6 is dissociated from activation of the sympathetic efferent fibers or sprouting and is thought to engage the IL-1 prostaglandin pathway (Cunha et al. 1992). A recent study showed that the neuronal effects of IL-6 depend on the presence of the soluble IL-6 receptor (Obreja et al. 2005). IL-6 application to DRG neurons caused an increase of intracellular calcium in about one-third of the neurons, suggesting functional IL-6 receptors in a subpopulation of these neurons (von Banchet et al. 2005).

ANTI-INFLAMMATORY CYTOKINES

Anti-inflammatory cytokines such as IL-4 and IL-10 have antihyperalgesic actions in animal models of neuropathic pain (Wagner et al. 1998). IL-10 pretreatment also reduces hyperalgesic responses to intraplantar injections of carrageenan, IL-1β, IL-6, and TNF-α (Poole et al. 1995). Intrathecally applied human IL-2 has a short-lived antinociceptive effect in the CCI model (Yao et al. 2002).

RETROGRADE AND ANTEROGRADE SIGNALING

Communication between cells is a fundamental requirement of a multicellular organism. The DRG contain the first-order sensory neurons that respond immediately and directly to axonal injuries; their supporting satellite cells respond concurrently. The neuronal soma must receive accurate and timely information as to the site and extent of axonal damage to allow upregulation of transcription factors, cytoskeletal proteins, cell adhesion and axon guidance molecules, and trophic factors and their receptors.

PRINCIPLES OF COMMUNICATIONS BETWEEN NERVE FIBERS AND DRG CELLS

Two principal mechanisms of communication link peripheral nerve fibers with DRG cells: electrophysiological communication and chemical axonal transport. The initial signal from the injury site to the cell body is thought to be a rapid depolarization-induced burst of action potentials (Berdan et al. 1993; Ziv and Spira 1993; Mandolesi et al. 2004); this electrical effect can immediately influence both neurons and satellite cells of the DRG and can be blocked by preemptive local anesthesia.

Later on, signals dependent on axonal transport are thought to impinge on the cell body. Neurons can specifically internalize macromolecules such as trophic factors, lectins, toxins, and other pathogens (for review, see von Bartheld 2003). Factors released from injured tissue may be internalized at peripheral terminals, whereas other proteins produced by Schwann cells or by infiltrating immune cells as a result of nerve or deep tissue injury are picked up mid-axonally; these agents are transported retrogradely along the axons until they reach the level of the cell body. Some factors may stay and influence transcription of new proteins at the nucleus, while others continue along the axon and are transported anterogradely along the dorsal root toward the central terminal in the spinal cord.

TROPHIC CURRENCIES IN NEURAL NETWORKS

Previous investigations have revealed that retrograde axonal transport of proteins (Redshaw and Bisby 1984, 1987), including neurotrophins (DiStefano and Curtis 1994), is increased after injury to the peripheral nerve. For neurotrophins, an increase in retrograde transport represents a relatively rapid and transient response to sensory nerve injury; by day 7 following the lesion, transport of NGF, brain-derived neurotrophic factor (BDNF), glial-cell-line-derived neurotrophic factor (GDNF), neurotrophin (NT)-3, and NT-4 returns to basal levels (Curtis et al. 1998; Tonra et al. 1998; Leitner et al. 1999; Mufson et al. 1999). The continuous supply of neurotrophic factors from axon terminals to the cell body under basal conditions has an important role in the maintenance and survival of specific populations of adult neurons. The increased retrograde transport of neurotrophins following nerve injury suggests that a loss of trophic factors might act as an injury signal for the cell body. With the exception of NGF, which exhibits exclusively retrograde transport, neurotrophins are also known to undergo anterograde trafficking (for review, see Yano and Chao 2004).

SIGNALING OF CYTOKINES

At the peripheral injury site, different immunomodulatory factors such as TNF-α, leukemia inhibitory factor (LIF) (Curtis et al. 1994), and ciliary neurotrophic factor (CNTF) (Curtis et al. 1993) are induced within hours of injury. All undergo retrograde transport to the DRG. In contrast, although IL-6 undergoes significant upregulation after nerve transection, it is not transported (Kurek et al. 1996).

Endogenous TNF-α transport is induced after CCI of the sciatic nerve (Shubayev and Myers 2001; Schäfers et al. 2002), and it returns to basal levels by day 7 post-injury. This observation is temporally similar to increases in axonal transport observed for neurotrophins (Curtis et al. 1998; Leitner et al. 1999; Mufson et al. 1999). Using exogenous biotinylated TNF-α, Shubayev and Myers (2001, 2002) observed fast retrograde transport of TNF-α tracer from the injury site to the DRG, followed by anterograde transport from the DRG to the spinal cord. This transport is believed to be selective to certain classes of nerve fibers and may be dependent on injury-specific signals and on packaging of the TNF-transporting complex (Myers et al. 2006). TNF-α and TNFR activation and retrograde cotransport from the injury site could represent a mechanism for cellular activation and TNF-α upregulation in the DRG and spinal cord. Uptake and transport by uninjured axons suggest mechanisms leading to changes in levels of TNF-α, TNFR2, phosphorylated p38 MAPK (p-p38 MAPK), and phosphorylated extracellular signal-regulated protein kinase (p-ERK) in adjacent soma with structurally intact axons (DeLeo et al. 2000; Schäfers et al. 2003b,c; Obata et al. 2004; Ohtori et al. 2004).

However, other studies using radiolabeled TNF-α support a predominantly anterograde TNF-α transport from the nerve injury site to the innervated muscle (Schäfers et al. 2002) (Fig. 1). Intraneural injection of radiolabeled TNF-α resulted in early accumulation in the gastrocnemius muscle. Endogenous sources of TNF-α after nerve injury include axonal uptake from Schwann cells or sensory neurons in the DRG that increase their TNF-α expression after nerve injury.

SIGNALING OF MAP KINASES AND TRANSCRIPTION FACTORS

Kinases such as p38 MAPK, ERK, and c-Jun N-terminal kinase (JNK) are activated downstream of TNF-α. Several of these kinases have also been implicated in retrograde signaling. Phosphorylated ERK is retrogradely transported following nerve injury (Reynolds et al. 2001; Perlson et al. 2005). Phosphorylated JNK is also retrogradely transported in the injured sciatic nerve (Lindwall and Kanje 2005), apparently together with the JNK-interacting protein (JIP) and other upstream kinases. JNK3 (the JNK isoform that is expressed primarily in the nervous system) is capable of both anterograde and retrograde transport along the sciatic nerve (Cavalli et al. 2005). Receptor-mediated NGF transport activates retrograde transport of p-ERK, p38, and of a serine/threonine kinase termed p-Akt (protein kinase B) in DRG neurons (Delcroix et al. 2003).

Peripheral nerve axotomy causes upregulation of the interleukins LIF, IL-6, and CNTF. These ligands activate the Janus kinase (JAK)-signal transducer and activator of transcription-3 (STAT3) signaling pathway, such that axonal phospho-STAT3 is a strong candidate as a retrograde injury signal (Lee et al. 2004; Qiu et al. 2005). Recent data indicate that activating transcription factors 2 and 3 are also transported retrogradely following sciatic nerve injury (Lindwall and Kanje 2005).

RETROGRADE INJURY SIGNALS: "NEW" AXOPLASMIC PROTEINS

Besides interruption of the arrival of macromolecules that are normally transported from terminals, the appearance of new axoplasmic proteins "activated" by modification at the injury site may impinge on the cell body. Evidence for this possibility has mainly been forthcoming from work by Ambron and colleagues in the invertebrate model *Aplysia*. Microinjection of *Aplysia* axoplasm, harvested from sites proximal to a nerve injury (retrogradely transported), into cultured neurons leads to uptake of microinjected proteins into the nuclei concomitant with growth and survival responses (Ambron and Walters 1996; Zhang and Ambron 2000). Retrograde transport of axoplasm components from lesioned nerves was suggested to be dependent on "nuclear localization signals" (NLS), a new function of NLS sequences in addition to their well-known role in

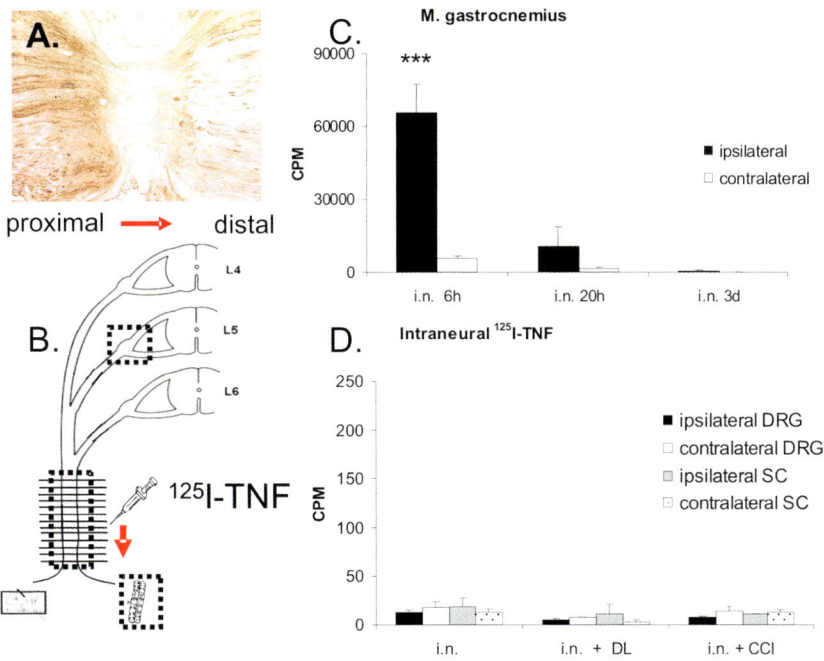

Fig. 1. Anterograde axonal transport of tumor necrosis factor (TNF) after nerve injury. (A) Immunohistochemical staining of endogenous TNF in the rat sciatic nerve 20 hours after place-ment of a double ligature; the area around the proximal ligature is shown. TNF accumulates proximally to the ligature, suggesting anterograde transport. (B) Schematic of experimental treatments to determine the axonal transport of exogenously applied 125-I-labeled TNF (Schäfers et al. 2002). Radiolabeled TNF was injected into the rat sciatic nerve. After dif-ferent time points, nerve segments, gastrocnemius muscle, plantar skin, and lumbar DRG were dissected for detection of radioactivity. (C) Distribution of I-125 in the gastrocnemius muscle after intraneural injection of 125-I-TNF. After 6 hours, the ipsilateral gastrocnemius muscle shows a significant increase of 125-I-TNF, suggesting fast anterograde transport. (D) There is no accumulation of 125-I-TNF in the plantar skin after injection of 125-I-TNF into the intact (i.n.), double-ligated (DL), or chronic constriction injury (CCI)-lesioned sciatic nerve. CPM = counts per minute.

mediating nuclear transport. Recently, it was shown that NLS-dependent retro-grade transport is contingent upon transport factors termed "importins." These nuclear import factors are believed to provide an additional mechanism for retrograde injury signaling (Hanz et al. 2003). Importins are found throughout axons and dendrites at significant distances from the cell body, and importin-β protein is increased after nerve lesion by local translation of axonal mRNA. This process leads to formation of high-affinity NLS-binding complexes that traffic retrogradely due to an interaction of importin-α with the motor protein dynein; these complexes thus may enable retrograde transport of signals that modulate the regeneration of injured neurons (for a more detailed review, see Hanz and Fainzilber 2006). A recent study showed that retrograde transport of p-ERK is mediated by importins (Perlson et al. 2005).

DORSAL ROOT GANGLION CHANGES
AFTER PERIPHERAL NERVE INJURY

Compelling evidence indicates that pain due to peripheral nerve injury is related to changes in primary afferent neuron function. Nerve-injury-induced hyperalgesia and allodynia reflect, at least in part, changes in the excitability and/or phenotype of primary afferent neurons. In this chapter, we emphasize DRG changes related to TNF-α as the basis for understanding changes in the DRG in response to nerve injury.

ALGESIC ROLE OF TNF-ALPHA IN NAIVE, NERVE-LESIONED, AND CHRONICALLY COMPRESSED DORSAL ROOT GANGLIA

After nerve injury, DRG neurons robustly increase their expression of TNF-α (Shubayev and Myers 2001; Schäfers et al. 2003c; Dubovy et al. 2006; Xu et al. 2006), and axotomized DRG show an increase of TNF-mRNA (Murphy et al. 1995). Injection or perfusion of TNF-α into or onto naive rat DRG in vivo induces allodynia (Homma et al. 2002; Schäfers et al. 2003d; Murata et al. 2006) and elicits neuronal discharge (Schäfers 2003c, Ozaktey 2006). After nerve injury, subthreshold quantities of TNF-α injected into DRG cells result in faster onset of allodynia and increased spontaneous pain behavior, suggesting an increased sensitivity of nerve-injured DRG to TNF (Schäfers et al. 2003d). Markedly increased sensitivity to exogenous TNF-α is also seen in DRG neuronal discharge in vitro, where not only are neurons responsive to lower concentrations of TNF-α, but firing frequencies are distinctly higher and the duration of the response is longer (Schäfers et al. 2003c). Similar results were obtained in a model of low back pain, in which TNF-α administered to compressed DRG enhanced ongoing allodynia (Homma et al. 2002); following mechanical compression of DRG, TNF-α-induced neuronal firing was enhanced. In another model of low back pain, TNF-α applied to nerve roots synergized with root traction to cause neuropathic pain behavior and neuropathological changes (Igarashi et al. 2000). Neutralizing the activity of endogenous TNF-α of the compressed DRG with soluble TNF receptors reduced allodynia (Homma et al. 2002).

Thus, there is strong in vivo and in vitro evidence that injured nerve fibers are sensitized to the excitatory effects of TNF-α. Application of TNF-α to the dorsal root (Onda et al. 2002, 2003) or administration of TNF-α-containing nucleus pulposus to the DRG (Cuellar et al. 2004) induces spontaneous discharges in dorsal horn wide-dynamic-range neurons.

THE ROLE OF INJURED AFFERENTS AND UNINJURED NEIGHBORING AFFERENTS

Many forms of nerve injury fail to fully transect an entire nerve fascicle, and many intact fibers are thus closely apposed to injured fibers and consequently share the same environmental consequences (for review, see McMahon et al. 2005). There are two ways in which these "spared" sensory neurons may be exposed to increased levels of neurotrophic or inflammatory factors. First, the peripheral targets they innervate are partially denervated. Given that the expression of target-derived factors does not seem to depend on innervation density, "spared" fibers will have less competition for these factors and receive a larger "share" than under basal conditions. Second, Schwann cells reacting to Wallerian degeneration, as well as other immune cells invading the nerve, start to express several of the factors normally expressed by peripheral targets, including neurotrophins such as NGF or GDNF or inflammatory mediators such as IL-1 or TNF-α. These factors bathe all nerve fibers equally.

After nerve injury, both injured afferents and their uninjured neighbors develop ectopic activity. Thus, both populations of afferents are theoretically capable of initiating or maintaining the behavioral changes observed after nerve injury. The role played by injured and uninjured axons in neuropathic pain is controversial; much attention has focused on the directly damaged primary afferents and their influence on the activity of dorsal horn neurons. For example, cutting the dorsal root of the injured spinal nerve eliminated or prevented SNL-induced pain behavior (Sheen and Chung 1993), and low-threshold ectopic activity occurs predominantly in injured A-fibers within 16–18 hours of injury and is sustained for as many as 10 weeks post-injury (Liu et al. 1999; Han et al. 2000). Injured sensory neurons with medium to large cell bodies upregulate expression of neurotransmitters implicated in nociceptive transmission such as substance P (Noguchi et al. 1994), BDNF (Michael et al. 1999), and ERK (Obata et al. 2004).

However, increasing evidence suggests that DRG neurons with intact axons also show an alteration of excitability and gene expression, and these changes might have functional roles in neuropathic pain. Cutting the dorsal root of the uninjured neighboring ganglion following SNL eliminates mechanical hyperalgesia and cold allodynia (Yoon et al. 1996; Li et al. 2000). A subpopulation of uninjured unmyelinated afferents also develops ongoing ectopic activity and alpha-adrenergic sensitivity (Ali et al. 1999), suggesting that in the presence of nerve injury changes in uninjured afferents are sufficient to initiate neuropathic pain behavior. Substance P, CGRP, BDNF, transient receptor potential vanilloid 1 (TRPV1), and p38 MAPK increase in uninjured neurons in several neuropathic pain models (Ma and Bisby 1998; Hudson et al. 2001; Fukuoka and Noguchi 2002; Obata et al. 2004). Given the mixed nature of most incomplete

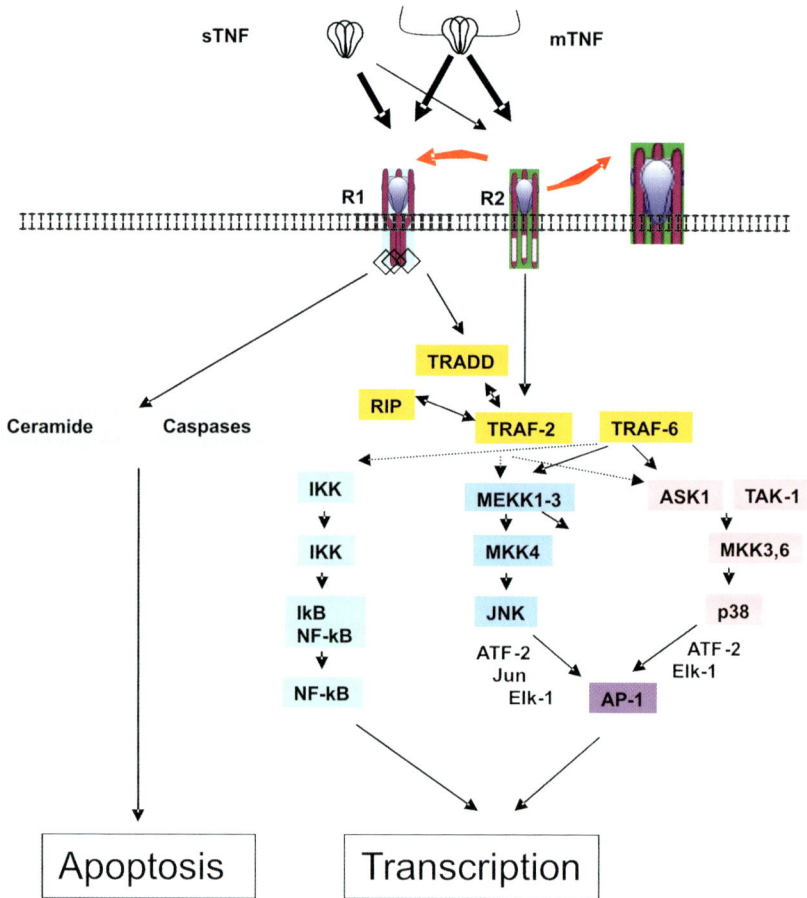

Fig. 2. Tumor necrosis factor (TNF) receptors and signaling molecules. Soluble TNF (sTNF) and membrane-bound TNF (mTNF) bind to both TNF receptor 1 (TNFR1) and TNF receptor 2 (TNFR2). TNFR1 has intrinsic tyrosine kinase activity, whereas TNFR2 lacks a cytoplasmic domain and initiates ligand-mediated signaling molecules via tumor necrosis factor receptor-associated factor 2 (TRAF-2). TNFR1 can induce an apoptosis cascade. IkB kinase (IKK) activity resides on a large multiprotein complex, which is activated by some MAP kinases (MKKs). TNF is able to activate both the Jun amino-terminal kinase (JNK) and p38 kinase cascades. AP-1 is directly activated through phosphorylation by JNK, and its expression is induced through JNK- and p38-kinase dependent activation of transcription factors. Abbreviations: ASK = apoptosis signal-regulating kinase 1; ATF2 = activating transcription factor 2; MKK = MAP kinase kinase; RIP = receptor interaction protein; TAK-1: transforming growth factor β-activated kinase 1; TRADD = TNF-receptor-1-associated death domain. (Adapted from Eder 1997.)

nerve lesions, it seems likely that changes in phenotype are associated both with injured axons and with intact axons that have been altered by the milieu generated by the injury.

Regarding TNF-α, it has been shown that small and medium, presumably low-threshold myelinated DRG neurons, whether injured or uninjured, display TNF-α immunoreactivity after CCI (Schäfers et al. 2003c). Both injured and intact DRG neurons are sensitized to exogenous TNF-α in vitro after L5 spinal nerve ligation (Schäfers et al. 2003d). However, other investigators have not observed increased TNF-α immunoreactivity in the cytoplasm of DRG neurons after sciatic or spinal nerve ligature (Dubovy et al. 2006), but showed instead a distinct elevation of TNF-α in satellite cells and neuronal nuclei.

In a manner similar to sensitization of the uninjured afferents after nerve injury, neuropathic pain is also induced by exclusive injury to motor axons. Transection of the L5 ventral root exposes the sensory axons to the milieu of Wallerian degeneration and results in bilateral mechanical allodynia that is rapid (within 24 hours), robust, and prolonged (lasting for 56 days), similar to the allodynia induced by L5 spinal nerve transsection (Li et al. 2000, Li et al. 2002, Xu et al. 2006). The postulated mechanism is exposure of the DRG neurons and their peripheral afferent fibers to products of degenerating efferent motor axons in the sciatic nerve and the denervated muscles (Li et al. 2002). Indeed, infiltration of the DRG by ED-1-positive macrophages and the immunoreactivity of TNF-α and TNFR1 are increased in ipsilateral L4 and L5 DRG following L5 ventral root dissection (Li et al. 2000; Xu et al. 2006).

POTENTIAL MECHANISMS FOR TNF-EVOKED DISCHARGES IN DORSAL ROOT GANGLION NEURONS

Although both injured and adjacent uninjured DRG display similar sensitization to TNF-α, different mechanisms may be involved. Response latencies of several minutes suggest the involvement of intracellular signal transduction pathways. Excitatory effects of TNF-α on DRG neurons are dependent on protein kinase A (Zhang et al. 2002). TNF-α exerts its effect through two known receptors, TNFR1 and TNFR2. Nerve injury leads to increased expression of both receptors by peripheral nerve axons (George et al. 2005; Dubovy et al. 2006) and by DRG (Schäfers et al. 2003b; Ohtori et al. 2004; Dubovy et al. 2006; Xu et al. 2006). Induction of hyperalgesia seems to be mediated by TNFR1, because pretreatment with neutralizing antibodies to TNFR1, but not to TNFR2, can reduce hyperalgesia (Sommer et al. 1998), and because antisense oligonucleotide to TNFR1 can block development of inflammatory hyperalgesia (Parada et al. 2003). In accordance with these findings, TNFR1 knockout mice, but not TNFR2 knockout mice, showed reduced thermal hyperalgesia after CCI and SNL (Vogel et al. 2006; Schäfers et al., in preparation).

TNF receptors activate multiple signaling pathways, including ceramide signaling and activation of several MAPK pathways (Fig. 2). It is now recognized that the p38 MAPK pathway is an important regulator in neuropathic pain. For example, TNF-α activates p38 MAPK in cultured DRG neurons (Pollock et al. 2002). Recently, it was shown that TNF-α acutely increases tetrodotoxin (TTX)-resistant Na$^+$ currents in small DRG neurons; this modulation occurs via activation of TNFR1 and induction of p38 activity (Jin and Gereau 2006). Acute application of TNF to cultured DRG neurons also increases p-JNK and p-p38 (Pollock et al. 2002), while topical application of TNF-α to rat nerve root increases p-ERK with on onset time of several hours (Takahashi et al. 2006). Taken together, this evidence suggests that other MAPK may also play a role in the activation of DRG cells in response to nerve injury.

TNF-α has been shown to regulate a variety of other ion channels in the nervous system; however, this activity has not been studied in the context of pain. For example, TNF-α decreases outward K$^+$ currents in retinal ganglion neurons (Diem et al. 2001) and increases L-type Ca^{2+} currents in hippocampal neurons (Furukawa and Mattson 1998) and in superior cervical ganglion neurons (Soliven and Albert 1992). In central neurons, TNF-α increases cell surface expression of the α-amino-3-hydroxy-5-methyl-4-isoxazolepropionate (AMPA) receptor subunit GluR1 in association with an increase in calcium-permeable AMPA/kainate receptors (see Beattie and Stellwagen, this volume). Through these and possibly other mechanisms, TNF-α can modulate the number of membrane ion channels, as well as their activity and protein phosphorylation, thereby affecting signal transduction pathways. TNF-α may also have TNFR-independent effects on cells. Previous in vitro studies suggested that TNF trimers insert into cell membranes and form cation channels (Kagan et al. 1992; Baldwin et al. 1996), resulting in increased Na$^+$ influx, although this phenomenon is currently not thought to play a major role. In addition, indirect actions of cytokines, mediated by other algogenic compounds, are likely in many paradigms. Prostaglandins, bradykinin, and neuropeptides may mediate TNF-α-induced hyperalgesia. TNF-α enhances the sensitivity to capsaicin of rat sensory neurons (Nicol et al. 1997), probably via the neuronal production of prostaglandins.

SUMMARY

Cytokine activation or dysregulation is implied in a variety of painful disease states. Recently, many studies have provided evidence that cytokines are also involved in the induction or facilitation of neuropathic as well as inflammatory pain. Cytokine levels are rapidly and markedly upregulated in peripheral nerves, in dorsal root ganglia, and in the spinal cord after peripheral nerve injuries. Whereas direct application of exogenous proinflammatory cytokines induces pain, blockade of these cytokines or application of anti-inflammatory cytokines reduces pain behavior in most experimental paradigms. Direct receptor-mediated actions of cytokines have been shown, as well as actions involving downstream mediators. Recent studies have also suggested that cytokines may additionally contribute to neuropathic pain by anterograde and/or retrograde signaling. Anticytokine agents currently on the market are effective for the treatment of mostly inflammatory pain conditions, and they are starting to be introduced for neuropathic pain states, but their use is limited by potential life-threatening complications. Agents that specifically target downstream signaling molecules may provide hope for safer and more specific therapies.

REFERENCES

Ali Z, Ringkamp M, Hartke TV, et al. Uninjured C-fiber nociceptors develop spontaneous activity and alpha-adrenergic sensitivity following L6 spinal nerve ligation in monkey. *J Neurophysiol* 1999; 81:455–466.

Ambron RT, Walters ET. Priming events and retrograde injury signals. A new perspective on the cellular and molecular biology of nerve regeneration. *Mol Neurobiol* 1996; 13:61–79.

Apfel SC, Zochodne DW. Thalidomide neuropathy: too much or too long? *Neurology* 2004; 62:2158–2159.

Baldwin RL, Stolowitz ML, Hood L, Wisnieski BJ. Structural changes of tumor necrosis factor alpha associated with membrane insertion and channel formation. *Proc Natl Acad Sci USA* 1996; 93:1021–1026.

Barnes PF, Chatterjee D, Brennan PJ, Rea TH, Modlin RL. Tumor necrosis factor production in patients with leprosy. *Infect Immun* 1992; 60:1441–1446.

Berdan RC, Easaw JC, Wang R. Alterations in membrane potential after axotomy at different distances from the soma of an identified neuron and the effect of depolarization on neurite outgrowth and calcium channel expression. *J Neurophysiol* 1993; 69:151–164.

Cavalli V, Kujala P, Klumperman J, Goldstein LS. Sunday Driver links axonal transport to damage signaling. *J Cell Biol* 2005; 168:775–787.

Copray JC, Mantingh I, Brouwer N, et al. Expression of interleukin-1 beta in rat dorsal root ganglia. *J Neuroimmunol* 2001; 118:203–211.

Cuellar JM, Montesano PX, Carstens E. Role of TNF-alpha in sensitization of nociceptive dorsal horn neurons induced by application of nucleus pulposus to L5 dorsal root ganglion in rats. *Pain* 2004; 110:578–587.

Cui JG, Holmin S, Mathiesen T, Meyerson BA, Linderoth B. Possible role of inflammatory mediators in tactile hypersensitivity in rat models of mononeuropathy. *Pain* 2000; 88:239–248.

Cunha FQ, Poole S, Lorenzetti BB, Ferreira SH. The pivotal role of tumour necrosis factor alpha in the development of inflammatory hyperalgesia. *Br J Pharmacol* 1992; 107:660–664.

Cunha TM, Verri WA Jr, Silva JS, et al. A cascade of cytokines mediates mechanical inflammatory hypernociception in mice. *Proc Natl Acad Sci USA* 2005; 102:1755–1760.

Curtis R, Adryan KM, Zhu Y, et al. Retrograde axonal transport of ciliary neurotrophic factor is increased by peripheral nerve injury. *Nature* 1993; 365:253–255.

Curtis R, Scherer SS, Somogyi R, et al. Retrograde axonal transport of LIF is increased by peripheral nerve injury: correlation with increased LIF expression in distal nerve. *Neuron* 1994; 12:191–204.

Curtis R, Tonra JR, Stark JL, et al. Neuronal injury increases retrograde axonal transport of the neurotrophins to spinal sensory neurons and motor neurons via multiple receptor mechanisms. *Mol Cell Neurosci* 1998; 12:105–118.

De Jongh RF, Vissers KC, Meert TF, et al. The role of interleukin-6 in nociception and pain. *Anesth Analg* 2003; 96:1096–1103.

Delcroix JD, Valletta JS, Wu C, et al. NGF signaling in sensory neurons: evidence that early endosomes carry NGF retrograde signals. *Neuron* 2003; 39:69–84.

DeLeo JA, Rutkowski MD, Stalder AK, Campbell IL. Transgenic expression of TNF by astrocytes increases mechanical allodynia in a mouse neuropathy model. *Neuroreport* 2000; 11:599–602.

Diem R, Meyer R, Weishaupt JH, Bähr M. Reduction of potassium currents and phosphatidylinositol 3-kinase-dependent AKT phosphorylation by tumor necrosis factor-alpha rescues axotomized retinal ganglion cells from retrograde cell death in vivo. *J Neurosci* 2001; 21:2058–2066.

DiStefano PS, Curtis R. Receptor mediated retrograde axonal transport of neurotrophic factors is increased after peripheral nerve injury. *Prog Brain Res* 1994; 103:35–42.

Dubovy P, Jancalek R, Klusakova I, Svizenska I, Pejchalova K. Intra- and extraneuronal changes of immunofluorescence staining for TNF- and TNFR1 in the dorsal root ganglia of rat peripheral neuropathic pain models. *Cell Mol Neurobiol* 2006; 26:1205–1217.

Eastgate JA, Symons JA, Wood NC, et al. Correlation of plasma interleukin 1 levels with disease activity in rheumatoid arthritis. *Lancet* 1988; 2:706–709.

Eder J. Tumour necrosis factor alpha and interleukin 1 signalling: do MAPKK kinases connect it all? *Trends Pharmacol Sci* 1997; 18:319–322.

Flatters SJ, Fox AJ, Dickenson AH. Spinal interleukin-6 (IL-6) inhibits nociceptive transmission following neuropathy. *Brain Res* 2003; 984:54–62.

Fukuoka H, Kawatani M, Hisamitsu T, Takeshige C. Cutaneous hyperalgesia induced by peripheral injection of interleukin-1 beta in the rat. *Brain Res* 1994; 657:133–140.

Fukuoka T, Noguchi K. Contribution of the spared primary afferent neurons to the pathomechanisms of neuropathic pain. *Mol Neurobiol* 2002; 26:57–67.

Furukawa K, Mattson MP. The transcription factor NF-kappaB mediates increases in calcium currents and decreases in NMDA- and AMPA/kainate-induced currents induced by tumor necrosis factor-alpha in hippocampal neurons. *J Neurochem* 1998; 70:1876–1886.

Genevay S, Guerne PA, Gabay C. Efficacy of tumor necrosis factor-alpha blockade for severe sciatica. *Rev Med Suisse Romande* 2004; 124:543–545.

George A, Schmidt C, Weishaupt A, Toyka KV, Sommer C. Serial determination of tumor necrosis factor-alpha content in rat sciatic nerve after chronic constriction injury. *Exp Neurol* 1999; 160:124–132.

George A, Marziniak M, Schäfers M, Toyka KV, Sommer C. Thalidomide treatment in chronic constrictive neuropathy decreases endoneurial tumor necrosis factor-alpha, increases interleukin-10 and has long-term effects on spinal cord dorsal horn met-enkephalin. *Pain* 2000; 88:267–275.

George A, Buehl A, Sommer C. Wallerian degeneration after crush injury of rat sciatic nerve increases endo- and epineurial tumor necrosis factor-alpha protein. *Neurosci Lett* 2004; 372:215–219.

George A, Buehl A, Sommer C. Tumor necrosis factor receptor 1 and 2 proteins are differentially regulated during Wallerian degeneration of mouse sciatic nerve. *Exp Neurol* 2005; 192:163–166.

Han HC, Lee DH, Chung JM. Characteristics of ectopic discharges in a rat neuropathic pain model. *Pain* 2000; 84:253–261.

Hanz S, Fainzilber M. Retrograde signaling in injured nerve—the axon reaction revisited. *J Neurochem* 2006;

Hanz S, Perlson E, Willis D, et al. Axoplasmic importins enable retrograde injury signaling in lesioned nerve. *Neuron* 2003; 40:1095–1104.

Homma Y, Brull SJ, Zhang JM. A comparison of chronic pain behavior following local application of tumor necrosis factor alpha to the normal and mechanically compressed lumbar ganglia in the rat. *Pain* 2002; 95:239–246.

Honore P, Wade CL, Zhong C, et al. Interleukin-1alphabeta gene-deficient mice show reduced nociceptive sensitivity in models of inflammatory and neuropathic pain but not post-operative pain. *Behav Brain Res* 2006; 167:355–364.

Hudson LJ, Bevan S, Wotherspoon G, et al. VR1 protein expression increases in undamaged DRG neurons after partial nerve injury. *Eur J Neurosci* 2001; 13:2105–2114.

Inoue A, Ikoma K, Morioka N, et al. Interleukin-1beta induces substance P release from primary afferent neurons through the cyclooxygenase-2 system. *J Neurochem* 1999; 73:2206–2213.

Jin X, Gereau RWT. Acute p38-mediated modulation of tetrodotoxin-resistant sodium channels in mouse sensory neurons by tumor necrosis factor-alpha. *J Neurosci* 2006; 26:246–255.

Junger H, Sorkin LS. Nociceptive and inflammatory effects of subcutaneous TNFalpha. *Pain* 2000; 85:145–151.

Kagan BL, Baldwin RL, Munoz D, Wisnieski BJ. Formation of ion-permeable channels by tumor necrosis factor-alpha. *Science* 1992; 255:1427–1430.

Kleinschnitz C, Brinkhoff J, Zelenka M, Sommer C, Stoll G. The extent of cytokine induction in peripheral nerve lesions depends on the mode of injury and NMDA receptor signaling. *J Neuroimmunol* 2004; 149:77–83.

Kurek JB, Austin L, Cheema SS, Bartlett PF, Murphy M. Up-regulation of leukaemia inhibitory factor and interleukin-6 in transected sciatic nerve and muscle following denervation. *Neuromuscul Disord* 1996; 6:105–114.

Lee N, Neitzel KL, Devlin BK, MacLennan AJ. STAT3 phosphorylation in injured axons before sensory and motor neuron nuclei: potential role for STAT3 as a retrograde signaling transcription factor. *J Comp Neurol* 2004; 474:535–545.

Leitner ML, Molliver DC, Osborne PA, et al. Analysis of the retrograde transport of glial cell line-derived neurotrophic factor (GDNF), neurturin, and persephin suggests that in vivo signaling for the GDNF family is GFRalpha coreceptor-specific. *J Neurosci* 1999; 19:9322–9331.

Li Y, Dorsi MJ, Meyer RA, Belzberg AJ. Mechanical hyperalgesia after an L5 spinal nerve lesion in the rat is not dependent on input from injured nerve fibers. *Pain* 2000; 85:493–502.

Liefner M, Siebert H, Sachse T, et al. The role of TNF-alpha during Wallerian degeneration. *J Neuroimmunol* 2000; 108:147–152.

Lindenlaub T, Sommer C. Cytokines in sural nerve biopsies from inflammatory and non-inflammatory neuropathies. *Acta Neuropathol (Berl)* 2003; 105:593–602.

Lindholm D, Heumann R, Meyer M, Thoenen H. Interleukin-1 regulates synthesis of nerve growth factor in non-neuronal cells of rat sciatic nerve. *Nature* 1987; 330:658–659.

Lindwall C, Kanje M. Retrograde axonal transport of JNK signaling molecules influence injury induced nuclear changes in p-c-Jun and ATF3 in adult rat sensory neurons. *Mol Cell Neurosci* 2005; 29:269–282.

Liu B, Li H, Brull SJ, Zhang JM. Increased sensitivity of sensory neurons to tumor necrosis factor alpha in rats with chronic compression of the lumbar ganglia. *J Neurophysiol* 2002; 88:1393–1399.

Liu X, Chung K, Chung JM. Ectopic discharges and adrenergic sensitivity of sensory neurons after spinal nerve injury. *Brain Res* 1999; 849:244–247.

Ma W, Bisby MA. Increase of calcitonin gene-related peptide immunoreactivity in the axonal fibers of the gracile nuclei of adult and aged rats after complete and partial sciatic nerve injuries. *Exp Neurol* 1998; 152:137–149.

Ma W, Quirion R. Increased calcitonin gene-related peptide in neuroma and invading macrophages is involved in the up-regulation of interleukin-6 and thermal hyperalgesia in a rat model of mononeuropathy. *J Neurochem* 2006; 98:180–192.

Mandolesi G, Madeddu F, Bozzi Y, Maffei L, Ratto GM. Acute physiological response of mammalian central neurons to axotomy: ionic regulation and electrical activity. *FASEB J* 2004; 18:1934–1936.

Michael GJ, Averill S, Shortland PJ, Yan Q, Priestley JV. Axotomy results in major changes in BDNF expression by dorsal root ganglion cells: BDNF expression in large trkB and trkC cells, in pericellular baskets, and in projections to deep dorsal horn and dorsal column nuclei. *Eur J Neurosci* 1999; 11:3539–3551.

Mufson EJ, Kroin JS, Sendera TJ, Sobreviela T. Distribution and retrograde transport of trophic factors in the central nervous system: functional implications for the treatment of neurodegenerative diseases. *Prog Neurobiol* 1999; 57:451–484.

Murata Y, Onda A, Rydevik B, et al. Changes in pain behavior and histologic changes caused by application of tumor necrosis factor-alpha to the dorsal root ganglion in rats. *Spine* 2006; 31:530–535.

Murphy PG, Grondin J, Altares M, Richardson PM. Induction of interleukin-6 in axotomized sensory neurons. *J Neurosci* 1995; 15:5130–5138.

Murphy PG, Ramer MS, Borthwick L, et al. Endogenous interleukin-6 contributes to hypersensitivity to cutaneous stimuli and changes in neuropeptides associated with chronic nerve constriction in mice. *Eur J Neurosci* 1999; 11:2243–2253.

Myers RR, Heckman HM, Rodriguez M. Reduced hyperalgesia in nerve-injured WLD mice: relationship to nerve fiber phagocytosis, axonal degeneration, and regeneration in normal mice. *Exp Neurol* 1996; 141:94–101.

Myers RR, Campana WM, Shubayev VI. The role of neuroinflammation in neuropathic pain: mechanisms and therapeutic targets. *Drug Discov Today* 2006; 11:8–20.

Nicol GD, Lopshire JC, Pafford CM. Tumor necrosis factor enhances the capsaicin sensitivity of rat sensory neurons. *J Neurosci* 1997; 17:975–982.

Noguchi K, Dubner R, De Leon M, Senba E, Ruda MA. Axotomy induces preprotachykinin gene expression in a subpopulation of dorsal root ganglion neurons. *J Neurosci Res* 1994; 37:596–603.

Obata K, Yamanaka H, Dai Y, et al. Differential activation of MAPK in injured and uninjured DRG neurons following chronic constriction injury of the sciatic nerve in rats. *Eur J Neurosci* 2004; 20:2881–2895.

Obreja O, Rathee PK, Lips KS, Distler C, Kress M. IL-1 beta potentiates heat-activated currents in rat sensory neurons: involvement of IL-1RI, tyrosine kinase, and protein kinase C. *Faseb J* 2002; 16:1497–1503.

Obreja O, Biasio W, Andratsch M, et al. Fast modulation of heat-activated ionic current by proinflammatory interleukin 6 in rat sensory neurons. *Brain* 2005; 128:1634–1641.

Ohtori S, Takahashi K, Moriya H, Myers RR. TNF-alpha and TNF-alpha receptor type 1 upregulation in glia and neurons after peripheral nerve injury: studies in murine DRG and spinal cord. *Spine* 2004; 29:1082–1088.

Okamoto K, Martin DP, Schmelzer JD, Mitsui Y, Low PA. Pro- and anti-inflammatory cytokine gene expression in rat sciatic nerve chronic constriction injury model of neuropathic pain. *Exp Neurol* 2001; 169:386–391.

Olmarker K, Nutu M, Storkson R. Changes in spontaneous behavior in rats exposed to experimental disc herniation are blocked by selective TNF-alpha inhibition. *Spine* 2003; 28:1635–1641.

Onda A, Hamba M, Yabuki S, Kikuchi S. Exogenous tumor necrosis factor-alpha induces abnormal discharges in rat dorsal horn neurons. *Spine* 2002; 27:1618–1624.

Onda A, Yabuki S, Kikuchi S. Effects of neutralizing antibodies to tumor necrosis factor-alpha on nucleus pulposus-induced abnormal nociresponses in rat dorsal horn neurons. *Spine* 2003; 28:967–972.

Opree A, Kress M. Involvement of the proinflammatory cytokines tumor necrosis factor-alpha, IL-1 beta, and IL-6 but not IL-8 in the development of heat hyperalgesia: effects on heat-evoked calcitonin gene-related peptide release from rat skin. *J Neurosci* 2000; 20:6289–6293.

Ozaktay AC, Kallakuri S, Takebayashi T, et al. Effects of interleukin-1 beta, interleukin-6, and tumor necrosis factor on sensitivity of dorsal root ganglion and peripheral receptive fields in rats. *Eur Spine J* 2006; 15:1529–1537

Parada CA, Yeh JJ, Joseph EK, Levine JD. Tumor necrosis factor receptor type-1 in sensory neurons contributes to induction of chronic enhancement of inflammatory hyperalgesia in rat. *Eur J Neurosci* 2003; 17:1847–1852.

Perkins MN, Kelly D, Davis AJ. Bradykinin B1 and B2 receptor mechanisms and cytokine-induced hyperalgesia in the rat. *Can J Physiol Pharmacol* 1995; 73:832–836.

Perlson E, Hanz S, Ben-Yaakov K, et al. Vimentin-dependent spatial translocation of an activated MAP kinase in injured nerve. *Neuron* 2005; 45:715–726.

Pollock J, McFarlane SM, Connell MC, et al. TNF-alpha receptors simultaneously activate Ca^{2+} mobilisation and stress kinases in cultured sensory neurones. *Neuropharmacology* 2002; 42:93–106.

Poole S, Cunha FQ, Selkirk S, Lorenzetti BB, Ferreira SH. Cytokine-mediated inflammatory hyperalgesia limited by interleukin-10. *Br J Pharmacol* 1995; 115:684–688.

Qiu J, Cafferty WB, McMahon SB, Thompson SW. Conditioning injury-induced spinal axon regeneration requires signal transducer and activator of transcription 3 activation. *J Neurosci* 2005; 25:1645–1653.

Ramer MS, Murphy PG, Richardson PM, Bisby MA. Spinal nerve lesion-induced mechanoallodynia and adrenergic sprouting in sensory ganglia are attenuated in interleukin-6 knockout mice. *Pain* 1998; 78:115–121.

Ramer MS, Thompson SW, McMahon SB. Causes and consequences of sympathetic basket formation in dorsal root ganglia. *Pain* 1999; Suppl 6:S111–120.

Redshaw JD, Bisby MA. Fast axonal transport in central nervous system and peripheral nervous system axons following axotomy. *J Neurobiol* 1984; 15:109–117.

Redshaw JD, Bisby MA. Proteins of fast axonal transport in regenerating rat sciatic sensory axons: a conditioning lesion does not amplify the characteristic response to axotomy. *Exp Neurol* 1987; 98:212–221.

Reynolds AJ, Hendry IA, Bartlett SE. Anterograde and retrograde transport of active extracellular signal-related kinase 1 (ERK1) in the ligated rat sciatic nerve. *Neuroscience* 2001; 105:761–771.

Ribeiro RA, Vale ML, Ferreira SH, Cunha FQ. Analgesic effect of thalidomide on inflammatory pain. *Eur J Pharmacol* 2000; 391:97–103.

Safieh-Garabedian B, Poole S, Allchorne A, Winter J, Woolf CJ. Contribution of interleukin-1 beta to the inflammation-induced increase in nerve growth factor levels and inflammatory hyperalgesia. *Br J Pharmacol* 1995; 115:1265–1275.

Schäfers M, Brinkhoff J, Neukirchen S, Marziniak M, Sommer C. Combined epineurial therapy with neutralizing antibodies to tumor necrosis factor-alpha and interleukin-1 receptor has an additive effect in reducing neuropathic pain in mice. *Neurosci Lett* 2001; 310:113–116.

Schäfers M, Geis C, Brors D, Yaksh TL, Sommer C. Anterograde transport of tumor necrosis factor-alpha in the intact and injured rat sciatic nerve. *J Neurosci* 2002; 22:536–545.

Schäfers M, Svensson CI, Sommer C, Sorkin LS. Tumor necrosis factor-alpha induces mechanical allodynia after spinal nerve ligation by activation of p38 MAPK in primary sensory neurons. *J Neurosci* 2003a; 23:2517–2521.

Schäfers M, Sorkin LS, Geis C, Shubayev VI. Spinal nerve ligation induces transient upregulation of tumor necrosis factor receptors 1 and 2 in injured and adjacent uninjured dorsal root ganglia in the rat. *Neurosci Lett* 2003b; 347:179–182.

Schäfers M, Geis C, Svensson CI, Luo ZD, Sommer C. Selective increase of tumour necrosis factor-alpha in injured and spared myelinated primary afferents after chronic constrictive injury of rat sciatic nerve. *Eur J Neurosci* 2003c; 17:791–804.

Schäfers M, Lee DH, Brors D, Yaksh TL, Sorkin LS. Increased sensitivity of injured and adjacent uninjured rat primary sensory neurons to exogenous tumor necrosis factor-alpha after spinal nerve ligation. *J Neurosci* 2003d; 23:3028–3038.

Shafer DM, Assael L, White LB, Rossomando EF. Tumor necrosis factor-alpha as a biochemical marker of pain and outcome in temporomandibular joints with internal derangements. *J Oral Maxillofac Surg* 1994; 52:786-791; discussion 791–782.

Shamash S, Reichert F, Rotshenker S. The cytokine network of Wallerian degeneration: tumor necrosis factor-alpha, interleukin-1alpha, and interleukin-1beta. *J Neurosci* 2002; 22:3052–3060.

Sheen K, Chung JM. Signs of neuropathic pain depend on signals from injured nerve fibers in a rat model. *Brain Res* 1993; 610:62–68.

Shubayev VI, Myers RR. Axonal transport of TNF-alpha in painful neuropathy: distribution of ligand tracer and TNF receptors. *J Neuroimmunol* 2001; 114:48–56.

Shubayev VI, Myers RR. Anterograde TNF alpha transport from rat dorsal root ganglion to spinal cord and injured sciatic nerve. *Neurosci Lett* 2002; 320:99–101.

Soliven B, Albert J. Tumor necrosis factor modulates Ca2+ currents in cultured sympathetic neurons. *J Neurosci* 1992; 12:2665–2671.

Sommer C, Myers RR. Thalidomide inhibition of TNF reduces hyperalgesia in neuropathic rats. *Reg Anesth* 1994; 19:1.

Sommer C, Schäfers M. Painful mononeuropathy in C57BL/Wld mice with delayed wallerian degeneration: differential effects of cytokine production and nerve regeneration on thermal and mechanical hypersensitivity. *Brain Res* 1998; 784:154–162.

Sommer C, Schmidt C, George A. Hyperalgesia in experimental neuropathy is dependent on the TNF receptor 1. *Exp Neurol* 1998; 151:138–142.

Sommer C, Petrausch S, Lindenlaub T, Toyka KV. Neutralizing antibodies to interleukin 1-receptor reduce pain associated behavior in mice with experimental neuropathy. *Neurosci Lett* 1999; 270:25–28.

Sommer C, Schäfers M, Marziniak M, Toyka KV. Etanercept reduces hyperalgesia in experimental painful neuropathy. *J Peripher Nerv Syst* 2001; 6:67–72.

Sorkin LS, Xiao WH, Wagner R, Myers RR. Tumour necrosis factor-alpha induces ectopic activity in nociceptive primary afferent fibres. *Neuroscience* 1997; 81:255–262.

Sweitzer S, Martin D, DeLeo JA. Intrathecal interleukin-1 receptor antagonist in combination with soluble tumor necrosis factor receptor exhibits an anti-allodynic action in a rat model of neuropathic pain. *Neuroscience* 2001; 103:529–539.

Tak PP, Smeets TJ, Daha MR, et al. Analysis of the synovial cell infiltrate in early rheumatoid synovial tissue in relation to local disease activity. *Arthritis Rheum* 1997; 40:217–225.

Takahashi N, Kikuchi S, Shubayev VI, Campana WM, Myers RR. TNF-alpha and phosphorylation of ERK in DRG and spinal cord: insights into mechanisms of sciatica. *Spine* 2006; 31:523–529.

Thompson SW, Priestley JV, Southall A. gp130 cytokines, leukemia inhibitory factor and interleukin-6, induce neuropeptide expression in intact adult rat sensory neurons in vivo: time-course, specificity and comparison with sciatic nerve axotomy. *Neuroscience* 1998; 84:1247–1255.

Tobinick EL, Britschgi-Davoodifar S. Perispinal TNF-alpha inhibition for discogenic pain. *Swiss Med Wkly* 2003; 133:170–177.

Tonra JR, Curtis R, Wong V, et al. Axotomy upregulates the anterograde transport and expression of brain-derived neurotrophic factor by sensory neurons. *J Neurosci* 1998; 18:4374–4383.

Vale ML, Benevides VM, Sachs D, et al. Antihyperalgesic effect of pentoxifylline on experimental inflammatory pain. *Br J Pharmacol* 2004; 143:833–844.

Vissers KC, De Jongh RF, Hoffmann VL, Meert TF. Exogenous interleukin-6 increases cold allodynia in rats with a mononeuropathy. *Cytokine* 2005; 30:154–159.

Vogel C, Stallforth S, Sommer C. Altered pain behavior and regeneration after nerve injury in TNF receptor deficient mice. *J Periph Nerv Syst* 2006; 11:294–303.

von Banchet GS, Kiehl M, Schaible HG. Acute and long-term effects of IL-6 on cultured dorsal root ganglion neurones from adult rat. *J Neurochem* 2005; 94:238–248.

von Bartheld CS. Axonal transport and neuronal transcytosis of trophic factors, tracers and pathogens. *J Neurobiol* 2003; 58:295–314.

Wagner R, Myers RR. Schwann cells produce tumor necrosis factor alpha: expression in injured and non-injured nerves. *Neuroscience* 1996a; 73:625–629.

Wagner R, Myers RR. Endoneurial injection of TNF-alpha produces neuropathic pain behaviors. *Neuroreport* 1996b; 7:2897–2901.

Wagner R, Janjigian M, Myers RR. Anti-inflammatory interleukin-10 therapy in CCI neuropathy decreases thermal hyperalgesia, macrophage recruitment, and endoneurial TNF-alpha expression. *Pain* 1998; 74:35–42.

Watkins LR, Hansen MK, Nguyen KT, Lee JE, Maier SF. Dynamic regulation of the proinflammatory cytokine, interleukin-1beta: molecular biology for non-molecular biologists. *Life Sci* 1999; 65:449–481.

Wolf G, Gabay E, Tal M, Yirmiya R, Shavit Y. Genetic impairment of interleukin-1 signaling attenuates neuropathic pain, autotomy, and spontaneous ectopic neuronal activity, following nerve injury in mice. *Pain* 2006; 120:315–324.

Woolf CJ, Allchorne A, Safieh-Garabedian B, Poole S. Cytokines, nerve growth factor and inflammatory hyperalgesia: the contribution of tumour necrosis factor alpha. *Br J Pharmacol* 1997; 121:417–424.

Xu JT, Xin WJ, Zang Y, Wu CY, Liu XG. The role of tumor necrosis factor-alpha in the neuropathic pain induced by Lumbar 5 ventral root transection in rat. *Pain* 2006; 123:306–321.

Yano H, Chao MV. Mechanisms of neurotrophin receptor vesicular transport. *J Neurobiol* 2004; 58:244–257.

Yao MZ, Gu JF, Wang JH, et al. Interleukin-2 gene therapy of chronic neuropathic pain. *Neuroscience* 2002; 112:409–416.

Yoon YW, Na HS, Chung JM. Contributions of injured and intact afferents to neuropathic pain in an experimental rat model. *Pain* 1996; 64:27–36.

Zelenka M, Schäfers M, Sommer C. Intraneural injection of interleukin-1beta and tumor necrosis factor-alpha into rat sciatic nerve at physiological doses induces signs of neuropathic pain. *Pain* 2005; 116:257–263.

Zhang JM, Li H, Liu B, Brull SJ. Acute topical application of tumor necrosis factor alpha evokes protein kinase A-dependent responses in rat sensory neurons. *J Neurophysiol* 2002; 88:1387–1392.

Zhang XP, Ambron RT. Positive injury signals induce growth and prolong survival in *Aplysia* neurons. *J Neurobiol* 2000; 45:84–94.

Ziv NE, Spira ME. Spatiotemporal distribution of Ca2+ following axotomy and throughout the recovery process of cultured *Aplysia* neurons. *Eur J Neurosci* 1993; 5:657–668.

Correspondence to: Maria Schäfers, MD, Department of Neurology, University of Duisburg-Essen, Hufelandstr. 55, 45147 Essen, Germany. Tel: 49-201-7232588; fax: 49-201-7235953; email: maria.schaefers@uni-due.de.

Immune and Glial Regulation of Pain, edited by Joyce
A. DeLeo, Linda S. Sorkin, and Linda R. Watkins,
IASP Press, Seattle, © 2007.

6

Analgesic Effects of Immune-Cell-Derived Opioids

Halina Machelska and Christoph Stein

*Department of Anesthesiology and Intensive Care Medicine,
Charité University Hospital, Campus Benjamin Franklin, Berlin, Germany*

Acute and chronic pain is frequently associated with inflammation resulting from tissue destruction, abnormal immune reactivity, or nerve injury. For many years research attention focused on proalgesic molecules such as protons, bradykinin, prostaglandins, excitatory amino acids, neuropeptides (e.g., calcitonin gene-related peptide and substance P), and proinflammatory cytokines (Woolf and Salter 2000; Watkins and Maier 2002; Cunha and Ferreira 2003; Marchand et al. 2005; Rittner et al. 2005). However, concurrently with pain generation, endogenous mechanisms develop to counteract pain. In the brain and spinal cord these mechanisms rely on descending pathways that use opioid peptides, norepinephrine, or serotonin and their receptors (Terman et al. 1984; Millan 2002; Fields 2004). Similar counterregulatory processes occur within peripheral inflamed tissue. Such effects can be brought about by anti-inflammatory cytokines (Cunha and Ferreira 2003) and by interactions between leukocyte-derived opioid peptides and peripheral sensory neurons carrying opioid receptors (Stein et al. 2003; Machelska and Stein 2006). In this chapter, we present an overview of current information on the anatomy and function of peripheral opioid receptors, on mechanisms of opioid-containing leukocyte migration to inflamed tissue, on the production and release of opioid peptides from immune cells, and on analgesia resulting from interactions between peripheral opioid peptides and their receptors.

PERIPHERAL OPIOID RECEPTORS

Three genes have been identified encoding the μ-, δ-, and κ-opioid receptors, respectively (Kieffer and Gaveriaux-Ruff 2002). All three receptors can

mediate pain inhibition, and they are all found throughout the central and peripheral nervous system. Recent interest has focused on the characterization of
opioid receptors on nociceptors because their activation can inhibit pain directly
at its origin without unwanted central side effects. Peripheral opioid receptors
are synthesized in dorsal root ganglia (DRG) and are intra-axonally transported
to the peripheral (and central) sensory nerve endings. Opioid receptors belong
to the family of seven transmembrane domain G-protein-coupled receptors.
Upon activation by opioid ligands they couple to inhibitory G proteins ($G_{i/o}$),
which leads to inhibition of calcium and/or sodium channels and to decreased
levels of cyclic adenosine monophosphate. As a result, opioids attenuate neuronal excitability and inhibit the propagation of action potentials and the release
of proinflammatory neuropeptides (e.g., substance P, calcitonin gene-related
peptide) from peripheral sensory nerve endings (references in Stein et al. 2003;
Wenk et al. 2006).

Tissue inflammation leads to increased synthesis, G-protein-coupling,
enhanced axonal transport, and inhibitory activity of peripheral opioid receptors (Jeanjean et al. 1995; Ji et al. 1995; Mousa et al. 2001; Zöllner et al. 2003;
Pühler et al. 2004, 2006; Wenk et al. 2006). Also, the number of nociceptors
increases and the perineural barrier is disrupted, which facilitates the access
of opioid agonists to their receptors (Antonijevic et al. 1995). All these effects
enhance the analgesic efficacy of opioids at their peripheral receptors in inflammation (Stein et al. 2003).

Opioid receptors have also been demonstrated in immune cells in studies
that reported opioid-mediated modulation of the proliferation of these cells and
of their functions (e.g., chemotaxis, superoxide and cytokine production, and
mast cell degranulation). These immunomodulatory actions can be stimulatory as well as inhibitory (Sacerdote et al. 2003; Sharp 2003). However, the
significance of such effects with regard to pain modulation has not yet been
investigated.

PRODUCTION OF OPIOID PEPTIDES IN IMMUNE CELLS

Three families of opioid peptides are well characterized in the nervous
and neuroendocrine systems (Akil et al. 1998). Each family derives from a
distinct gene and from one of the three precursor proteins: proopiomelanocortin
(POMC), proenkephalin, and prodynorphin. Appropriate processing yields their
representative opioid peptides, the endorphins, enkephalins, and dynorphins, respectively. These peptides exhibit different affinity and selectivity for the three
opioid receptors: μ (endorphins, enkephalins), δ (enkephalins, endorphins), and
κ (dynorphin). Two additional endogenous opioid peptides have been isolated

from bovine brain: endomorphin-1 and endomorphin-2. Both peptides are considered highly selective μ-receptor ligands, but their precursors are not yet known (Zadina et al. 1997; Akil et al. 1998).

POMC-related opioid peptides have been found in mononuclear and poly-morphonuclear leukocytes of many vertebrates and invertebrates (Przewlocki et al. 1992; Cabot et al. 1997; Machelska et al. 2003; Smith 2003). Although earlier studies described truncated POMC transcripts, a full-length transcript encoding all three POMC exons was shown in rat mononuclear leukocytes (Lyons and Blalock 1997). This POMC transcript contains the sequence for the signal peptide that is necessary for correct routing into the regulated secretory pathway. The POMC protein is then proteolytically processed in the endo-plasmic reticulum and the Golgi network. The enzymatic machinery includes carboxypeptidase E, the prohormone convertases PC1 and PC2, and the binding protein 7B2, and is expressed in leukocytes in the blood and within inflamed tissue in rats (Mousa et al. 2004).

Proenkephalin mRNA and enkephalins have been detected in lymphocytes, macrophages, and mast cells (Przewlocki et al. 1992; Cabot et al. 2001; Machelska et al. 2003). Deletion of the gene coding for proenkephalin resulted in the complete absence of Met-enkephalin both in the brain and in T-lympho-cytes, strongly indicating that this peptide derives from the same precursor in the nervous and immune systems (Hook et al. 1999). The enzymes necessary for posttranslational processing of proenkephalin have also been identified in immune cells (Vindrola et al. 1994; LaMendola et al. 1997). Dynorphin and endomorphins are also detectable in mononuclear and polymorphonuclear leukocytes (Cabot et al. 2001; Machelska et al. 2003; Chadzinska et al. 2005; Labuz et al. 2006).

MIGRATION OF OPIOID-PEPTIDE-CONTAINING IMMUNE CELLS TO INFLAMED TISSUE

The recruitment of leukocytes from the circulation into inflammatory sites involves a well-orchestrated sequence of events. This process begins with the rolling of leukocytes along the endothelial cell wall, an event that is mediated predominantly by L-, P-, and E-selectins. Leukocytes are then activated by chemokines, leading to the upregulation and increased avidity of integrins. Integrins mediate the firm adhesion of leukocytes to endothelia via molecules such as intercellular adhesion molecule-1 (ICAM-1). Finally, the transmigra-tion of leukocytes through the endothelium is mediated by molecules such as platelet-endothelial cell adhesion molecule-1 (PECAM-1) (von Andrian and Mackay 2000).

These events also regulate the migration of opioid-producing leukocytes. In inflamed rat paw tissue, L-selectin, integrins α_4 and β_2, and the chemokines CXCL1 (keratinocyte-derived chemokine) and CXCL2/3 (macrophage inflammatory protein-2) are expressed by leukocytes, while P- and E-selectins, ICAM-1, and PECAM-1 are upregulated on the endothelium (Mousa et al. 2000; Machelska et al. 2002, 2004; Brack et al. 2004c) (Fig. 1). Expression of CXCL1 and CXCL2/3 mRNA and protein significantly increases during the course of inflammation (Brack et al. 2004b,c), and L-selectin, integrin β_2, and the

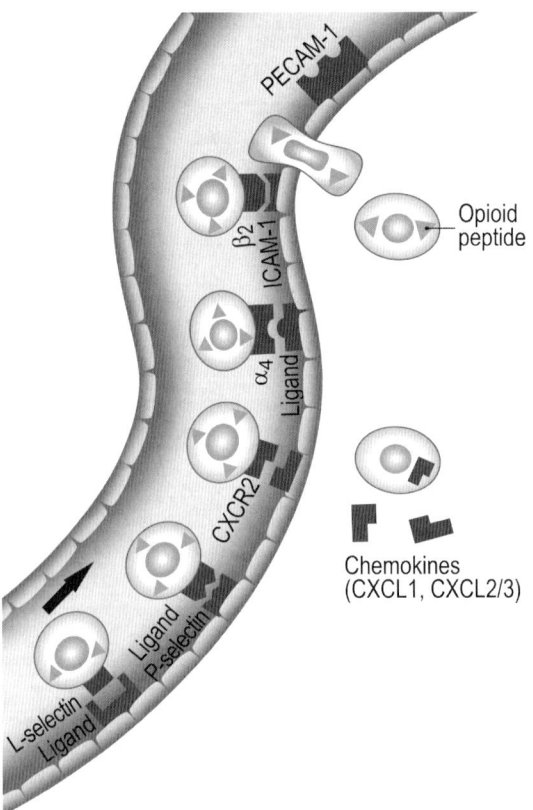

Fig. 1. Migration of opioid peptide-containing immune cells to inflamed tissue. P-selectin, intercellular adhesion molecule-1 (ICAM-1), and platelet-endothelial cell adhesion molecule-1 (PECAM-1) are upregulated on the vascular endothelium of blood vessels. L-selectin and integrins α_4 and β_2 are coexpressed by opioid peptide-containing circulating leukocytes. These cells also coexpress chemokine receptors (CXCR2). Chemokines (CXCL1 and CXCL2/3) are released from immune and endothelial cells. L- and P-selectin mediate rolling of opioid-containing cells along the vascular endothelium. These cells can then be activated by chemokines, which upregulate adhesion molecules. Alpha-4 and β_2 integrins and ICAM-1 mediate opioid-containing leukocyte adhesion to and migration through the endothelium. Adhesion molecules interact with their respective ligands expressed on leukocytes and on the endothelium. Arrow in the blood vessel indicates the direction of the events.

chemokine receptor CXCR2 are coexpressed by opioid-containing leukocytes (Mousa et al. 2000; Brack et al. 2004c; Machelska et al. 2004). Furthermore, pretreatment of rats with a selectin blocker (fucoidin), with selective antibodies against either ICAM-1, integrins α_4 and β_2, or CXCL1 and CXCL2/3 substantially decreases the number of opioid-containing immune cells accumulating in inflamed tissue (Machelska et al. 1998, 2002, 2004; Brack et al. 2004c). These findings suggest that circulating opioid-producing immune cells are directed to inflamed tissue by specific chemotactic and adhesive mechanisms.

SECRETION OF OPIOID PEPTIDES FROM IMMUNE CELLS

The regulated release of peptides requires secretory granules deriving from the Golgi network for transport to the cell membrane. As discussed above, immune cells in the blood and in inflamed tissue express the entire machinery required for POMC processing into functionally active β-endorphin (Mousa et al. 2004). Furthermore, in macrophages, monocytes, granulocytes, and lymphocytes, β-endorphin is present in secretory granules that are arranged at the cell periphery, ready for exocytosis (Mousa et al. 2004). Opioid-containing inflammatory cells carry receptors for several secretory agents such as corticotropin-releasing factor (CRF), interleukin (IL)-1β, and norepinephrine (Mousa et al. 1996, 2003; Binder et al. 2004). CRF is present in immune cells, fibroblasts, and the vascular endothelium, and its expression is enhanced in inflamed tissues of animals and humans (Schäfer 2003). CRF, IL-1β, and norepinephrine can stimulate the release of opioid peptides from leukocytes (Fig. 2) in a receptor-selective and calcium-dependent manner (Kavelaars et al. 1990; Schäfer et al. 1994; Cabot et al. 1997, 2001; Binder et al. 2004; Rittner et al. 2006b). In summary, consistent with the hitherto identified components of opioid peptide processing in immune cells, several agents (CRF, IL-1β, and norepinephrine) can release opioid peptides in a receptor-specific manner.

ANALGESIA PRODUCED BY IMMUNE-CELL-DERIVED OPIOID PEPTIDES

EFFECTS OF CORTICOTROPIN-RELEASING FACTOR, CYTOKINES, AND NOREPINEPHRINE

CRF-, IL-1β-, and norepinephrine-induced release of opioids from immune cells also occurs in vivo (Fig. 2). When injected into inflamed paws, these agents produce CRF-, IL-1β-, adrenergic-, and opioid-receptor-specific analgesia. Beta-endorphin plays a major role, but Met-enkephalin, dynorphin

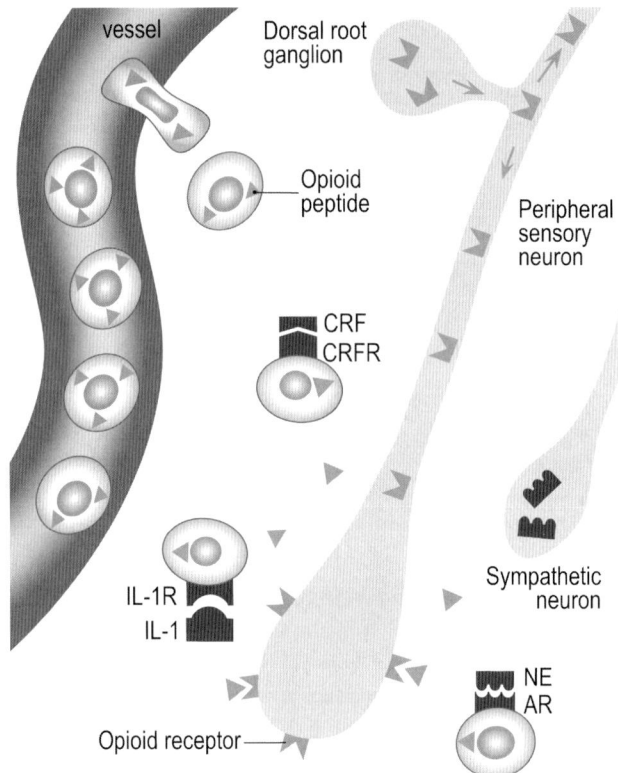

Fig. 2. Secretion of opioid peptides from immune cells in inflamed tissue. Extravasated leukocytes can be stimulated by releasing agents such as corticotropin-releasing factor (CRF), interleukin-1β (IL-1), and norepinephrine (NE). CRF, IL-1, and sympathetic neuron-derived NE elicit opioid peptide release by activating CRF receptors (CRFR), IL-1 receptors (IL-1R), and adrenergic receptors (AR) on leukocytes, respectively. Opioids bind to peripheral opioid receptors (which are produced in dorsal root ganglia and transported to peripheral endings of sensory neurons) and produce analgesia by inhibiting the excitability of these neurons.

and endomorphins can also be involved (Schäfer et al. 1994; Machelska et al. 2003; Mousa et al. 2003; Labuz et al. 2006). Under these conditions leukocytes are indeed the target for CRF and IL-1β because immunosuppression with cyclosporine A, depletion of granulocytes, blockade of chemokines (CXCL1 and CXCL2/3), or pretreatment with anti-selectin and anti-ICAM-1 result in a significant reduction of opioid-containing cells and of CRF- or IL-1β-induced analgesia (Schäfer et al. 1994; Machelska et al. 1998, 2002; Brack et al. 2004c; Labuz et al. 2006). Moreover, cyclosporine-A-induced attenuation of CRF-mediated analgesia can be restored by transfer of activated lymphocytes (Hermanussen et al. 2004), and the selective chemotaxis of activated granulocytes by CXCL1 and CXCL2/3 does not produce hyperalgesia (Rittner et al. 2006a).

These findings are in line with other studies on local analgesic effects of CRF (Hargreaves et al. 1989; McLoon et al. 2002), IL-6, and tumor necrosis factor-α (Czlonkowski et al. 1993), and with the contribution of endogenous CRF and IL-1β to electroacupuncture-induced analgesia in inflammation (Sekido et al. 2004). However, the findings are in contrast to reports showing pronociceptive effects of cytokines (Cunha and Ferreira 2003) or chemokines (Oh et al. 2001; Szabo et al. 2002). Importantly, however, most of these studies were performed in the absence of fully developed inflammation or employed significant painful stimuli rather than detection thresholds in behavioral testing (discussed in Rittner et al. 2005).

Norepinephrine administered into inflamed tissue produces analgesia that is reversible by α_1-, α_2-, and β_2-adrenergic receptor antagonists, by μ- and δ-opioid receptor antagonists, and by an antibody against β-endorphin (Binder et al. 2004). These data suggest that this catecholamine produces analgesia via release of opioid peptides that activate peripheral opioid receptors. In a study comparing inflamed with noninflamed tissue, norepinephrine did not influence pain behavior without inflammation, which is consistent with the lack of opioid-containing immune cells and with the scarcity of adrenergic receptors (Binder et al. 2004). Again, the role of peripheral adrenergic receptors in pain modulation appears controversial. In other studies examining noninflamed tissue, norepinephrine has been shown to produce pain, and it has been postulated that pain is mediated via α_{2B} receptors while analgesia is mediated via α_{2C} receptors (references in Binder et al. 2004). Thus, different receptor subtypes, receptor localization, microenvironment, the presence or absence of inflammation, the presence of opioid peptide-containing inflammatory cells, and the coexpression of the respective stimulatory receptors are important parameters to be considered.

ENDOGENOUS OPIOID ANALGESIA

Stress is a natural stimulus triggering inhibition of pain (Terman et al. 1984; Fields 2004). In rats with paw inflammation, stress induced by cold water (4°C) swim (for 1 minute) elicits potent analgesia in inflamed paws but not in contralateral noninflamed paws (Stein et al. 1990a; Machelska et al. 2003). Whereas at early stages of the inflammatory reaction (6 hours), both peripheral and central opioid receptors contribute, at later stages (4–6 days) endogenous analgesia is mediated exclusively by peripheral opioid receptors (Stein et al. 1990a,b; Machelska et al. 2003). Thus, peripheral opioid mechanisms of pain control become more prevalent with the duration and severity of inflammation. The most prominent opioid peptide involved is β-endorphin, but Met-enkephalin, dynorphin, and endomorphins also contribute (Stein et al. 1990a; Machelska et

al. 2003; Labuz et al. 2006). Endogenous triggers of this stress-induced analgesia are locally produced CRF and sympathetic nerve-derived catecholamines
(Fig. 2), because this effect is abolished by local neutralization of CRF and by
sympathetic blockade (Schäfer et al. 1996; Machelska et al. 2003; Binder et
al. 2004). The source of opioid peptides is various types of immune cells, as
demonstrated by the abolishment of this effect by immunosuppression with
cyclosporine A or whole-body irradiation, and by depletion of granulocytes
and monocytes/macrophages (Stein et al. 1990b; Przewlocki et al. 1992; Brack
et al. 2004a; Labuz et al. 2006). Moreover, this endogenous analgesic effect is
extinguished by inhibiting the extravasation of β-endorphin-containing immune
cells via blockade of L- and P-selectins, of α_4 and β_2 integrins, or of ICAM-1
(Machelska et al. 1998, 2002, 2004), consistent with the regulated migration of
opioid-containing cells described above (Fig. 1). In the visceral system, T-lymphocytes are postulated to mediate antinociception by induction of β-endorphin
expression in the myenteric nervous system (Verma-Gandhu et al. 2006).

A future challenge is to identify factors that will increase migration of
opioid-containing cells to injured tissue and inhibit pain. Initial studies have
shown that the systemic administration of hematopoietic growth factors did not
significantly increase the number of opioid-containing leukocytes in peripheral
inflamed tissue and did not change CRF- or stress-induced analgesia (Brack et
al. 2004b). Increasing the migration of opioid-containing cells to inflamed tissue with local injections of CXCL2/3 did not result in stronger analgesia either.
This result may have been due to the relatively small number of neuronal opioid
receptors at this very early (2-hour) stage of inflammation (Brack et al. 2004d).
Indeed, our previous studies had shown that intrinsic opioid analgesia increases
with the duration of inflammation (2 hours–4 days), in parallel with the number
of opioid-containing leukocytes, with the number of peripheral opioid receptors,
and with the efficacy of opioid receptor-G-protein coupling in sensory neurons
(Mousa et al. 2001; Rittner et al. 2001; Zöllner et al. 2003).

CLINICAL IMPLICATIONS

Peripheral opioid analgesia is of clinical relevance. Opioid receptors have
been demonstrated on peripheral terminals of sensory nerves in human synovia
(Stein et al. 1996), and activation of these receptors mediates analgesia in patients with various types of pain (e.g., chronic rheumatoid arthritis, osteoarthritis, bone pain, and pain after dental, laparoscopic, and urinary bladder surgery)
(Stein et al. 2003; Likar et al. 2004; Hanna et al. 2005). The most extensively
studied clinical situation is the intra-articular application of opioids for pain
control after knee surgery (reviewed in Kalso et al. 1997, 2002; Reuben and

Sklar 2000; Gupta et al. 2001; Stein et al. 2001, 2003; Sawynok 2003; Rosseland 2005). The majority of the reviews agree on the analgesic efficacy of intra-articular morphine (Reuben and Sklar 2000; Gupta et al. 2001; Kalso et al. 2002; Sawynok 2003; Stein et al. 2003). Not surprisingly, there are reports showing a lack of such effects (reviewed in Kalso et al. 1997; Stein et al. 2001, 2003; Rosseland 2005). Most commonly, the negative findings have been attributed to lack of assay sensitivity (e.g., low intensity of baseline pain), lack of tissue inflammation, and the superimposition of general or local anesthetic effects (Kalso et al. 2002; Stein et al. 2001, 2003; Rosseland 2005). Controversial conclusions from reviews are likely to result from different criteria used for the selection of studies and for evaluation of their validity. For example, out of over 60 published studies, only 25 were considered "evaluable" by Kalso et al. (2002), while 43 were selected by Rosseland (2005). An important deduction is that, similar to the animal studies, the analgesic efficacy of intra-articular opioids is low immediately after surgical injury but increases with the duration and extent of tissue inflammation (Kalso et al. 2002).

Opioid peptides are found in human synovial lining cells, mast cells, lymphocytes, and macrophages. The prevailing peptides are β-endorphin and Met-enkephalin, while only minor amounts of dynorphin are detectable (Stein et al. 1993, 1996). Consistently, in patients who have had knee surgery, the blockade of intra-articular opioid receptors by the local administration of naloxone results in significantly increased postoperative pain (Stein et al. 1993). These findings suggest that in a stressful clinical situation, such as surgery, opioids are tonically released from inflammatory cells and activate peripheral opioid receptors to attenuate pain. Importantly, these endogenous opioids do not interfere with exogenous morphine, i.e., intra-articular morphine is an equally potent analgesic in patients with and without opioid-producing inflammatory synovial cells (Stein et al. 1996; Likar et al. 2004). This finding suggests that immune-cell-derived opioid peptides do not readily produce cross-tolerance to morphine at peripheral opioid receptors.

FUTURE DIRECTIONS

Effective control of inflammatory pain can result from interactions between leukocyte-derived opioid peptides and their receptors on peripheral endings of sensory neurons. These findings provide new insights into intrinsic mechanisms of pain control and open strategies for development of new drugs and alternative approaches to the treatment of pain. Immunocompromised patients (such as those with AIDS, cancer, or diabetes) frequently suffer from painful neuropathies that can be associated with intra- and perineural inflammation, with reduced intraepidermal nerve fiber density, and with low CD4[+] lympho-cyte counts (Polydefkis et al. 2002). Thus, it may be interesting to investigate the production and release of opioids and the migration of opioid-containing leukocytes in these patients. The important role of certain adhesion molecules and chemokines in the trafficking of opioid-containing cells to injured tissues indicates that antiadhesion or antichemokine strategies for the treatment of inflammatory diseases may in fact carry a significant risk for exacerbation of pain. It would be highly desirable to identify stimulating factors and strategies that would selectively attract opioid-producing cells and increase peripheral opioid receptor numbers in damaged tissue. A further interesting aspect is to in-vestigate whether immune-derived opioid peptides and exogenous peripherally acting opioids interact in an additive or synergistic fashion. Additional targets for research may emerge from recent findings that T-lymphocytes might induce expression of β-endorphin in peripheral neurons to produce analgesia (Verma-Gandhu et al. 2006) and that opioids trigger integrin-mediated monocyte rolling and adhesion in vitro and in vivo in animals (Pello et al. 2006).

Importantly, opioid analgesia resulting from neuroimmune interactions oc-curs in peripheral tissues. Therefore, it is devoid of central opioid side effects (such as respiratory depression, nausea, dysphoria, and addiction) and of typical side effects produced by cyclooxygenase inhibitors (such as gastric erosions, ulcers, bleeding, diarrhea, thromboembolic complications, and renal toxicity). Many efforts are currently underway to develop peripherally acting analgesics by aiming at individual excitatory receptors or channels on sensory neurons (Simonin and Kieffer 2002). The major advantage of targeting opioid receptors is their mechanism of action: the inhibition of calcium (and possibly sodium) channels simply renders the nociceptor less excitable by the plethora of stimu-lating molecules expressed in damaged tissue. Thus, peripherally acting opioids can prevent and reverse the action of multiple excitatory agents simultaneously, in contrast to blocking only one single noxious agent. Uncovering mechanisms that can enhance the availability of endogenous opioids within injured tissue and increase the signal transduction of peripheral opioid receptors will open exciting possibilities for pain research and therapy.

ACKNOWLEDGMENTS

Supported by the grants from Deutsche Forschungsgemeinschaft (KFO 100) and Bundesministerium für Bildung und Forschung (No. 01GZ0311). We thank Christine Voigts for the preparation of illustrations.

REFERENCES

Akil H, Owens C, Gutstein H, et al. Endogenous opioids: overview and current issues. *Drug Alcohol Depend* 1998; 51:127–140.

Antonijevic I, Mousa SA, Schäfer M, Stein C. Perineurial defect and peripheral opioid analgesia in inflammation. *J Neurosci* 1995; 15:165–172.

Binder W, Mousa SA, Sitte N, et al. Sympathetic activation triggers endogenous opioid release and analgesia within peripheral inflamed tissue. *Eur J Neurosci* 2004; 20:92–100.

Brack A, Labuz D, Schiltz A, et al. Tissue monocytes/macrophages in inflammation: hyperalgesia versus opioid-mediated peripheral antinociception. *Anesthesiology* 2004a; 101:204–211.

Brack A, Rittner HL, Machelska H, et al. Mobilization of opioid-containing polymorphonuclear cells by hematopoietic growth factors and influence on inflammatory pain. *Anesthesiology* 2004b; 100:149–157.

Brack A, Rittner HL, Machelska H, et al. Control of inflammatory pain by chemokine-mediated recruitment of opioid-containing polymorphonuclear cells. *Pain* 2004c; 12:229–238.

Brack A, Rittner HL, Machelska H, et al. Endogenous peripheral antinociception in early inflammation is not limited by the number of opioid-containing leukocytes but by opioid receptor expression. *Pain* 2004d; 108:67–75.

Cabot PJ, Carter L, Gaiddon C, et al. Immune cell-derived β-endorphin: production, release and control of inflammatory pain in rats. *J Clin Invest* 1997; 100:142–148.

Cabot PJ, Carter L, Schäfer M, Stein C. Methionine-enkephalin-and Dynorphin A-release from immune cells and control of inflammatory pain. *Pain* 2001; 93:207–212.

Chadzinska M, Starowicz K, Scislowska-Czarnecka A, et al. Morphine-induced changes in the activity of proopiomelanocortin and prodynorphin systems in zymosan-induced peritonitis in mice. *Immunol Lett* 2005; 101:185–192.

Cunha FQ, Ferreira SH. Peripheral hyperalgesic cytokines. *Adv Exp Med Biol* 2003; 521:22–39.

Czlonkowski A, Stein C, Herz A. Peripheral mechanisms of opioid antinociception in inflammation: involvement of cytokines. *Eur J Pharmacol* 1993; 242:229–235.

Fields H. State-dependent opioid control of pain. *Nat Rev Neurosci* 2004; 5:565–575.

Gupta A, Bodin L, Holmstrom B, Berggren L. A systematic review of the peripheral analgesic effects of intraarticular morphine. *Anesth Analg* 2001; 93:761–770.

Hanna MH, Elliott KM, Fung M. Randomized, double-blind study of the analgesic efficacy of morphine-6-glucuronide versus morphine sulfate for postoperative pain in major surgery. *Anesthesiology* 2005; 102:815–821.

Hargreaves KM, Dubner R, Costello AH. Corticotropin releasing factor (CRF) has a peripheral site of action for antinociception. *Eur J Pharmacol* 1989; 170:275–279.

Hermanussen S, Do M, Cabot PJ. Reduction of beta-endorphin-containing immune cells in inflamed paw tissue corresponds with a reduction in immune-derived antinociception: reversible by donor activated lymphocytes. *Anesth Analg* 2004; 98:723–729.

Hook S, Camberis M, Prout M, et al. Preproenkephalin is a Th2 cytokine but is not required for Th2 differentiation in vitro. *Immunol Cell Biol* 1999; 77:385–390.

Jeanjean AP, Moussaoui SM, Maloteaux J-M, Laduron PM. Interleukin-1β induces long-term increase of axonally transported opiate receptors and substance P. *Neuroscience* 1995; 68:151–157.

Ji RR, Zhang Q, Law PY, et al. Expression of μ-, δ-, and κ-opioid receptor-like immunoreactivities in rat dorsal root ganglia after carrageenan-induced inflammation. *J Neurosci* 1995; 15:8156–8166.

Kalso E, Tramer MR, Carroll D, McQuay HJ, Moore RA. Pain relief from intra-articular morphine after knee surgery: a qualitative systematic review. *Pain* 1997; 71:127–134.

Kalso E, Smith L, McQuay HJ, Moore RA. No pain, no gain: clinical excellence and scientific rigour—lessons learned from IA morphine. *Pain* 2002; 98:269–275.

Kavelaars A, Ballieux RE, Heijnen CJ. In vitro beta-adrenergic stimulation of lymphocytes induces the release of immunoreactive beta-endorphin. *Endocrinology* 1990; 126:3028–3032.

Kieffer BL, Gaveriaux-Ruff C. Exploring the opioid system by gene knockout. *Prog Neurobiol* 2002; 66:285–306.

Labuz D, Berger S, Mousa SA, et al. Peripheral antinociceptive effects of exogenous and immune cell-derived endomorphins in prolonged inflammatory pain. *J Neurosci* 2006; 26:4350–4358.

LaMendola J, Martin SK, Steiner DF. Expression of PC3, carboxypeptidase E and enkephalin in human monocyte-derived macrophages as a tool for genetic studies. *FEBS Lett* 1997; 404:19–22.

Likar R, Mousa SA, Philippitsch G, et al. Increased numbers of opioid expressing inflammatory cells do not affect intra-articular morphine analgesia. *Br J Anaesth* 2004; 93:375–80.

Lyons PD, Blalock JE. Pro-opiomelanocortin gene expression and protein processing in rat mononuclear leukocytes. *J Neuroimmunol* 1997; 78:47–56.

Machelska H, Stein C. Leukocyte-derived opioid peptides and inhibition of pain. *J Neuroimmune Pharmacol* 2006; 1:90–97.

Machelska H, Cabot PJ, Mousa SA, Zhang Q, Stein C. Pain control in inflammation governed by selectins. *Nat Med* 1998; 4:1425–1428.

Machelska H, Mousa SA, Brack A, et al. Opioid control of inflammatory pain regulated by intercellular adhesion molecule-1. *J Neurosci* 2002; 22:5588–5596.

Machelska H, Schopohl JK, Mousa SA, et al. Different mechanisms of intrinsic pain inhibition in early and late inflammation. *J Neuroimmunol* 2003; 141:30–39.

Machelska H, Brack A, Mousa SA, et al. Selectins and integrins but not platelet-endothelial cell adhesion molecule-1 regulate opioid inhibition of inflammatory pain. *Br J Pharmacol* 2004; 142:772–780.

Marchand F, Perretti M, McMahon B. Role of the immune system in chronic pain. *Nat Rev Neurosci* 2005; 6:521–532.

McLoon LK, Sandnas AM, Nockleby KJ, Wirtschafter JD. Reduction in vesicant-induced cellular inflammation and hyperalgesia by local injection of corticotropin releasing factor in rabbit eyelid. *Inflamm Res* 2002; 51:16–23.

Millan MJ. Descending control of pain. *Prog Neurobiol* 2002; 66:355–474.

Mousa SA, Schäfer M, Mitchell WM, Hassan AHS, Stein C. Local upregulation of corticotropin-releasing hormone and interleukin-1 receptors in rats with painful hindlimb inflammation. *Eur J Pharmacol* 1996; 311:221–231.

Mousa SA, Machelska H, Schäfer M, Stein C. Co-expression of beta-endorphin with adhesion molecules in a model of inflammatory pain. *J Neuroimmunol* 2000; 108:160–170.

Mousa SA, Zhang Q, Sitte N, Ji R, Stein C. beta-Endorphin-containing memory-cells and mu-opioid receptors undergo transport to peripheral inflamed tissue. *J Neuroimmunol* 2001; 115:71–78.

Mousa SA, Bopaiah CP, Stein C, Schäfer M. Involvement of corticotropin-releasing hormone receptor subtypes 1 and 2 in peripheral opioid-mediated inhibition of inflammatory pain. *Pain* 2003; 106:297–307.

Mousa SA, Shakibaei M, Sitte N, Schäfer M, Stein C. Subcellular pathways of beta-endorphin synthesis, processing, and release from immunocytes in inflammatory pain. *Endocrinology* 2004; 145:1331–1341.

Oh SB, Tran PB, Gillard SE, et al. Chemokines and glycoprotein120 produce pain hypersensitivity by directly exciting primary nociceptive neurons. *J Neurosci* 2001; 21:5027–5035.

Pello OM, Duthey B, Garcia-Bernal D, et al. Opioids trigger alpha 5 beta 1 integrin-mediated monocyte adhesion. *J Immunol* 2006; 176:1675–1685.

Polydefkis M, Yiannoutsos CT, Cohen BA, et al. Reduced intraepidermal nerve fiber density in HIV-associated sensory neuropathy. *Neurology* 2002; 58:115–119.

Przewlocki R, Hassan AHS, Lason W, et al. Gene expression and localization of opioid peptides in immune cells of inflamed tissue. Functional role in antinociception. *Neuroscience* 1992; 48:491–500.

Pühler W, Zöllner C, Brack A, et al. Rapid upregulation of mu opioid receptor mRNA in dorsal root ganglia in response to peripheral inflammation depends on neuronal conduction. *Neuroscience* 2004; 129:473–479.

Pühler W, Rittner HL, Mousa SA, et al. Interleukin-1 beta contributes to the upregulation of kappa opioid receptor mRNA in dorsal root ganglia in response to peripheral inflammation. *Neuroscience* 2006; 141:989–998.

Reuben SS, Sklar J. Pain management in patients who undergo outpatient arthroscopic surgery of the knee. *J Bone Joint Surg Am* 2000; 82A:1754–1766.

Rittner HL, Brack A, Machelska H, et al. Opioid peptide expressing leukocytes-identification, recruitment and simultaneously increasing inhibition of inflammatory pain. *Anesthesiology* 2001; 95:500–508.

Rittner HL, Machelska H, Stein C. Leukocytes in the regulation of pain and analgesia. *J Leukoc Biol* 2005; 78:1215–1222.

Rittner HL, Mousa SA, Labuz D, et al. Selective local PMN recruitment by CXCL1 or CXCL2/3 injection does not cause inflammatory pain. *J Leukoc Biol* 2006a; 79:1022–1032.

Rittner HL, Labuz D, Schaefer M, et al. Pain control by CXCR2 ligands through Ca^{2+}-regulated release of opioid peptides from polymorphonuclear cells. *FASEB J* 2006b; 20:2627–2629.

Rosseland LA. No evidence for analgesic effect of intra-articular morphine after knee arthroscopy: a qualitative systematic review. *Reg Anesth Pain Med* 2005; 30:83–98.

Sacerdote P, Limiroli E, Gaspani L. Experimental evidence for immunomodulatory effects of opioids. *Adv Exp Med Biol* 2003; 521:106–116.

Sawynok J. Topical and peripherally acting analgesics. *Pharmacol Rev* 2003; 55:1–20.

Schäfer M. Cytokines and peripheral analgesia. *Adv Exp Med Biol* 2003; 521:40–50.

Schäfer M, Carter L, Stein C. Interleukin-1β and corticotropin-releasing-factor inhibit pain by releasing opioids from immune cells in inflamed tissue. *Proc Natl Acad Sci USA* 1994; 91:4219–4223.

Schäfer M, Mousa SA, Zhang Q, Carter L, Stein C. Expression of corticotropin-releasing factor in inflamed tissue is required for intrinsic peripheral opioid analgesia. *Proc Natl Acad Sci USA* 1996; 93:6096–6100.

Sekido R, Ishimaru K, Sakita M. Corticotropin-releasing factor and interleukin-1beta are involved in the electroacupuncture-induced analgesic effect on inflammatory pain elicited by carrageenan. *Am J Chin Med* 2004; 32:269–279.

Sharp BM. Opioid receptor expression and intracellular signaling by cells involved in host defence and immunity. *Adv Exp Med Biol* 2003; 521:8–105.

Simonin F, Kieffer BL. Two faces for an opioid peptide—and more receptors for pain research. *Nat Neurosci* 2002; 5:185–186.

Smith EM. Opioid peptides in immune cells. *Adv Exp Med Biol* 2003; 521:51–68.

Stein C, Gramsch C, Herz A. Intrinsic mechanisms of antinociception in inflammation. Local opioid receptors and beta-endorphin. *J Neurosci* 1990a; 10:1292–1298.

Stein C, Hassan AHS, Przewlocki R, et al. Opioids from immunocytes interact with receptors on sensory nerves to inhibit nociception in inflammation. *Proc Natl Acad Sci USA* 1990b; 87:5935–5939.

Stein C, Hassan AHS, Lehrberger K, Giefing J, Yassouridis A. Local analgesic effect of endogenous opioid peptides. *Lancet* 1993; 342:321–324.

Stein C, Pflüger M, Yassouridis A, et al. No tolerance to peripheral morphine analgesia in presence of opioid expression in inflamed synovia. *J Clin Invest* 1996; 98:793–799.

Stein C, Machelska H, Schäfer M. Peripheral analgesic and antiinflammatory effects of opioids. *Z Rheumatol* 2001; 60:416–424.

Stein C, Schäfer M, Machelska H. Attacking pain at its source: new perspectives on opioids. *Nat Med* 2003; 9:1003–1008.

Szabo I, Chen X-H, Xin L, et al. Heterologous desensitization of opioid receptors by chemokines inhibits chemotaxis and enhances the perception of pain. *Proc Natl Acad Sci USA* 2002; 99:10276–10281.

Terman GW, Shavit Y, Lewis JW, Cannon JT, Liebeskind JC. Intrinsic mechanisms of pain inhibition: activation by stress. *Science* 1984; 14:1270–1277.

Verma-Gandhu M, Bercik P, Motomura Y, et al. CD4+ T-cell modulation of visceral nociception in mice. *Gastroenterology* 2006; 130:1721–1728.

Vindrola O, Mayer AM, Citera G, Spitzer JA, Espinoza LR. Prohormone convertases PC2 and PC3 in rat neutrophils and macrophages. Parallel changes with proenkephalin-derived peptides induced by LPS in vivo. *Neuropeptides* 1994; 27:235–244.

von Andrian UH, Mackay CR. T-cell function and migration. Two sides of the same coin. *N Engl J Med* 2000; 343:1020–1034.

Watkins LR, Maier SF. Beyond neurons: evidence that immune and glial cells contribute to pathological pain states. *Physiol Rev* 2002; 82:981–1011.

Wenk HN, Brederson JD, Honda CN. Morphine directly inhibits nociceptors in inflamed skin. *J Neurophysiol* 2006; 95:2083–2097.

Woolf CJ, Salter MW. Neuronal plasticity: increasing the gain in pain. *Science* 2000; 288:1765–1769.

Zadina JE, Hackler L, Ge LJ, Kastin AJ. A potent and selective endogenous agonist for the mu-opiate receptor. *Nature* 1997; 386:499–502.

Zöllner C, Shaqura MA, Bopaiah CP, et al. Painful inflammation-induced increase in mu-opioid receptor binding and G-protein coupling in primary afferent neurons. *Mol Pharmacol* 2003; 64:202–210.

Correspondence to: Halina Machelska, PhD, Klinik für Anaesthesiologie und operative Intensivmedizin, Charité-Universitätsmedizin Berlin, Campus Benjamin Franklin, Hindenburgdamm 30, D-12200 Berlin, Germany. Tel: 49-30-8445-3851; fax: 49-30-8445-4469; email: halina.machelska@charite.de.

Part III

Immune/Glial-Pain Interactions: Dorsal Root Ganglia

Immune and Glial Regulation of Pain, edited by Joyce A. DeLeo, Linda S. Sorkin, and Linda R. Watkins, IASP Press, Seattle, © 2007.

7

Chemokines and Their Receptors in the Nervous System: A Link to Neuropathic Pain

Fletcher A. White,[a,b] Patrick E. Monahan,[a] and Robert H. LaMotte[c]

[a]Department of Cell Biology, Neurobiology and Anatomy, Loyola University, Chicago, Maywood, Illinois, USA; [b]Department of Anesthesiology, Loyola University Health System, Maywood, Illinois, USA; [c]Department of Anesthesiology, Yale University School of Medicine, New Haven, Connecticut, USA

INJURY-INDUCED CHANGES IN THE PERIPHERAL NERVOUS SYSTEM

Peripheral nerve injury can trigger pain and initiate a wide variety of cellular changes in sensory neurons. It has been proposed that neuropathic pain following peripheral nerve injury is due to the enhanced excitability or the chronic sensitization of nociceptive neurons in the peripheral and central nervous system. For example, following a peripheral nerve injury, a subset of injured and neighboring intact peripheral sensory neurons may exhibit spontaneous ectopic discharges (Tal and Devor 1992; Sheth et al. 2002; Ma et al. 2003; Obata et al. 2003; Xie et al. 2005). These pathophysiological discharges may trigger neuroplastic changes resulting in the sensitization (enhanced excitability) of second-order and perhaps higher-order neurons in the somatovisceral afferent pathway (Woolf 1983). In turn, signal amplification by central sensitization allows afferent input arriving in the spinal cord dorsal horn along low-threshold mechanoreceptive Aβ fibers to have a nociceptive effect (Campbell et al. 1988; Torebjork et al. 1992), thus contributing to tactile allodynia (nociceptive responses to innocuous stimuli). Although it is clear that molecular and possibly anatomical changes in the spinal cord dorsal horn are responsible for some attributes of chronic pain, it remains a mystery as to what events and which anatomical sites are critical in the development and maintenance of neuropathic pain.

PERIPHERAL NERVE INJURY AND INFLAMMATION

Acute pain is a normal response to injury. It is an immediate and typically short-lived state, and the cause can usually be identified and treated. Chronic pain, in contrast, persists beyond the normal time for healing. Neuropathic pain is a type of chronic pain that occurs after trauma or pathologies that directly affect the nervous system. The inflammatory response to injury plays a prominent role in both acute and chronic pain and injuries, whether or not they involve the nervous system. Persistent inflammation of the nervous system may lead to altered gene expression, abnormal processing of pain signals, and enhanced pain states. In this way, signaling pathways designed to facilitate a protective response to tissue injury become, instead, sources of chronic pathological pain.

Possible sources of inflammatory pain include the production and release of proinflammatory mediators including bradykinin, tachykinins, serotonin, histamine, ATP, and cytokines such as tumor necrosis factor alpha (TNF-α), interleukin 1-β (IL-1β), and interleukin-6 (IL-6) (for a review, see Verri et al. 2006). Data to support this theory are derived from studies on the effects of the direct application of pro-inflammatory cytokines to peripheral neurons. The outcome of such studies demonstrate that cytokines can increase nociceptive neuronal responses to stimuli (thermal, mechanical, and chemical) applied either directly to neurons or to their peripheral receptive fields (Nicol et al. 1997; Sorkin et al. 1997; Junger and Sorkin 2000; Homma et al. 2002; Liu et al. 2002; Ozaktay et al. 2006).

A family of cytokines that have recently come to light as playing a role in the induction and maintenance of chronic pain are the chemotactic cytokines, known as chemokines. Cellular production and release of chemokines are normally associated with the immune response to infection or to localized injury or trauma. Chemokines typically have a relatively rapid onset and short duration of action, resulting in extravasation and control of leukocyte mobilization (Yabe et al. 2004; Chessell et al. 2005; Fulgenzi et al. 2005; Nakayama et al. 2006). Although chemokines usually have a beneficial effect in limiting responses to cellular and organ damage, a breakdown in the regulation of the inflammatory response may result in a wide range of chronic diseases including chronic pain. The pathogenesis and course of many chronic inflammatory conditions such as atherosclerosis, arthritis, and inflammatory bowel disease are mediated in large part by chemokines (Charo and Ransohoff 2006). In addition, a multitude of neurological conditions that are marked by inflammation during the onset or progression of disease (multiple sclerosis, cerebral ischemic injury, and Alzheimer's disease) as well as virus-based diseases (related to HIV or herpes simplex infection) are known to include a strong chemokine component (Cartier et al. 2005). This chemokine-mediated component is also likely to extend to the pathogenesis and maintenance of chronic pain in both disease-related conditions (e.g., multiple sclerosis HIV-1 infection, and herpes simplex infection) and following trauma, leading to de novo and/or prolonged expression of chemokines and their receptors (White et al. 2005a). Interference with chemokine function is a promising approach for the development of both novel anti-inflammatory medication and new analgesic treatments for chronic pain conditions.

CHEMOKINES AND THEIR RECEPTORS AND INTRACELLULAR SIGNALING

Chemokines constitute a large family of relatively low-molecular mass proteins classified by the presence of a cysteine motif in the N-terminal region of the protein. Initial characterization of chemokines divided the family into alpha and beta chemokines. In alpha chemokines, one amino acid separates the first two cysteine residues (cysteine–X amino acid–cysteine or CXC), whereas in beta chemokines, the first two cysteine residues are adjacent to each other (cysteine-cysteine, or CC). Two additional classes were added for the chemokines, lymphotactin (single cysteine, XC) and fractalkine (first two cysteines are separated by three amino acids, CX3C). The chemokine nomenclature herein utilizes both the original ligand name and the systematic name. The systematic name uses XC, CC, CXC and CX3C, indicating the class to which the chemokine belongs, followed by the letter "L" (for ligand) and then a number. The numbering system corresponds to that already in use to designate the genes encoding each chemokine (see Table I).

All chemokines exert their biological effects through the activation of an extended family of seven-transmembrane G-protein-coupled receptors (GP-CRs). Nineteen chemokine receptors have been cloned including six CXC receptors (CXCR1-6), 10 CC receptors (CCR1-10), and two single receptors each for lymphotactin (XCR1) and fractalkine (CX3CR1). Chemokine receptors are notoriously promiscuous, i.e., single chemokines can activate several different chemokine receptors. There are, however, instances when a chemokine receptor is uniquely activated by a single chemokine. For example, the CXCR4 receptor has only one known ligand, stromal-derived factor-1 alpha (SDF1α/CXCL12).

The common response of all non-excitable cells to chemokine stimulation is chemotaxis. Activation of chemokines and their receptors also triggers downstream signaling cascades via dissociation of G proteins, which induces the phosphoinositide 3-kinase pathway (PI3K) and activates phospholipase C, resulting in Ca^{2+} influx and protein kinase C activation (Murphy 1994). Knockout experiments in mice have revealed the central role played by PI3K

Table I
Chemokine nomenclature

Receptor	Systematic Name	Original Name
CCR1	CCL3	Macrophage inflammatory protein-1 alpha (MIP-1α)
	CCL5	Regulated on activation normal T-cell expressed and secreted (RANTES)
	CCL 7	Monocyte chemoattractant protein-3 (MCP-3)
	CCL14	Hemofiltrate CC chemokine-1 (HCC-1)
	CCL15	Hemofiltrate CC chemokine-2 (HCC-2)
	CCL16	Hemofiltrate CC chemokine-4 (HCC-4)
	CCL23	Myeloid progenitor inhibitory factor-1 (MIPF-1)
CCR2	CCL2	Monocyte chemoattractant protein-1 (MCP-1)
	CCL7	Monocyte chemoattractant protein-3 (MCP-3)
	CCL13	Monocyte chemoattractant protein-4 (MCP-4)
	CCL16	Hemofiltrate CC chemokine-4 (HCC-4)
CCR3	CCL3	Macrophage inflammatory protein-1 alpha (MIP-1α)
	CCL4	Macrophage inflammatory protein-1 beta (MIP-1β)
	CCL5	Regulated on activation normal T-cell expressed and secreted (RANTES)
	CCL8	Monocyte chemoattractant protein-2 (MCP-2)
	CCL14	Hemofiltrate CC chemokine-1 (HCC-1)
CCR4	CCL17	Thymus and activation-regulated chemokine (TARC)
	CCL22	Macrophage-derived chemokine (MDC)
CCR5	CCL3	Macrophage inflammatory protein-1 alpha (MIP-1α)
	CCL4	Macrophage inflammatory protein-1 beta (MIP-1β)
	CCL5	Regulated on activation normal T-cell expressed and secreted (RANTES)
	CCL8	Monocyte chemoattractant protein-2 (MCP-2)
CCR6	CCL20	Macrophage inflammatory protein-1 alpha (MIP-1α)
CCR7	CCL19	Macrophage inflammatory protein-1 beta (MIP-1β)
	CCL21	Secondary lymphoid tissue chemokine (SLC)
CCR8	CCL1	I-309 (TCA-3, SIS-f)
CCR9	CCL25	Thymus-expressed chemokine (TECK)
CCR10	CCL27	Cutaneous T-cell-attracting chemokine (CTACK)
	CCL28	Mucosae-associated epithelial chemokine (MEC)
CCR11	CCR19	Macrophage inflammatory protein-1 beta (MIP-1β)
	CCR21	Secondary lymphoid tissue chemokine (SLC)
	CCR25	Thymus-expressed chemokine (TECK)
CXCR1	CXCL1	Growth-related oncogene-alpha (GRO-α)
	CXCL6	Granulocyte chemotactic protein-2 (GCP-2)
	CXCL8	Interleukin-8 (IL-8)

Table I (Continued)

Receptor	Systematic Name	Original Name
CXCR2	CXCL1	Growth-related oncogene-alpha (GRO-α)
	CXCL2	Growth-related oncogene-beta (GRO-β)
	CXCL3	Growth-related oncogene-gamma (GRO-γ)
	CXCL5	Epithelial cell-derived neutrophil activating factor-78 (ENA-78)
	CXCL6	Granulocyte chemotactic protein-2 (GCP-2)
	CXCL7	Neutrophil-activating protein-2 (NAP-2)
	CXCL8	Interleukin-8 (IL-8)
CXCR3	CXCL9	Monokine induced by gamma-interferon (MIG)
	CXCL10	Gamma-interferon-inducible protein 10 (IP-10)
	CXCL11	Interferon inducible T-cell alpha chemoattractant (I-TAC)
CXCR4	CXCL12	Stromal cell-derived factor-1 alpha/beta (SDF-1α/β)
CXCR5	CXCL13	B-cell-activating chemokine-1 (BCA-1)
CXCR6	CXCL16	Scavenger receptor for phosphatidylserine and oxidized LDLs (SRPSOX)
CX3CR1	CX3CL1	Fractalkine (neurotactin)
XCR1	XCL1	Lymphotactin-alpha (SCM-1α)
	XCL2	Lymphotactin-beta (SCM-1β)

in cellular responses to chemokines (Hirsch et al. 2000; Sasaki et al. 2000), and transient Ca^{2+} elevations are one of the most well-characterized effects of chemokines (Oh et al. 2001; Gillard et al. 2002). It is important to note that many cellular responses to chemokines can be blocked with pertussis toxin, indicating that many G proteins involved in chemokine signaling are members of the $G_{i/o}$ protein family. Recent functional characterizations of chemokine receptors suggest that these proteins form dimers or other higher-order structures that are bound to lipid rafts (Mellado et al. 2001; Rodriguez-Frade et al. 2001). This dimerization of receptors potentially leads to the recruitment of Janus-activated kinase (JAK) signaling and to the activation of signal transducers and activators of transcription (STATS) (Maurer and von Stebut 2004). In addition, evidence also suggests that chemokines may activate mitogen-activated protein kinase (MAPK) by either G_a or G-independent signaling (Ganju et al. 1998; Rodriguez-Frade et al. 2001).

Chemokine influences in the immune system can be largely separated into two functional roles; they act as chemoattractants during inflammation and as traffickers of hematopoietic stem cells during development and differentiation (Lapidot et al. 2005; Charo and Ransohoff 2006). Chemokines associated with inflammation control the recruitment of effector leukocytes during infection, inflammation, tissue injury, and tumors. Many of the inflammatory chemokines have broad target cell selectivity and act on cells of the innate and the adaptive immune system. Chemokines that influence hematopoiesis, in contrast, enable immature myeloid cells and leukocytes to navigate through the bone marrow and thymus. These hematopoietic chemokines also act during initiation of adaptive immune responses in the spleen and lymph nodes, and in immune surveillance of healthy peripheral tissues. Some chemokines also have recognized angiogenic properties during the neovascularization that follows trauma and disease (Ceradini and Gurtner 2005; Kakinuma and Hwang 2006).

FUNCTION OF CHEMOKINES IN THE DEVELOPING NERVOUS SYSTEM

The role of chemokines in the nervous system, similar to their role in the immune system, can be largely divided into two functional roles—the regulation of neural development and the modulation of glial and neuronal responses to injury and disease. Much of the data reporting chemokine modulation in the nervous system are derived from studies of neural development in both the central (CNS) and peripheral (PNS) nervous systems. Among the first findings was the ability of RANTES/CCL5 (regulated on activation of normal T-cell expressed and secreted) to produce, in vitro, both the migration of mouse embryonic sensory neurons and their differentiation into a nociceptive neuron phenotype independent of nerve growth factor (Bolin et al. 1998).

Chemokines can also provide trophic support for neurons. IL-8/CXCL8 and growth-related oncogene (GRO-β/CXCL2) promote the survival of cultured hippocampal pyramidal neurons and cerebellar granule cells, respectively (Araujo and Cotman 1993; Horuk et al. 1997; Limatola et al. 2000). Under conditions of neurotrophin deprivation, monokine induced by gamma-interferon (MIG/CXCL9), an agonist of CXCR3, acts as a neurotrophic factor for both PC12 and cultured sympathetic neurons (Uwabe et al. 2005). Under neurotoxic conditions, the chemokine/receptor interaction of fractalkine/CX3CL1 and CX3CR1 can also promote survival of hippocampus pyramidal neurons (Meucci et al. 2000).

Another chemokine/receptor pairing, SDF1α/CXCL12 acting via CXCR4, has been found to be essential for neural crest cell migration and pathfinding in both cranial and somatic sensory ganglia of the zebrafish and mouse, respectively, and for the initial trajectory of murine ventral motor neurons and retinal ganglion cell axons (Chalasani et al. 2003a; Belmadani et al. 2005; Knaut et al. 2005; Lieberam et al. 2005). SDF1α/CXCL12 also appears to be important as a trophic factor both for embryonic retinal ganglion cells (Chalasani et al. 2003b) and for subpopulations of TrkA and TrkC somatic dorsal root ganglion (DRG) neurons (Belmadani et al. 2005).

In the CNS, in vitro studies of SDF1α/CXCL12 have revealed the necessity of this chemokine for the successful migration of cerebellar granule neurons and neuronal precursor cells (Bajetto and Bonavia 1999; Lazarini et al. 2000; Klein et al. 2001; Belmadani et al. 2005). The most telling revelation of the effects of SDF1α/CXCL12 on CNS development came from mice lacking genes for either the ligand (SDF1α/CXCL12) or its receptor (CXCR4). These knockout mice exhibited profound abnormalities in the organization of cerebellar neuronal layers and distinctly smaller dentate gyri in the hippocampus compared to wild-type mice (Ma et al. 1998; Zou et al. 1998; Bagri et al. 2002; Lu et al. 2002).

Additional evidence of a role for chemokines in neural progenitor cell migration was recently revealed using an elegant in vitro model of neuroinflammation in the CNS. Playing on the concept that neural progenitors or bone marrow stem cells transplanted into the brain will migrate into areas of brain damage, Belmadani and colleagues (2006) used an in vitro hippocampal slice culture to determine whether factors associated with damaged areas of the slice culture (cytokines and/or chemokines) can direct the migration of neural progenitor cells. Subsequently, this group demonstrated that unlike wild-type neural progenitor cells, neural progenitor cells derived from CCR2 knockout mice exhibited little migration toward sites of inflammation in the hippocampal slice paradigm. Taken together, these data strongly support a central role for chemokines in a number of attributes associated with neural development.

CHEMOKINE CONTRIBUTIONS TO CNS DISEASE

Chemokines are likely to play a major role in the pathogenesis of many diseases of the nervous system. The enormous importance of chemokines in diseases of the CNS is perhaps best illustrated by the autoimmune disease, multiple sclerosis, and by HIV-1-associated dementia. The case for a chemokine influence on multiple sclerosis is most notable because there is a strong and consistent relationship between chemokine expression in the CNS and clinical symptoms of the disease. Evidence of a chemokine role in the pathogenic process of both multiple sclerosis and the animal model experimental autoimmune encephalomyelitis (EAE), a CD4[+] Th1-mediated demyelinating disease, stems from the finding that chemokines are produced in the endothelial cells of the CNS vasculature and expressed by infiltrating leukocytes in inflammatory foci and in the perivascular space as well as by associated astrocytes (Ubogu et al. 2006). The importance of chemokines in EAE is emphasized by the further demonstration that CCR1 and CCR2 knockout mice exhibit significantly lower incidences of EAE and that the blocking of macrophage inflammatory protein-1 alpha (MIP-1α/CCL3, a ligand of both CCR1 and CCR5) with an antibody prevents clinical signs of the disease and CNS infiltration by monocytes (Karpus

et al. 1995; Fife et al. 2000, 2001). Perhaps paradoxically, production of constitutively low levels of monocyte chemoattractant protein-1 (MCP-1/CCL2)
in the transgenic murine CNS culminates in significantly increased numbers of
macrophages in the parenchyma of the nervous tissue, yet milder clinical signs
of EAE. This effect may be due to impaired T-cell proliferation and interferon
gamma (IFN-γ) production (Elhofy et al. 2005).

Another aspect of chemokine function in the diseased nervous system is
illustrated by chemokine receptor facilitation of HIV-1 infection. Although only
microglia and perivascular macrophages are capable of viral replication in the
nervous system, exposure of hippocampal and cerebellar granule cells to the
HIV-1 viral envelope glycoprotein, gp120, produces dose-dependent neuronal
apoptosis. The ability of gp120 to kill neurons is facilitated either directly, by
the presence of either neuronal CCR5 or CXCR4, which act as coreceptors for
the viral coat protein (Horuk 1999), or indirectly via the presence of chemokine-
receptor-bearing microglial cells, which release neurotoxic substances when
infected or activated by gp120 (Kaul et al. 2001). During early pathogenesis of
the disease, macrophage-specific HIV-1 predominates and CCR5 is the major
target. Later in the pathogenesis of the disease, CXCR4-specific viruses emerge.
Subsequently, either CCR5 and/or CXCR4 may be central to the development
of AIDS-related dementia (Kaul et al. 2001).

CHEMOKINES AS NEUROMODULATORS

Not all chemokine receptor expression contributes to disease conditions in
the adult nervous system. A third functional role can be defined by the selective
distribution of chemokines and their receptors throughout the normal nervous
system (including the hypothalamus, nucleus accumbens, limbic system, hippocampus, thalamus, cortex, cerebellum, spinal cord, and peripheral sensory
ganglia (van der Meer et al. 2000; Banisadr et al. 2002a,b; Bhangoo et al. 2006).
A multitude of chemokine receptors are present in the naive CNS including
CCR1, CCR2, CCR5, CXCR3, CXCR4, and CX3CR1 (van der Meer et al.
2000; Banisadr et al. 2002a,b; Abbadie et al. 2003; Cowell and Silverstein 2003;
Verge et al. 2004; Bhangoo et al. 2006, 2007). There is also ample evidence
that receptor/ligand binding modifies synaptic activity, modulates transmission,
and evokes second-messenger systems within neurons and glia (Mizuno et al.
2003; Ambrosini and Aloisi 2004). Moreover, individual neurons can coexpress
multiple functional chemokine receptors and chemokines (Coughlan et al. 2000;
Banisadr et al. 2002b; Bhangoo et al. 2006).

A prime example of a functional role for chemokines in the CNS is the
chemokine-receptor-regulated neurotransmission effects by IFN-γ-producing
protein-10 (IP-10/CXCL10) acting via CXCR3 on intracellular Ca^{2+} dynamics

and on the production of electrical activity in hippocampal neurons (Nelson and Gruol 2004). Another example is the dose-dependent ability of SDF1/CXCL12 to reduce the amplitude of evoked excitatory postsynaptic currents in Purkinje neurons (Ragozzino et al. 2002). Neurons of the rodent hippocampus and cerebellum also exhibit Ca^{2+} transients following stimulation with GROα/CXCL2, IL-8/CXCL8, RANTES/CCL5, macrophage-derived chemokine (MDC/CCL22), and fractalkine/CX3CL1 (Giovannelli et al. 1998; Meucci et al. 1998; Gillard et al. 2002). Chemokines such as SDF1/CXCL12 acting via CXCR4 on neurons and/or astrocytes are also thought to affect the release of glutamate, potentially affecting neuronal excitability (Limatola et al. 2000; Bezzi et al. 2001) and/or neuronal apoptosis (Bajetto et al. 2002). In addition, the chemokine GROα/CXCL2 is thought to provoke the release of gamma-aminobutyric acid (GABA) at central synapses (Giovannelli et al. 1998), whereas MCP-1/CCL2 negatively modulates GABA-induced currents and/or facilitates excitotoxic events in the neonatal rat CNS (Galasso et al. 2000; Gosselin et al. 2005).

Chemokine induction of excitatory effects in rodent neurons is not limited to cells in the CNS, because chemokines also produce changes in intracellular Ca^{2+} dynamics of neurons and glia in the PNS (Oh et al. 2001, 2002; Bhangoo et al. 2006, 2007) and generate action potentials in postnatal and adult sensory neurons (Oh et al. 2001; White et al. 2005c; Sun et al. 2006). Moreover, application of RANTES/CCL5 or MCP-1/CCL2 to neonatal DRG cultures produces excitation in nociceptive sensory neurons, resulting in the release of substance P (Oh et al. 2001) or calcitonin gene-related peptide (Qin et al. 2005).

Another means by which chemokines potentially alter neuronal signaling in the nervous system is via heterologous desensitization between chemokines and opioids. This phenomenon was first discovered in vitro and confirmed in vivo (Szabo et al. 2002; Zhang et al. 2004). Injections of the individual chemokines RANTES/CCL5, SDF1α/CXCL12, and fractalkine/CX3CL1, but not MCP-1/CCL2, into the periaqueductal gray 30 minutes prior to administration of morphine or the mu-opioid agonist DAMGO effectively blocked the expected analgesic effect on a rodent tail subjected to a cold-water bath. These authors further determined that the effects of the chemokines were both dose- and time-dependent. Given that the receptor for MCP-1/CCL2, CCR2, is not found normally in the periaqueductal gray (whereas those for the other aforementioned chemokine receptors are present), a distinct lack of opioid receptor cross-sensitization by MCP-1/CCL2 prior to morphine administration comes as no surprise (Szabo et al. 2002).

CHEMOKINES AND THEIR RECEPTORS
IN ACUTE AND CHRONIC PAIN

Several lines of evidence have demonstrated that the cellular release of cytokines and nerve growth factors contribute to both nociception and the development of neuropathic pain. While many of these factors may be key to the process of neuropathic pain induction, information about the mechanisms of neuropathic pain maintenance is seriously lacking.

There is adequate evidence demonstrating that like other cytokines, chemokines and their receptors facilitate acute pain as well as chronic pain. For example, Oh and colleagues (2001) demonstrated that the simple injection of SDF1α/CXCL12, RANTES/CCL5, or MIP1α/CCL3 into the noninflamed adult rat hindpaw produces dose-dependent tactile allodynia. Presumably, these ligands are acting directly on CXCR4, CCR5, and CCR1 on sensory neurons to elicit pain behavior in rats, although the authors did not rule out the possibility of indirect effects via non-neuronal cells. Assuming a direct neuronal effect, the allodynia may be due to receptor activation and downstream signaling or perhaps due to a sensitization of a mechanosensitive transient receptor potential (TRP) ion channel, such as TRPA1 in primary sensory neurons (Nagata et al. 2005; Kwan et al. 2006). MIP-1α/CCL3, although not associated with mechanotransduction, can enhance thermal sensitivity of another TRP ion channel, the heat-sensitive capsaicin receptor TRPV1 (Zhang et al. 2005). The receptor for MIP-1α, CCR1, is found both on leukocytes and on >85% of sensory neurons bearing TRPV1 (Zhang et al. 2005).

Evidence for a role for chemokines and their receptors in chronic pain is illustrated by data derived from several accepted models of rodent neuropathic pain. These models include partial ligation of the sciatic nerve (Abbadie et al. 2003; Tanaka et al. 2004; Lindia et al. 2005), chronic constriction injury of the sciatic nerve (Milligan et al. 2004; Zhang and De Koninck 2006; Kleinschnitz et al. 2005), chronic compression of the L4–L5 dorsal root ganglion (CCD, a rodent model of spinal stenosis; White et al. 2005c; Sun et al. 2006), lysophosphatidylcholine-induced focal nerve demyelination (White et al. 2005b), bone cancer pain (Vit et al. 2006), and zymosan-induced inflammatory pain (Milligan et al. 2004; Verge et al. 2004; Xie et al. 2006). Each of these models has revealed an upregulation of the chemokine receptors CX3CR1 or CCR2 and/or the CCR2 ligand, MCP-1/CCL2, in neural tissue associated with the injury.

The potential importance of the chemokine receptor CCR2 in neuropathic pain states following peripheral nerve injury was first demonstrated in genetically engineered mice lacking CCR2. These receptor knockout mice failed to display mechanical hyperalgesia following partial ligation of the sciatic nerve without a detectable change in acute pain behavior (Abbadie et al. 2003). A more recent study demonstrated that following chronic compression of the

DRG, exogenous administration of MCP-1/CCL2 produced both membrane threshold depolarization and action potentials in a subpopulation of small, medium, and large neuronal cell bodies in the intact DRG (Sun et al. 2005, 2006; White et al. 2005c) (see Fig. 1). Subsequently, two ionic mechanisms contributing to the excitatory effects of MCP-1 were identified in acutely dissociated small-diameter neurons in animals previously subjected to CCD. MCP-1 activated a non-voltage-dependent, depolarizing current with properties of a nonselective cation conductance, and it also inhibited a voltage-dependent outward current (Sun et al. 2006).

These chemokine-induced excitatory effects on sensory neurons may further facilitate the axonal transport and, as noted above, the release of the neuropeptide, calcitonin gene-related peptide (Qin et al. 2005). The presence of MCP-1/CCL2 is not limited to the DRG soma. Zhang and De Koninick (2006) recently demonstrated that MPC-1/CCL2 is also present in central afferent fibers in the spinal cord. In addition, electrical activity due to peripheral nerve injury may also stimulate central afferent release of MCP-1/CCL2 into the spinal cord dorsal horn, further activating CCR2-bearing glial cells or neurons (DeLeo et al. 2002; Abbadie et al. 2003; Zhang and De Koninck 2006).

Although the duration and degree to which chemokines and their receptors upregulate in sensory neurons following peripheral injury are relatively unknown, mRNA and protein for some chemokines/receptors exhibit an exceptionally prolonged upregulation in the injury-associated DRG (White et al. 2005b; Zhang and De Koninck 2006), and in the trigeminal ganglion following herpes simplex virus infection (Theil et al. 2003; Cook et al. 2004; Wickham et al. 2005). Taken together, prolonged chemokine/receptor expression in sensory ganglia may be a central facet of many injury-induced and virus-associated neuropathic pain syndromes.

CHEMOKINES, GLIA, AND CHRONIC PAIN

It has been proposed that activated glial cells—astrocytes and microglia—are central to chronic neuropathic pain (Watkins and Maier 2003). As astrocytes and microglial cells are in the vicinity of the central terminations of primary afferent neurons, these cells can become activated by the presynaptic release of glutamate and ATP.

Chemokines may be released from neurons and from activated glial cells. There are at least two ways in which activated glia may contribute to persistent pain. One manner is the activity-dependent release of a factor by an injured neuron. Alternatively, a receptor present on glial cells is upregulated in a time-sensitive manner. Either mechanism may contribute to the development and maintenance of neuropathic pain.

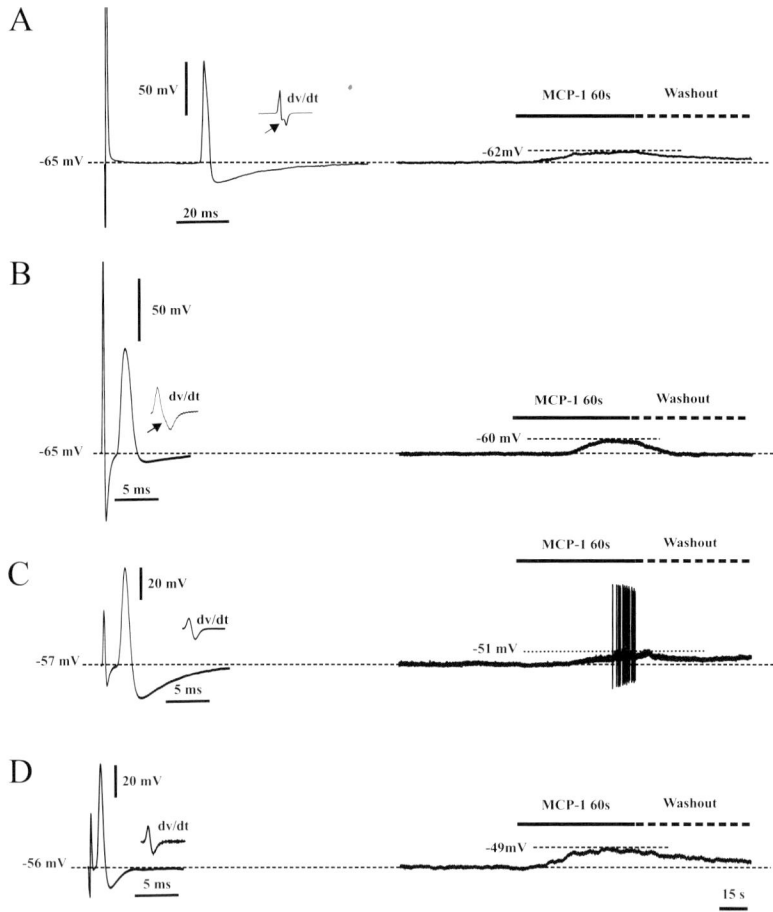

Fig. 1. Responses of DRG neurons to monocyte chemoattractant protein-1 (MCP-1/CCL2) applied to somata on the surface of the formerly compressed ganglion at POD5. The neurons were classified visually by somal size as small (A), medium (B and C), or large (D). Each neuron was further classified by axonal conduction velocity (action potential preceded by an artifact electrically evoked from the dorsal root, on the left) and by the presence or absence of a "hump" on the falling phase of the action potential causing an extra deflection in the first derivative (arrows, A and B left inset). The hump is typical for nociceptive neurons.

The chemokine MCP-1/CCL2 is upregulated and presumably released by sensory neurons in response to peripheral nerve injury (Tanaka et al. 2004; White et al. 2005c; Xie et al. 2006; Zhang and De Koninck 2006). Although there is no evidence for injury-induced upregulation in sensory neurons, fractalkine/CX3CL1 does exhibit increased release following peripheral nerve injury (Verge et al. 2004). Both MCP-1/CCL2 and fractalkine/CX3CL1 are likely to contribute to glial activation after peripheral nerve injury (Milligan et al. 2004; Zhang and De Koninck 2006). Upregulation of chemokines following nerve injury is not limited to the PNS because cells in the spinal cord also upregulate IP-10/CXCL10 (Glaser et al. 2004) and MCP-1/CCL2 (Zhang and De Koninck 2006).

Concurrent with peripheral nerve injury is the upregulation of the chemokine receptors, CCR1 in central neurons and CCR2 (Abbadie et al. 2003) and CX3CR1 in microglial cells (Verge et al. 2004). An excellent example of the direct contribution of chemokine receptors to persistent pain following peripheral injury has been demonstrated in CCR2 knockout mice (Abbadie et al. 2003). Perhaps more intriguing is the prospect that CX3CR neutralization can both prevent and attenuate neuropathic pain behavior (Milligan et al. 2004).

RELATIONSHIP OF CHEMOKINES TO DISEASE-RELATED CHRONIC PAIN

Neuropathic pain is a topic of some concern for individuals with autoimmune or life-threatening diseases because the pain syndromes are difficult to treat and significantly detract from the patients' quality of life. A prime example is the pain syndrome called distal symmetrical polyneuropathy (DSP), which affects as many as one-third of all HIV-infected individuals (Skopelitis et al. 2006). This painful sensory neuropathy frequently begins with paresthesias in the fingers and toes progressing over weeks to months, followed by the development of pain, often of a burning and lancinating nature, which can make walking very difficult. Measurements of pain hypersensitivity have demonstrated allodynia and hyperalgesia in HIV-1-infected individuals. Interestingly, as is the case for HIV-1-associated effects on the CNS (noted previously), there is no productive infection of peripheral neurons by the virus. Thus, indirect effects of HIV-1 must lead to the development of this pain state (e.g., gp120 binding to either CCR5 or CXCR4).

There are at least two ways in which HIV-1-induced DSP may occur: (1) Viral protein shedding in the PNS enables gp120 to produce painful neuropathy via glial/neuronal signaling in the DRG and/or spinal cord (Milligan et al. 2000; Keswani et al. 2003) or (2) gp120 directly activates sensory neurons (Herzberg and Sagen 2001; Oh et al. 2001).

To complicate matters further, AIDS patients who are treated with highly active antiretroviral therapeutic (HAART) agents can also develop a painful sensory neuropathy. Intriguingly, the symptoms of this syndrome are clinically indistinguishable from those of HIV-induced DSP, including a burning sensation in the hands and feet and hypersensitivity to pain. The fact that the two syndromes are usually seen in association with one another makes diagnosis more difficult.

Recent studies have shed new light on the mechanisms of HAART-induced DSP (Bhangoo et al., 2007). The authors found that the HAART drug, 2',3'-dideoxycytidine (zalcitabine or ddC), produced neuropathic pain behavior, increased CXCR4 mRNA expression in the DRG, and significantly increased SDF1/CXCL12-dependent neuronal activation. Moreover, ddC-induced rodent pain behavior could be attenuated using the highly specific CXCR4 antagonist, AMD3100 (Bhangoo et al. 2007).

PNS and CNS inflammatory demyelinating diseases such as Guillain-Barré syndrome (acute idiopathic polyneuritis), Charcot-Marie-Tooth disease types 1 and 4, and multiple sclerosis can also be accompanied by neuropathic pain (Carter et al. 1998). Epidemiological studies suggest that chronic pain syndromes afflict 50–80% of patients with multiple sclerosis and 70–90% of individuals with Guillain-Barré syndrome (Moulin 1998). Disease-related components that may be central to this neuropathic pain symptomatology may include axonal degeneration and the resulting Wallerian degeneration (Bruck 2005) and the upregulation and chronic expression of chemokines and their cognate receptors (Mahad et al. 2002; Charo and Ransohoff 2006).

There is presently little direct evidence of chemokines contributing to neuropathic pain in acute and chronic inflammatory demyelinating disorders in humans. However, direct study in several rodent models of demyelinating diseases known to elicit neuropathic pain behavior may be instrumental in determining the possible role of chemokine-influenced chronic pain. These models include late-developing peripheral axon demyelination in periaxin knockout mice (Gillespie et al. 2000); lysophosphatidylcholine-induced transient focal demyelination of the sciatic nerve in mice and rats (Wallace et al. 2003; White et al. 2005b; Bhangoo et al. 2006); and the late, acute clinical phase of experimental autoimmune neuritis (Moalem-Taylor et al. 2007; unpublished observations). Rats and mice subjected to transient focal demyelination of the sciatic nerve exhibit chronic upregulation of MCP-1/CCL2 and IP-10/CXCL10 and the receptors CCR2, CCR5, and CXCR4 in primary sensory neurons (White et al. 2005b; Bhangoo et al. 2006). These chemokines/receptors may effectively modulate the accompanying chronic pain behavior by modifying the manner in which these sensory neurons respond to peripheral stimuli.

CONCLUSIONS

Chemokines are responsible for specific recruitment of leukocytes during inflammation and disease. Besides the well-established role of chemokines in the immune system, a number of chemokines and their receptors exert their activity in neural stem cells and are constitutively expressed by adult neurons and glial cells, where they are involved in intercellular communication. Chemokines exhibit de novo expression in the nervous system following the induction of disease and nerve injury, and they may be central to neurodegeneration or neuroprotection. Recently, it has been shown that chemokine/receptor interactions are also associated with modification of the physiological properties of sensory neurons following peripheral nerve injury, including hyperalgesia and allodynia. There is uncertainty about the exact mechanism by which chemokines act in these states, because they could affect neurons either directly or indirectly. Nonetheless, the data suggest that strategies aimed at limiting the actions of chemokines may result an important new direction of therapy.

ACKNOWLEDGMENTS

F.A. White: NIH grant NS049136, Illinois Excellence in Medicine, State of Illinois; R.H. LaMotte: NIH grant NS14624.

REFERENCES

Abbadie C, Lindia JA, Cumiskey AM, et al. Impaired neuropathic pain responses in mice lacking the chemokine receptor CCR2. *Proc Natl Acad Sci USA* 2003; 100:7947–7952.

Ambrosini E, Aloisi F. Chemokines and glial cells: a complex network in the central nervous system. *Neurochem Res* 2004; 29:1017–1038.

Araujo DM, Cotman CW. Trophic effects of interleukin-4, -7 and -8 on hippocampal neuronal cultures: potential involvement of glial-derived factors. *Brain Res* 1993; 600:49–55.

Bagri A, Marin O, Plump AS, et al. Slit proteins prevent midline crossing and determine the dorsoventral position of major axonal pathways in the mammalian forebrain. *Neuron* 2002; 33:233–248.

Bajetto A, Bonavia RBS, Piccioli P, et al. Glial and neuronal cells express functional chemokine receptor CXCR4 and its natural ligand stromal cell-derived factor 1. *J Neurochem* 1999; 73:2348–2357.

Bajetto A, Bonavia R, Barbero S, Schettini G. Characterization of chemokines and their receptors in the central nervous system: physiopathological implications. *J Neurochem* 2002; 82:1311–1329.

Banisadr G, Fontanges P, Haour F, et al. Neuroanatomical distribution of CXCR4 in adult rat brain and its localization in cholinergic and dopaminergic neurons. *Eur J Neurosci* 2002a; 16:1661–1671.

Banisadr G, Queraud-Lesaux F, Boutterin MC, et al. Distribution, cellular localization and functional role of CCR2 chemokine receptors in adult rat brain. *J Neurochem* 2002b; 81:257–269.

Belmadani A, Tran PB, Ren D, et al. The chemokine stromal cell-derived factor-1 regulates the migration of sensory neuron progenitors. *J Neurosci* 2005; 25:3995–4003.

Belmadani A, Tran PB, Ren D, Miller RJ. Chemokines regulate the migration of neural progenitors to sites of neuroinflammation. *J Neurosci* 2006; 26:3182–3191.

Bezzi P, Domercq M, Brambilla L, et al. CXCR4-activated astrocyte glutamate release via TNFalpha: amplification by microglia triggers neurotoxicity. *Nat Neurosci* 2001; 4:702–710.

Bhangoo S, Jung H, Chan DM, et al. Peripheral demyelination injury induces upregulation of chemokine/receptor expression and neuronal signaling in a model of neuropathic pain. *Soc Neurosci Abstracts* 2006; 250.3.

Bhangoo SK, Ren D, Miller RJ, et al. CXCR4 chemokine receptor signaling mediates pain hypersensitivity in association with antiretroviral toxic neuropathy. *Brain Behav Immun* 2007; 21:581–591.

Bolin LM, Murray R, Lukacs NW, et al. Primary sensory neurons migrate in response to the chemokine RANTES. *J Neuroimmunol* 1998; 81:49–57.

Bruck W. The pathology of multiple sclerosis is the result of focal inflammatory demyelination with axonal damage. *J Neurol* 2005; 252(Suppl 5):3–9.

Campbell JN, Raja SN, Meyer RA, Mackinnon SE. Myelinated afferents signal the hyperalgesia associated with nerve injury. *Pain* 1988; 32:89–94.

Carter H, McKenna C, MacLeod R, Green R. Health professionals' responses to multiple sclerosis and motor neurone disease. *Palliat Med* 1998; 12:383–394.

Cartier L, Hartley O, Dubois-Dauphin M, Krause K-H. Chemokine receptors in the central nervous system: role in brain inflammation and neurodegenerative diseases. *Brain Res Rev* 2005; 48:16–42.

Ceradini DJ, Gurtner GC. Homing to hypoxia: HIF-1 as a mediator of progenitor cell recruitment to injured tissue. *Trends Cardiovasc Med* 2005; 15:57–63.

Chalasani SH, Sabelko KA, Sunshine MJ, et al. Chemokine, SDF-1, Reduces the effectiveness of multiple axonal repellents and is required for normal axon pathfinding. *J Neurosci* 2003a; 23:1360–1371.

Chalasani SH, Baribaud F, Coughlan CM, et al. The chemokine stromal cell-derived factor-1 promotes the survival of embryonic retinal ganglion cells. *J Neurosci* 2003b; 23:4601–4612.

Charo IF, Ransohoff RM. The many roles of chemokines and chemokine receptors in inflammation. *N Engl J Med* 2006; 354:610–621.

Chessell IP, Hatcher JP, Bountra C, et al. Disruption of the P2X7 purinoceptor gene abolishes chronic inflammatory and neuropathic pain. *Pain* 2005; 114:386–396.

Cook WJ, Kramer MF, Walker RM, et al. Persistent expression of chemokine and chemokine receptor RNAs at primary and latent sites of herpes simplex virus 1 infection. *Virol J* 2004; 1:5.

Coughlan CM, McManus CM, Sharron M, et al. Expression of multiple functional chemokine receptors and monocyte chemoattractant protein-1 in human neurons. *Neuroscience* 2000; 97:591–600.

Cowell RM, Silverstein FS. Developmental changes in the expression of chemokine receptor CCR1 in the rat cerebellum. *J Comp Neurol* 2003; 457:7–23.

DeLeo J, Rutkowski M, Winkelstein B. The modulatory role of spinal chemokine activation in neuropathic pain. *Soc Neurosci Abstracts* 2002; 655.16.

Elhofy A, Wang J, Tani M, et al. Transgenic expression of CCL2 in the central nervous system prevents experimental autoimmune encephalomyelitis. *J Leukoc Biol* 2005; 77:229–237.

Fife B, Huffnagle G, Kuziel W, Karpus WJ. CC chemokine receptor 2 is critical for induction of experimental autoimmune. *J Exp Med* 2000; 192:899–906.

Fife BT, Paniagua MC, Lukacs NW, Kunkel SL, Karpus WJ. Selective CC chemokine receptor expression by central nervous system-infiltrating encephalitogenic T cells during experimental autoimmune encephalomyelitis. *J Neurosci Res* 2001; 66:705–714.

Fulgenzi A, Dell'Antonio G, Foglieni C, et al. Inhibition of chemokine expression in rat inflamed paws by systemic use of the antihyperalgesic oxidized ATP. *BMC Immunol* 2005; 6:18.

Galasso JM, Liu Y, Szaflarski J, Warren JS, Silverstein FS. Monocyte chemoattractant protein-1 is a mediator of acute excitotoxic injury in neonatal rat brain. *Neuroscience* 2000; 101:737–744.

Ganju RK, Brubaker SA, Meyer J, et al. The alpha-chemokine, stromal cell-derived factor-1alpha, binds to the transmembrane G-protein-coupled CXCR-4 receptor and activates multiple signal transduction pathways. *J Biol Chem* 1998; 273:23169–23175.

Gillard SE, Lu M, Mastracci RM, Miller RJ. Expression of functional chemokine receptors by rat cerebellar neurons. *J Neuroimmunol* 2002; 124:16–28.

Gillespie CS, Sherman DL, Fleetwood-Walker SM, et al. Peripheral demyelination and neuropathic pain behavior in periaxin-deficient mice. *Neuron* 2000; 26:523–531.

Giovannelli A, Limatola C, Ragozzino D, et al. CXC chemokines interleukin-8 (IL-8) and growth-related gene product alpha (GROalpha) modulate Purkinje neuron activity in mouse cerebellum. *J Neuroimmunol* 1998; 92:122–132.

Glaser J, Gonzalez R, Perreau VM, Cotman CW, Keirstead HS. Neutralization of the chemokine CXCL10 enhances tissue sparing and angiogenesis following spinal cord injury. *J Neurosci Res* 2004; 77:701–708.

Gosselin RD, Varela C, Banisadr G, et al. Constitutive expression of CCR2 chemokine receptor and inhibition by MCP-1/CCL2 of GABA-induced currents in spinal cord neurones. *J Neurochem* 2005; 95:1023–1034.

Herzberg U, Sagen J. Peripheral nerve exposure to HIV viral envelope protein gp120 induces neuropathic pain and spinal gliosis. *J Neuroimmunol* 2001; 116:29–39.

Hirsch E, Katanaev VL, Garlanda C, et al. Central role for G protein-coupled phosphoinositide 3-kinase gamma in inflammation. *Science* 2000; 287:1049–1053.

Homma Y, Brull SJ, Zhang JM. A comparison of chronic pain behavior following local application of tumor necrosis factor alpha to the normal and mechanically compressed lumbar ganglia in the rat. *Pain* 2002; 95:239–246.

Horuk R. Chemokine receptors and HIV-1: the fusion of two major research fields. *Immunol Today* 1999; 20:89–94.

Horuk R, Martin AW, Wang Z, et al. Expression of chemokine receptors by subsets of neurons in the central nervous system. *J Immunol* 1997; 158:2882–2890.

Junger H, Sorkin LS. Nociceptive and inflammatory effects of subcutaneous TNFalpha. *Pain* 2000; 85:145–151.

Kakinuma T, Hwang ST. Chemokines, chemokine receptors, and cancer metastasis. *J Leukoc Biol* 2006; 79:639–651.

Karpus W, Lukacs N, McRae B, et al. An important role for the chemokine macrophage inflammatory protein-1 alpha in the pathogenesis of the T cell-mediated autoimmune disease, experimental autoimmune encephalomyelitis. *J Immunol* 1995; 155:5003–5010.

Kaul M, Garden GA, Lipton SA. Pathways to neuronal injury and apoptosis in HIV-associated dementia. *Nature* 2001; 410:988–994.

Keswani SC, Polley M, Pardo CA, et al. Schwann cell chemokine receptors mediate HIV-1 gp120 toxicity to sensory neurons. *Ann Neurol* 2003; 54:287–296.

Klein RS, Rubin JB, Gibson HD, et al. SDF-1 alpha induces chemotaxis and enhances Sonic hedgehog-induced proliferation of cerebellar granule cells. *Development* 2001; 128:1971–1981.

Kleinschnitz C, Brinkhoff J, Sommer C, Stoll G. Contralateral cytokine gene induction after peripheral nerve lesions: dependence on the mode of injury and NMDA receptor signaling. *Brain Res Mol Brain Res* 2005; 136:23–28.

Knaut H, Blader P, Strahle U, Schier AF. Assembly of trigeminal sensory ganglia by chemokine signaling. *Neuron* 2005; 47:653–666.

Kwan KY, Allchorne AJ, Vollrath MA, et al. TRPA1 contributes to cold, mechanical, and chemical nociception but is not essential for hair-cell transduction. *Neuron* 2006; 50:277–289.

Lapidot T, Dar A, Kollet O. How do stem cells find their way home? *Blood* 2005; 106:1901–1910.

Lazarini F, Casanova P, Tham TN, et al. Differential signalling of the chemokine receptor CXCR4 by stromal cell-derived factor 1 and the HIV glycoprotein in rat neurons and astrocytes. *Eur J Neurosci* 2000; 12:117–125.

Lieberam I, Agalliu D, Nagasawa T, Ericson J, Jessell TM. A CXCL12-CXCR4 chemokine signaling pathway defines the initial trajectory of mammalian motor axons. *Neuron* 2005; 47:667–679.

Limatola C, Ciotti MT, Mercanti D, et al. The chemokine growth-related gene product beta protects rat cerebellar granule cells from apoptotic cell death through alpha-amino-3-hydroxy-5-methyl-4-isoxazolepropionate receptors. *Proc Natl Acad Sci USA* 2000; 97:6197–6201.

Lindia JA, McGowan E, Jochnowitz N, Abbadie C. Induction of CX3CL1 expression in astrocytes and CX3CR1 in microglia in the spinal cord of a rat model of neuropathic pain. *J Pain* 2005; 6:434–438.

Liu B, Li H, Brull SJ, Zhang J-M. Increased sensitivity of sensory neurons to tumor necrosis factor alpha in rats with chronic compression of the lumbar ganglia. *J Neurophysiol* 2002; 88:1393–1399.

Lu M, Grove EA, Miller RJ. Abnormal development of the hippocampal dentate gyrus in mice lacking the CXCR4 chemokine receptor. *Proc Natl Acad Sci USA* 2002; 99:7090–7095.

Ma C, Shu Y, Zheng Z, et al. Similar electrophysiological changes in axotomized and neighboring intact dorsal root ganglion neurons. *J Neurophysiol* 2003; 89:1588–1602.

Ma Q, Jones D, Borghesani PR, et al. Impaired B-lymphopoiesis, myelopoiesis, and derailed cerebellar neuron migration in CXCR4- and SDF-1-deficient mice. *Proc Natl Acad Sci USA* 1998; 95:9448–9453.

Mahad DJ, Howell SJL, Woodroofe MN. Expression of chemokines in the CSF and correlation with clinical disease activity in patients with multiple sclerosis. *J Neurol Neurosurg Psychiatry* 2002; 72:498–502.

Maurer M, von Stebut E. Macrophage inflammatory protein-1. *Int J Biochem Cell Biol* 2004; 36:1882–1886.

Mellado M, Rodriguez-Frade JM, Manes S, Martinez AC. Chemokine signaling and functional responses: the role of receptor dimerization and TK pathway activation. *Annu Rev Immunol* 2001; 19:397–421.

Meucci O, Fatatis A, Simen AA, et al. Chemokines regulate hippocampal neuronal signaling and gp120 neurotoxicity. *Proc Natl Acad Sci USA* 1998; 95:14500–14505.

Meucci O, Fatatis A, Simen AA, Miller RJ. Expression of CX3CR1 chemokine receptors on neurons and their role in neuronal survival. *Proc Natl Acad Sci USA* 2000; 97:8075–8080.

Milligan ED, Mehmert KK, Hinde JL, et al. Thermal hyperalgesia and mechanical allodynia produced by intrathecal administration of the human immunodeficiency virus-1 (HIV-1) envelope glycoprotein, gp120. *Brain Res* 2000; 861:105–116.

Milligan ED, Zapata V, Chacur M, et al. Evidence that exogenous and endogenous fractalkine can induce spinal nociceptive facilitation in rats. *Eur J Neurosci* 2004; 20:2294–2302.

Mizuno T, Kawanokuchi J, Numata K, Suzumura A. Production and neuroprotective functions of fractalkine in the central nervous system. *Brain Res* 2003; 979:65–70.

Moalem-Taylor G, Allbutt HN, Iordanova MD, Tracey DJ. Pain hypersensitivity in rats with experimental autoimmune neuritis, an animal model of human inflammatory demyelinating neuropathy. *Brain Behav Immun* 2007; 21:699–710.

Moulin DE. Pain in central and peripheral demyelinating disorders. *Neurol Clin* 1998; 16:889–898.

Murphy PM. The molecular biology of leukocyte chemoattractant receptors. *Annu Rev Immunol* 1994; 12:593–633.

Nagata K, Duggan A, Kumar G, Garcia-Anoveros J. Nociceptor and hair cell transducer properties of TRPA1, a channel for pain and hearing. *J Neurosci* 2005; 25:4052–4061.

Nakayama T, Mutsuga N, Yao L, Tosato G. Prostaglandin E2 promotes degranulation-independent release of MCP-1 from mast cells. *J Leukoc Biol* 2006; 79:95–104.

Nelson TE, Gruol DL. The chemokine CXCL10 modulates excitatory activity and intracellular calcium signaling in cultured hippocampal neurons. *J Neuroimmunol* 2004; 156:74–87.

Nicol GD, Lopshire JC, Pafford CM. Tumor necrosis factor enhances the capsaicin sensitivity of rat sensory neurons. *J Neurosci* 1997; 17:975–982.

Obata K, Yamanaka H, Fukuoka T, et al. Contribution of injured and uninjured dorsal root ganglion neurons to pain behavior and the changes in gene expression following chronic constriction injury of the sciatic nerve in rats. *Pain* 2003; 101:65–77.

Oh SB, Tran PB, Gillard SE, et al. Chemokines and glycoprotein120 produce pain hypersensitivity by directly exciting primary nociceptive neurons. *J Neurosci* 2001; 21:5027–5035.

Oh SB, Endoh T, Simen AA, Ren D, Miller RJ. Regulation of calcium currents by chemokines and their receptors. *J Neuroimmunol* 2002; 123:66–75.

Ozaktay AC, Kallakuri S, Takebayashi T, et al. Effects of interleukin-1 beta, interleukin-6, and tumor necrosis factor on sensitivity of dorsal root ganglion and peripheral receptive fields in rats. *Eur Spine J* 2006; 15:1529–1537.

Qin X, Wan Y, Wang X. CCL2 and CXCL1 trigger calcitonin gene-related peptide release by exciting primary nociceptive neurons. *J Neurosci Res* 2005; 82:51–62.

Ragozzino D, Renzi M, Giovannelli A, Eusebi F. Stimulation of chemokine CXC receptor 4 induces synaptic depression of evoked parallel fibers inputs onto Purkinje neurons in mouse cerebellum. *J Neuroimmunol* 2002; 127:30–36.

Rodriguez-Frade JM, Mellado M, Martinez AC. Chemokine receptor dimerization: two are better than one. *Trends Immunol* 2001; 22:612–617.

Sasaki S, Hirata I, Maemura K, et al. Prostaglandin E2 inhibits lesion formation in dextran sodium sulphate-induced colitis in rats and reduces the levels of mucosal inflammatory cytokines. *Scand J Immunol* 2000; 51:23–28.

Sheth RN, Dorsi MJ, Li Y, Murinson BB, et al. Mechanical hyperalgesia after an L5 ventral rhizotomy or an L5 ganglionectomy in the rat. *Pain* 2002; 96:63–72.

Skopelitis EE, Kokotis PI, Kontos AN, et al. Distal sensory polyneuropathy in HIV-positive patients in the HAART era: an entity underestimated by clinical examination. *Int J STD AIDS* 2006; 17:467–472.

Sorkin LS, Xiao WH, Wagner R, Myers RR. Tumour necrosis factor-alpha induces ectopic activity in nociceptive primary afferent fibres. *Neuroscience* 1997; 81:255–262.

Sun J, Yang B, Ma C, Donnelly DF, LaMotte RH. Monocyte chemoattractant protein-1 (MCP-1) depolarizes acutely dissociated nociceptive neurons from chronically compressed dorsal root ganglia by activating a nonselective cationic conductance. *Soc Neurosci Abstracts* 2005; 35:511.

Sun JH, Yang B, Donnelly DF, Ma C, LaMotte RH. MCP-1 enhances excitability of nociceptive neurons in chronically compressed dorsal root ganglia. *J Neurophysiol* 2006; 96:2189–2199.

Szabo I, Chen XH, Xin L, et al. Heterologous desensitization of opioid receptors by chemokines inhibits chemotaxis and enhances the perception of pain. *Proc Natl Acad Sci USA* 2002; 99:10276–10281.

Tal M, Devor M. Ectopic discharge in injured nerves: comparison of trigeminal and somatic afferents. *Brain Res* 1992; 579:148–151.

Tanaka T, Minami M, Nakagawa T, Satoh M. Enhanced production of monocyte chemoattractant protein-1 in the dorsal root ganglia in a rat model of neuropathic pain: possible involvement in the development of neuropathic pain. *Neurosci Res* 2004; 48:463–469.

Theil D, Derfuss T, Paripovic I, et al. Latent herpesvirus infection in human trigeminal ganglia causes chronic immune response. *Am J Pathol* 2003; 163:2179–2184.

Torebjork HE, Lundberg LE, LaMotte RH. Central changes in processing of mechanoreceptive input in capsaicin-induced secondary hyperalgesia in humans. *J Physiol* 1992; 448:765–780.

Ubogu EE, Cossoy MB, Ransohoff RM. The expression and function of chemokines involved in CNS inflammation. *Trends Pharmacol Sci* 2006; 27:48–55.

Uwabe K, Matsumoto M, Nagata K. Monokine induced by interferon-gamma acts as a neurotrophic factor on PC12 cells and rat primary sympathetic neurons. *J Biol Chem* 2005; 280:34268–34277.

van der Meer P, Ulrich AM, Gonzalez-Scarano F, Lavi E. Immunohistochemical analysis of CCR2, CCR3, CCR5, and CXCR4 in the human brain: potential mechanisms for HIV dementia. *Exp Mol Pathol* 2000; 69:192–201.

Verge GM, Milligan ED, Maier SF, et al. Fractalkine (CX3CL1) and fractalkine receptor (CX3CR1) distribution in spinal cord and dorsal root ganglia under basal and neuropathic pain conditions. *Eur J Neurosci* 2004; 20:1150–1160.

Verri WA Jr, Cunha TM, Parada CA, et al. Hypernociceptive role of cytokines and chemokines: targets for analgesic drug development? *Pharmacol Ther* 2006; 112:116–138.

Vit JP, Ohara PT, Tien DA, et al. The analgesic effect of low dose focal irradiation in a mouse model of bone cancer is associated with spinal changes in neuro-mediators of nociception. *Pain* 2006; 120:188–201.

Wallace VCJ, Cottrell DF, Brophy PJ, Fleetwood-Walker SM. Focal lysolecithin-induced de-myelination of peripheral afferents results in neuropathic pain behavior that is attenuated by cannabinoids. *J Neurosci* 2003; 23:3221–3233.

Watkins LR, Maier SF. Glia: a novel drug discovery target for clinical pain. *Nat Rev Drug Discov* 2003; 2:973–985.

White FA, Bhangoo SK, Miller RJ. Chemokines: integrators of pain and inflammation. *Nat Rev Drug Discov* 2005a; 4:834–844.

White FA, Ripsch M, Bhangoo S, et al. Regulation of chemokines/receptors in the dorsal root ganglion following focal demyelination of the sciatic nerve. *Soc Neurosci Abstracts* 2005b; 748.49.

White FA, Sun J, Waters SM, et al. Excitatory monocyte chemoattractant protein-1 signaling is up-regulated in sensory neurons after chronic compression of the dorsal root ganglion. *Proc Natl Acad Sci USA* 2005c; 102:14092–14097.

Wickham S, Lu B, Ash J, Carr DJ. Chemokine receptor deficiency is associated with increased chemokine expression in the peripheral and central nervous systems and increased resistance to herpetic encephalitis. *J Neuroimmunol* 2005; 162:51–59.

Woolf CJ. Evidence for a central component of post-injury pain hypersensitivity. *Nature* 1983; 306:686–688.

Xie W, Strong JA, Meij JT, Zhang JM, Yu L. Neuropathic pain: early spontaneous afferent activity is the trigger. *Pain* 2005; 116:243–256.

Xie WR, Deng H, Li H, et al. Robust increase of cutaneous sensitivity, cytokine production and sympathetic sprouting in rats with localized inflammatory irritation of the spinal ganglia. *Neuroscience* 2006; 142:809–822.

Yabe T, Herbert J, Takanohashi A, Schwartz J. Treatment of cerebellar granule cell neurons with the neurotrophic factor pigment epithelium-derived factor in vitro enhances expression of other neurotrophic factors as well as cytokines and chemokines. *J Neurosci Res* 2004; 77:642–652.

Zhang J, De Koninck Y. Spatial and temporal relationship between monocyte chemoattractant protein-1 expression and spinal glial activation following peripheral nerve injury. *J Neurochem* 2006; 97:772–783.

Zhang N, Rogers TJ, Caterina M, Oppenheim JJ. Proinflammatory chemokines, such as C-C che-mokine ligand 3, desensitize mu-opioid receptors on dorsal root ganglia neurons. *J Immunol* 2004; 173:594–599.

Zhang N, Inan S, Cowan A, et al. A proinflammatory chemokine, CCL3, sensitizes the heat- and capsaicin-gated ion channel TRPV1. *Proc Natl Acad Sci USA* 2005; 102:4536–4541.

Zou YR, Kottmann AH, Kuroda M, Taniuchi I, Littman DR. Function of the chemokine receptor CXCR4 in haematopoiesis and in cerebellar development. *Nature* 1998; 393:595–599.

Correspondence to: Fletcher A. White, PhD, Department of Cell Biology, Neu-robiology and Anatomy, Loyola University Medical Center, 2160 S First Street, Maywood, IL 60153, USA. Tel: 1-708-216-6728; fax: 1-708-216-6731; email: fwhite@lumc.edu.

Immune and Glial Regulation of Pain, edited by Joyce A. DeLeo, Linda S. Sorkin, and Linda R. Watkins, IASP Press, Seattle, © 2007.

8

Electrophysiological Evidence of Enhanced Nociceptive Transmission in Response to Dorsal Root Exposure to Nucleus Pulposus

Jason M. Cuellar[a] and E. Carstens[b]

[a]Department of Anesthesia, Stanford University Medical Center, Stanford, California, USA; [b]Section of Neurobiology, Physiology and Behavior, University of California, Davis, California, USA

The intervertebral disk is a remarkable anatomic structure located at each vertebral column segment, distributing load while enabling incredible range of motion and enduring relatively enormous forces throughout our various activities of daily living (Wilke et al. 1999; Setton and Chen 2004). Each disk consists of an outer concentric fibrous lamella, the anulus fibrosus, and an inner gelatinous matrix of proteoglycans and collagens, known as the nucleus pulposus (NP) (Setton and Chen 2004). Failure of anulus fibrosus integrity can allow herniation of the NP, resulting in various clinical sequelae, such as radiculopathic pain in the arm or buttock and/or leg (sciatica), first described over 70 years ago (Mixter and Barr 1934). Symptoms often persist, resulting in surgery in an increasingly substantial percentage of cases (Deyo et al. 2005), yet despite decades of study, the actual mechanism by which herniated NP (HNP) causes pain remains unknown.

It was originally concluded that mechanical compression by NP of the dorsal root ganglion (DRG) or of the nerve root exiting or traversing the intervertebral foramen at the level of herniation was the source of the pain (Mixter and Barr 1934), and many animal models support this conclusion (Chatani et al. 1995; Cornefjord et al. 1997; Hu and Xing 1998; Song et al. 1999; Tabo et al. 1999; Zhang et al. 1999; Winkelstein et al. 2002; Ma et al. 2006). However, nerve root compression is often asymptomatic (Hitselberger and Witten 1968; Wiesel et al. 1984; Boden et al. 1990; Carragee et al. 2005), mechanical nerve root stimulation is only painful following NP exposure (Smyth and Wright

1958; Kuslich et al. 1991) and radiculopathy has been reported in the absence of nerve root compression (Fernstrom 1960). This evidence supports the hypothesis that leakage of the NP may cause symptoms of sciatica in the absence of nerve root compression (Lindahl 1966; Marshall et al. 1977; McCarron et al. 1987). Animal models have demonstrated that experimental herniation of NP or application of NP to nerve roots can induce histological changes and reduce nerve conduction velocity in evoked potentials of cauda equina nerve root (McCarron et al. 1987; Olmarker et al. 1993, 1996, 1997; Kayama et al. 1996, 1998; Otani et al. 1997; Kawakami et al. 1998), causing mechanical allodynia (Kawakami et al. 1996, 1998, 1999, 2000b, 2001, 2003) or thermal hyperalgesia (Kawakami et al. 1996, 2000a). Although these studies provide evidence of HNP-induced nerve root damage, they do not address the mechanism of radiculopathic pain, i.e., enhanced or pathological nociceptive transmission. This chapter reviews electrophysiological recordings from first- and second-order sensory neurons that have been performed to study the pathophysiological mechanisms of HNP-induced radiculopathy in greater detail.

DORSAL ROOT GANGLION NEURONS

Takeyabashi et al. (2001) performed multiunit recordings from the fifth lumbar (L5) dorsal root in rats, comparing responses evoked by mechanical stimulation of the receptive field area (hindpaw) or direct DRG stimulation before and up to 6 hours after the subdural application of NP to the L5 DRG. A gradual increase in spontaneous firing rate was observed after NP application compared to the subcutaneous fat control, which became significant 150 minutes post-NP and remained elevated to the 6-hour endpoint. Although the reduction in mechanical thresholds for hindpaw stimulation did not become statistically significant, that of direct mechanical DRG stimulation was significantly reduced. These findings are interesting because they provide a possible explanation for the spontaneous pain experienced by HNP-induced radiculopathy patients. If the threshold is lowered to mechanically evoke action potentials in DRG neurons, contact of the DRG with surrounding structures, such as those that form the intervertebral foramen (Cohen et al. 1990; Aota et al. 2001), could induce abnormal afferent neuronal discharges that might be interpreted as noxious stimulation or paresthesia (Nordin et al. 1984). The concept of the DRG as a source of aberrant neuronal discharge underlying neuropathic pain states has been proposed previously (Howe et al. 1977; Wall and Devor 1983; Nordin et al. 1984; Weinstein 1986; Devor and Wall 1990).

Ma et al. (2006) have recently shown that following chronic compression of the DRG (CCD model; Hu and Xing 1998; Zhang et al. 1999), an "inflammatory soup" containing bradykinin, serotonin, prostaglandin E_2, and histamine at equimolar concentrations (each 10^{-6} M) was more effective at inducing electrophysiological changes in both nociceptive and non-nociceptive DRG neurons. In this elegant and thorough study, recordings were made not only from dissociated rat DRG neurons but also from somata of intact DRG neurons and from single DRG fibers proximal to the somata, following CCD or in nonsurgical controls (Ma et al. 2006). Inflammatory soup applied to the intact DRG evoked action potential discharges following CCD but not in control neurons. In addition, following CCD, DRG neurons had a reduced threshold for evoked action potentials and an increased spontaneous firing rate, and inflammatory soup caused an increase in the CCD-induced spontaneous firing that was not observed in control neurons. Furthermore, the authors concluded that because results were similar for dissociated DRGs, which lack their associated satellite cells, as for intact DRGs, the inflammatory soup-induced excitability increases were (mechanistically) intrinsic to the DRG neurons (Ma et al. 2006). The authors did not, however, overlook the likelihood that during CCD, the DRG neurons may be surrounded by inflammatory mediators released from injured tissue and immune cells (Fig. 1). Although this study did not investigate the effects of NP, it does provide important insight into the possibility that HNP-induced sensory changes result from a combination of mechanical and inflammatory insult (Kawakami et al. 1994; Olmarker and Myers 1998). Herniated NP not only protrudes through the anulus fibrosus, disrupting the tissue layers, but may also compress the nerve roots and/or DRG, possibly causing edema of the DRG (Rydevik et al. 1989; Yabuki et al. 1998; Aota et al. 2001).

It remains unknown whether the cause of HNP-induced radiculopathic pain is an autoimmune reaction directed against the NP (Bobechko and Hirsch 1965; Elves et al. 1975; Gertzbein et al. 1975, 1977; Naylor et al. 1975) that affects the nearby nervous tissue via cytokines released from recruited and activated immune cells, such as macrophages (Gronblad et al. 1994; Haro et al. 1996; Ito et al. 1996; Murata et al. 2004b) and leukocytes (Kawakami et al. 2000b), or activated glial cells (Watkins and Maier 2005) (Fig. 1). However, evidence is growing for the involvement of an inflammatory component in this process (Marshall et al. 1977; McCarron et al. 1987; Olmarker et al. 1995), and the findings of Ma et al. (2006) may help corroborate the idea that compression of the DRG by a herniated disk may render the DRG more susceptible to the sensitizing effects of various inflammatory mediators and may be partly responsible for some clinically significant sensory effects due to spontaneous discharges of the DRG (Howe et al. 1977).

In addition to compressing the DRG and inducing local inflammatory changes around the DRG, NP exposure can directly damage DRG neurons (Kayama et al. 1996; Olmarker et al. 1996), inducing cellular apoptosis (Murata

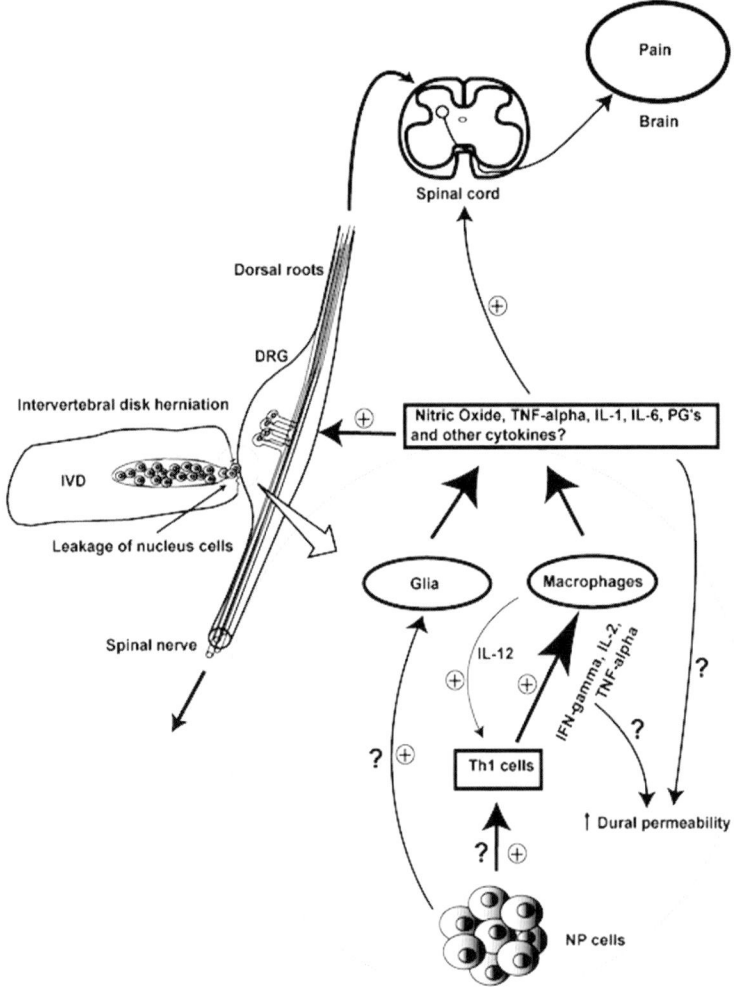

Fig. 1. Schematic diagram showing possible mechanisms of disk-herniation-induced sensitization of dorsal horn and/or dorsal root ganglion (DRG) neurons, ultimately resulting in spontaneous pain (sciatica). A representative intervertebral disk (IVD) is shown at left. Upon disk herniation, the nucleus pulposus (NP) extrudes out through the anulus fibrosus, compressing the DRG. NP cells may also leak out, possibly causing an autoimmune inflammatory reaction. The classic cellular immune response is mediated by T-helper type 1 (Th1) cells, which release interferon-gamma (IFN-γ), interleukin-2 (IL-2), and tumor necrosis factor alpha (TNF-α), activating macrophages. Upon activation, macrophages can release various inflammatory cytokines, some of which might induce sensitization of DRG and spinal cord dorsal horn neurons, resulting in aberrant nociceptive signals. Dural permeability may be compromised after exposure to NP cells (Murata et al. 2005); however, the mediator of this process remains unknown. Although it has not yet been demonstrated that glial cell activation is a mediator of disk-herniation-induced sensitization, there is growing evidence of a role for glial cells in inflammatory pain (Watkins and Maier 2005).

et al. 2006) and enhanced localization of TNF-α (Murata et al. 2004a; Weiler et al. 2005). Nucleus pulposus may also affect the DRG capsule, increasing its permeability to allow abnormal passage of even very large biomolecules (Murata et al. 2005), which could allow local and infiltrated cytokines to gain access to the DRG (Fig. 1).

SPINAL DORSAL HORN NEURONS

Two studies have shown enhanced responses of L5 wide-dynamic-range (WDR) neurons of the spinal dorsal horn after L5 nerve root exposure to NP. The first of these studies observed a prolonged firing of WDR neurons after hindpaw pinch 1–2 hours after epidural NP application, but not after control application of fat tissue (Anzai et al. 2002). Innocuous mechanical stimulation was not enhanced after NP application. However, statistical analyses were not performed to compare responses between or within groups. The second study reported statistically significant increases in WDR neuronal firing in response to pinch 1–2 hours after NP was harvested from a tail disk and placed onto the L5 nerve root (Onda et al. 2003). The authors made a distinction between the firing during the noxious stimulation—the "response"—and that which continued after the stimulation ceased—the "afterdischarge" (AD). The number of action potentials during the 60-second AD period was enhanced 2 hours after NP application to a much greater extent than during the response period. Importantly, coadministration of a rat monoclonal tumor necrosis factor (TNF) antibody (10 μL of 50 μg/mL in phosphate-buffered saline) with the NP prevented the enhanced AD firing. Responses to innocuous brushing of the hindpaw were not enhanced 2 hours after NP application.

Two other recent rat studies have shown enhanced responses of L5 WDR dorsal horn neurons after autologous NP from the tail was applied epidurally to the L5 DRG, rather than to the nerve root. Cuellar et al. (2004) observed a statistically significant enhancement of WDR neurons in response to a 10-second 46°C and a 50°C hindpaw stimulus with a Peltier thermode 1–3 hours after NP application. Although statistical analysis to compare the response and AD periods (as reported by Onda et al. 2003) was not performed (action potentials for 60 seconds after the stimulus onset were summed), it appears that the AD was the greatest contributor to the enhanced responses following NP application. Responses to mechanical von Frey stimulation with innocuous and noxious forces were also significantly enhanced 1–3 hours post-NP application. Coapplication of soluble TNF-α receptor type 1 (0.013 μg in 5 μL 0.9% saline) to the DRG with NP prevented the enhanced thermal and mechanical WDR neuronal responses. Although it might be tempting to implicate TNF-α as the cause of HNP-induced neuronal sensitization and thus pain, the finding that TNF-α blockade attenuates the process only implicates its involvement in what might be a complex inflammatory cascade. The finding that doxycycline is more effective than TNF-α blockade alone at preventing HNP-induced neuropathy suggests that several cytokines might be involved (Olmarker and Larsson 1998).

Wind-up is the progressive increase in nociceptive neuronal responses to repetitive C-fiber stimulation at a constant intensity (Mendell and Wall 1965), and its enhancement might be an indicator of central sensitization (Cook et al. 1987; Woolf 1996). Wind-up of L5 dorsal horn WDR neurons before and 1–3 hours after autologous epidural NP application to the L5 DRG was recently studied (Cuellar et al. 2005). The hindpaw receptive field area was stimulated at 0.1, 0.3, and 1.0 Hz with subcutaneous bipolar needle electrodes, using an intensity three times greater than that which elicited action potentials at latencies consistent with C-fiber input (100–400 ms). No windup was elicited at any time point before or after application of saline (control) during 0.1 Hz stimulation. However, wind-up of the late AD period (1–3.3 seconds following each stimulus) was observed 3 hours after NP application (Fig. 2). Wind-up was induced by 0.3 Hz stimulation before NP application and was significantly enhanced as early as 1 hour after NP application. Although the C-fiber response was enhanced 2–3 hours following NP, the AD period was the greatest contributor to the NP-induced enhancement, showing significant increases as early as 1 hour after NP application. These results are comparable to those of Onda et al. (2003) mentioned above, who reported that NP-induced enhancement of nociceptive dorsal horn neuronal responses was predominately due to increased action potentials during the AD period. Cuellar et al. (2005) also found that, in addition to enhanced wind-up during 1Hz stimulation, the initial (i.e., the first of the 20 consecutive stimuli) C-fiber response was also enhanced 1–2 hours post-NP application (Fig. 2). This finding is consistent with an increase in general

---

Fig. 2. Mean responses of wide-dynamic range (WDR) dorsal horn neurons to electrical stimulation (at 3 times the C-fiber threshold; 0.5-ms pulses) of the receptive field area on the hindpaw before (open symbols) vs. 3 hours after application (filled symbols) of saline or nucleus pulposus (NP) to the L5 dorsal root ganglion. The paw was electrically stimulated at frequencies of 0.1 Hz (A–D), 0.3 Hz (not shown), or 1 Hz (E–H). Graphs A and B display 0.1-Hz stimulus-induced responses following NP application during the C-fiber period (A; 100–400 ms latency) or afterdischarge period (B; 1–3.33 s latency). Graphs C and D similarly display responses for the same stimulation following saline control. Graphs E and F show responses during 1-Hz stimulation following NP application during the C-fiber period (E; 100–400 ms latency) or afterdischarge (AD) period (B; 400–1000 ms latency). Graphs G and H similarly display responses for the same stimulation following saline control. Error bars denote SEM. Asterisks indicate that the total number of spikes is significantly different than pretreatment (*P < 0.05, **P < 0.005; post hoc least significant difference test). Adapted from Cuellar et al. (2005). ⟶

0.1 Hz stimulation, NP treatment

A. C-fiber period

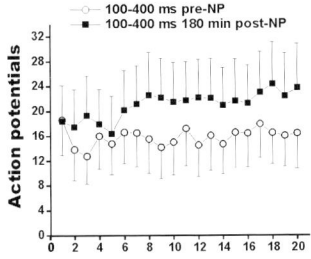

B. AD period

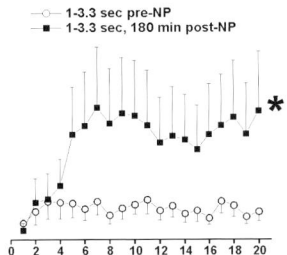

0.1 Hz stimulation, saline control

C. C-fiber period

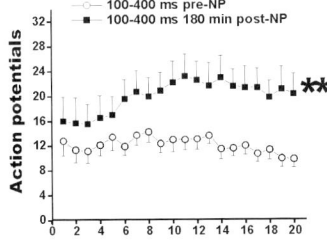

D. AD period

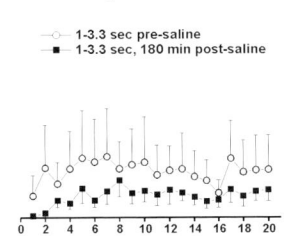

1 Hz stimulation, NP treatment

E. C-fiber period

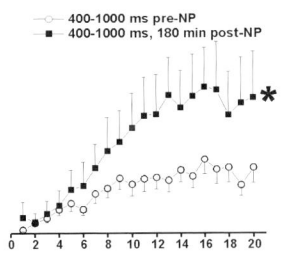

F. AD period

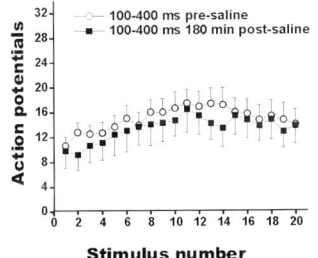

1 Hz stimulation, saline control

G. C-fiber period

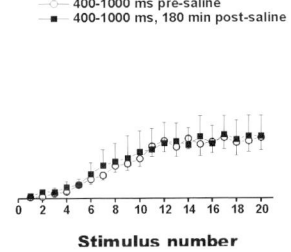

H. AD period

excitability of the dorsal horn neuron and/or with nociceptor sensitization. Al-though the observed enhancement of wind-up following epidural NP application supports an NP-induced central sensitization, the study design did not absolutely rule out the possibility that NP caused peripheral sensitization (i.e., sensitiza-tion of DRG neurons), increasing the excitability of these nociceptors. In that case, the observed increase in dorsal horn neuronal firing could have been a reflection of enhanced firing of sensitized nociceptors rather than of sensitized dorsal horn neurons. However, two observations argue against this possibility: (1) DRG neurons have not been observed to wind up (Herrero et al. 2000), and (2) an enhanced spontaneous firing rate was not observed. To completely rule out peripheral sensitization, the study must be repeated with direct sciatic nerve stimulation rather than stimulation of the cutaneous receptive field.

That the AD period was the most affected component of windup in these studies is interesting. What is the significance of this AD period? It might be a function of the slow removal of peptide neurotransmitters from the synap-tic cleft (Urban and Randic 1984; Gerber and Randic 1989; De Koninck and Henry 1991; Gerber et al. 1991; Radhakrishnan and Henry 1991). Exposure of the DRG neurons to NP enabled wind-up of dorsal horn neurons during 0.1-Hz stimulation, which does not normally occur (Sivilotti et al. 1993; Cuellar et al. 2005), suggesting an inability of the cell to completely repolarize within the normal time-course. This might result either from an increased release of neurotransmitters from the primary afferent (DRG) neurons (Urban and Ran-dic 1984; Baranauskas and Nistri 1998; Gardell et al. 2003) or from enhanced sensitivity or a prolonged response of the secondary (dorsal horn) neuron to the same amount of neurotransmitter, or from a combination of the two.

FUTURE STUDIES

The recent failure of TNF-α inhibition by infliximab (a monoclonal TNF-α antibody) to reduce sciatic pain more than an intravenous saline placebo in a human randomized control trial (Korhonen et al. 2005) highlights our mechanis-tic ignorance of this complex disease. More studies are needed to elucidate the detailed mechanisms by which nucleus pulposus exerts its neurophysiological changes in patients who sustain herniations. Human cytokine studies in patients with intervertebral disk herniations must be carefully performed with better con-trols than have been used in the past. If we are to elucidate future drug targets, electrophysiological studies such as that of Ma and colleagues must incorporate the simultaneous blockade of various mediators in the inflammatory cascade. Pending the realization of such studies, HNP-induced radiculopathy will most likely remain a disease treated surgically rather than pharmacologically.

REFERENCES

Anzai H, Hamba M, Onda A, Konno S, Kikuchi S. Epidural application of nucleus pulposus enhances nociresponses of rat dorsal horn neurons. *Spine* 2002; 27:E50–55.

Aota Y, Onari K, An HS, Yoshikawa K. Dorsal root ganglia morphologic features in patients with herniation of the nucleus pulposus: assessment using magnetic resonance myelography and clinical correlation. *Spine* 2001; 26:2125–2132.

Baranauskas G, Nistri A. Sensitization of pain pathways in the spinal cord: cellular mechanisms. *Prog Neurobiol* 1998; 54:349–365.

Bobechko W, Hirsch C. Auto-immune response to nucleus pulposus in the rabbit. *J Bone Joint Surg* 1965; 47B:574–580.

Boden SD, Davis DO, Dina TS, Patronas NJ, Wiesel SW. Abnormal magnetic-resonance scans of the lumbar spine in asymptomatic subjects. A prospective investigation. *J Bone Joint Surg Am* 1990; 72:403–408.

Carragee EJ, Alamin TF, Miller JL, Carragee JM. Discographic, MRI and psychosocial determinants of low back pain disability and remission: a prospective study in subjects with benign persistent back pain. *Spine J* 2005; 5:24–35.

Chatani K, Kawakami M, Weinstein JN, Meller ST, Gebhart GF. Characterization of thermal hyperalgesia, c-fos expression, and alterations in neuropeptides after mechanical irritation of the dorsal root ganglion. *Spine* 1995; 20:277–289; discussion 290.

Cohen MS, Wall EJ, Brown RA, Rydevik B, Garfin SR. 1990 AcroMed Award in basic science. Cauda equina anatomy. II: Extrathecal nerve roots and dorsal root ganglia. *Spine* 1990; 15:1248–1251.

Cook AJ, Woolf CJ, Wall PD, McMahon SB. Dynamic receptive field plasticity in rat spinal cord dorsal horn following C-primary afferent input. *Nature* 1987; 325:151–153.

Cornefjord M, Sato K, Olmarker K, Rydevik B, Nordborg C. A model for chronic nerve root compression studies. Presentation of a porcine model for controlled, slow-onset compression with analyses of anatomic aspects, compression onset rate, and morphologic and neurophysiologic effects. *Spine* 1997; 22:946–957.

Cuellar JM, Montesano PX, Carstens E. Role of TNF-alpha in sensitization of nociceptive dorsal horn neurons induced by application of nucleus pulposus to L5 dorsal root ganglion in rats. *Pain* 2004; 110:578–587.

Cuellar JM, Montesano PX, Antognini JF, Carstens E. Application of nucleus pulposus to L5 dorsal root ganglion in rats enhances nociceptive dorsal horn neuronal windup. *J Neurophysiol* 2005; 94:35–48.

De Koninck Y, Henry JL. Substance P-mediated slow excitatory postsynaptic potential elicited in dorsal horn neurons in vivo by noxious stimulation. *Proc Natl Acad Sci USA* 1991; 88:11344–11348.

Devor M, Wall PD. Cross-excitation in dorsal root ganglia of nerve-injured and intact rats. *J Neurophysiol* 1990; 64:1733–1746.

Deyo RA, Gray DT, Kreuter W, Mirza S, Martin BI. United States trends in lumbar fusion surgery for degenerative conditions. *Spine* 2005; 30:1441–1445; discussion 1446–1447.

Elves MW, Bucknill T, Sullivan MF. In vitro inhibition of leucocyte migration in patients with intervertebral disc lesions. *Orthop Clin North Am* 1975; 6:59–65.

Fernstrom V. Disk rupture with surgical observations. *Acta Chir Scand Suppl* 1960; 258.

Gardell LR, Vanderah TW, Gardell SE, et al. Enhanced evoked excitatory transmitter release in experimental neuropathy requires descending facilitation. *J Neurosci* 2003; 23:8370–8379.

Gerber G, Randic M. Participation of excitatory amino acid receptors in the slow excitatory synaptic transmission in the rat spinal dorsal horn in vitro. *Neurosci Lett* 1989; 106:220–228.

Gerber G, Cerne R, Randic M. Participation of excitatory amino acid receptors in the slow excitatory synaptic transmission in rat spinal dorsal horn. *Brain Res* 1991; 561:236–251.

Gertzbein SD, Tile M, Gross A, Falk R. Autoimmunity in degenerative disc disease of the lumbar spine. *Orthop Clin North Am* 1975; 6:67–73.

Gertzbein SD, Tait JH, Devlin SR. The stimulation of lymphocytes by nucleus pulposus in patients with degenerative disk disease of the lumbar spine. *Clin Orthop* 1977:149–154.

Gronblad M, Virri J, Tolonen J, et al. A controlled immunohistochemical study of inflammatory cells in disc herniation tissue. *Spine* 1994; 19:2744–2751.

Haro H, Shinomiya K, Komori H, et al. Upregulated expression of chemokines in herniated nucleus pulposus resorption. *Spine* 1996; 21:1647–1652.

Herrero JF, Laird JM, Lopez-Garcia JA. Wind-up of spinal cord neurones and pain sensation: much ado about something? *Prog Neurobiol* 2000; 61:169–203.

Hitselberger WE, Witten RM. Abnormal myelograms in asymptomatic patients. *J Neurosurg* 1968; 28:204–206.

Howe JF, Loeser JD, Calvin WH. Mechanosensitivity of dorsal root ganglia and chronically injured axons: a physiological basis for the radicular pain of nerve root compression. *Pain* 1977; 3:25–41.

Hu SJ, Xing JL. An experimental model for chronic compression of dorsal root ganglion produced by intervertebral foramen stenosis in the rat. *Pain* 1998; 77:15–23.

Ito T, Yamada M, Ikuta F, et al. Histologic evidence of absorption of sequestration-type herniated disc. *Spine* 1996; 21:230–234.

Kawakami M, Weinstein JN, Chatani K, et al. Experimental lumbar radiculopathy. Behavioral and histologic changes in a model of radicular pain after spinal nerve root irritation with chromic gut ligatures in the rat. *Spine* 1994; 19:1795–1802.

Kawakami M, Tamaki T, Weinstein JN, et al. Pathomechanism of pain-related behavior produced by allografts of intervertebral disc in the rat. *Spine* 1996; 21:2101–2107.

Kawakami M, Tamaki T, Hayashi N, Hashizume H, Nishi H. Possible mechanism of painful radiculopathy in lumbar disc herniation. *Clin Orthop* 1998; 23:241–251.

Kawakami M, Matsumoto T, Kuribayashi K, Tamaki T. mRNA expression of interleukins, phospholipase A2, and nitric oxide synthase in the nerve root and dorsal root ganglion induced by autologous nucleus pulposus in the rat. *J Orthop Res* 1999; 17:941–946.

Kawakami M, Tamaki T, Hayashi N, et al. Mechanical compression of the lumbar nerve root alters pain-related behaviors induced by the nucleus pulposus in the rat. *J Orthop Res* 2000a; 18:257–264.

Kawakami M, Tamaki T, Matsumoto T, et al. Role of leukocytes in radicular pain secondary to herniated nucleus pulposus. *Clin Orthop* 2000b; 26:268–277.

Kawakami M, Matsumoto T, Tamaki T. Roles of thromboxane A2 and leukotriene B4 in radicular pain induced by herniated nucleus pulposus. *J Orthop Res* 2001; 19:472–477.

Kawakami M, Hashizume H, Nishi H, et al. Comparison of neuropathic pain induced by the application of normal and mechanically compressed nucleus pulposus to lumbar nerve roots in the rat. *J Orthop Res* 2003; 21:535–539.

Kayama S, Konno S, Olmarker K, Yabuki S, Kikuchi S. Incision of the anulus fibrosus induces nerve root morphologic, vascular, and functional changes. An experimental study. *Spine* 1996; 21:2539–2543.

Kayama S, Olmarker K, Larsson K, et al. Cultured, autologous nucleus pulposus cells induce functional changes in spinal nerve roots. *Spine* 1998; 23:2155–2158.

Korhonen T, Karppinen J, Paimela L, et al. The treatment of disc herniation-induced sciatica with infliximab: results of a randomized, controlled, 3-month follow-up study. *Spine* 2005; 30:2724–2728.

Kuslich SD, Ulstrom CL, Michael CJ. The tissue origin of low back pain and sciatica: a report of pain response to tissue stimulation during operations on the lumbar spine using local anesthesia. *Orthop Clin North Am* 1991; 22:181–187.

Lindahl O. Hyperalgesia of the lumbar nerve roots in sciatica. *Acta Orthop Scand* 1966; 37:367–374.

Ma C, Greenquist KW, Lamotte RH. Inflammatory mediators enhance the excitability of chronically compressed dorsal root ganglion neurons. *J Neurophysiol* 2006; 95:2098–2107.

Marshall LL, Trethewie ER, Curtain CC. Chemical radiculitis. A clinical, physiological and immunological study. *Clin Orthop* 1977; 129:61–67.

McCarron RF, Wimpee MW, Hudkins PG, Laros GS. The inflammatory effect of nucleus pulposus. A possible element in the pathogenesis of low-back pain. *Spine* 1987; 12:760–764.

Mendell LM, Wall PD. Responses of single dorsal cord cells to peripheral cutaneous unmyelinated fibres. *Nature* 1965; 206:97 99.

Mixter WJ, Barr JS. Rupture of the intervertebral disc with involvement of the spinal canal. *N Engl J Med* 1934; 211:210–215.

Murata Y, Onda A, Rydevik B, Takahashi K, Olmarker K. Distribution and appearance of tumor necrosis factor-alpha in the dorsal root ganglion exposed to experimental disc herniation in rats. *Spine* 2004a; 29:2235–2241.

Murata Y, Rydevik B, Takahashi K, Takahashi I, Olmarker K. Macrophage appearance in the epineurium and endoneurium of dorsal root ganglion exposed to nucleus pulposus. *J Peripher Nerv Syst* 2004b; 9:158–164.

Murata Y, Rydevik B, Takahashi K, Larsson K, Olmarker K. Incision of the intervertebral disc induces disintegration and increases permeability of the dorsal root ganglion capsule. *Spine* 2005; 30:1712–1716.

Murata Y, Nannmark U, Rydevik B, Takahashi K, Olmarker K. Nucleus pulposus-induced apoptosis in dorsal root ganglion following experimental disc herniation in rats. *Spine* 2006; 31:382–390.

Naylor A, Happey F, Turner RL, et al. Enzymic and immunological activity in the intervertebral disk. *Orthop Clin North Am* 1975; 6:51–58.

Nordin M, Nystrom B, Wallin U, Hagbarth KE. Ectopic sensory discharges and paresthesiae in patients with disorders of peripheral nerves, dorsal roots and dorsal columns. *Pain* 1984; 20:231–245.

Olmarker K, Larsson K. Tumor necrosis factor alpha and nucleus-pulposus-induced nerve root injury. *Spine* 1998; 23:2538–2544.

Olmarker K, Rydevik B, Nordborg C. Autologous nucleus pulposus induces neurophysiologic and histologic changes in porcine cauda equina nerve roots. *Spine* 1993; 18:1425–1432.

Olmarker K, Blomquist J, Strömberg J, et al. Inflammatogenic properties of nucleus pulposus. *Spine* 1995; 20:665–669.

Olmarker K, Nordborg C, Larsson K, Rydevik B. Ultrastructural changes in spinal nerve roots induced by autologous nucleus pulposus. *Spine* 1996; 21:411–414.

Olmarker K, Brisby H, Yabuki S, Nordborg C, Rydevik B. The effects of normal, frozen, and hyaluronidase-digested nucleus pulposus on nerve root structure and function. *Spine* 1997; 22:471–475; discussion 476.

Olmarker K, Myers RR. Pathogenesis of sciatic pain: role of herniated nucleus pulposus and deformation of spinal nerve root and dorsal root ganglion. *Pain* 1998; 78:99–105.

Onda A, Yabuki S, Kikuchi S. Effects of neutralizing antibodies to tumor necrosis factor-alpha on nucleus pulposus-induced abnormal nociresponses in rat dorsal horn neurons. *Spine* 2003; 28:967–972.

Otani K, Arai I, Mao GP, et al. Experimental disc herniation: evaluation of the natural course. *Spine* 1997; 22:2894–2899.

Radhakrishnan V, Henry JL. Novel substance P antagonist, CP-96,345, blocks responses of cat spinal dorsal horn neurons to noxious cutaneous stimulation and to substance P. *Neurosci Lett* 1991; 132:39–43.

Rydevik BL, Myers RR, Powell HC. Pressure increase in the dorsal root ganglion following mechanical compression. Closed compartment syndrome in nerve roots. *Spine* 1989; 14:574–576.

Setton LA, Chen J. Cell mechanics and mechanobiology in the intervertebral disc. *Spine* 2004; 29:2710–2723.

Sivilotti LG, Thompson SW, Woolf CJ. Rate of rise of the cumulative depolarization evoked by repetitive stimulation of small-caliber afferents is a predictor of action potential windup in rat spinal neurons in vitro. *J Neurophysiol* 1993; 69:1621–1631.

Smyth MJ, Wright V. Sciatica and the intervertebral disc: An experimental study. *J Bone Joint Surg* 1958; 40–A:1401–1418.

Song XJ, Hu SJ, Greenquist KW, Zhang JM, LaMotte RH. Mechanical and thermal hyperalgesia and ectopic neuronal discharge after chronic compression of dorsal root ganglia. *J Neurophysiol* 1999; 82:3347–3358.

Tabo E, Jinks SL, Eisele JH Jr, Carstens E. Behavioral manifestations of neuropathic pain and mechanical allodynia, and changes in spinal dorsal horn neurons, following L4-L6 dorsal root constriction in rats. *Pain* 1999; 80:503–520.

Takebayashi T, Cavanaugh JM, Cuneyt Ozaktay A, Kallakuri S, Chen C. Effect of nucleus pulposus on the neural activity of dorsal root ganglion. *Spine* 2001; 26:940–945.

Urban L, Randic M. Slow excitatory transmission in rat dorsal horn: possible mediation by peptides. *Brain Res* 1984; 290:336–341.

Wall PD, Devor M. Sensory afferent impulses originate from dorsal root ganglia as well as from the periphery in normal and nerve injured rats. *Pain* 1983; 17:321–339.

Watkins LR, Maier SF. Immune regulation of central nervous system functions: from sickness responses to pathological pain. *J Intern Med* 2005; 257:139–155.

Weiler C, Nerlich AG, Bachmeier BE, Boos N. Expression and distribution of tumor necrosis factor alpha in human lumbar intervertebral discs: a study in surgical specimen and autopsy controls. *Spine* 2005; 30:44–53; discussion 54.

Weinstein J. Report of the 1985 ISSLS Traveling Fellowship. Mechanisms of spinal pain. The dorsal root ganglion and its role as a mediator of low-back pain. *Spine* 1986; 11:999–1001.

Wiesel SW, Tsourmas N, Feffer HL, Citrin CM, Patronas N. A study of computer-assisted tomography. I. The incidence of positive CAT scans in an asymptomatic group of patients. *Spine* 1984; 9:549–551.

Wilke HJ, Neef P, Caimi M, Hoogland T, Claes LE. New in vivo measurements of pressures in the intervertebral disc in daily life. *Spine* 1999; 24:755–762.

Winkelstein BA, Weinstein JN, DeLeo JA. The role of mechanical deformation in lumbar radiculopathy: an in vivo model. *Spine* 2002; 27:27–33.

Woolf CJ. Windup and central sensitization are not equivalent. *Pain* 1996; 66:105–108.

Yabuki S, Kikuchi S, Olmarker K, Myers RR. Acute effects of nucleus pulposus on blood flow and endoneurial fluid pressure in rat dorsal root ganglia. *Spine* 1998; 23:2517–2523.

Zhang JM, Song XJ, LaMotte RH. Enhanced excitability of sensory neurons in rats with cutaneous hyperalgesia produced by chronic compression of the dorsal root ganglion. *J Neurophysiol* 1999; 82:3359–3366.

Correspondence to: Earl Carstens, PhD, Section of Neurobiology, Physiology and Behavior, University of California, Davis, 1 Shields Avenue, Davis, CA 95616, USA. Email: eecarstens@ucdavis.edu.

Immune and Glial Regulation of Pain, edited by Joyce
A. DeLeo, Linda S. Sorkin, and Linda R. Watkins,
IASP Press, Seattle, © 2007.

9

Peripheral Nerve Injury and Protection by Erythropoietin: Dorsal Root Ganglion Signaling Cascades and Chronic Pain

W. Marie Campana

*Department of Anesthesiology, University of California,
San Diego, La Jolla, California, USA*

Erythropoietin (Epo) is a hematopoietic cytokine best known for its production in the kidney and for its essential effects on the survival, proliferation, and differentiation of erythroid progenitor cells (Krantz 1991). The development of recombinant Epo as a biopharmaceutical for the treatment of anemia and its approval by the U.S. Food and Drug Administration have dramatically improved the quality of life of patients suffering from chronic kidney disease (Ludwig and Strasser 2001). In addition to its function in hematopoiesis, Epo has been identified as a potent neuroprotective factor (Sakanaka et al. 1998; Siren et al. 2001; Campana and Myers 2003) and more recently, as an anti-inflammatory agent (Agnello et al. 2002; Genc et al. 2004; Campana et al. 2006; Savino et al. 2006). These activities are demonstrable in both the central and peripheral nervous systems.

Epo elicits its effects by binding to the predimerized Epo receptor (EpoR). The EpoR is a member of the cytokine receptor superfamily, characterized by conserved cysteines and a WSXWS motif in the extracellular domain, but it has more limited similarities in the cytoplasmic region (Bazan 1990). Binding of Epo to its receptor results in the formation of a high-affinity complex (K_D ~ 0.1–10 nM) in various cell types (Wojchowski et al. 1999). This process causes conformational changes in the EpoR and results in recruitment of the tyrosine kinase, Janus kinase-2 (JAK2), to the receptor. JAK2 plays a vital role in mediating signals downstream of the EpoR (Witthuhn et al. 1993). JAK2-specific antisense oligonucleotides and dominant-negative forms of JAK2 block the biological activities of Epo (Ihle et al. 1994). Signaling proteins activated downstream of JAK2 include signal transducer and activator of transcription-5

(STAT5) (Bittorf et al. 2000), phosphoinositide-3-kinase (PI3K), and protein kinase B (Akt) (Bao et al. 2005), as well as the Ras-extracellular regulated kinase (ERK)/mitogen-activated protein (MAP) kinase pathway (Arai et al. 2002).

The presence of the Epo receptor in mouse brain was first demonstrated by the binding of radiolabeled Epo to brain slices (Digicaylioglu et al. 1995). Intense Epo binding was observed in the hippocampus, cortex, and midbrain areas. In human adult brain, the Epo receptor is present in neurons, astrocytes, and microglia, but not in oligodendrocytes (Nagai et al. 2001). It is also located in the spinal cord and may be most abundant in nociceptive neurons (Sekiguchi et al. 2003). We established the presence of the EpoR in the peripheral nervous system (PNS) by identifying it in the cell bodies of dorsal root ganglion (DRG) primary sensory neurons by immunohistochemistry and by immunoprecipitation from tissue extracts (Campana and Myers 2001, 2003). Expression of the EpoR is developmentally regulated. In humans, Epo receptors are most abundant in both the brain and spinal cord by 16 weeks (Juul et al. 1999). Whether age-dependent expression of the EpoR is related to the ability of neurons to survive injury is an important question.

We are rapidly learning a number of facts regarding the biochemistry of the EpoR in the nervous system, but the significance of these data remains to be determined. The apparent molecular mass of the EpoR varies depending upon cell type (Masuda et al. 1993); this variability probably reflects glycosylation and may regulate receptor affinity for Epo. In addition to the membrane-anchored form, soluble EpoR may be generated (Nagao et al. 1992). The soluble receptor retains Epo-binding activity and may neutralize endogenously produced or exogenous Epo (Sakanaka et al. 1998). The former effect would serve to counteract autocrine or paracrine pathways within the nerve. The functional significance of the EpoR in the central nervous system (CNS) was demonstrated in studies of EpoR gene knockout mice. EpoR gene deficiency is lethal to the embryo; however, prior to death (day E12), a significant number of neuronal progenitor cells showed increased sensitivity to low oxygen tension and underwent extensive apoptosis (Yu et al. 2002). These results suggested that EpoR-dependent cell signaling might be neuroprotective. Additional evidence for this hypothesis came from a study by Sakanaka et al. (1998), in which recombinant human erythropoietin (rhEpo) was infused for 7 days at 0.5–25 units/day into the lateral ventricles of gerbils, with or without occlusion of the common carotid artery. Epo prevented ischemic damage and improved the function of the animals in learning tests, compared with vehicle-treated controls. Epo treatment rescued neurons that otherwise would have degenerated. The same investigators also showed that infusion of soluble EpoR, under conditions of mild ischemia, induces neuronal damage, increases terminal deoxynucleotidyl transferase biotin dUTP nick end labeling (TUNEL)-positive hippocampal neurons, and impairs learning ability. In more recent studies, Epo has proven to be neuroprotective in animal models of spinal cord compression injury (Grasso et al. 2005), autoimmune encephalomyelitis (Agnello et al. 2002), schizophrenia (Ehrenreich et al. 2004), and traumatic brain injury (Brines et al. 2000). Collectively, these findings suggest that Epo and the EpoR are potent neuroprotective factors within the CNS.

The potential activity of Epo in counteracting neuropathic pain after peripheral nerve injury was first established using an L5 spinal nerve crush (L5 SNC) injury model in rats (Campana and Myers 2003). This type of injury results in chronic mechanical allodynia (Winkelstein et al. 2001). Because the injury is in close proximity to the DRG, this model also is associated with effects on DRG neuronal viability (Degn et al. 1999). We treated rats with Epo systemically because Epo readily crosses the blood-brain barrier, apparently using a saturable, receptor-mediated mechanism (Brines et al. 2000). Others have demonstrated that systemically delivered Epo protects against metabolic stress and neuronal death in the CNS (Siren et al. 2001). In our studies, Epo given as a daily subcutaneous injection of 2680 units/kg, beginning one day prior to injury, did not initially protect against pain-related behaviors, compared with vehicle-treated controls; however, Epo treatment substantially improved the rate of recovery (Campana and Myers 2003). We tried a number of procedures to improve the response of animals in the early course of our studies, including pretreatment with Epo or using a higher dose (5000 units/kg); however, again, Epo did not alleviate initial pain-related behaviors. We observed similar results with Epo in the chronic constriction injury (CCI) model (Campana et al. 2006). Thus, these results suggested that Epo is effective at counteracting processes that lead to the maintenance of chronic pain states, but not the development of pain. We speculate that the activity demonstrated by Epo in these early studies may be most relevant to chronic pain states in human patients.

More recently, Epo has been identified as a potential therapeutic for peripheral neuropathies associated with pain in diabetes (Bianchi et al. 2004), HIV (Keswani et al. 2004), and chemotherapy-induced neuropathies (Bianchi et al. 2006). Epo specifically rescues cultured DRG neurons from axonal degeneration and death induced by the HIV-1 envelope protein gp120 and by the antiretroviral drug zalcitabine (Keswani et al. 2004); this axonal damage may be responsible for pain in HIV neuropathy. In diabetic and chemotherapy-induced neuropathies, there is a significant loss of C-fiber innervation of the epidermis and a concurrent elevation of thermal withdrawal latency (hypoalgesia). In an animal model of diabetic neuropathy (induced by streptozotocin), systemic, thrice-weekly treatments with rhEpo prevented the loss of these nociceptive fibers, which corresponded with reduction of the hypoalgesia; thermal withdrawal latencies returned toward basal levels. RhEpo also reduced mechanical hyperalgesia in diabetic rats after 5 weeks of treatment. Similar to what we have observed in models of mechanical nerve injury, treatment with Epo had no nociceptive effects in uninjured animals (Campana and Myers 2003; Bianchi et al. 2004). Collectively, our data demonstrate that Epo modulates pain-related behaviors associated with abnormal changes in C- and Aβ-fiber functions. In addition, the persistence of pain in peripheral neuropathies can be associated with changes in the viability of primary sensory neurons (Feldman et al. 2003). Thus, the neuroprotective effects of Epo may minimize nociceptive alterations that lead to chronic pain states.

Recent studies from our laboratory and from the laboratories of others suggest that the neuroprotective activity of Epo and EpoR in the PNS probably reflects receptors expressed not only by neurons, but also by Schwann cells. Peripheral nerve injury (crush or CCI) induces rapid upregulation of Epo mRNA and its receptor at the site of injury and distal to the injury site (Li et al. 2005). By contrast, increased Epo mRNA is not observed in the DRG. We localized the source of Epo production in the injured nerve to activated Schwann cells; the Epo receptor was present in both axons and Schwann cells. Schwann-cell-produced Epo may function in an autocrine/paracrine fashion, activating Schwann cell EpoR. However, Epo protein may be transported retrogradely from the injury site to the cell bodies of primary sensory neurons. In activated Schwann cells, Epo stimulates phosphorylation of the EpoR and of JAK2 and ERK/MAP kinase (Li et al. 2005). ERK1/2 phosphorylation occurs downstream of JAK2, given that pharmacological antagonism of JAK2 with AG490 blocks ERK1/2 phosphorylation. In Schwann cells, activation of the JAK2-ERK/MAP kinase pathway leads to cell proliferation in vitro and in vivo.

In the injured nerve, Schwann cells play an essential role in both degeneration of injured axons and in regeneration. This regulatory activity is mediated in part by secreted growth factors and cytokines (Myers 1997). Epo-induced cell signaling in Schwann cells decreases injury-induced expression of mRNA for the proinflammatory cytokine tumor necrosis factor-α (TNF-α) (Campana et al. 2006). TNF-α is a major orchestrator of Wallerian degeneration and initiator of chronic neuropathic pain states (Wagner and Myers 1996a,b; Sorkin et al. 1997). The ability of Epo to limit Schwann-cell-produced TNF-α within the first 5 days after injury correlates with reduced axonal degeneration and a facilitated rate of recovery from chronic pain states (Campana et al. 2006). We propose that Epo balances the inflammatory cytokine milieu and thereby protects axons and glia from further damage. This model is supported by the work of Keswani et al. (2004), who demonstrated that exogenously administered Epo prevents limb weakness and neuropathic pain behaviors in a rat model of distal axonopathy. Furthermore, Epo downregulates production of inflammatory infiltrates in animal models of autoimmune encephalomyelitis (Savino et al. 2006). In this study, TNF-α and interleukin (IL)-6 expression were both reduced by more than 50%.

Autocrine and paracrine pathways occurring locally at the site of peripheral nerve injury are probably complemented by a process in which Epo and its receptor communicate signals from the injury site to the cell bodies of primary sensory neurons. Understanding these pathways that connect the sciatic nerve to the dorsal horn is the focus of much attention in our laboratory. Evidence indicates that blocking retrograde transport of inflammatory signals produced at the site of peripheral nerve injury may inhibit the development of pain states (Yamamoto and Yaksh 1993). However, there is no prior evidence that agents such as Epo, which are upregulated at the peripheral nerve injury site and alleviate pain, may also be transported in a retrograde manner like TNF-α and other factors that produce pain (DiStefano et al. 1992; Shubayev and Myers 2001). To address this problem, we injected rhEpo directly into the sciatic nerve at a CCI site as shown in Fig. 1. The photomicrographs in Fig. 1 show DRG isolated from animals that received Epo at the injury site and from animals that were injected with vehicle. No apparent change in DRG morphology was observed. However, in immunohistochemistry studies, we observed a substantial decrease in TNF-α protein immunopositivity in the DRG of Epo-treated animals within 1 day. To confirm this observation, we isolated RNA and performed real-time quantitative PCR. In the vehicle-treated animals, CCI significantly increased TNF-α mRNA in the DRG. However, in rats that were treated with Epo, the injury-induced increase in TNF-α mRNA in the DRG was blocked. A number of explanations may account for this result. First, Epo functions at the injury site to reduce transport of inflammatory signals that lead to increased TNF-α expression in the DRG. Alternatively, Epo and its receptor may be transported from the CCI site to the DRG and directly block increased TNF-α expression.

To determine whether endogenously produced Epo is transported from an injury site retrogradely to the DRG, we performed a double-ligation study. Double ligatures were placed on the sciatic nerve of rats with and without CCI. Ligatures were tied 1 and 2 cm proximal to the CCI site immediately after loose ligature placement. Nerve tissue was collected 24 hours later, fixed in 4% paraformaldehyde, and processed in paraffin. Longitudinal sections were analyzed by immunofluorescence using anti-Epo and/or anti-EpoR. Sections were taken from between the CCI injury site (or the corresponding site in animals that did not undergo CCI) and the first tight ligature (to test the accumulation of retrogradely transported material), between the ligatures (to control for injury from tight ligatures), and proximal to the second tight ligature nearest the DRG (to test the accumulation of anterograde material from the cell body). This procedure allowed us to assay the material on either side of, and between, the ligatures to determine the bulk flow of Epo and EpoR. In uninjured animals, there

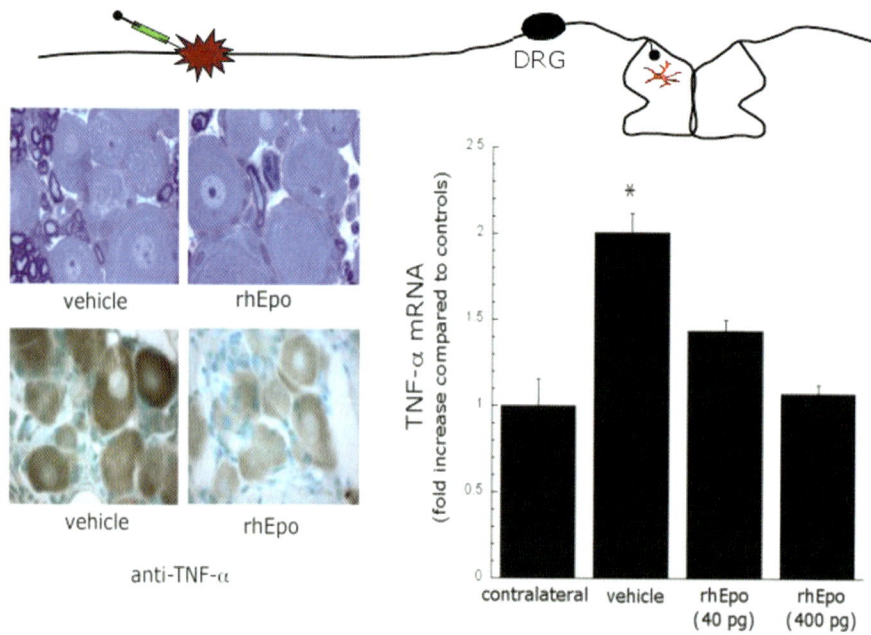

Fig. 1. The photomicrographs in Fig. 1 show dorsal root ganglia (DRG) isolated from rats that received local injection of recombinant human erythropoietin (rhEpo) at the injury site and from animals that were injected with vehicle. Tumor necrosis factor α (TNF-α) mRNA was reduced in DRG of rhEpo-treated compared to vehicle-treated animals. Thus, injection of rhEpo into the injury site reduces TNF expression in primary sensory neurons. No change in DRG morphology was apparent.

was minimal accumulation of Epo or EpoR around either ligature (Fig. 2A–C). In animals with CCI, Epo and EpoR were clearly colocalized in the nerve (Fig. 2D–F). The greatest level of Epo and EpoR accumulated between the CCI injury and the distal ligature, suggesting retrograde transport. Less antigen was observed between the proximal ligature and the DRG, suggesting only modest anterograde transport from the DRG. Because Epo and its receptor are clearly neuroprotective, it follows that retrograde transport of Epo in the sciatic nerve could serve a neuroprotective function, acting as a positive signal in regulating synthesis of proteins associated with protection and repair of nerve tissue.

We conducted additional experiments using the CCI model and double-ligation system to assess transport. In these experiments, tissue extracts were prepared for analysis of phosphorylated JAK2 by Western blotting. Fig. 3 shows Western blots of nerve sections using commercially available antibodies specific for phosphorylated JAK2 and total JAK2. Our results demonstrate that phosphorylated JAK2 is highest between the CCI injury and the most distal

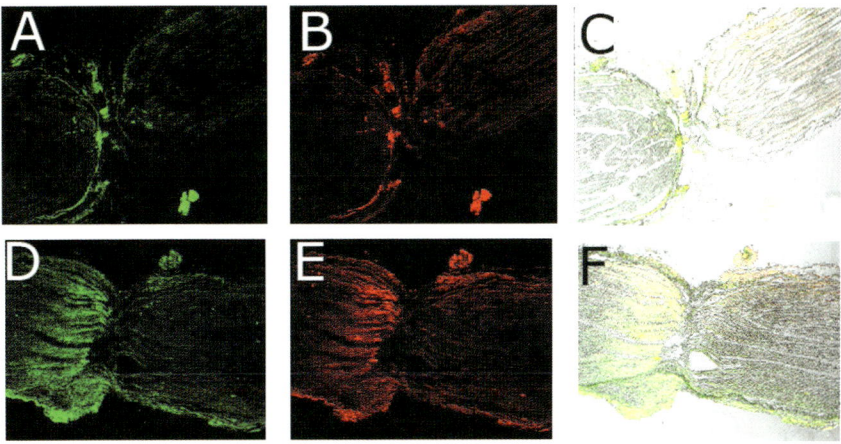

Fig. 2. Retrograde transport of erythropoietin (Epo) and its receptor (EpoR) from the site of chronic constriction injury (CCI). Double-labeled immunofluorescence of Epo (A,D; green), EpoR (B,E; red), and colocalization of Epo/EpoR (C,F; yellow) are shown under phase contrast in a longitudinal nerve section between the CCI site (not shown) and the most distal ligature (shown) in control animals without CCI (A,B,C) and in CCI-treated animals (D,E,F). Green-colored fluorescence was obtained by Alexa 488 (FITC) conjugated secondary antibody, and red-colored fluorescence was obtained by Alexa 564 (rhodamine) conjugated secondary antibody. Micrographs are representative of five animals per group.

tight ligature 24 hours after injury (lane 3). Epo and the EpoR were located in this area, apparently due to retrograde transport. This accumulation was not a result of local injury from the ligatures, because nerve segments between the ligatures did not show enhanced JAK2 phosphorylation (lane 2). Thus, we conclude that JAK2 may be transported in a retrograde fashion from the injury site to the cell bodies of injured neurons and is likely to be associated with the Epo-EpoR complex. Alternatively, and perhaps more intriguingly, the EpoR may continue to signal from within intracellular transported vesicles, as has been demonstrated for the epidermal growth factor receptor (Gruenberg and Stenmark 2004).

The beneficial activities of endogenously produced Epo may be therapeutically exploited by administering Epo systemically, as we and others have described (Siren et al. 2001; Campana and Myers 2003; Kewani et al. 2004; Campana et al. 2006). Systemically delivered Epo induces the phosphorylation of JAK2 in both primary sensory neurons and surrounding satellite cells after L5 SNC and to a lesser extent in sham-operated animals (Campana and Myers 2003). This finding is associated with a reduced number of TUNEL-positive neurons and satellite cells in the DRG, indicating that JAK2-mediated signaling protects diverse DRG cells from death. Similarly, in cortical neurons, activation of JAK2 is associated with neuroprotection from both TNF-α and glutamate ex-citotoxicity (Digicaylioglu and Lipton 2001). Phosphorylated JAK2 antagonizes TNF-mediated signaling by deactivating the nuclear factor (NF)-κB inhibitor, leading to the production of neuroprotective genes. Epo also increases calcium influx into neurons, by direct interaction of the EpoR with voltage-independent calcium channels (Miller et al. 1999). Increased calcium influx into neurons has multiple functions, including activating MAP kinases (Koshimura et al. 1999) and enhancing resistance to glutamate toxicity (Morishita et al. 1997). However, Epo does not increase JAK2 phosphorylation universally in neurons; the regulated populations include large TrkA/NF200-immunopositive neurons associated with large, low-threshold Aβ fibers and small neurons (most of which are nociceptive) that are negative for isolectin B4 (derived from *Griffonia simplicifolia*) (Snider and McMahon 1998). After peripheral nerve injury, small neurons are lost more quickly (Degn et al. 1999), and upregulation of JAK2 phosphorylation in this surviving subset of neurons may prevent their demise. This possibility may also explain why Epo is effective in protecting cutaneous innervation (C-fibers) in peripheral neuropathies. Another mechanism whereby Epo may protect primary sensory neurons from death is by blocking nitric-oxide-induced death. Cultured hippocampal and cerebral cortical neurons exposed to nitric oxide in the presence of Epo (100 pg/mL) show decreased cell death (Calapai et al. 2000).

Developing Epo mimetics that have neuroprotective, but not hematopoietic, effects is of great interest given the cost of recombinant protein therapy and the problematic long-term side effects of Epo itself. We reported on a novel Epo-mimetic peptide that showed promise in inducing neurite sprouting and

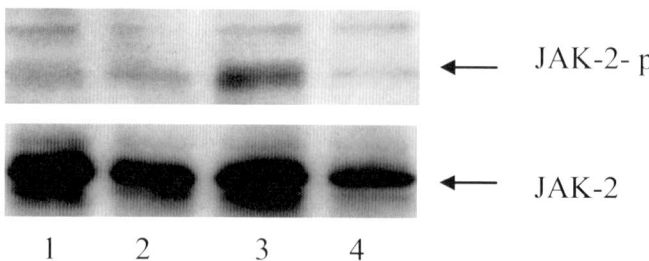

Fig. 3. Retrograde transport of phosphorylated Janus kinase 2 (JAK2) after chronic constriction injury (CCI). Western blots using (A) anti-phosphorylated JAK2 were stripped and reprobed with (B) JAK2. Equal loading of nerve lysates was resolved in a 7.5% sodium dodecyl sulfate-polyacrylamide gel electrophoresis. Lane 1, nerve from the site of CCI; lane 2, nerve from between the distal and proximal tight ligatures; lane 3, nerve from between CCI and the distal ligature; lane 4, nerve from the area proximal to the proximal ligature. Blots were developed by enhanced chemiluminescence. Each Western blot is representative of three animals.

neuroprotection in vitro (Campana et al. 1998), but its stability in the plasma was extremely limited. Another candidate is carbamylated Epo, which has potent tissue protective activities while not possessing erythropoietic activities (Leist et al. 2004). This modified protein does not appear to function by binding to the EpoR, but stimulates the common beta subunit heteroreceptor (Brines et al. 2004). Whether carbamylated Epo is effective in the treatment of chronic neuropathic pain has not yet been examined. The effects we observed with rhEpo on pain behaviors, apoptosis, TNF-α mRNA levels, and JAK2 signaling were not influenced by changes in blood pressure, because no significant differences between rhEpo and vehicle were observed with the doses we studied (Campana et al. 2006). However, we observed a significant increase in hematocrit after 14 days of Epo treatment. Increased erythrocytes contain high amounts of antioxidants that are capable of scavenging free or nitric oxide radicals; this mechanism has been implicated in reducing pain behavior (Wagner et al. 1998) and in protecting cells from death (Ravati et al. 1999; Asanuma et al. 2001).

Currently, pharmacological therapies used to treat neuropathic pain, including opioids, nonsteroidal anti-inflammatory drugs, antidepressants and local anesthetic agents, are generally ineffective or have substantial drawbacks due to side effects. Generally, these treatments do not protect neurons from "stress" or death. In fact, there have been reports that chronic morphine treatment, leading to "morphine tolerance," may indeed induce the death of neurons (Mao et al. 2002). Thus, developing therapeutics that have analgesic, protective, and restorative properties would be fruitful. Neurotrophic factors, such as nerve growth factor (NGF)-β and neurotrophin-4 (NT-4), possess potent neuroprotective activity (Meakin and Shooter 1992; Deckworth and Johnson 1993); however, these factors are limited as therapeutics because of their tendency to induce hyperalgesia (Shu and Mendell 1999).

CONCLUSIONS

Epo is a novel neuroprotective factor that is effective in facilitating recovery from chronic neuropathic pain states. It does not prevent the initiation of chronic pain states, but in several animal models of neuropathic pain (L5 SNC, CCI, and spinal nerve root ligation), it alleviates chronically maintained pain states. Two mechanisms are proposed: (1) Epo protects both primary sensory neurons and peripheral glia from degeneration, dysfunction, and death after damage to nerves; and (2) Epo antagonizes pain-producing proinflammatory cytokines, such as TNF-α and IL-1β, that are induced by Schwann cells at the site of peripheral nerve injury and in the DRG. We have established that Epo induces phosphorylation of JAK2 and activates downstream signaling pathways, known to be anti-apoptotic. In Schwann cells, ERK/MAP kinase may be one of these pathways. Further elucidation of cross-talk between the pathways activated by inflammatory and neuroprotective cytokines in nerve injury offers the potential for identification of novel therapeutic strategies.

ACKNOWLEDGMENTS

The author would like to thank Jenny Dolkas, Xiaoqing Li, Mila Angert, and Heidi Heckman for their outstanding technical support. This work was supported by NIH grant R01 NS041983 to W.M. Campana.

REFERENCES

Agnello D, Bigini P, Villa P, et al. Erythropoietin exerts an anti-inflammatory effect on the CNS in a model of experimental autoimmune encephalomyelitis. *Brain Res* 2002; 952:128–134.

Asanuma M, Nishibayashi-Asanuma S, Miyazaki I, Kohno M, Ogawa N. 2001. Neuroprotective effects of non-steroidal anti-inflammatory drugs by direct scavenging of nitric oxide radicals. *J Neurochem* 2001; 76:1895–1909.

Arai A, Kanda E, Miura O. Rac is activated by erythropoietin or interleukin-3 and is involved in activation of the ERK signaling pathway. *Oncogene* 202; 21:2641–2651.

Bao S, Wang Y, Sweeney P, et al. Keratinocyte growth factor induces Akt kinase activity and inhibits Fas-mediated apoptosis in A549 lung epithelial cells. *Am J Physiol Lung Cell Mol Physiol* 2005; 288:L36–42.

Bazan JF. Haemopoietic receptors and helical cytokines. *Immunol Today* 1990; 11:350–354.

Bianchi R, Buyukakilli B, Brines M, et al. Erythropoietin both protects and reverses experimental diabetic neuropathy. *Proc Natl Acad Sci USA* 2004; 101:823–828.

Bianchi R, Brines M, Lauria G, et al. Protective effect of erythropoietin and its carbamylated derivative in experimental Cisplatin peripheral neurotoxicity. *Clin Cancer Res* 2006; 12:2607–2612.

Bittorf T, Jaster R, Soares MJ, et al. Induction of erythroid proliferation and differentiation by a trophoblast-specific cytokine involves activation of the JAK/STAT pathway. *J Mol Endocrinol* 2000; 25:253–262.

Brines ML, Ghezzi P, Keenan S, et al. Erythropoietin crosses the blood-brain barrier to protect against experimental brain injury. *Proc Natl Acad Sci USA* 2000; 97:10526–10531.

Brines M, Grasso G, Fiordaliso F. Erythropoietin mediates tissue protection through an erythropoietin and common beta-subunit heteroreceptor. *Proc Natl Acad Sci USA* 2004; 101:14907–14912.

Calapai G, Marciano MC, Corica F, et al. Erythropoietin protects against brain ischemic injury by inhibition of nitric oxide formation. *Eur J Pharmacol* 2000; 401:349–356.

Campana WM, Myers RR. Erythropoietin and erythropoietin receptors in the peripheral nervous system: changes after nerve injury. *FASEB J* 2001; 15:1804–1806.

Campana WM, Myers RR. Exogenous erythropoietin protects against dorsal root ganglion apoptosis and pain following peripheral nerve injury. *Eur J Neurosci* 2003; 18:1497–1506.

Campana WM, Misasi R, O'Brien JS. Identification of a neurotrophic sequence in erythropoietin. *Int J Mol Med* 1998; 1:235–241.

Campana WM, Li X, Shubayev VI, et al. Erythropoietin reduces Schwann cell TNF-alpha, Wallerian degeneration and pain-related behaviors after peripheral nerve injury. *Eur J Neurosci* 2006; 23:617–626.

Deckworth TL, Johnson EM. Neurotrophic factor deprivation-induced death. *Ann NY Acad Sci* 1993; 28:121–131.

Degn J, Tandrup T, Jakobsen J. Effect of nerve Crush on Perikaryal number and volume of neurons in adult dorsal root ganglion. *J Comp Neurol* 1999; 412:186–192.

Digicaylioglu M, Lipton SA. Erythropoietin-mediated neuroprotection involves cross-talk between JAK2 and NF-κB signaling cascades. *Nature* 2001; 412:641–647.

Digicaylioglu M, Bichet S, Marti HH, et al. Localization of specific erythropoietin binding sites in defined areas of the mouse brain. *Proc Natl Acad Sci USA* 1995; 92:3717–3720.

DiStefano PS, Friedman B, Radziejewski C. The neurotrophins BDNF, NT-3 and NGF display distinct patterns of retrograde axonal transport in peripheral and central neurons. *Neuron* 1992; 8:983–993.

Ehrenreich H, Degner D, Meller J, et al. Erythropoietin: a candidate compound for neuroprotection in schizophrenia. *Mol Psychiatry* 2004; 9:42–54.

Feldman EL. Oxidative stress and diabetic neuropathy: a new understanding of an old problem. *J Clin Invest* 2003; 111:431–433.

Genc S, Koroglu TF, Genc K. Erythropoietin and the nervous system. *Brain Res* 2004; 1000:19–31.

Grasso G, Sfacteria A, Passalacqua M, et al. Erythropoietin and erythropoietin receptor expression after experimental spinal cord injury encourages therapy by exogenous erythropoietin. *Neurosurgery* 2005; 56:821–827.

Gruenberg J, Stenmark H. The biogenesis of multivesicular endosomes. *Nat Rev Mol Cell Biol* 2004; 5:317–323.

Ihle JN, Witthuhn BA, Quelle FW, et al. Signaling by the cytokine receptor superfamily: JAKs and STATs. *Trends Biochem Sci* 1994; 19:222–227.

Juul SE, Yachnis AT, Rojiani AM, Christensen RD. Immunohistochemical localization of erythropoietin and its receptor in the developing human brain. *Pediatr Dev Pathol* 1999; 2:148–158.

Keswani SC, Buldanlioglu U, Fischer A, et al. A novel endogenous erythropoietin mediated pathway prevents axonal degeneration. *Ann Neurol* 2004; 56:815–826.

Koshimura K, Murakami Y, Sohmiya M, Tanaka J, Kato Y. Effects of erythropoietin on neuronal activity. *J Neurochem* 1999; 72:2565–2572.

Krantz SB. Erythropoietin. *Blood* 1991; 77:419–434.

Li X, Gonias SL, Campana WM. Schwann cells express erythropoietin receptor and represent a major target for Epo in peripheral nerve injury. *Glia* 2005; 51:254–265.

Liest M, Ghexxi P, Grasso G, et al. Derivatives of erythropoietin that are tissue protective but not erythropoietic. *Science* 2004; 305:239–242.

Ludwig H, Strasser K. Symptomatology of anemia. *Semin Oncol* 2001; 28:7–14.

Mao J, Sung B, Ji RR, Lim G. Neuronal apoptosis associated with morphine tolerance: evidence for an opioid-induced neurotoxic mechanism. *J Neurosci* 2002; 22:7650–7661.

Masuda S, Nagao M, Takahata K, et al. Functional erythropoietin receptor of cells with neural characteristics. Comparison with receptor properties of erythroid cells. *J Biol Chem* 1993; 268:11208–11216.

Meakin SO, Shooter EM. The nerve growth factor family of receptors. *Trends Neurosci* 1992; 15:323–331.

Miller BA, Barber DL, Bell LL, et al. Identification of the erythropoietin receptor domain required for calcium channel activation. *J Biol Chem* 1999; 274:20465–20472.

Morishita E, Masuda S, Nagao M, Yasuda Y, Sasaki R. Erythropoietin receptor is expressed in rat hippocampal and cerebral cortical neurons, and erythropoietin prevents in vitro glutamate-induced neuronal death. *Neuroscience* 1997; 76:105–116.

Myers RR. Morphology of the peripheral nervous system and its relationship to neuropathic pain. In: Yaksh TL, Lynch C, Zapol WM, et al. (Eds). *Anesthesia: Biologic Foundations*. Philadelphia: Lippincott-Raven, 1997, pp 483–514.

Nagai A, Nakagawa E, Choi HB, et al. Erythropoietin and erythropoietin receptors in human CNS neurons, astrocytes, microglia, and oligodendrocytes grown in culture. *J Neuropathol Exp Neurol* 2001; 60:386–392.

Nagao M, Masuda S, Abe S, Ueda M, Sasaki R. Production and ligand-binding characteristics of the soluble form of murine erythropoietin receptor. *Biochem Biophys Res Commun* 1992; 188:888–897.

Ravati A, Junker V, Kouklei M, et al. Enalapril and moexipril protect from free radical-induced neuronal damage in vitro and reduce ischemic brain injury in mice and rats. *Eur J Pharmacol* 1999; 373:21–33.

Sakanaka M, Wen TC, Matsuda S, et al. In vivo evidence that erythropoietin protects neurons from ischemic damage. *Proc Natl Acad Sci USA* 1998; 95:4635–4640.

Savino C, Pedotti R, Baggi F, et al. Delayed administration of erythropoietin and its non-erythropoietic derivatives ameliorates chronic murine autoimmune encephalomyelitis. *J Neuroimmunol* 2006; 172:27–37.

Sekiguchi Y, Kikuchi S, Myers RR, Campana WM. ISSLS prize winner: Erythropoietin inhibits spinal neuronal apoptosis and pain following nerve root crush. *Spine* 2003; 28:2577–2584.

Shu XQ, Mendell LM. Neurotrophins and hyperalgesia. *Proc Natl Acad Sci* 1999; 96:7693–7696.

Shubayev VI, Myers RR. Axonal transport of TNF-alpha in painful neuropathy: distribution of ligand tracer and TNF receptors. *J Neuroimmunol* 2001; 114:48–56.

Siren AL, Fratelli M, Brines M. Erythropoietin prevents neuronal apoptosis after cerebral ischemia and metabolic stress. *Proc Natl Acad Sci USA* 2001; 98:4044–4049.

Snider WD, McMahon SB. Tackling pain at the source: new ideas about nociceptors. *Neuron* 1998; 20:629–632.

Sorkin LS, Xiao WH, Wagner R, Myers RR. Tumor necrosis factor-alpha induces ectopic activity in nociceptive primary afferent fibres. *Neuroscience* 1997; 81:255–262.

Wagner R, Myers RR. Schwann cells produce tumor necrosis factor alpha: expression in injured and non-injured nerves. *Neuroscience* 1996a; 73:625–629.

Wagner R, Myers RR. Endoneurial injection of TNF-alpha produces neuropathic pain behaviors. *NeuroReport* 1996b; 7:2897–2901.

Wagner R, Myers RR, O'Brien JS. Prosaptide prevents hyperalgesia and reduces peripheral TNFR1 expression following TNF-alpha nerve injection. *NeuroReport* 1998; 9:2827–2831.

Winkelstein BA, Rutkowski MD, Sweitzer SM, Pahl JL, DeLeo JA. Nerve injury proximal or distal to the DRG induces similar spinal glial activation and selective cytokine expression but differential behavioral responses to pharmacologic treatment. *J Comp Neurol* 2001; 439:127–139.

Witthuhn BA, Quelle FW, Silvennoinen O, et al. JAK2 associates with the erythropoietin receptor and is tyrosine phosphorylated and activated following stimulation with erythropoietin. *Cell* 1993; 74:227–236.

Wojchowski DM, Gregory RC, Miller CP, Pandit AK, Pircher TJ. Signal transduction in the erythropoietin receptor system. *Exp Cell Res* 1999; 253:143–156.

Yamamoto T, Yaksh TL. Effects of colchicine applied to the peripheral nerve on the thermal hyperalgesia evoked with chronic nerve constriction. *Pain* 1993; 55:227–233.

Yu X, Shacka JJ, Eells JB. et al. Erythropoietin receptor signalling is required for normal brain development. *Development* 2002; 129:505–516.

Correspondence to: W. Marie Campana, PhD, Department of Anesthesiology, University of California, San Diego, 9500 Gilman Drive, La Jolla, CA 92093-0629, USA. Email: wcampana@ucsd.edu.

Immune and Glial Regulation of Pain, edited by Joyce
A. DeLeo, Linda S. Sorkin, and Linda R. Watkins,
IASP Press, Seattle, © 2007.

10

Inflammation of Dorsal Root Ganglia: Satellite Cell Activation and Immune Cell Recruitment after Nerve Injury

Elspeth M. McLachlan and Ping Hu

*Prince of Wales Medical Research Institute, Randwick,
New South Wales, Australia*

Inflammation in the nervous system plays a major role in the generation of pain—both the pain that is initiated by inflammation at the peripheral terminals of nociceptors and the neuropathic pain that may develop when injured nervous tissue is invaded by immune cells. Neuropathic pain generally follows lesions that disrupt the blood-nerve barrier in the periphery, i.e., partial nerve injuries or injuries in which local inflammation is induced by an irritant chemical or by constriction, which leads to compression, edema, and disruption of many axons. Hematogenous monocytes and lymphocytes, as well as resident macrophages, migrate to and intermingle in and around the lesion when the vascular barrier is opened. In addition, however, immune cells are also recruited to the area around the cell bodies of origin of these axons (motor, sympathetic, and sensory) that lie far from the injury. The inflammatory reaction around these somata is probably triggered by a retrograde axonal signal that causes the surrounding glia (satellite cells in the ganglia and astrocytes in the ventral horn) to release chemokines.

Numerous studies in rodent models of nerve injuries that produce pain behavior—licking and guarding the foot, paw withdrawal to low-threshold stimuli (allodynia) or to non-noxious heat and cold (thermal hyperalgesia)—have described the activation of both microglia and astrocytes in the dorsal horn around the central terminals of primary afferent neurons affected by the lesion. Although the role of these glia in pain is controversial, with opinions ranging from responsible (Tsuda et al. 2005) to unrelated (Colburn et al. 1997), the question of why inflammation occurs around the central terminals of sensory neurons has not been answered. One possibility is that a signal arises in the somata of lesioned sensory neurons and is transmitted to the central terminals, causing them to release a chemokine that activates glia in the local environment. The release of proinflammatory cytokines is thought to be important in producing neuronal hyperexcitability and ectopic activity in pain pathways (Wieseler-Frank et al. 2005). The generation of spontaneous activity by intact but sensitized nociceptors and/or by injured and uninjured large-diameter neurons (presumed to be low-threshold mechanoreceptors) (Campbell and Meyer 2006) provides a basis for the clinical observations of spontaneous pain. Inflammation is clearly a major factor in the excitation of intact and damaged axons. Other relevant changes are the overt plasticity in the central connections of mechano-sensitive pathways, while neuronal excitability increases in both the dorsal horn and the thalamus.

This chapter reviews what is known about the inflammation that occurs within dorsal root ganglia (DRG) following sciatic nerve injuries that transect peripheral axons that arise from these ganglia. Most of the work has been done in rats with sciatic transection and ligation. This lesion axotomizes ~65% of neurons in the L4 and L5 DRG and prevents their regeneration. Some data are also available for other lesions, including transection of the L5 spinal nerve, transection and ligation of the sural nerve, freezing of the sciatic nerve to permit rapid regeneration (Mira 1971), and chronic constriction injury of the sciatic nerve (Bennett and Xie 1988), only some of which induce pain behavior. Here we describe the recruitment of inflammatory cells to the DRG after lesions that either do or do not expose their axons to the products of Wallerian degeneration. In the context of this volume, the focus will be on differences between the responses to axotomy and those to injuries that may generate pain.

THE INTERFACE BETWEEN DORSAL ROOT GANGLIA AND THE IMMUNE SYSTEM

In peripheral nerve trunks, as in the central nervous system (CNS), a blood-nerve barrier largely isolates the endoneurial space from the blood. The population of resting macrophages is similar to that in the DRG (Hu and McLachlan 2003a), and these cells have slow turnover rates, with life cycles of about 3 months (Vass et al. 1993). A few T lymphocytes survey the endoneurial compartment.

In contrast, in DRG and sympathetic ganglia, the barrier separating the neuronal somata and their satellite glia from the blood is very permeable compared to those of the CNS and the peripheral nerve trunks (Jacobs et al. 1976). This permeability not only permits the neurons to be exposed to circulating proteins, but also enables blood leukocytes to move readily into and out of the ganglia through the vasculature.

Another site at which immune cells come into close proximity to the DRG is at the subarachnoid angle, where the arachnoid and pia connect to the perineurium near the central pole of the ganglion. Here, invaginating venous vessels are exposed to the cerebrospinal fluid (CSF) where the spinal root emerges into the spinal canal from the DRG (McCabe and Low 1969). In this region, macrophages and lymphocytes that have been in contact with the CSF accumulate (Morse and Low 1972) and may move into the DRG (Hu and McLachlan 2002).

THE NEUROGLIAL RESPONSE TO PERIPHERAL NERVE INJURY

Following injury to a peripheral nerve, retrograde signals produce changes in the neuronal cell bodies of the DRG within 12 hours (Cajal 1928; Holtzman et al. 1967; Lieberman 1971). During the next few days, the neuron's metabolism changes so that protein synthesis increases to support regeneration, and enzymes involved in transmitter secretion are downregulated. Examples of this redirection of protein synthesis are the expression of activating transcription factor 3 (ATF3; Tsujino et al. 2000) and c-Jun (Herdegen et al. 1997) after axotomy.

The cell body reaction is rapidly followed by changes in the satellite glia adjacent to the reacting neurons. Glial fibrillary acidic protein (GFAP) is upregulated around axotomized DRG neurons within 24 hours, as occurs in astrocytes around axotomized motor neurons (Aldskogius and Kozlova 1998). The satellite cells begin to divide, leading to gliosis throughout the DRG, particularly around the larger-diameter somata, where perineuronal rings several cells thick become prominent (Zhou et al. 1999). The gliosis is more marked if the axons cannot regenerate, and GFAP remains upregulated for months unless the neurons reinnervate their targets (Aldskogius and Kozlova 1998).

IMMUNE CELLS IN THE NORMAL DORSAL ROOT GANGLIA

The immune cell population in the normal rat DRG consists of resident macrophages expressing the macrophage scavenger receptor CD163 (detected by the antibody/marker ED2). This protein plays a role in the production of pro-inflammatory mediators, including nitric oxide, interleukin-1β (IL-1β), IL-6, and tumor necrosis factor-α (TNF-α) (Polfliet et al. 2006). Most of these macrophages contain a few small intracellular organelles that are positive for CD68 (ED1 antibody), and about half of them also express major histocompatibility complex type II (MHC II) (Hu and McLachlan 2003a). ED1 is generally considered a marker of phagocytic macrophages (Graeber et al. 1990; Al-Shatti et al. 2005).

MHC II is expressed by at least as many ED2– cells that are also ED1– (Fig. 1, top row). A small population of cells express CD11b, the complement type 3 receptor (detected using OX-42), some of which are MHC II+; a population with similar frequency and distribution are CD4+. Occasional T lymphocytes within the DRG parenchyma are almost exclusively CD8+ αβ T-cell-receptor-

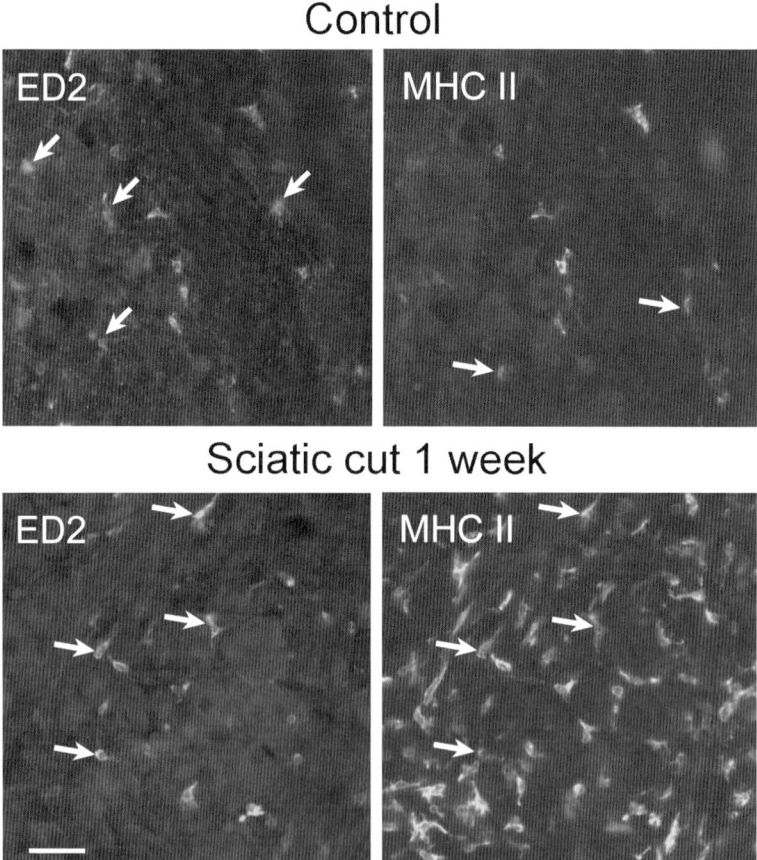

Fig. 1. The effect of sciatic transection on resident and hematogenous macrophages in rat dorsal root ganglia (DRG). Micrographs from L5 DRG of adult rat 1 week after sciatic transection show sections from contralateral (Control, above) and operated (Sciatic cut 1 week, below) sides. ED2 (on left): resident macrophages immunopositive for CD163 do not change their density or distribution after the nerve lesion. MHC II (on right): another population of cells within the control DRG is positive for major histocompatibility complex type II (MHC II), and the density of these cells increases dramatically after transection (below). In the control DRG, some resident macrophages express MHC II (arrows on left), but other MHC II+ cells lack ED2 (arrows on right). After transection, most ED2+ cells are MHC II+ (colocalization indicated by arrows), but a large population of MHC II+ macrophages have invaded the ganglion. Calibration at lower left represents 50 μm and applies throughout.

positive (TCR+) cells. Equivalent populations have been reported in normal human DRG (Graus et al. 1990).

INVASION BY BLOOD-DERIVED MACROPHAGES AFTER NERVE TRANSECTION

Following peripheral nerve injury (e.g., to the sciatic nerve), macrophages accumulate at the site of the lesion within 24 hours. The earliest sign of macrophage activation in the DRG that project axons in the ligated and transected sciatic nerve is an increase in the expression of ED1 (Hu and McLachlan 2003a), detectable after 3 days. Given that total macrophage density is hardly changed at this stage, the increase in ED1 probably results from its increased expression by activated ED2+ resident macrophages.

After a week, the total number of macrophages in the DRG has dramatically increased, with a fivefold increase in the number of cells expressing only MHC II+. At this stage, the ED2+ population within the attached spinal nerve is unchanged, and the density of MHC II+/ED2– macrophages in the nerve has only doubled. Clusters of MHC II+ cells are present within the DRG around blood vessels and near the subarachnoid angle (Hu and McLachlan 2002), from which location they spread throughout the parenchyma, filling the spaces between the neuronal somata (Figs. 1, 2A,C). ED1 is expressed in many MHC II+ cells, with and without ED2, indicating that both recruited and resident macrophages are activated and may become phagocytic. Additional OX-42+ and CD4+ macrophages appear, but their density is much lower than that of MHC II+ cells (Hu et al. 2007). MHC I is expressed on macrophages and possibly on neurons and glia, but it does not have the same distribution as OX-42 immunoreactivity. Although double labeling to confirm the extent of colocalization is incomplete, several distinct types of macrophages that invade the DRG after nerve injury can be identified (Table I).

The number of macrophages seems to peak about 1 week after the lesion and gradually falls over the next few months (Hu and McLachlan 2002, 2003a). By 4 weeks, clusters of monocytes around blood vessels are rarely detected, implying that influx is transient, in contrast to observations after the same lesions in sympathetic ganglia, where clusters of both T cells and macrophages are still present after 3 months (Hu and McLachlan 2004). Over the ensuing weeks, many small-diameter sensory neurons die if regeneration is prevented (Tandrup et al. 2000; Hu and McLachlan 2003b). If the axotomized neurons have been labeled retrogradely with FluoroGold at the time of transection, the dye can be identified within ED2+ or MHC II+ macrophages (Fig.2D; see Hu and McLachlan 2003a). If the neurons are allowed to regenerate, macrophage

Table I

Non-neuronal cells within dorsal root ganglia before and after nerve lesions that axotomize sensory neurons

Cell Type	Primary Antibody/ Clone	Major Antigen	Other Markers, Especially after Injury	Increased Density after Injury	Likely Mechanism	Comments
Satellite glia	GFAP	GFAP	p75	Yes	Proliferation	p75 and trkA/trkB present NGF/BDNF to attract sprouting sympathetic and peptidergic axons
			S100B			More marked upregulation in Schwann cells
Macrophages	ED2	CD163	CD68, MHC II	No		Upregulate CD163 and express CD68 and MHC II but no increase in density
	OX-6	MHC II	CD68	Yes	Recruitment	Predominant; a subpopulation expresses CD68
	OX-42	CD11b	CD4, MHC II, CD68	Yes	Recruitment	Perineuronal rings, especially after CCI
	ED1	CD68	ED2, MHC II, OX-42	Yes	Expression	Intracellular organelles expressed after activation
	OX-18	MHC I	?	Yes	Expression	Also on neurons
Lymphocytes	OX-8	CD8			Recruitment	Predominant, almost all within parenchyma
	W3/25	CD4		Rare		Only in blood vessels and meninges
	OX-39	CD25		Only after spinal nerve lesion		Mainly in meninges, rare in parenchyma

Abbreviations: BDNF = brain-derived neurotrophic factor, CCI = chronic constriction injury, GFAP = glial fibrillary acidic protein, MHC = major histocompatibility complex, NGF = nerve growth factor, trkA = tyrosine kinase A, trkB = tyrosine kinase B.

density peaks at only 65% of that 1 week after transection, but returns to control levels over a similar time course (P. Hu, unpublished data); the extent of cell death under these conditions is not clear.

If the spinal nerve is cut close to the L5 DRG, axotomizing the great majority of sensory neurons (except those projecting in the dorsal ramus), then the number of MHC II+ cells rises even higher than after sciatic transection, with a much larger proportion expressing ED1. However, there is again no change

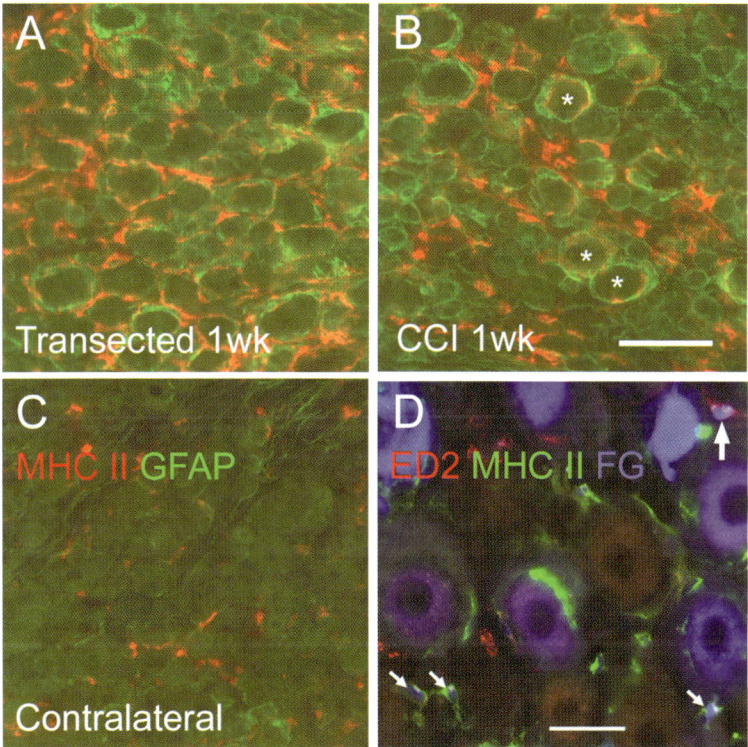

Fig. 2. Distinct functions of MHC II+ macrophages after different nerve lesions. Micrographs from rat L4 dorsal root ganglia (DRG) 1 week after (A) sciatic transection, (B) chronic constriction injury (CCI), and (C) contralateral to the CCI, showing the distribution of MHC II+ cells (red) between the DRG neuron somata and the upregulation of glial fibrillary acidic protein (GFAP, green) in satellite glia on the lesioned side. After CCI, fewer MHC II+ cells invade the DRG than after transection, but some of them penetrate the glial sheath of medium- to large-diameter neuron somata (asterisks in B), forming perineuronal rings. Calibration in B represents 100 μm and applies to A, B, C. (D) Ten weeks after sciatic transection, many small neurons have died. Retrograde labeling with FluoroGold (FG, blue) from the lesion reveals the surviving (mainly larger-diameter) neuron somata but also some macrophages (arrows) that have phagocytosed FG. Large vertical arrow indicates a phagocytic ED2+ cell (red); small oblique arrows indicate MHC II+ cells (green) that contain FG. Note MHC II+ cells close to the surface of the neuron in the center. Calibration in D represents 50 μm.

in the number of ED2+ cells (Hu and McLachlan 2003a), confirming that ED2 is restricted to resident macrophages that do not proliferate after injury. After spinal nerve transection, many more neurons die, including some with myelinated axons (Lekan et al. 1997).

An inflammatory state that is qualitatively similar to that found after peripheral nerve transection is produced in DRG by exposure to paclitaxel, an anticancer drug that produces dysesthesias and spontaneous (sometimes chronic) pain in patients. Clinically relevant doses in rats lead to mechanical/thermal hyperalgesia, motor deficits, and infiltration into DRG of macrophages, including those expressing CD68 and CD11b, reflecting direct axon damage as indicated by ATF3 expression (Peters et al. 2007).

INFLAMMATION AROUND UNDAMAGED SENSORY NEURONS

Most macrophage aggregations are found around neurons axotomized by the lesion, as demonstrated by retrograde labeling from the lesion site (Hu and McLachlan 2002) or by the expression of ATF3 (Hu et al. 2007). Although some undamaged neurons are involved, axotomized neurons are also the main targets for the axons of sympathetic and peptidergic neurons, which form perineuronal baskets of terminals (McLachlan et al. 1993; McLachlan and Hu 1998) that sprout in response to production of neurotrophin by proliferated glia (Zhou et al. 1999).

However, there are other lesions that produce inflammation of DRG with little or no direct damage to sensory neurons. Transection or ligation of the L5 spinal nerve is followed by degeneration of its axons in the distal branches of the sciatic nerve. The intact axons of L4 spinal nerve travel in these same branches of the sciatic nerve to the periphery. The L4 DRG shows mild but distinct inflammatory responses with invasion by macrophages and lymphocytes (Hu and McLachlan 2002). Although this response might result from irritation of the L4 spinal nerve at the lesion site, or from unintentional damage to a few axons during L5 transection (Shortland et al. 2006), this possibility seems remote because the response is similar to that seen in L5 DRG after transection of the sural nerve (P. Hu, unpublished data), which axotomizes ~40% of the sciatic population.

A slightly different situation follows transection of one ventral root with subsequent degeneration of only motor axons in the peripheral nerve trunks. This lesion produces pain behavior, upregulation of ED1 in macrophages, and expression of TNF-α and neurotrophins, which are among the changes seen after other sciatic nerve injuries (Li et al. 2002; Wu et al. 2002; Obata et al. 2004, 2006).

These two injuries that lead to both DRG inflammation and pain behavior leave intact axons that travel to the periphery surrounded by a population of immune cells involved in clearing the debris of degenerated axons and myelin. This finding indicates that DRG inflammation can be triggered by signals that are independent of axotomy of its sensory neurons. It is surprising how few myelinated axons need to be transected to produce this response.

INVASION BY MACROPHAGES AFTER
CHRONIC CONSTRICTION INJURY

One of the most thoroughly studied injury models that produces pain behavior is chronic constriction injury (CCI) of the sciatic nerve using several loose chromic gut ligatures that irritate the nerve and compromise the vascular supply. Although the perineurium is left intact, it becomes inflamed, and over several days, edema develops within the nerve, leading to disruption of many axons, particularly myelinated ones (Basbaum et al. 1991). In such partial nerve injuries, axons that remain intact are exposed to an orchestrated inflammatory response that clears axonal debris and degenerating myelin.

Following CCI of the sciatic nerve (Hu et al. 2007), most of the effects of transection are evident in L4 and L5 DRG, with macrophage density a little lower after a week compared to that achieved after transection of the nerve, reflecting the smaller number of axotomized neurons (demonstrated by ATF3 expression). A major difference from the response to transection is the targeting of larger-diameter neurons by OX-42+ macrophages, which encircle the somata beneath the GFAP+ glial sheath (Fig. 3A). Further, similar rings of macrophages are positive for CD4 (Figs. 3B, 4E) and MHC II (Fig. 3C), while some of the OX-42+ cells in the rings also express ED1 (Fig. 3D). It appears likely that some of these macrophages express all four of these markers (Table I). Although some of these perineuronal rings also appear after nerve transection, they are less complete, and their frequency is much lower than after CCI. However, 10 weeks after transection, MHC II+ rings are still present beneath the glial sheath (Hu and McLachlan 2002).

The function of these OX-42+ macrophages is unclear, although their apparent contact with neuronal somata is highly suggestive of a direct interaction. There is significant plasticity after nerve injury in low-threshold mechanoreceptors that project in the dorsal columns. Larger-diameter neurons (with myelinated axons) are those that bear thick layers of GFAP+ glia after sciatic transection and can receive perineuronal baskets of sympathetic or peptidergic terminals. They are the population that is targeted by OX-42+/CD4+ macrophages, particularly after CCI, and may be part of the population that projects to the dorsal column nuclei (gracile) and is involved in the potentiation of responses of thalamic neurons to noxious stimuli following peripheral nerve injury (Miki et al. 2000). Plasticity in this pathway seems to be triggered by activation of extracellular signal-regulated protein kinase and p38 mitogen-activated protein kinase and by expression of brain-derived neurotrophic factor in DRG neurons (Obata and Noguchi 2006).

INVASION BY T LYMPHOCYTES AFTER NERVE INJURIES

T lymphocytes invade the lesion site (Jander et al. 2001) and adjacent neural tissue within 1–2 days after sciatic transection and are detectable at increased density within the DRG by 3 days (Hu and McLachlan 2002), suggesting that

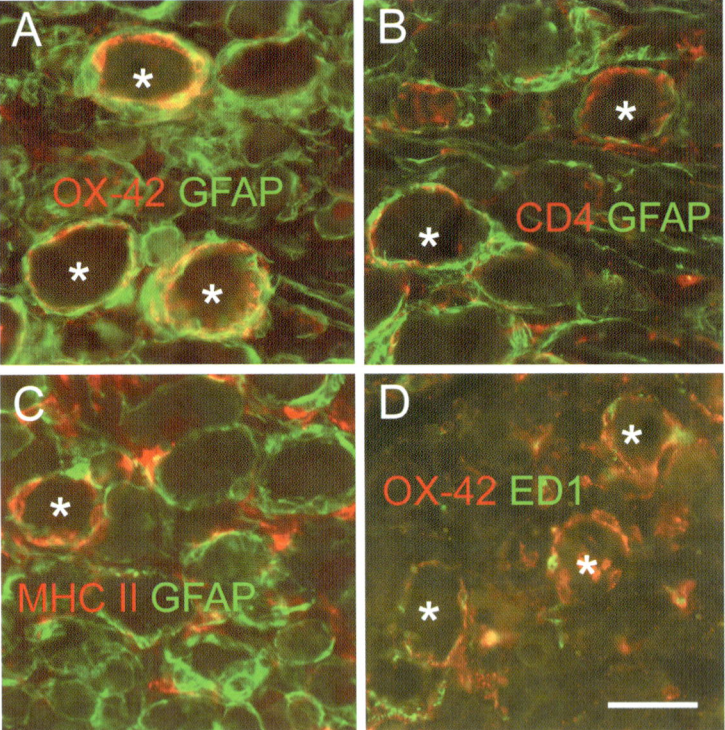

Fig. 3. Macrophages encircling larger-diameter neuron somata after chronic constriction injury of the sciatic nerve. Micrographs showing examples of perineuronal rings of macrophages (asterisks indicate neurons surrounded by rings) one week after CCI. The rings are positive for (A) CD11b (indicated by OX-42, red), (B) CD4 (red), and (C) less frequently MHC II (red), lying beneath the sheaths of glial fibrillary acidic protein-positive (GFAP+) satellite glia (green) apparently abutting the neuronal surface. (D) Three OX-42+ (red) perineuronal rings (asterisks) in which some OX-42+ cells contain granules positive for CD68 (indicated by ED1, green). These rings of macrophages positive for OX-42, CD4, MHC II, and/or ED1 encircle only larger-diameter neurons and appear in much higher numbers after CCI than after transection. Calibration in D represents 50 μm and applies throughout.

T cells are the first immune cells to be attracted by the changes in the neuronal cell bodies. After a week, the density of T lymphocytes is markedly increased (reaching 5–10 times greater than control). As for MHC II+ macrophages (Fig. 4B), the sites of entry are implied by clusters near blood vessels and the subarachnoid angle (Figs. 4A,C), from which they appear to be distributed throughout the parenchyma (Fig. 4D). The αβ TCR+ cells within the parenchyma are virtually all positive for the macrophage marker CD8.

While macrophage density declines, T-cell density remains elevated over several months, whether or not the axons can regenerate (P. Hu, unpublished data). Particularly at later stages, occasional very dense clusters of T cells and MHC II+/ED1+ macrophages appear around isolated neuron somata (Hu and McLachlan 2003a). Why these cells target particular neurons and whether they are protective or destructive remain mysteries.

The density of T cells rises many times higher after spinal nerve transection than after sciatic transection, although there is some decline over the ensuing months. In the unlesioned DRG adjacent to the spinal nerve lesion, a small number of invading T cells persist undiminished over the same period (Hu and McLachlan 2002). Following L5 spinal nerve transection, a small proportion of T cells are CD25+ (i.e., they bear the IL-2 receptor), particularly among those in the subarachnoid angle (Hu and McLachlan 2002). As CD25+ T cells are not seen within the parenchyma after sciatic transection, this sign of activation is not necessary for recruitment of T cells into the DRG.

After CCI, there is greater recruitment of αβ T lymphocytes into the DRG and the spinal cord than after transection (Hu et al. 2007). Again, almost all are CD8+, although rare CD4+ T cells were detected in blood vessels or the meninges (Fig. 4E). The determinants of T-cell recruitment are not known. Monocyte chemoattractant protein-1 (MCP-1), which is produced by both DRG neurons and glia after injury (Tanaka et al. 2004; Zhang and De Koninck 2006), also attracts T cells (Carr et al. 1994), but how much MCP-1 is generated after each lesion is not known. MHC class I, a prerequisite for antigen presentation to CD8+ T cells, and for the cytotoxic effects of these cells, is expressed to a similar extent after both CCI and transection, although with a different distribution. The greater recruitment around fewer axotomized sensory neurons implies that differences associated with the lesion site are important in triggering immune involvement after CCI (Hu et al. 2007).

RECRUITMENT OF IMMUNE CELLS INTO THE DORSAL ROOT GANGLIA

While there is little barrier to the movement of monocytes out of the vasculature into the DRG, details of the processes involved in attracting and facilitating the entry of hematogenous monocytes have not been worked out. An immune reaction initiated by macrophages that carry antigen from the site of peripheral myelin degeneration to the lymphoid organs has been suggested to explain T-cell infiltration of the facial nucleus after axotomy of its motor axons (Olsson et al. 1992). Such an immune reaction might be involved in triggering inflammation in the DRG. It is assumed that chemokines, such as MCP-1, are produced by DRG neurons and satellite glia after nerve injury, particularly in

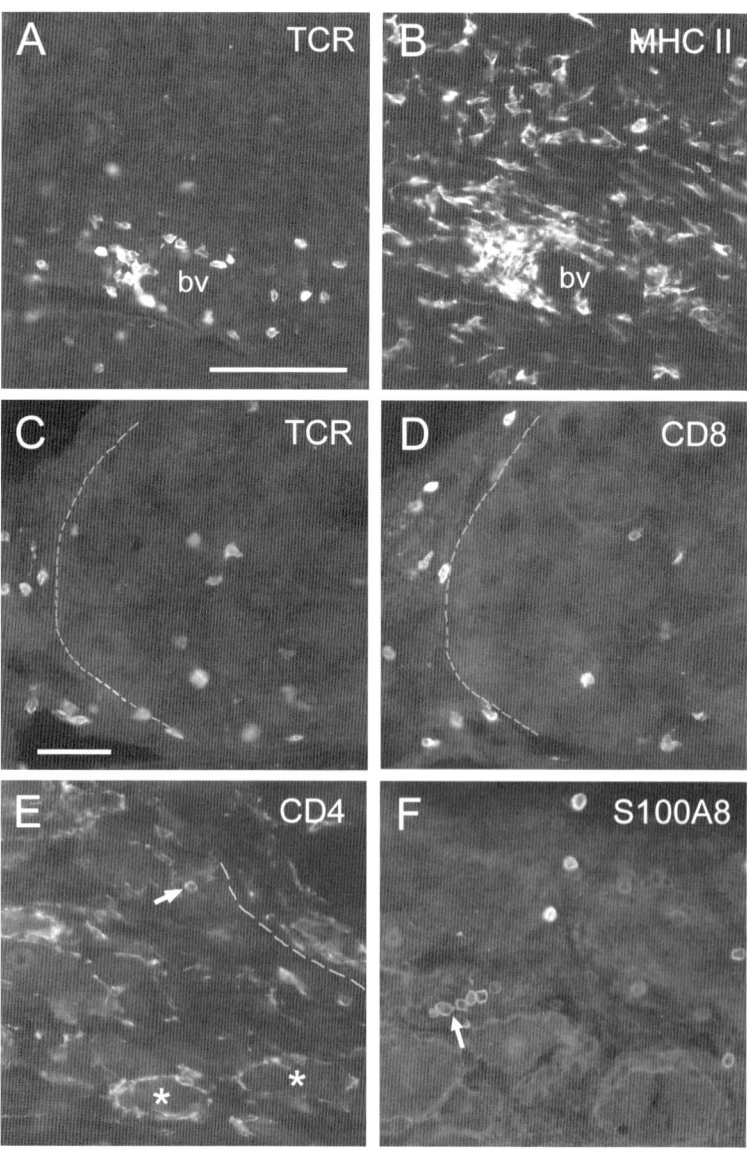

the first few days. The early influx of T lymphocytes would subsequently attract macrophages.

Adhesion molecules, such as intercellular adhesion molecule-1 (ICAM-1; Rodriguez Parkitna et al. 2006) and/or vascular cell adhesion molecule-1 (VCAM-1; Engelhardt and Ransohoff 2005), would have to be expressed on the vascular endothelium in order to trap the passing monocytes. Unless T cells and macrophages in the subarachnoid angle are intravascular, penetration of the capsule is likely to require the upregulation of chondroitin sulfate proteoglycan-degrading enzymes such as matrix metalloproteinases, as has been shown in sympathetic ganglia (Leone et al. 2005).

A feature of the clumps of cells in and around blood vessels, and of the cells that gather in the subarachnoid angle, is that they include immune cells that are not seen inside the parenchyma. Neutrophils do not invade the ganglia, although a few appear in blood vessels and the meninges (Fig. 4F). Some CD4+ lymphocytes appear around the outer sheath of the DRG, particularly associated with blood vessels, but they do not invade the parenchyma. Brightly immuno-fluorescent ED2+ cells on the meninges that do not appear within the DRG are probably dendritic cells (McMenamin 1999). These cell types must either be unresponsive to the chemokines produced within the DRG or be repelled by a chemical barrier, perhaps the high concentration of some of the chemoattractants (Vianello et al. 2005).

POSSIBLE FUNCTIONS OF IMMUNE CELLS IN DORSAL ROOT GANGLIA

The most likely effect of inflammation within the DRG seems to be the reduction of threshold for discharge of both injured and uninjured neurons that project centrally in pain pathways (Kim et al. 1998; Ali et al. 1999; DeLeo et al.

⟵ **Fig. 4.** Localization of lymphocytes and neutrophils in dorsal root ganglia (DRG) after nerve injury. (A, B) Micrographs from rat L5 DRG 1 week after sciatic transection showing clusters of (A) T cells and (B) MHC II+ cells around the wall of a blood vessel (bv) in adjacent sections. Calibration in A represents 100 μm and also applies to B. (C, D) Micrographs from rat L5 DRG 1 week after CCI near the subarachnoid angle (edge of DRG parenchyma shown as dashed lines to the left), with clusters of lymphocytes immunopositive for (C) αβ T-cell receptor (TCR) and (D) CD8 in adjacent sections. T cells appear to penetrate the DRG in this region because their density in the rest of the parenchyma is much lower. (E) CD4+ macrophages within the DRG 1 week after CCI forming two perineuronal rings (asterisks), while a CD4+ T cell lies on the edge of the ganglion (small arrow), probably within a superficial blood vessel near the surface of the DRG (dashed line); such cells were extremely rare within the DRG parenchyma. (F) Neutrophils immunopositive for S100A8 associated with the vascular sheath of the DRG 1 week after CCI, including a rouleau of S100A8+ cells within a small blood vessel (arrow). Calibration in C represents 50 μm and also applies to D–F.

2004; Wieseler-Frank et al. 2005). The sensation of pain generated after nerve injury has usually been associated with spontaneous activity that develops in uninjured Aδ- and C- nociceptive axons (Wu et al. 2001), probably in response to the expression of cytokines, such as TNF-α, IL-1β, and IL-6, released by inflammatory cells in the degenerating nerve trunk (Sorkin et al. 1997; Stoll et al. 2002). However, DRG somata (Kim et al. 1998; Dib-Hajj et al. 1999; Stebbing et al. 1999), as well as dorsal horn neurons (Hains et al. 2004) and thalamic neurons (Zhao et al. 2006), become hyperexcitable and can discharge spontaneously due to modified sodium channel expression. Inflammation is therefore associated with raised excitability at many sites along the pain pathways. While this process could be related, at least in part, to cytokine release from macrophages and glia in the DRG and spinal cord, it is not known whether microglia in the thalamus are activated after peripheral nerve injury. Another factor that might raise neuronal excitability and initiate discharge is the relative ischemia resulting from the higher metabolic activity associated with activation and proliferation of non-neuronal cells at these sites.

While it is tempting to suggest that the outcome of monocyte recruitment may be the neuronal production of a signal that passes to their central terminals in the dorsal horn, initiating the activation of microglia and astrocytes in the territory of the lesioned nerve (Wieseler-Frank et al. 2005), this suggestion is incompatible with the rapidity with which the microglia within the dorsal horn respond to peripheral axotomy (within 2 days) (Aldskogius and Kozlova 1998). Activation of microglia has been attributed to degeneration of primary afferent axons (Aldskogius et al. 1985) or to the release of substances such as interferon-γ (Vikman et al. 2003) or adenosine triphosphate (Tsuda et al. 2005) from the terminals of injured neurons. Glial activation is significantly greater after CCI than after transection (Hu et al. 2007) and extends well beyond the superficial layers where most cutaneous nociceptive axons terminate. While the subset of nociceptors that survive the inflammatory lesion is presumably responsible for thermal hyperalgesia, mechanical allodynia is difficult to attribute to myelinated axons after this lesion, which indicates that sensitized nociceptors in the periphery may be involved (Campbell and Meyer 2006).

Invading macrophages and lymphocytes may be either protective or destructive within the DRG. The earliest reports showed that a conditioning lesion of the ventral root that exposes intact sensory axons to the products of Wallerian degeneration potentiates their regeneration following subsequent transection (Rich and Johnson 1985). Similarly, central sensory axons were "primed" to regenerate following bacterial inflammation of DRG (Lu and Richardson 1991). These effects are thought to be triggered by production of neurotrophins by macrophages and glia. Microglia are primarily involved in maintenance and protection in the CNS (Streit 2002), and DRG macrophages may play a similar role, although "excessive" activation is potentially damaging through the complement system. There is no direct evidence of T-cell function in lesioned DRG. In the CNS, a protective role of CD4+, CD25+ T cells in regulating autoimmune reactions normally and following injury has been advocated (Schwartz and Kipnis 2005), and CD4+ T cells have been shown to protect facial motor neurons against axotomy-induced cell death (Jones et al. 2005). Protective functions are also suggested by the expression of B7.2 costimulatory molecules on microglia in the dorsal horn after peripheral nerve lesions (Rutkowski et al. 2004). In contrast, both CD4+ and CD8+ T cells in the CNS have been implicated in demyelinating inflammatory disease (McDole et al. 2006), and there is evidence for a similar destructive role after spinal cord injury (Jones et al. 2004).

While there is good evidence that excitatory cytokines such as TNF-α released from macrophages are involved in generating pain (Schäfers et al. 2003), it has been reported that thalidomide treatment did not abolish pain behavior after CCI, whereas treatment with cyclosporin A, an inhibitor of lymphocyte activation, was effective (Bennett 2000). It is also notable that mechanical/thermal hyperalgesia is reduced in athymic nude rats (Moalem et al. 2004), suggesting a more important contribution to neuropathic pain by T lymphocytes than has been considered so far.

ACKNOWLEDGMENTS

Work in the authors' laboratory has been funded by the National Health & Medical Research Council of Australia (grant numbers 222751 and 400918) and the Wellcome Trust (055627). We are grateful to Carolyn Geczy for helpful discussion and provision of antibody to S100A8 and to Emma Kettle, Kim Dilati, and Rathi Ramasamy for excellent technical assistance. All work in the authors' laboratory was approved by the University of New South Wales Animal Care and Ethics Committee.

REFERENCES

Al-Shatti T, Barr AE, Safadi FF, Amin M, Barbe MF. Increase in inflammatory cytokines in median nerves in a rat model of repetitive motion injury. *J Neuroimmunol* 2005; 167:13–22.

Aldskogius H, Kozlova EN. Central neuron-glial and glial-glial interactions following axon injury. *Prog Neurobiol* 1998; 55:1–26.

Aldskogius H, Arvidsson J, Grant G. The reaction of primary sensory neurons to peripheral nerve injury with particular emphasis on transganglionic changes. *Brain Res* 1985; 357:27–46.

Ali Z, Ringkamp M, Hartke TV, et al. Uninjured C-fiber nociceptors develop spontaneous activity and α-adrenergic sensitivity following L6 spinal nerve ligation in monkey. *J Neurophysiol* 1999; 81:455–466.

Basbaum AI, Gautron M, Jazat F, Mayes M, Guilbaud G. The spectrum of fiber loss in a model of neuropathic pain in the rat: an electron microscopic study. *Pain* 1991; 47:359–367.

Bennett GJ. A neuroimmune interaction in painful peripheral neuropathy. *Clin J Pain* 2000; 16: S139–143.

Bennett GJ, Xie Y-K. A peripheral mononeuropathy in rat that produces disorders of pain sensation like those seen in man. *Pain* 1988; 33:87–107.

Cajal SR. *Degeneration and Regeneration of the Nervous System*. London: Oxford University Press, 1928.

Campbell JN, Meyer RA. Mechanisms of neuropathic pain. *Neuron* 2006; 52:77–92.

Carr MW, Roth SJ, Luther E, Rose SS, Springer TA. Monocyte chemoattractant protein 1 acts as a T-lymphocyte chemoattractant. *Proc Natl Acad Sci USA* 1994; 91:3652–3656.

Colburn RW, DeLeo JA, Rickman AJ, et al. Dissociation of microglial activation and neuro-pathic pain behaviors following peripheral nerve injury in the rat. *J Neuroimmunol* 1997; 79:163–175.

DeLeo JA, Tanga FY, Tawfik VL. Neuroimmune activation and neuroinflammation in chronic pain and opioid tolerance/hyperalgesia. *Neuroscientist* 2004; 10:40–52.

Dib-Hajj SD, Fjell J, Cummins TR, et al. Plasticity of sodium channel expression in DRG neurons in the chronic constriction model of neuropathic pain. *Pain* 1999; 83:591–600.

Engelhardt B, Ransohoff RM. The ins and outs of T-lymphocyte trafficking to the CNS: anatomical sites and molecular mechanisms. *Trends Immunol* 2005; 26:485–495.

Graeber MB, Streit WJ, Kiefer R, Schoen SW, Kreutzberg GW. New expression of myelomonocytic antigen by microglia and perivascular cells following lethal motor neuron injury. *J Neuroim-munol* 1990; 27:121–132.

Graus F, Campo E, Cruz-Sanchez F, Ribalta T, Palacin A. Expression of lymphocyte, macrophage and class I and II major histocompatibility complex antigens in normal human dorsal root ganglia. *J Neurol Sci* 1990; 98:203–211.

Hains BC, Saab CY, Klein JP, Craner MJ, Waxman SG. Altered sodium channel expression in second-order spinal sensory neurons contributes to pain after peripheral nerve injury. *J Neurosci* 2004; 24:4832–4839.

Herdegen T, Skene P, Bähr M. The c-Jun transcription factor—bipotential mediator of neuronal death, survival and regeneration. *Trends Neurosci* 1997; 20:227–231.

Holtzman E, Novikoff AB, Villaverde H. Lysosomes and GERL in normal and chromatolytic neurones of the rat ganglion nodosum. *J Cell Biol* 1967.

Hu P, McLachlan EM. Macrophage and lymphocyte invasion of dorsal root ganglia after peripheral nerve lesions in the rat. *Neuroscience* 2002; 112:23–38.

Hu P, McLachlan EM. Distinct functional types of macrophage in dorsal root ganglia and spinal nerve proximal to sciatic and spinal nerve transections in the rat. *Exp Neurol* 2003a; 184:590–605.

Hu P, McLachlan EM. Selective reactions of cutaneous and muscle afferent neurons to peripheral nerve transection in rats. *J Neurosci* 2003b; 23:10559–10567.

Hu P, McLachlan EM. Inflammation in sympathetic ganglia proximal to sciatic nerve transection in rats. *Neurosci Lett* 2004; 365:39–42.

Hu P, Bembrick AL, Keay KA, McLachlan EM. Immune cell involvement in dorsal root ganglia and spinal cord after chronic constriction or transection of the rat sciatic nerve. *Brain Behav Immun* 2007; in press.

Jacobs JM, Macfarlane RM, Cavanagh JB. Vascular leakage in the dorsal root ganglia of the rat, studied with horseradish peroxidase. *J Neurol Sci* 1976; 29:95–107.

Jander S, Lausberg F, Stoll G. Differential recruitment of CD8+ macrophages during Wallerian degeneration in the peripheral and central nervous system. *Brain Pathol* 2001; 11:27–38.

Jones KJ, Serpe CJ, Byram SC, DeBoy CA, Sanders VM. Role of the immune system in the maintenance of mouse facial motoneuron viability after nerve injury. *Brain Behavior Immunity* 2005; 19:12–19.

Jones TB, Ankeny DP, Guan Z, et al. Passive or active immunization with myelin basic protein impairs neurological function and exacerbates neuropathology after spinal cord injury in rats. *J Neurosci* 2004; 24:3752–3761.

Kim HJ, Na HS, Kim SH, et al. Cell type-specific changes of the membrane properties of peripherally-axotomized dorsal root ganglion neurons in a rat model of neuropathic pain. *Neuroscience* 1998; 86:301–309.

Lekan HA, Chung K, Yoon YW, Chung JM, Coggeshall RE. Loss of dorsal root ganglion cells concomitant with dorsal root axon sprouting following segmental nerve lesion. *Neuroscience* 1997; 81:527–534.

Leone L, De Stefano ME, Del Signore A, Petrucci TC, Paggi P. Axotomy of sympathetic neurons activates the metalloproteinase-2 enzymatic pathway. *J Neuropath Exp Neurol* 2005; 64:1007–1017.

Li L, Xian CJ, Zhong J-H, Zhou X-F. Effect of lumbar 5 ventral root transection on pain behaviors: a novel rat model for neuropathic pain without axotomy of primary sensory neurons. *Exp Neurol* 2002; 175:23–34.

Lieberman AR. The axon reaction: a review of the principal features of perikaryal responses to axon injury. *Int Rev Neurobiol* 1971; 14:49–124.

Lu X, Richardson PM. Inflammation near the nerve cell body enhances axonal regeneration. *J Neurosci* 1991; 11:972–978.

McCabe JS, Low FN. The subarachnoid angle: an area of transition in peripheral nerve. *Anat Rec* 1969; 164:15–34.

McDole J, Johnson AJ, Pirko I. The role of CD8+ T-cells in lesion formation and axonal dysfunction in multiple sclerosis. *Neurol Res* 2006; 28:256–261.

McLachlan EM, Hu P. Axonal sprouts containing calcitonin gene-related peptide and substance P form pericellular baskets around large diameter neurones after sciatic nerve transection in the rat. *Neuroscience* 1998; 84:961–965.

McLachlan EM, Jänig W, Devor M, Michaelis M. Peripheral nerve injury triggers noradrenergic sprouting within dorsal root ganglia. *Nature* 1993; 363:543–546.

McMenamin PC. Distribution and phenotype of dendritic cells and resident tissue macrophages in the dura mater, leptomeninges, and choroid plexus of the rat brain as demonstrated in wholemount preparations. *J Comp Neurol* 1999; 405:553–562.

Miki K, Iwata K, Tsuboi Y, et al. Dorsal column-thalamic pathway is involved in thalamic hyperexcitability following peripheral nerve injury: a lesion study in rats with experimental mononeuropathy. *Pain* 2000; 85:263–271.

Mira JC. Maintien de la continuité de la lame basale des fibres nerveuses périphériques après "section" des axones par congélation localisée. [Maintenance of the continuity of the basal lamina of peripheral nerve fibers after "section" of the axons by localized congelation.] *C R Acad Sci Hebd Seances Acad Sci D* 1971; 273:1836–1839.

Moalem G, Xu K, Yu L. T lymphocytes play a role in neuropathic pain following peripheral nerve injury in rats. *Neuroscience* 2004; 129:767–777.

Morse DE, Low FN. The fine structure of subarachnoid macrophages in the rat. *Anat Rec* 1972; 174:469–475.

Obata K, Noguchi K. BDNF in sensory neurons and chronic pain. *Neurosci Res* 2006; 55:1–10.

Obata K, Yamanaka H, Dai Y, et al. Contribution of degeneration of motor and sensory fibers to pain behavior and the changes in neurotrophic factors in rat dorsal root ganglion. *Exp Neurol* 2004; 188:149–160.

Obata K, Yamanaka H, Kobayashi K, et al. The effect of site and type of nerve injury on the expression of brain-derived neurotrophic factor in the dorsal root ganglion and on neuropathic pain behavior. *Neuroscience* 2006; 137:961–970.

Olsson T, Diener P, Ljungdahl A, et al. Facial nerve transection causes expansion of myelin autoreactive T cells in regional lymph nodes and T cell homing to the facial nucleus. *Autoimmunity* 1992; 13:117–126.

Peters CM, Jimenez-Andrade JM, Jonas BM, et al. Intravenous paclitaxel administration in the rat induces a peripheral sensory neuropathy characterized by macrophage infiltration and injury to sensory neurons and their supporting cells. *Exp Neurol* 2007; 203:42–54.

Polfliet MM, Fabriek BO, Daniels WP, Dijkstra CD, van den Berg TK. The rat macrophage scavenger receptor CD163: expression, regulation and role in inflammatory mediator production. *Immunobiology* 2006; 211:419–425.

Rich KM, Johnson EM. Ventral rhizotomy enhances regeneration of uninjured sensory neurons. *Brain Res* 1985; 335:182–187.

Rodriguez Parkitna J, Korostynski M, Kaminska-Chowaniec D, et al. Comparison of gene expression profiles in neuropathic and inflammatory pain. *J Physiol Pharmacol* 2006; 57:401–414.

Rutkowski MD, Lambert F, Raghavendra V, DeLeo JA. Presence of spinal B7.2 (CD86) but not B7.1 (CD80) co-stimulatory molecules following peripheral nerve injury: role of nondestructive immunity in neuropathic pain. *J Neuroimmunol* 2004; 146:94–98.

Schäfers M, Geis C, Svensson CI, Luo ZD, Sommer C. Selective increase of tumor necrosis factor-alpha in injured and spared myelinated primary afferents after chronic constrictive injury of rat sciatic nerve. *Eur J Neurosci* 2003; 17:791–804.

Schwartz M, Kipnis J. Therapeutic T cell-based vaccination for neurodegenerative disorders: the role of CD4+CD25+ regulatory T cells. *Ann NY Acad Sci* 2005; 1051:701–708.

Shortland PJ, Baytug B, Krzyzanowska A, et al. ATF3 expression in L4 dorsal root ganglion neurons after L5 spinal nerve transection. *Eur J Neurosci* 2006; 23:365–373.

Sorkin LS, Xiao WH, Wagner R, Myers RR. Tumour necrosis factor-alpha induces ectopic activity in nociceptive primary afferent fibres. *Neuroscience* 1997; 81:255–262.

Stebbing MJ, Eschenfelder S, Häbler HJ, et al. Changes in the action potential in sensory neurones after peripheral axotomy in vivo. *Neuroreport* 1999; 10:201–206.

Stoll G, Jander S, Myers RR. Degeneration and regeneration of the peripheral nervous system: from Augustus Waller's observations to neuroinflammation. *J Periph Nerv Syst* 2002; 7:13–27.

Streit WJ. Microglia as neuroprotective, immunocompetent cells of the CNS. *Glia* 2002; 40:133–139.

Tanaka T, Minami M, Nakagawa T, Satoh M. Enhanced production of monocyte chemoattractant protein-1 in the dorsal root ganglia in a rat model of neuropathic pain: possible involvement in the development of neuropathic pain. *Neurosci Res* 2004; 48:463–469.

Tandrup T, Woolf CJ, Coggeshall RE. Delayed loss of small dorsal root ganglion cells after transection of the rat sciatic nerve. *J Comp Neurol* 2000; 422:172–180.

Tsuda M, Inoue K, Salter MW. Neuropathic pain and spinal microglia: a big problem from molecules in "small" glia. *Trends Neurosci* 2005; 28:101–107.

Tsujino H, Kondo E, Fukuoka T, et al. Activating transcription factor 3 (ATF3) induction by axotomy in sensory and motoneurons: a novel neuronal marker of nerve injury. *Mol Cell Neurosci* 2000; 15:170–182.

Vass K, Hickey WF, Schmidt RE, Lassmann H. Bone marrow-derived elements in the peripheral nervous system. *Lab Invest* 1993; 69:275–282.

Vianello F, Olszak IT, Poznansky MC. Fugetaxis: active movement of leukocytes away from a chemokinetic agent. *J Mol Med* 2005; 83:752–763.

Vikman KS, Hill RH, Backstrom E, Robertson B, Kristensson K. Interferon-gamma induces characteristics of central sensitization in spinal dorsal horn neurons in vitro. *Pain* 2003; 106:241–251.

Wieseler-Frank J, Maier SF, Watkins LR. Central proinflammatory cytokines and pain enhancement. *Neurosignals* 2005; 14:166–174.

Wu G, Ringkamp M, Hartke TV, et al. Early onset of spontaneous activity in uninjured C-fiber nociceptors after injury to neighboring nerve fibers. *J Neurosci* 2001; 21:RC140.

Wu G, Ringkamp M, Murinson BB, et al. Degeneration of myelinated efferent fibers induces spontaneous activity in uninjured C-fiber afferents. *J Neurosci* 2002; 22:7746–7753.

Zhang J, De Koninck Y. Spatial and temporal relationship between monocyte chemoattractant protein-1 expression and spinal glial activation following peripheral nerve injury. *J Neurochem* 2006; 97:772–783.

Zhao P, Waxman SG, Hains BC. Sodium channel expression in the ventral posterolateral nucleus of the thalamus after peripheral nerve injury. *Mol Pain* 2006; 2:27.

Zhou XF, Deng Y-S, Chie E, et al. Satellite cell-derived nerve growth factor and neurotrophin-3 are involved in noradrenergic sprouting in the dorsal root ganglia following peripheral nerve injury in the rat. *Eur J Neurosci* 1999; 11:1711–1722.

Correspondence to: Prof. Elspeth M. McLachlan, Prince of Wales Medical Research Institute, Gate 1, Barker Street, Randwick, NSW 2031, Australia. Tel: 61-2-9399-1031; fax: 61-2-9399-1034; email: e.mclachlan@unsw.edu.au.

Part IV

Glial Regulation of Neuronal Functions Relevant to Pain

Immune and Glial Regulation of Pain, edited by Joyce
A. DeLeo, Linda S. Sorkin, and Linda R. Watkins,
IASP Press, Seattle, © 2007.

11

Cytokine Regulation of Ion Channels in the Pain Pathway

Maria Elena P. Morales and Robert W. Gereau IV

*Washington University Pain Center, Department of Anesthesiology,
and Department of Anatomy and Neurobiology, Washington University School
of Medicine, St. Louis, Missouri, USA*

Cytokines are a diverse group of small proteins that are critical for communication between cells. They are released by various cell types and can act both systemically and regionally within an organism. Cytokines have been extensively studied in the field of immunology because they have critical functions in immune responses. Cytokines are integral to acquired and innate immune responses and are important in inflammation, infection, and development. They elicit responses in target cells by binding to specific receptors on the cell surface. Cytokines are being recognized as important players in many different biological processes, and their roles extend far beyond their traditional function in immune responses.

Over the past few decades, many studies have identified critical roles for cytokines in the induction and modulation of pain. Cytokines have long been known to be integral components of the inflammatory response to injury or infection (for review, see Lin et al. 2000). As such, they induce the release in the periphery of other inflammatory mediators, which can then activate or sensitize primary afferent nociceptors. It is becoming increasingly clear however, that cytokines play a more direct role in pain induction. After nerve injury, interleukin-6 (IL-6), IL-1β, and tumor necrosis factor-α (TNF-α) mRNA transcripts increase in the spinal cord and the dorsal root ganglia (DRG) (Murphy et al. 1995; Winkelstein et al. 2001). In a number of neuropathic pain models, TNF-α, IL-1β, and IL-6 protein levels increase in the spinal cord and the DRG after nerve injury (Murphy et al. 1995; DeLeo et al. 1997; Saldanha et al. 2000; Winkelstein et al. 2001; Schafers et al. 2002). Altered levels of these cytokines are found at sites far-removed from the primary insult, suggesting that these molecules may have roles beyond simple involvement in the inflammatory response at the injury site.

The increased expression of cytokines in the periphery, spinal cord, and DRG after nerve injury provides evidence of their potential involvement in neuronal activation and thus in nociception. However, the possibility remains that the role of these cytokines is not one of direct induction of pain but rather of communication among non-neuronal cells that are activated in these regions as a result of the injury. In short, the increased expression of these cytokines could occur in parallel with another mechanism that induces pain. Although it is certainly true that cytokines mediate communication among immune cells in these regions, extensive data have shown that they also have a more direct role in pain induction. Cytokines such as TNF-α, IL-1β, IL-8, IL-12, IL-18, and RANTES (regulated on activation normal T-cell expressed and secreted/CCL5), as well as the chemokines macrophage inflammatory protein-1α (MIP-1α/CCL3), stromal cell-derived factor-1α (SDF-1α/CXCL12), and macrophage-derived chemokine (MDC/CCL22), induce mechanical and/or thermal hypersensitivity after intraplantar injection (Ferreira et al. 1988; Cunha et al. 1991, 1992; Woolf et al. 1997; Oh et al. 2001; Verri et al. 2004, 2005; Zhang et al. 2005; Jin and Gereau 2006). In addition, direct application of TNF-α and IL-1β to the DRG and to the sciatic nerve results in mechanical allodynia (Homma et al. 2002; Schafers et al. 2003; Zelenka et al. 2005).

Consistent with the findings that application of cytokines induces pain, treatments that block the action of these cytokines have also been shown to reduce pain. Intrathecal pretreatment with soluble TNF receptor alone or in combination with IL-1 receptor antagonist reduces mechanical allodynia after injury (Sweitzer et al. 2001). Direct application of anti-TNF-α antibody to the sciatic nerve at the time of chronic constriction injury induction results in decreased thermal and mechanical hypersensitivity compared to animals treated with control sheep IgG (Lindenlaub et al. 2000; Sommer et al. 2001). These approaches have not only been effective in reducing nociceptive responses in animal models; they have also been used in patients as effective treatments for painful clinical conditions. The soluble TNF-α receptor (etanercept), a monoclonal antibody to TNF-α (infliximab), and an IL-1 receptor antagonist (anakinra) are examples of cytokine-targeted drugs currently used to treat painful clinical conditions such as rheumatoid arthritis and inflammatory bowel disease (Ardizzone and Bianchi Porro 2005; Atzeni et al. 2005; Konttinen et al. 2005; Ranganathan 2005).

Collectively, these data show that cytokines have a definitive role in pain induction. However, the mechanisms by which these cytokines modulate the transduction of nociceptive signals are still being uncovered. There are many potential targets in cytokine modulation of pain sensitivity. Cytokines could activate transcriptional pathways leading to upregulation of receptors or channels, resulting in increased sensitivity to peripheral stimuli. Alternatively, they could initiate protein synthesis directed at increasing sites of synaptic connectivity between primary afferents and second-order neurons, thus enhancing synaptic strength at these connections. While there are many potential targets in cytokine-induced modulation of pain sensitivity, in this chapter we will focus on cytokine modulation of ion channels and the implications of that interaction in altering pain sensitivity.

ION CHANNELS INVOLVED IN PAIN

Cytokines clearly have many diverse actions capable of regulating a plethora of cellular processes, but their specific modulation of pain sensitivity could be linked to changes in ion channel physiology. Distinct ion channels that are known to be critical to nociceptor function are potential targets in cytokine modulation of pain sensitivity. Here, we will briefly describe some of these ion channels and summarize their potential and identified involvement in pain mechanisms.

SODIUM CHANNELS

Several sodium channels have been identified as integral components of nociceptor function. The sodium channel family consists of nine subtypes of voltage-gated channels ($Na_V1.1$–1.9) that vary in localization, kinetics, and sensitivity to tetrodotoxin (TTX). Arguably, the most prominent sodium channels studied in relation to pain are the TTX-resistant (TTX-R) subunits termed $Na_V1.8$ (Akopian et al. 1996) and $Na_V1.9$ (Dib-Hajj et al. 1998). Although these subunits are very similar, they are functionally distinct. Both are slowly inactivating compared to TTX-sensitive subunits, but $Na_V1.8$ mediates a relatively transient current while $Na_V1.9$ mediates a more persistent current that is more slowly inactivating (Tate et al. 1998). Interest in these channels with reference to pain mechanisms arose from the fact that their expression is restricted to the DRG, and within the DRG, they are restricted to small- and medium-diameter nociceptors (Sangameswaran et al. 1996; Tate et al. 1998). Functionally, the roles of $Na_V1.8$ and $Na_V1.9$ in nociception seem to be very different, as identified through knockout of the respective genes. $Na_V1.8$ null mice have impaired development of inflammatory hyperalgesia and deficits in their response to noxious thermal and mechanical stimuli (Akopian et al. 1999). They also have impaired responses to sensitizing noxious visceral stimuli as well as a complete absence of referred hyperalgesia after intracolonic capsaicin (Laird et al. 2002). Although $Na_V1.9$ null mice have no apparent impairment in their response to acute nociceptive stimuli, they do have significant deficits in nociceptive responses to inflammation. They have a significantly attenuated second phase in the formalin test as well as truncated responses to inflammatory stimuli, indicating a role for $Na_V1.9$ in the maintenance of these nociceptive responses (Priest et al. 2005). Clearly, these channels have a significant role in inflammatory hyperalgesia, a condition in which cytokines are integral.

TTX-sensitive sodium channels are also implicated in alterations in nociception. Specifically, changes in $Na_V1.3$ and $Na_V1.7$ expression in the DRG have been identified in animal models of neuropathy (Black et al. 1999; Dib-Hajj et al. 1999; Hong et al. 2004). Both of these channels mediate currents with fast inactivation rates. In addition, unlike the TTX-R Na^+ channels, their localization is not restricted to nociceptors. Although expression of $Na_V1.3$ is almost absent in the naïve adult rat, its increased expression after injury has been linked to a role in ectopic discharge from nociceptors (Cummins and Waxman 1997; Black et al. 1999). $Na_V1.7$ is expressed in all neuronal subtypes in the DRG, and mutations in the gene for this channel have been linked to clinical neuropathy (Yang et al. 2004).

Although the few channels discussed here have been the focus of research on sodium channel involvement in nociception, there are certainly others that could play critical roles in the induction and modulation of nociception (for review, see Lai et al. 2004). It is apparent from the data discussed here that these sodium channels have integral roles in various pain states, and all can be important sites of cytokine-induced induction and modulation of pain.

POTASSIUM CHANNELS

Since modulation of K^+ channel activity can directly affect neuronal firing, K^+ channels are likely suspects in any search for mechanisms of modulation of neuronal excitability. Opening of K^+ channels leads to decreases in excitability, whereas blocking them can lead to enhanced excitability. K^+ channels have also been identified as potential targets in the modulation of nociception. For example, activation of K^+ channels is one mechanism by which many opioids (Ocana et al. 1996; Ikeda et al. 2000) and tricyclic antidepressants (Galeotti et al. 2001) produce antinociceptive effects, and inhibition of K^+ channel function has been shown to enhance nociceptive responses (Hu et al. 2006).

There are at least five different classes of K^+ channels (Gutman et al. 2003), of which several subtypes have been implicated in pain. Here, we will discuss the voltage-gated K^+ (K_V) channels, the two-pore K^+ (K_{2p}) channels, and the inward rectifying K^+ (K_{IR}) channels. Each of these classes of channels includes several different subtypes. We will focus on those that have been identified as important players in nociception.

The K_V channel family consists of several different subtypes that are expressed throughout the body. Of this group, the K_V1, K_V4, and K_V7 subfamilies are of particular importance in pain transmission (for review, see Ocana et al. 2004). From the K_V1 subfamily, $K_V1.1$ has been shown to have a role in nociception because knockout of the gene encoding this subunit results in hypersensitivity to thermal and inflammatory stimuli (Clark and Tempel 1998), and $K_V1.4$ has been localized to primary afferent nociceptors where it could contribute to nociception (Rasband et al. 2001). From the K_V4 subfamily, $K_V4.1$, $K_V4.2$, and $K_V4.3$ channel subunits produce A-type currents that regulate neuronal excitability (for review, see Song 2002). These transient outward currents are activated at subthreshold membrane potentials, inactivate rapidly, and quickly recover from inactivation. They can regulate neuronal excitability by counteracting small depolarizations, thereby maintaining the cell at more hyperpolarized potentials. Therefore, inhibition of these A-type currents results in increased neuronal firing (Hu and Gereau 2003; Hu et al. 2006; Takeda et al. 2006). After chronic constriction injury, K^+ channel α-subunit mRNA decreases in injured DRG compared to contralateral uninjured controls (Kim et al. 2002). Among the transcripts that decrease are those encoding the K_V subunits 4.2 and 4.3, which provides a potential mechanism for the increased excitability of DRG neurons after chronic constriction injury that leads to enhanced nociception. In addition, knockout of the $K_V4.2$ subunit results in hypersensitivity to thermal and mechanical stimuli (Hu et al. 2006), indicating an integral role of this subunit in regulating excitability in the pain neuraxis. Finally, in models of persistent and neuropathic pain, the K_V7 channel opener, retigabine, has been shown to reduce nociceptive behavior (Blackburn-Munro and Jensen 2003). Compounds that specifically activate these channels are potential therapeutic agents for nociception. Further investigation is necessary to fully elucidate the roles of these K_V subfamilies in nociception.

The two-pore K^+ channel family includes 15 channel subtypes (Gutman et al. 2003; Franks and Honore 2004), of which the mRNA for at least six has been identified in the DRG (Kang and Kim 2006). K_{2P} channels produce a background leak conductance that influences resting membrane potential, excitability and action potential duration (Franks and Honore 2004). One channel in particular, TREK-1, has been identified as a potential polymodal pain sensor, because knockout of this channel results in deficits in behavioral responses to nociceptive osmotic, thermal, and mechanical stimuli (Alloui et al. 2006). Although research on the role of the K_{2P} channel family in nociception is sparse, the family's biophysical properties, as well as localization, implicate these channels as potentially critical modulators of nociceptive responses.

Finally, the K_{IR} channels are a group of channels characterized by conduction of larger inward K^+ currents at potentials below the equilibrium potential for K^+ (E_K) than the outward K^+ currents elicited at potentials above E_K, and thus they are termed "inward rectifiers." These channels are responsible for maintaining the resting membrane potential and for action potential repolarization, among many other functions (for review, see Lu 2004). The K_{IR} family comprises seven subfamilies (Gutman et al. 2003), of which two will be discussed here because of their known involvement in nociception.

The G-protein-regulated inward rectifier K^+ channels (GIRKs) and the ATP-sensitive K^+ (K_{ATP}) channels have both been extensively studied in relation to nociception. Research has mainly focused on the role of these channels in morphine-induced antinociception. Block of K_{ATP} channels prevents the antinociception induced by morphine administration, and deletion of GIRKs also impairs morphine-induced analgesia in a number of behavioral tests of nociception (reviewed by Ocana et al. 2004). The antinociception produced by morphine administration is thought to be mediated in part by activation of G proteins that open these K^+ channels, leading to decreased cell excitability (reviewed by Ocana et al. 2004). These channels represent an intriguing possible target for chemokine modulation of nociceptive mechanisms because all chemokine receptors are G-protein-coupled receptors; thus, chemokines could potentially activate these K_{IR} channels and affect processing of nociceptive stimuli.

Taken together, the data regarding K^+ channel involvement in pain identify an integral role for these channels in regulating behavioral responses to nociceptive stimuli. K^+ channel activity can be modulated by a number of intracellular signaling molecules including kinases and G proteins; activation of these intermediates is a potential mechanism by which cytokines can alter nociceptive processing.

TRP CHANNELS

Alterations in nociception can also occur at the level of stimulus detection (see Bhave and Gereau 2004). The transient receptor potential (TRP) channel family comprises six subfamilies of homologous six transmembrane domain proteins that form nonselective cation channels specializing in the detection of thermal and chemical stimuli (Story 2006). Some of these channels have been the focus of intense study over the past decade, and significant progress has been made in identifying their roles in pain sensation.

The transient receptor potential vanilloid (TRPV) subfamily is one such subset of channels that has been identified as integral to many pain mechanisms. Specifically, TRPV1, TRPV2, TRPV3, and TRPV4 are known to act as thermoreceptors throughout the spectrum of warm or hot temperatures, with TRPV1 and TRPV2 acting in the noxious heat range and TRPV3 and 4 in the innocuous warmth range (for review, see Patapoutian et al. 2003). Study of TRPV1 has dominated the literature on TRP channels and pain. It was the first vanilloid receptor cloned and has been identified to be responsive to heat at temperatures ≥42°C (Welch et al. 2000); to capsaicin, the pungent component of chili peppers (Caterina et al. 1997); and to low pH (Tominaga et al. 1998). Knockout of TRPV1 results in decreases in thermal hypersensitivity after inflammation, complete loss of capsaicin sensitivity, and greatly attenuated responses to low pH (Caterina et al. 2000).

Of the remaining TRP channel subfamilies, two are of particular interest in pain sensation. From the melastatin (TRPM) and ankyrin (TRPA) families, respectively, TRPM8 and TRPA1 have been identified as cold sensors, with TRPA1 acting in the noxious cold range (<17°C) (Story et al. 2003) and TRPM8 in the innocuous cold range (25–28°C) (Peier et al. 2002). Both are expressed in primary afferent sensory neurons, with TRPM8 localized to small-diameter neurons of the DRG and TRPA1 colocalized with calcitonin gene-related peptide and substance P, two markers of nociceptors. In addition to temperature, these channels are activated to varying degrees by a number of ligands. TRPM8 is activated by menthol and the synthetic peptide icilin (McKemy et al. 2002). TRPA1 is activated by a number of pungent compounds found in cinnamon oil, mustard oil, clove oil, wintergreen oil, and ginger, as well as by bradykinin, a key mediator of peripheral inflammation (Bandell et al. 2004).

These channels have important roles in various mechanisms of nociception. TRPM8 has been identified in Aδ and C fibers expressing tyrosine kinase A (TrkA) receptors (Kobayashi et al. 2005). In addition, TRPM8 is abundantly expressed in the trigeminal ganglion, where it could contribute to the mechanism of tooth pain induced by temperature changes.

Two separate groups have characterized the nociceptive responses of TRPA1 knockout mice to a variety of stimuli. Both groups identified deficits in the nociceptive response to mustard oil, indicating that TRPA1 is the only receptor activated by this compound, but they observed different responses to mechanical and cold stimuli. In one study, knockout of TRPA1 results in deficits in the detection of noxious cold. TRPA1 knockout animals exhibited decreased withdrawal from a cold surface maintained at 0–1°C, as well as diminished sensitivity to acetone on the dorsal surface of the hindpaw as compared to wild-type animals. The study also showed that knockout of the receptor results in deficits in mechanical nociception (Kwan et al. 2006). In contrast, the other group did not note any deficits in responses to cold or mechanical stimuli (Bautista et al. 2006). Although the controversy remains unsolved, in a recent study using antisense knockdown of TRPA1 in the DRG, a significant decrease in cold hyperalgesia after spinal nerve ligation was observed at 3, 5, and 7 days after injury (Katsura et al. 2006). In addition, a recent study investigating genetic predictors for pain sensitivity in humans points to a potential link between TRPA1 and decreased sensitivity to noxious cold in a gender-specific manner (Kim et al. 2006).

EVIDENCE OF CYTOKINE REGULATION
OF ION CHANNELS IN PAIN

Much is known about the importance of cytokines in pain induction and maintenance, and although many ion channels have been identified as potential targets of these cytokines in pain induction, research aimed at characterizing a functional interaction between these two components of the pain pathway is sparse and only deals with a small subset of cytokines. Here, we will discuss the evidence that indicates a functional role of cytokine modulation of ion channels in nociception.

TNF-α and TRPV1 are both widely studied in the field of pain, and as such, it is no surprise that of the few studies investigating cytokine modulation of ion channels in pain, most investigate the roles of one or both of these proteins. Nicol et al. (1997) examined the ability of TNF-α to modulate capsaicin sensitivity in rat DRG. As mentioned earlier, knockout experiments have shown that capsaicin sensitivity is solely mediated by TRPV1. Therefore, it is a reasonable hypothesis that the effects of TNF-α on capsaicin sensitivity can only occur through a TRPV1-mediated mechanism. Twenty-four-hour pretreatment of cultured embryonic rat DRG with TNF-α resulted in a dose-dependent increase in the percentage of capsaicin-responsive cells (Nicol et al. 1997). A maximal effect was observed after only 4 hours of pretreatment. It is very unlikely that the capsaicin-sensitive neurons are undergoing mitotic division in this preparation, and thus it appears that the TNF-α treatment can alter the protein expression profiles or receptor surface expression of these neurons from being completely unresponsive to capsaicin to being significantly sensitive to the compound. It is not known whether TNF-α exerts this effect by initiating transcription of mRNA encoding TRPV1, by inducing the trafficking of internalized receptors to the membrane, or by another means.

TNF-α was also shown to increase capsaicin-evoked currents in these neurons. Application of TNF-α for 4, 12, and 24 hours evoked a twofold increase in current amplitudes elicited by capsaicin application. This increase was not observed after a 10-minute application of TNF-α, indicating that the time-course of TNF-α modulation of TRPV1 currents observed in this study is on the order of hours rather than minutes. However, the behavioral data regarding TNF-α and TRPV1 indicate that TNF-α can induce thermal hyperalgesia mediated by TRPV1 in just 30 minutes, the earliest time point tested after TNF administration (Jin and Gereau 2006). Although the time-course of TNF-α-induced modulation of TRPV1 still requires direct analysis, evidence has shed light on the mechanism by which this modulation occurs. The increase in capsaicin sensitivity seen after TNF-α application was blocked by the nonselective cyclooxygenase (COX) inhibitor indomethacin, as well as by the specific COX-2 inhibitor SC-236, indicating that the mechanism of TNF-α-induced enhancement of capsaicin-evoked currents involves prostaglandin synthesis (Nicol et al. 1997).

In addition to TNF-α, the chemokine CCL3, also known as macrophage inflammatory protein 1α (MIP-1α), has also been shown to potentiate cellular responses to capsaicin (Zhang et al. 2005). In human embryonic kidney (HEK) cells transfected with CCR1, one of the receptors for CCL3/MIP-1α, and TRPV1, pretreatment with CCL3/MIP-1α resulted in an approximately threefold increase in capsaicin-elicited calcium influx as measured by fura-2 emission. CCR1 is expressed in the DRG, predominantly in small- and medium-diameter neurons identified as nociceptors. Furthermore, the majority of neurons expressing TRPV1 also express CCR1. In dissociated DRG cultures, pretreatment with CCL3/MIP-1α sensitized the calcium response to capsaicin such that lower concentrations of capsaicin were able to elicit calcium responses indistinguishable from those elicited by higher concentrations of capsaicin applied alone. This effect was further potentiated by the addition of CCL8, another proinflammatory chemokine, indicating that the sensitization seen after CCL3/MIP-1α pretreatment is not saturated and that application of multiple chemokines can enhance the effect (Zhang et al. 2005). Pretreatment with CCL8 or CCL5 alone resulted in sensitization similar to that seen with CCL3/MIP-1α pretreatment, pointing to a more general role of chemokines in the modulation of TRPV1. The effect of CCL3/MIP-1α pretreatment was abolished by pretreatment with pertussis toxin, an inhibitor of the G_i protein. As expected, inhibition of the G_i protein interfered with the effects of CCL3/MIP-1α, because, as mentioned above, all chemokine receptors, including CCR1, are G-protein-coupled receptors; in this case, CCR1 is specifically coupled to G_i. Additionally, pretreatment with a phospholipase C (PLC) inhibitor and a protein kinase C (PKC) inhibitor were both able to impair the sensitization by CCL3/MIP-1α pretreatment, identifying these intracellular mediators as critical components of the pathway by which CCL3/MIP-1α activation of CCR1 potentiates the calcium response of DRG neurons to capsaicin (Zhang et al. 2005). Consistent with these findings, TRPV1 is a known target of phosphorylation by PKC, and this phosphorylation enhances the capsaicin-evoked activation of TRPV1 (Numazaki et al. 2002; Bhave et al. 2003).

Recently, our laboratory has identified a mechanism for TNF-α-induced thermal hypersensitivity mediated by TRPV1 and for TNF-α-induced mechanical hypersensitivity mediated by p38 mitogen-activated protein kinase

(MAPK) modulation of TTX-R Na^+ currents (Jin and Gereau 2006). Intraplantar TNF-α injection elicited a hyperalgesic response to thermal stimuli in wild-type mice. However, responses of TRPV1 knockout mice were indistinguishable from those seen prior to TNF-α treatment, and TNF-α-induced mechanical allodynia remained intact. This finding clearly identifies a link between TNF-α and TRPV1 in thermal hyperalgesia, and it also points to a distinct mechanism to account for mechanical allodynia induced by TNF-α. In dissociated mouse DRG cultures, TNF-α application, through TNF-α receptor 1 (TNFR1), induced increases in TTX-R Na^+ currents, and treatment with SB202190, a p38 MAPK inhibitor, prevented this increase. This p38-mediated increase in TTX-R Na^+ currents was proposed to be the mechanism by which TNF-α induces mechanical allodynia in vivo. In support of this role, in vivo pretreatment with the p38 inhibitor SB202190 inhibited the mechanical allodynia observed after TNF-α injection.

The TTX-R Na^+ currents observed in these experiments exhibited a relatively transient current characteristic of the currents produced by the $Na_V1.8$ channel subunit. While it is known that $Na_V1.8$ has a role in nociception (Akopian et al. 1999), its specific function in TNF-α-induced hypersensitivity remains unknown. Experiments using $Na_V1.8$ knockout mice should assist in deciphering the role of this ion channel in cytokine-induced nociception. If the channel is necessary for the mechanical hypersensitivity observed previously, it might also mediate increased excitability of primary afferent DRG, which is proposed to lead to hyperalgesia. Further study will be required to fully outline the role of $Na_V1.8$ in the hypersensitivity induced by TNF-α treatment.

In addition to TNF-α, IL-1β has also been shown to modulate the responses of TRPV1-positive sensory neurons to heat stimuli in vitro (Obreja et al. 2002). IL-1β application to dissociated rat DRG resulted in an increase in heat-activated current amplitudes and a decrease in the heat threshold for activation of these currents. These changes were prevented by treatment with protein kinase inhibitors specific to protein tyrosine kinases and to PKC, a known modulator of TRPV1 (Bhave et al. 2003). In addition, through RT-PCR, the receptor mediating these effects was identified as IL-1 receptor I (IL-1 RI), because IL-1 receptor II was not detected in this cell population. This study nicely shows a complete mechanism by which IL-1β can act upon TRPV1 to alter neuronal responses to heat in DRG.

Furthermore, in capsaicin-sensitive trigeminal nociceptors, IL-1β was shown to modulate Na^+ currents in a time- and dose-dependent manner (Liu et al. 2006). Interestingly, after a 5-minute incubation with IL-1β, Na^+ current amplitude decreased with increasing doses of IL-1β, while conductance-voltage and inactivation-voltage relationships were shifted to more hyperpolarized potentials at the highest dose. However, after 24-hour incubation with IL-1β,

Na$^+$ current amplitude increased significantly by approximately 67%, with no effect on conductance- or inactivation-voltage relationships. These effects were reversed by treatment with the IL-1β receptor antagonist, and they were independent of changes in TTX-R Na$^+$ currents, which did not significantly change when measured alone in the presence of TTX. Since these trigeminal ganglion neurons express IL-1 receptor I and not II, the effect of IL-1β is through an IL-1RI-mediated and G-protein-dependent mechanism that was also verified through the use of a G-protein inhibitor. The effects of long-term exposure to IL-1β could partially explain the hyperalgesia observed after chronic inflammation where cytokines and other inflammatory mediators are exposed to the primary afferents for longer durations.

Finally, in an act of defiance, someone has actually set out to study a cytokine other than TNF-α in combination with a cell population including, but not restricted to, TRPV1-expressing DRG. White et al. (2005) examined the effect of the chemokine, monocyte chemoattractant protein-1/CCL2 (MCP-1/CCL2), on DRG excitability in the context of chronic compression of the DRG. After chronic compression, expression of MCP-1/CCL2 and its receptor CCR2 increased in both injured and adjacent uninjured DRG. In addition, application of MCP-1/CCL2 to explanted, intact, formerly compressed DRG resulted in increased depolarization, whereas uncompressed DRG were unresponsive. While this selective activation of compressed DRG can be explained by the increase in CCR2 protein expression, it does raise the question of what mechanism, initiated by injury, causes this apparent shift in the DRG protein expression profile. Nevertheless, these data indicate that through a G-protein-mediated mechanism, MCP-1/CCL2 is able to induce excitation of chronically compressed DRG neurons. G-protein components are known to activate a number of intracellular kinases with the potential to phosphorylate ion channels, including TRPV1, and to increase DRG excitability. Additionally, using whole-cell voltage-clamp of previously compressed DRG neurons, Sun et al. (2006) found that local application of MCP-1/CCL2 to the cell soma inhibited voltage-dependent non-inactivating K$^+$ current without affecting A-type currents. Furthermore, in support of the role of MCP-1/CCL2 in nociception, CCR2 knockouts have a significantly attenuated second phase of the formalin test, indicating an impairment in their processing of inflammatory stimuli (Abbadie et al. 2003). In addition, these mice have a dramatic absence of mechanical allodynia after nerve injury. These data show that MCP-1/CCL2 and its receptor CCR2 have a functional role in nociceptive processing after injury and are potentially involved in inflammatory mechanisms of nociception.

Cytokines definitely have the ability to directly modulate neuronal excitability by altering ion channel activity. It appears that this role is not specific to TNF-α and TRPV1-positive neurons. As the field continues to recognize the importance of these molecules in pain induction and maintenance, our knowledge of cytokine modulation of ion channels in pain will certainly increase. Until then, perhaps we can look to other fields for direction in identifying cytokines involved in pain through the modulation of ion channel activity. We will briefly review the data from similar systems where cytokines have been shown to alter ion channel function not only in the central nervous system, but also throughout the body.

HINTS FROM BEYOND THE PAIN NEURAXIS: CYTOKINE REGULATION OF ION CHANNELS IN SIMILAR SYSTEMS

Since cytokines are capable of eliciting a variety of responses in a variety of cell types, and since they are so widely expressed, it is no surprise that they have integral roles in other non-immune functions. Cytokine modulation of ion channels in the nervous system is not restricted to pathways involved in pain transmission. In addition, outside the nervous system, examples of cytokine modulation of ion channels are found in the liver and the heart. We will briefly review this literature to establish a greater framework with which to understand cytokine modulation of ion channels.

First, a group of articles published over the past few years have described the effects of TNF-α on AMPA (α-amino-3-hydroxy-5-methyl-4-isoxazole propionate) receptor trafficking in the central nervous system and the role of this phenomenon in synaptic scaling in the hippocampus (Beattie et al. 2002; Stellwagen et al. 2005; Stellwagen and Malenka 2006). Synaptic scaling refers to global changes in the strength of all the synapses of a neuron due to chronic changes in neuronal activity. It is a homeostatic mechanism by which neurons can recalibrate the overall strength of connectivity to maintain activity-induced changes yet remain within a dynamic range of function. There are many potential mechanisms by which synaptic scaling can occur, one of which involves alterations in glutamate receptor trafficking and expression (Burrone and Murthy 2003).

TNF-α has been shown to increase AMPA-receptor surface expression in cultured hippocampal neurons as well as in slices, and this effect also coincided with an increased frequency of miniature excitatory postsynaptic currents, an effect presumably mediated by increased receptor expression (Beattie et al. 2002). The TNF-α-induced increase in AMPA-receptor surface expression was mediated by glial TNF-α binding to TNFR1 and by the subsequent activation of phosphatidylinositol 3 kinase (PI3K) (Stellwagen et al. 2005; Stellwagen and Malenka 2006). Interestingly, the increased expression was specific to glutamate receptor 2 (GluR2)-lacking AMPA receptors, which have an important role in synaptic scaling (Sutton et al. 2006). Finally, in both dissociated hippocampal cultures and acute slices, TNF-α was shown to be necessary for synaptic scaling (Stellwagen and Malenka 2006), identifying another mechanism by which cytokine modulation of ion channels can lead to long-term changes in neuronal connectivity. This mechanism could hold true for neurons along the pain neuraxis, where TNF-α has profound effects on pain sensitization.

In addition to regulation of glutamate receptor (GluR) trafficking, cytokine-induced changes in neuronal function are also mediated by modulation of GluR function. In dissociated hippocampal neurons, IL-1β pretreatment potentiated *N*-methyl-D-aspartate (NMDA)-induced increases in intracellular Ca^{2+} concentration through Src tyrosine kinase phosphorylation of NR2A/B subunits (Viviani et al. 2003). The increases in intracellular Ca^{2+} were blocked by treatment with MK801, the NMDA-receptor open channel blocker, and not by block of ryanodine receptors or IP3 receptors, supporting the role of the NMDA receptor as the channel mediating Ca^{2+} elevation. This is just another mechanism by which cytokines can affect neuronal transmission along the pain neuraxis; the molecular mechanisms of these effects still need to be determined in these regions.

Recently, Kawada et al. (2006) and Hatada et al. (2006) have determined the effects of TNF-α on K^+ channel activity in cardiomyocytes. In cultured cardiomyocytes, TNF-α, through a pertussis toxin-sensitive G-protein- and ceramidase-mediated mechanism, inhibits K^+ currents activated by protein kinase A (PKA). TNF-α acts by decreasing intracellular levels of cyclic adenosine monophosphate (cAMP), which in turn inhibits delayed rectifier K^+ channels (Hatada et al. 2006). In addition, TNF-α application to cultured rat cardiomyocytes decreased A-type K^+ currents, as well as delayed outward K^+ currents, concurrent with a reduction in $K_v4.2$ mRNA (Kawada et al. 2006). As mentioned earlier, inhibition of A-type K^+ currents can result in increased neuronal excitability of spinal dorsal horn neurons and has been linked to increases in hypersensitivity to thermal and mechanical stimuli (Hu et al. 2006). Although no study to date has specifically examined the effects of TNF-α on K^+ currents in neurons of the pain neuraxis, it is reasonable to hypothesize that an effect similar to that seen in cardiomyocytes may also be exhibited in these neurons. This possibility reveals another potential mechanism by which TNF-α and other similar cytokines could alter neuronal excitability and thus behavior.

Additionally, in dissociated preoptic/anterior hypothalamic neurons, IL-1β inhibited spontaneous firing by hyperpolarizing the cells and also resulted in a reversible increase in small inhibitory postsynaptic potentials (Tabarean et al. 2006). Moreover, within 2 minutes of application of IL-1β, delayed rectifier and A-type K^+ current amplitudes were significantly reduced. These results show that IL-1β modulation of K^+ currents may underlie the changes in neuronal excitability observed after inflammation. Further work in the pain neuraxis could outline the role of K$^+$ channels in IL-1β modulation of neuronal firing.

The chemokine SDF-1α/CXCL12 modulates action potential firing in neurons of the substantia nigra and the hypothalamus (Guyon et al. 2005a,b; 2006). It inhibits neuronal excitability, most likely via activation of GIRK channels as well as inhibition of both Na$^+$ and K$^+$ currents. As expected for any chemokine, this effect is blocked by inhibition of G proteins. This modulation of neuronal excitability could be involved in nociception after nerve injury and during regeneration.

Finally, in a rat liver cell line, TNF-α was shown to modulate K$^+$ and Cl$^-$ current activity (Nietsch et al. 2000). This effect was mediated by the intracellular signaling molecule PKC because treatment with a specific PKC inhibitor blocked TNF-α-induced increases in membrane currents. These data from rat liver cells identify PKC as a potential intermediary in the TNF-α-induced modulation of neuronal excitability.

The studies described in this chapter are a subset of those identifying potential roles for cytokines in the alteration of neuronal processes as well as those in other cell types. Specifically, we have discussed some of the studies that have identified a connection between cytokine treatment and modulation of ion channel activity. Although these instances are not along the pain neuraxis, they do involve similar systems. Intracellular signaling pathways and cytokine receptors are ubiquitous to many cell types, including neurons, and although the final effects may be different, as in modulation of cardiomyocyte or hepatocyte activity, these mechanisms may function similarly throughout the pain pathway. Therefore, this knowledge base should be a starting point from which to design further studies of cytokine modulation of ion channels in pain and should provide clues to how we can expect those relationships to function.

DISCUSSION AND CONCLUSIONS

Cytokines are integral components of the inflammatory response, and as such, they have also been shown to be key players in nociception. The mechanisms by which cytokines produce hypersensitivity are still being elucidated, but as discussed here, cytokine modulation of ion channels provides a vital first-step in alteration of neuronal activity. Whether by increasing Na$^+$ currents, decreasing K$^+$ currents, modulating TRP channel activity, or by an as yet unknown process, cytokines can impose critical changes in neuronal excitability and sensitization that result in increased sensitivity to nociceptive stimuli.

The field of cytokine modulation of ion channels in pain is in its infancy, as only a few papers truly delve into the function of these molecules in this complex process. With the insight provided by studies in other fields, we can systematically and actively undertake the challenge of increasing our understanding of cytokine modulation of ion channels in nociception. This effort will only aid in the increasing recognition of the importance of cytokines in pain and could lead to more directed therapies that target specific sites of cytokine modulation of ion channels involved in pain.

REFERENCES

Abbadie C, Lindia JA, Cumiskey AM, et al. Impaired neuropathic pain responses in mice lacking the chemokine receptor CCR2. *Proc Natl Acad Sci USA* 2003; 100:7947–7952.

Akopian AN, Sivilotti L, Wood JN. A tetrodotoxin-resistant voltage-gated sodium channel expressed by sensory neurons. *Nature* 1996; 379:257–262.

Akopian AN, Souslova V, England S, et al. The tetrodotoxin-resistant sodium channel SNS has a specialized function in pain pathways. *Nat Neurosci* 1999; 2:541–548.

Alloui A, Zimmermann K, Mamet J, et al. TREK-1, a K+ channel involved in polymodal pain perception. *EMBO J* 2006; 25:2368–2376.

Ardizzone S, Bianchi Porro G. Biologic therapy for inflammatory bowel disease. *Drugs* 2005; 65:2253–2286.

Atzeni F, Turiel M, Capsoni F, et al. Autoimmunity and anti-TNF-alpha agents. *Ann NY Acad Sci* 2005; 1051:559–569.

Bandell M, Story GM, Hwang SW, et al. Noxious cold ion channel TRPA1 is activated by pungent compounds and bradykinin. *Neuron* 2004; 41:849–857.

Bautista DM, Jordt SE, Nikai T, et al. TRPA1 mediates the inflammatory actions of environmental irritants and proalgesic agents. *Cell* 2006; 124:1269–1282.

Beattie EC, Stellwagen D, Morishita W, et al. Control of synaptic strength by glial TNFalpha. *Science* 2002; 295:2282–2285.

Bhave G, Gereau RW. Posttranslational mechanisms of peripheral sensitization. *J Neurobiol* 2004; 61:88–106.

Bhave G, Hu HJ, Glauner KS, et al. Protein kinase C phosphorylation sensitizes but does not activate the capsaicin receptor transient receptor potential vanilloid 1 (TRPV1). *Proc Natl Acad Sci USA* 2003; 100:12480–12485.

Black JA, Cummins TR, Plumpton C, et al. Upregulation of a silent sodium channel after peripheral, but not central, nerve injury in DRG neurons. *J Neurophysiol* 1999; 82:2776–2785.

Blackburn-Munro G, Jensen BS. The anticonvulsant retigabine attenuates nociceptive behaviours in rat models of persistent and neuropathic pain. *Eur J Pharmacol* 2003; 460:109–116.

Burrone J, Murthy VN. Synaptic gain control and homeostasis. *Curr Opin Neurobiol* 2003; 13:560–567.

Caterina MJ, Schumacher MA, Tominaga M, et al. The capsaicin receptor: a heat-activated ion channel in the pain pathway. *Nature* 1997; 389:816–824.

Caterina MJ, Leffler A, Malmberg AB, et al. Impaired nociception and pain sensation in mice lacking the capsaicin receptor. *Science* 2000; 288:306–313.

Clark JD, Tempel BL. Hyperalgesia in mice lacking the Kv1.1 potassium channel gene. *Neurosci Lett* 1998; 251:121–124.

Cummins TR, Waxman SG. Downregulation of tetrodotoxin-resistant sodium currents and up-regulation of a rapidly repriming tetrodotoxin-sensitive sodium current in small spinal sensory neurons after nerve injury. *J Neurosci* 1997; 17:3503–3514.

Cunha FQ, Lorenzetti BB, Poole S, Ferreira SH. Interleukin-8 as a mediator of sympathetic pain. *Br J Pharmacol* 1991; 104:765–767.

Cunha FQ, Poole S, Lorenzetti BB, Ferreira SH. The pivotal role of tumour necrosis factor alpha in the development of inflammatory hyperalgesia. *Br J Pharmacol* 1992; 107:660–664.

DeLeo JA, Colburn RW, Rickman AJ. Cytokine and growth factor immunohistochemical spinal profiles in two animal models of mononeuropathy. *Brain Res* 1997; 759:50–57.

Dib-Hajj SD, Tyrrell L, Black JA, Waxman SG. NaN, a novel voltage-gated Na channel, is expressed preferentially in peripheral sensory neurons and down-regulated after axotomy. *Proc Natl Acad Sci USA* 1998; 95:8963–8968.

Dib-Hajj SD, Fjell J, Cummins TR, et al. Waxman SG. Plasticity of sodium channel expression in DRG neurons in the chronic constriction injury model of neuropathic pain. *Pain* 1999; 83:591–600.

Ferreira SH, Lorenzetti BB, Bristow AF, Poole S. Interleukin-1 beta as a potent hyperalgesic agent antagonized by a tripeptide analogue. *Nature* 1988; 334:698–700.

Franks NP, Honore E. The TREK K2P channels and their role in general anaesthesia and neuroprotection. *Trends Pharmacol Sci* 2004; 25:601–608.

Galeotti N, Ghelardini C, Bartolini A. Involvement of potassium channels in amitriptyline and clomipramine analgesia. *Neuropharmacology* 2001; 40:75–84.

Gutman GA, Chandy KG, Adelman JP, et al. International Union of Pharmacology. XLI. Compendium of voltage-gated ion channels: potassium channels. *Pharmacol Rev* 2003; 55:583–586.

Guyon A, Banisadr G, Rovere C, et al. Complex effects of stromal cell-derived factor-1 alpha on melanin-concentrating hormone neuron excitability. *Eur J Neurosci* 2005a; 21:701–710.

Guyon A, Rovere C, Cervantes A, Allaeys I, Nahon JL. Stromal cell-derived factor-1alpha directly modulates voltage-dependent currents of the action potential in mammalian neuronal cells. *J Neurochem* 2005b; 93:963–973.

Guyon A, Skrzydelsi D, Rovere C, et al. Stromal cell-derived factor-1alpha modulation of the excitability of rat substantia nigra dopaminergic neurones: presynaptic mechanisms. *J Neurochem* 2006; 96:1540–1550.

Hatada K, Washizuka T, Horie M, et al. Tumor necrosis factor-alpha inhibits the cardiac delayed rectifier K current via the asphingomyelin pathway. *Biochem Biophys Res Comm* 2006; 344:189–193.

Homma Y, Brull SJ, Zhang JM. A comparison of chronic pain behavior following local application of tumor necrosis factor alpha to the normal and mechanically compressed lumbar ganglia in the rat. *Pain* 2002; 95:239–246.

Hong S, Morrow TJ, Paulson PE, Isom LL, Wiley JW. Early painful diabetic neuropathy is associated with differential changes in tetrodotoxin-sensitive and -resistant sodium channels in dorsal root ganglion neurons in the rat. *J Biol Chem* 2004; 279:29341–29350.

Hu HJ, Gereau RW. ERK Integrates PKA and PKC Signaling in superficial dorsal horn neurons. II. Modulation of neuronal excitability. *J Neurophysiol* 2003; 90:1680–1688.

Hu HJ, Carrasquillo Y, Karim F, et al. The Kv4.2 potassium channel subunit is required for pain plasticity. *Neuron* 2006; 50:89–100.

Ikeda K, Kobayashi T, Kumanishi T, Niki H, Yano R. Involvement of G-protein-activated inwardly rectifying K (GIRK) channels in opioid-induced analgesia. *Neurosci Res* 2000; 38:113–116.

Jin X, Gereau RW. Acute p38-mediated modulation of tetrodotoxin-resistant sodium channels in mouse sensory neurons by tumor necrosis factor-alpha. *J Neurosci* 2006; 26:246–255.

Kang D, Kim D. TREK-2 (K2P10.1) and TRESK (K2P18.1) are major background K$^+$ channels in dorsal root ganglion neurons. *Am J Physiol* 2006; 291:C138–146.

Katsura H, Obata K, Mizushima T, et al. Antisense knock down of TRPA1, but not TRPM8, alleviates cold hyperalgesia after spinal nerve ligation in rats. *Exp Neurol* 2006; 200:112–123.

Kawada H, Niwano S, Niwano H, et al. Tumor necrosis factor-alpha downregulates the voltage gated outward K$^+$ current in cultured neonatal rat cardiomyocytes: a possible cause of electrical remodeling in diseased hearts. *Circ J* 2006; 70:605–609.

Kim DS, Choi JO, Rim HD, Cho HJ. Downregulation of voltage-gated potassium channel alpha gene expression in dorsal root ganglia following chronic constriction injury of the rat sciatic nerve. *Brain Res Mol Brain Res* 2002; 105:146–152.

Kim H, Mittal DP, Iadarola MJ, Dionne RA. Genetic predictors for acute experimental cold and heat pain sensitivity in humans. *J Med Genet* 2006; 43:e40.

Kobayashi K, Fukuoka T, Obata K, et al. Distinct expression of TRPM8, TRPA1, and TRPV1 mRNAs in rat primary afferent neurons with adelta/c-fibers and colocalization with trk receptors. *J Comp Neurol* 2005; 493:596–606.

Konttinen YT, Seitsalo S, Lehto M, Santavirta S. Current management: Management of rheumatic diseases in the era of biological anti-rheumatic drugs. *Acta Orthop* 2005; 76:614–619.

Kwan KY, Allchorne AJ, Vollrath MA, et al. TRPA1 contributes to cold, mechanical, and chemical nociception but is not essential for hair-cell transduction. *Neuron* 2006; 50:277–289.

Lai J, Porreca F, Hunter JC, Gold MS. Voltage-gated sodium channels and hyperalgesia. *Annu Rev Pharmacol Toxicol* 2004; 44:371–397.

Laird JM, Souslova V, Wood JN, Cervero F. Deficits in visceral pain and referred hyperalgesia in Nav1.8 (SNS/PN3)-null mice. *J Neurosci* 2002; 22:8352–8356.

Lin E, Calvano SE, Lowry SF. Inflammatory cytokines and cell response in surgery. *Surgery* 2000; 127:117–126.

Lindenlaub T, Teuteberg P, Hartung T, Sommer C. Effects of neutralizing antibodies to TNF-alpha on pain-related behavior and nerve regeneration in mice with chronic constriction injury. *Brain Res* 2000; 866:15–22.

Liu L, Yang TM, Liedtke W, Simon SA. Chronic IL-1beta signaling potentiates voltage-dependent sodium currents in trigeminal nociceptive neurons. *J Neurophysiol* 2006; 95:1478–1490.

Lu Z. Mechanism of rectification in inward-rectifier K$^+$ channels. *Annu Rev Physiol* 2004; 66:103–129.

McKemy DD, Neuhausser WM, Julius D. Identification of a cold receptor reveals a general role for TRP channels in thermosensation. *Nature* 2002; 416:52–58.

Murphy PG, Grondin J, Altares M, Richardson PM. Induction of interleukin-6 in axotomized sensory neurons. *J Neurosci* 1995; 15:5130–5138.

Nicol GD, Lopshire JC, Pafford CM. Tumor necrosis factor enhances the capsaicin sensitivity of rat sensory neurons. *J Neurosci* 1997; 17:975–982.

Nietsch HH, Roe MW, Fiekers JF, Moore AL, Lidofsky SD. Activation of potassium and chloride channels by tumor necrosis factor alpha. Role in liver cell death. *J Biol Chem* 2000; 275:20556–20561.

Numazaki M, Tominaga T, Toyooka H, Tominaga M. Direct phosphorylation of capsaicin receptor VR1 by protein kinase Cepsilon and identification of two target serine residues. *J Biol Chem* 2002; 277:13375–13378.

Obreja O, Rathee PK, Lips KS, Distler C, Kress M. IL-1 beta potentiates heat-activated currents in rat sensory neurons: involvement of IL-1RI, tyrosine kinase, and protein kinase C. *FASEB J* 2002; 16:1497–1503.

Ocana M, Barrios M, Baeyens JM. Cromakalim differentially enhances antinociception induced by agonists of alpha(2)adrenoceptors, gamma-aminobutyric acid(B), mu and kappa opioid receptors. *J Pharmacol Exp Ther* 1996; 276:1136–1142.

Ocana M, Cendan CM, Cobos EJ, Entrena JM, Baeyens JM. Potassium channels and pain: present realities and future opportunities. *Eur J Pharmacol* 2004; 500:203–219.

Oh SB, Tran PB, Gillard SE, et al. Chemokines and glycoprotein 120 produce pain hypersensitivity by directly exciting primary nociceptive neurons. *J Neurosci* 2001; 21:5027–5035.

Patapoutian A, Peier AM, Story GM, Viswanath V. ThermoTRP channels and beyond: mechanisms of temperature sensation. *Nat Rev Neurosci* 2003; 4:529–539.

Peier AM, Moqrich A, Hergarden AC, et al. A TRP channel that senses cold stimuli and menthol. *Cell* 2002; 108:705–715.

Priest BT, Murphy BA, Lindia JA, et al. Contribution of the tetrodotoxin-resistant voltage-gated sodium channel NaV1.9 to sensory transmission and nociceptive behavior. *Proc Natl Acad Sci USA* 2005; 102:9382–9387.

Ranganathan P. Pharmacogenomics of tumor necrosis factor antagonists in rheumatoid arthritis. *Pharmacogenomics* 2005; 6:481–490.

Rasband MN, Park EW, Vanderah TW, et al. Distinct potassium channels on pain-sensing neurons. *Proc Natl Acad Sci USA* 2001; 98:13373–13378.

Saldanha G, Bar KJ, Yiangou Y, et al. Marked Increase of interleukin-6 in injured human nerves and dorsal root ganglia. *J Neurol Neurosurg Psychiatry* 2000; 69:693–694.

Sangameswaran L, Delgado SG, Fish LM, et al. Structure and function of a novel voltage-gated, tetrodotoxin-resistant sodium channel specific to sensory neurons. *J Biol Chem* 1996; 271:5953–5956.

Schafers M, Geis C, Brors D, Yaksh TL, Sommer C. Anterograde transport of tumor necrosis factor-alpha in the intact and injured rat sciatic nerve. *J Neurosci* 2002; 22:536–545.

Schafers M, Lee DH, Brors D, Yaksh TL, Sorkin LS. Increased sensitivity of injured and adjacent uninjured rat primary sensory neurons to exogenous tumor necrosis factor-alpha after spinal nerve ligation. *J Neurosci* 2003; 23:3028–3038.

Sommer C, Lindenlaub T, Teuteberg P, et al. Anti-TNF-neutralizing antibodies reduce pain-related behavior in two different mouse models of painful mononeuropathy. *Brain Res* 2001; 913:86–89.

Song WJ. Genes responsible for native depolarization-activated K^+ currents in neurons. *Neurosci Res* 2002; 42:7–14.

Stellwagen D, Malenka RC. Synaptic scaling mediated by glial TNF-alpha. *Nature* 2006; 440:1054–1059.

Stellwagen D, Beattie EC, Seo JY, Malenka RC. Differential regulation of AMPA receptor and GABA receptor trafficking by tumor necrosis factor-alpha. *J Neurosci* 2005; 25:3219–3228.

Story G. The emerging role of TRP channels in mechanisms of temperature and pain sensation. *Curr Neuropharmacol* 2006; 4:183–196.

Story GM, Peier AM, Reeve AJ, et al. ANKTM1, a TRP-like channel expressed in nociceptive neurons, is activated by cold temperatures. *Cell* 2003; 112:819–829.

Sun JH, Yang B, Donnelly DF, Ma C, Lamotte RH. MCP-1 enhances excitability of nociceptive neurons in chronically compressed dorsal root ganglia. *J Neurophysiol* 2006; 96:2189–2199.

Sutton MA, Ito HT, Cressy P, et al. Miniature neurotransmission stabilizes synaptic function via tonic suppression of local dendritic protein synthesis. *Cell* 2006; 125:785–799.

Sweitzer S, Martin D, DeLeo JA. Intrathecal interleukin-1 receptor antagonist in combination with soluble tumor necrosis factor receptor exhibits an anti-allodynic action in a rat model of neuropathic pain. *Neuroscience* 2001; 103:529–539.

Tabarean IV, Korn H, Bartfai T. Interleukin-1beta induces hyperpolarization and modulates synaptic inhibition in preoptic and anterior hypothalamic neurons. *Neuroscience* 2006; 141:1685–1695.

Takeda M, Tanimoto T, Ikeda M, et al. Enhanced excitability of rat trigeminal root ganglion neurons via decrease in A-type potassium currents following temporomandibular joint inflammation. *Neuroscience* 2006; 138:621–630.

Tate S, Benn S, Hick C, et al. Two sodium channels contribute to the TTX-R sodium current in primary sensory neurons. *Nat Neurosci* 1998; 1:653–655.

Tominaga M, Caterina MJ, Malmberg AB, et al. The cloned capsaicin receptor integrates multiple pain-producing stimuli. *Neuron* 1998; 21:531–543.

Verri WA Jr, Schivo IR, Cunha TM, et al. Interleukin-18 induces mechanical hypernociception in rats via endothelin acting on ETB receptors in a morphine-sensitive manner. *J Pharmacol Exp Ther* 2004; 310:710–717.

Verri WA Jr, Molina RO, Schivo IR, et al. Nociceptive effect of subcutaneously injected interleukin-12 is mediated by endothelin (ET) acting on ETB receptors in rats. *J Pharmacol Exp Ther* 2005; 315:609–615.

Viviani B, Bartesaghi S, Gardoni F, et al. Interleukin-1beta enhances NMDA receptor-mediated intracellular calcium increase through activation of the Src family of kinases. *J Neurosci* 2003; 23:8692–8700.

Welch JM, Simon SA, Reinhart PH. The activation mechanism of rat vanilloid receptor 1 by capsaicin involves the pore domain and differs from the activation by either acid or heat. *Proc Natl Acad Sci USA* 2000; 97:13889–13894.

White FA, Sun J, Waters SM, et al. Excitatory monocyte chemoattractant protein-1 signaling is up-regulated in sensory neurons after chronic compression of the dorsal root ganglion. *Proc Natl Acad Sci USA* 2005; 102:14092–14097.

Winkelstein BA, Rutkowski MD, Sweitzer SM, Pahl JL, DeLeo JA. Nerve injury proximal or distal to the DRG induces similar spinal glial activation and selective cytokine expression but differential behavioral responses to pharmacologic treatment. *J Comp Neurol* 2001; 439:127–139.

Woolf CJ, Allchorne A, Safieh-Garabedian B, Poole S. Cytokines, nerve growth factor and inflammatory hyperalgesia: the contribution of tumour necrosis factor alpha. *Br J Pharmacol* 1997; 121:417–424.

Yang Y, Wang Y, Li S, et al. Mutations in SCN9A, encoding a sodium channel alpha subunit, in patients with primary erythermalgia. *J Med Genet* 2004; 41:171–174.

Zelenka M, Schafers M, Sommer C. Intraneural injection of interleukin-1beta and tumor necrosis factor-alpha into rat sciatic nerve at physiological doses induces signs of neuropathic pain. *Pain* 2005; 116:257–263.

Zhang N, Inan S, Cowan A, et al. A proinflammatory chemokine, CCL3, sensitizes the heat- and capsaicin-gated ion channel TRPV1. *Proc Natl Acad Sci USA* 2005; 102:4536–4541.

Correspondence to: Robert W. Gereau IV, PhD, Washington University Pain Center, Department of Anesthesiology, Washington University School of Medicine, 660 S Euclid, Campus Box 8054, St. Louis, MO 63110, USA. Tel: 1-314-362-8312; fax: 1-314-362-8334; email: gereaur@wustl.edu.

Immune and Glial Regulation of Pain, edited by Joyce
A. DeLeo, Linda S. Sorkin, and Linda R. Watkins,
IASP Press, Seattle, © 2007.

12

AMPAR Synaptic and Surface Localization Is Altered by Glial-Derived Tumor Necrosis Factor Alpha: Relevance to Hyperalgesia and Central Sensitization

Eric C. Beattie[a] and David Stellwagen[b]

*[a]Department of Neurosciences, California Pacific Medical Center Research
Institute, San Francisco, California, USA; [b]Department of Psychiatry,
Stanford Medical School, Palo Alto, California, USA*

Tumor necrosis factor alpha (TNF-α) is an inflammatory cytokine that was recently identified as a regulator of glutamatergic synaptic function during health and disease. A central control point of synaptic strength or efficacy is the surface and synaptic localization of postsynaptic α-amino-3-hydroxy-5-methylisoxazole-4-propionic acid (AMPA)-type ionotropic glutamate receptors (AMPARs). In this chapter, we review the basic mechanisms of AMPAR trafficking in normal neuronal function and in the context of TNF-α supplied by neighboring glia. The goal is to reexamine our current thinking of the underlying mechanisms of hyperalgesia, an increased sensation of pain after painful peripheral stimuli that suggests the inappropriate strengthening of synaptic connections. We utilize a model where increased activation of primary afferent signals activates glia, which then release TNF-α onto the postsynaptic dorsal horn's nociceptive neurons. The missing link in this model is the mechanism of action between glial activation and dorsal horn neuron hypersensitization. We hypothesize a model based on our recent observations that TNF-α released by glia directly increases AMPAR surface localization, strengthening excitatory synapses (Beattie et al. 2002a; Stellwagen et al. 2005). If future studies continue to support such a model, this information will provide new drug targets for the reduction of hypernociceptive pain rooted in central sensitization.

EXCITATORY POSTSYNAPTIC FUNCTION: BASIC MECHANISMS

Glutamate is the major excitatory neurotransmitter in the mammalian central nervous system (CNS). It exerts its effects via a number of both pre-and postsynaptic receptors with differing physiological properties. The ionotropic glutamate receptors are ligand-gated ion channels that bind glutamate and allow cations to cross the neuronal membrane. These receptors, the major mediators of synaptic transmission, have been further subdivided based upon their biophysical and pharmacological properties into the N-methyl-D-aspartate (NMDA), AMPA, and kainate receptors (Hollmann and Heinemann 1994; Chittajallu et al. 1999). Each of these receptor classes has been demonstrated to have differential anatomical and cellular localizations, and each contributes to normal synaptic function. Proper regulation of synaptic strength is essential for the normal function of the CNS, including the formation and maintenance of memory. The mechanisms underlying both basic synaptic transmission and synaptic plasticity have been a major focus of the neuroscience field. Synaptic transmission is a highly regulated process, the strength of which is determined by changes in release of glutamate from presynaptic terminals and the localization and activity of receptors on the postsynaptic membrane.

Postsynaptic glutamate receptors are of particular interest because the surface localization of these receptors is highly dynamic and directly relevant to synaptic function (for reviews see Carroll et al. 2001; Malinow and Malenka 2002; Song and Huganir 2002; Bredt and Nicoll 2003). Dominating this field are the AMPA receptors that mediate the major component of fast excitatory synaptic transmission and are expressed exclusively at the postsynaptic membrane. Recent evidence demonstrates that NMDA receptors (reviewed in Carroll and Zukin 2002) as well as kainate receptors (Hirbec et al. 2003) are also dynamically trafficked to affect synaptic function. Changes in postsynaptic sensitivity to presynaptically released glutamate may be mediated by changes in the conductance of preexisting surface-expressed receptors or by a change in receptor density at the postsynaptic membrane. Although glutamate receptor subunit phosphorylation can lead to important changes in channel conductance (Benke et al. 1998), a wealth of data has demonstrated that surface expression of AMPARs is highly regulated, and the amount of this surface expression is directly related to synaptic efficacy (reviewed in Malinow and Malenka 2002; Collingridge et al. 2004). The rapid mobility of AMPARs occurs in a constitutive fashion, mediated by exocytosis and endocytosis and facilitating a continual turnover of AMPARs at the synaptic membrane (Luscher et al. 1999; Lin et al. 2000). AMPAR trafficking is also mediated by patterned synaptic activity and subsequent receptor activation (Carroll et al. 1999a; Lissin et al. 1999; Beattie et al. 2000; Ehlers 2000; Lin et al. 2000). These activity-dependent changes in

AMPAR trafficking have been linked to the modulation of synaptic strength, as occurs during specific forms of long-term potentiation (LTP; Malenka and Nicoll 1999) and long-term depression (LTD; Carroll et al. 2001). The molecular mechanisms underlying the delivery of receptors to the postsynaptic membrane and their removal have been productive areas of research.

Increases in AMPAR surface expression have been correlated with the development of LTP through both the awakening of "silent synapses" (insertion of AMPARs into synapses previously lacking them) (Isaac et al. 1995; Liao et al. 1995) and the increase in AMPARs at preexisting synapses (Shi et al. 1999; Hayashi et al. 2000). AMPAR phosphorylation is an important regulatory process involved in AMPAR-mediated delivery to the postsynaptic membrane through the activity of kinases including calcium/calmodulin-dependent protein kinase II (CaMKII) and protein kinase A (PKA) (Hayashi et al. 2000; Lee et al. 2000; Esteban et al. 2003). Interaction with intracellular proteins has also proven to be important. Disruption of AMPAR binding to proteins containing the PDZ domain or overexpression of such interacting proteins perturbs receptor surface expression (Hayashi et al. 2000; Rumbaugh et al. 2003). Additionally, transmembrane proteins such as stargazin or related transmembrane AMPAR regulatory proteins (TARPs; Chen et al. 2000; Tomita et al. 2003) are required for the delivery of AMPARs to synaptic membranes. Inhibition of phosphoinositide-3 (PI3) kinase by wortmanin also inhibits the surface delivery of AMPARs induced by glycine application, an in vitro model of LTP (Passafaro et al. 2001). Finally, synaptic localization of AMPARs and the development of LTP depend upon activation of AMPAR-associated PI3 kinase (Man et al. 2003). These studies are especially interesting in the context of our recent data showing that PI3 kinase signaling is needed for the TNF-α-induced surface expression of AMPARs (Stellwagen et al. 2005), as discussed in more detail below.

Endocytosis of receptors from the synaptic membrane is dependent on dynamin, an intracellular protein that tethers membrane receptors to endocytic vesicles (Carroll et al. 1999b). This process requires protein phosphorylation and interactions with other intracellular proteins. An increase in postsynaptic calcium levels has been linked with the physiological process of LTD (Mulkey and Malenka 1992) and with the regulated internalization of AMPARs (Beattie et al. 2000). The calcium-sensitive phosphatase calcineurin has also been linked to both of these processes (Mulkey and Malenka 1992; Beattie et al. 2000), suggesting a role for AMPAR dephosphorylation in the processes of receptor internalization and LTD. In addition, ample evidence has demonstrated that AMPAR-interacting proteins—including N-ethylmaleimide-sensitive fusion protein (NSF), glutamate receptor interacting protein (GRIP), and protein interacting with C-kinase (PICK)—regulate the internalization of AMPARs (reviewed in Braithwaite et al. 2000; Passafaro et al. 2001; Malinow and Malenka

2002; Xia et al. 2006). TARPs may also regulate the endocytosis of AMPARs, because dissociation of these two proteins is necessary for removal of AMPARs from the synaptic membrane (Tomita et al. 2003).

These studies have been based on a variety of techniques, including electrophysiological measurements of acute or cultured hippocampal slices, biochemical analysis of neuron cultures and tissue, and microscopy of fixed neurons. Live imaging of neurons is beginning to provide us with new details about the rapid movements of neuronal receptors in and on the surface of neurons (Adesnik et al. 2005; Bouschet et al. 2005; Ashby et al. 2006; Yudowski et al. 2006).

The delivery and removal of receptors to and from the postsynaptic membrane is dependent on a variety of highly regulated mechanisms. These mechanisms have profound effects on the diverse array of receptors at the postsynaptic membrane and allow for precise control of synaptic transmission and the formation of synaptic plasticity. These mechanisms controlling AMPAR trafficking have recently been confirmed to be vital to processes of living experience in an elegant model of whisker-stimulated synaptic potentiation in the mouse barrel cortex (Clem and Barth 2006). Control over transcription and translation of AMPAR subunit protein levels has been demonstrated to change the amount and subtype specificity of AMPAR surface expression over a time period of hours (Aronica et al. 1997; Pellegrini-Giampietro et al. 1997; Tanaka et al. 2000). New data shows that translation of resident messenger RNAs encoding AMPARs occurs in the dendrites (Ju et al. 2004). Nevertheless, the speed of these regulated changes in synaptic transmission and the necessity for the appropriate contingent of synaptic substructure proteins make it likely that trafficking mechanisms (along with degradation) are major contributors to the dynamic regulation of postsynaptic function (O'Brien et al. 1998; Ehlers 2000; Man et al. 2000; Stein et al. 2003; Tao et al. 2003; Ehrlich and Malinow 2004). Clearly, abnormalities in any of these trafficking systems will lead to dysfunction in synaptic transmission and subsequent progression of neuronal disorders.

EXCESSIVE SURFACE LOCALIZATION OF AMPARS AS A MECHANISM FOR NEURONAL DYSFUNCTION

Precise control of synaptic efficacy is important for the normal functioning of the CNS; therefore, the development of abnormalities in synaptic function can lead to neurological disorders or toxicity. Many experiments have indicated that overactivation of ionotropic glutamate receptors can lead to neurotoxicity, primarily through excessive neuronal calcium influx that initiates a cascade of apoptotic processes (Choi 1992; Lee et al. 1999; Mattson et al. 2000; Weiss and Sensi 2000; Mattson and Chan 2003). This glutamate-receptor-mediated neurotoxicity has been implicated in the neuronal death associated with acute traumas to the CNS and in the early stages of neurodegenerative disorders such as Alzheimer's and Parkinson's disease. Furthermore, hyperactivity of glutamate receptors may lead to seizures such as occurs in epilepsy without leading to neurotoxicity. Conversely, glutamate receptor hypoactivity can lead to neurological deficits such as schizophrenia (Tsai and Coyle 2002) and may contribute to cognitive decline in disorders such as Alzheimer's disease (Kamenetz et al. 2003). Addictive behavior has been demonstrated to involve inappropriate plasticity of glutamatergic transmission (Tzschentke and Schmidt 2003), highlighting the fact that imbalances in synaptic glutamate receptors can have serious neurobiological consequences. Since trafficking of AMPARs to the postsynaptic membrane is a major mechanism for normal neuronal function, it is clear that abnormal trafficking could lead to these conditions of neuronal dysfunction. Most AMPARs are not permeable to Ca^{2+}, the major intracellular mediator of cell death, because the GluR2 glutamate receptor subunit determines the selectivity of the channel and excludes Ca^{2+}. However, a subset of AMPA receptors exist at synaptic sites that contain no GluR2 subunits, making them Ca^{2+} permeable (Ogoshi and Weiss 2003). In addition, activation of AMPARs is required to relieve the voltage-dependent block of NMDA receptors, the major glutamate receptors that allow Ca^{2+} entry into neurons (Herron et al. 1986). Therefore, abnormal trafficking of AMPARs can both directly and indirectly lead to excitotoxicity and neuron death.

REGULATION OF AMPAR TRAFFICKING IN NEURONS BY GLIAL-RELEASED TNF-ALPHA

The theory that AMPAR trafficking plays a critical role in neuronal function and dysfunction has led to the search for regulators of such trafficking outside the classical glutamatergic realm. Several lines of evidence suggest that TNF-α may be a rapid regulator of glutamatergic synaptic function. Bath application of TNF-α led to a rapid, slight increase in basal (AMPAR-mediated) synaptic transmission in hippocampal slices (Tancredi et al. 1992). In cultures, brief applications of TNF-α increased the frequency of spontaneous miniature synaptic responses (Grassi et al. 1994). Moreover, extremely small (femtomolar) doses of TNF-α rapidly potentiated brainstem neuron responses to glutamatergic afferent activation (Emch et al. 2000), and TNF-α treatment potentiated neuronal sensitivity to glutamatergic excitotoxicity (Miller et al. 2005). These data, taken together, suggest that TNF-α could regulate synaptic transmission by influencing glutamate release and/or sensitivity.

Direct electrophysiological examination of glutamatergic synapses as well as microscopic evaluation of hippocampal neurons revealed that exogenous TNF-α application causes the exocytosis of AMPARs into synaptic sites, leading to an increase in synaptic strength (Beattie et al. 2002a). Fig. 1 shows representative data of the rapid increase in surface AMPARs induced by TNF-α application. TNF-α binds to neuronal TNF-R1 receptors and, through a PI3-kinase-dependent process, dramatically increases the surface expression of AMPARs (Stellwagen et al. 2005). The majority of these newly exocytosed AMPARs lack the GluR2 subunit and are therefore calcium permeable; under basal conditions, such receptors are not found in significant amounts on the cell surface (Ogoshi et al. 2005; Stellwagen et al. 2005). TNF-α does not appear to alter the trafficking of NMDA receptors, as acute TNF-α treatment did not alter their synaptic localization (Beattie et al. 2002a), nor does chronic TNF-α change NMDA-receptor protein levels (Glazner and Mattson 2000). All of these studies were done using hippocampal neurons, and so it is unclear whether these observations are translatable to other neuron classes. In vitro studies involving TNF-α application to cortical neurons (Leonoudakis et al. 2004) produce results very similar to those obtained in hippocampal neurons.

The effects of TNF-α are not restricted to AMPARs, however. Curiously, TNF-α treatment leads to the endocytosis of $GABA_A$ receptors, the major receptors mediating fast inhibitory transmission (Stellwagen et al. 2005). Therefore, addition of TNF-α leads to an increase in excitatory synaptic strength combined with a decrease in inhibitory synaptic strength, resulting in a large shift in the excitatory-to-inhibitory ratio (Stellwagen et al. 2005).

Acute application of exogenous TNF-α alters the trafficking of AMPARs, but TNF-α is generally thought of as a pro-inflammatory cytokine released by activated lymphocytes. However, the acute regulation of neurotransmitter receptor trafficking suggests a constitutive role for TNF-α in the normal functioning of the nervous system. There is evidence for the constitutive release of TNF-α in both neuronal cell culture and intact hippocampal slice preparations, as reduction of TNF-α signaling in either preparation results in a decrease in the number of AMPARs at the synapse and a weakening of synaptic strength (Beattie et al. 2002a). Further, TNF-α is constitutively released by the glia, suggesting a glial-neuronal signaling loop, where glia actively regulate the strength of nearby synapses (Beattie et al. 2002a). Fig. 2 shows a representative micrograph of astrocytes and neurons in mixed hippocampal culture. These data suggest that TNF-α may have an endogenous neuronal function separate from its role in immune signaling. In a form of synaptic plasticity that matches the effects of TNF-α—known as homeostatic synaptic plasticity, or sometimes referred to as synaptic scaling (Turrigiano and Nelson 2004; Wierenga et al.

2005)—excitatory and inhibitory inputs are inversely regulated to maintain a median firing rate. Thus, if activity is chronically blocked in a neural circuit, excitatory synapses become stronger and inhibitory synapses become weaker (Wierenga et al. 2005), a change dependent on the increase of TNF-α release from nearby glia (Stellwagen and Malenka 2006). Therefore, TNF-α regulates neurotransmitter receptor trafficking in the context of mediating a normal form of adaptive synaptic plasticity. Ongoing TNF-α release from glia is slowly modified in response to changes in the activity levels of neighboring neurons. However, the levels of constitutively released TNF-α are quite low (Stellwagen and Malenka 2006). Higher levels of TNF-α and other pro-inflammatory cytokines released during neuronal insults or pathologies could disrupt the normal glial feedback to neurons, resulting in abnormally strong excitation, weakened inhibition, and extra postsynaptic calcium intake due to the increased surface expression of GluR2-lacking, calcium-permeable AMPARs.

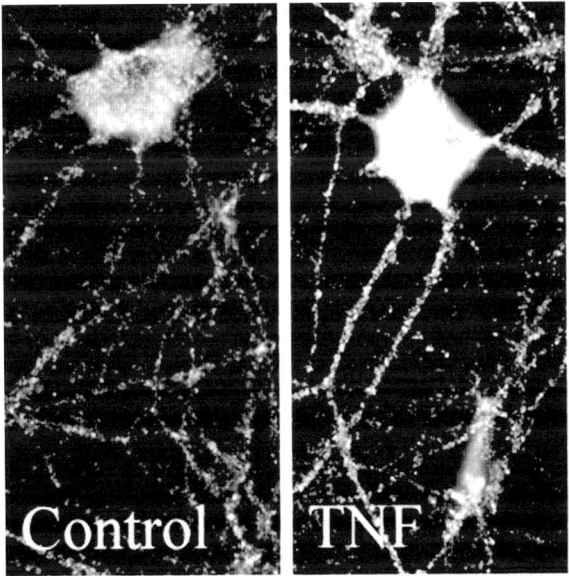

Fig. 1. Tumor necrosis factor (TNF) applied to cultured hippocampal neurons increases surface localization of AMPA receptors (AMPARs). Rat hippocampal neurons (18–21 days in vitro) were stained for exclusively surface AMPARs with an antibody to AMPAR subunit GluR1 under unpermeabilized membrane conditions. Panels show representative neurons with and without 15 minutes of pretreatment of 6 nM TNF-α. TNF-α induced a rapid and dramatic increase in surface AMPARs.

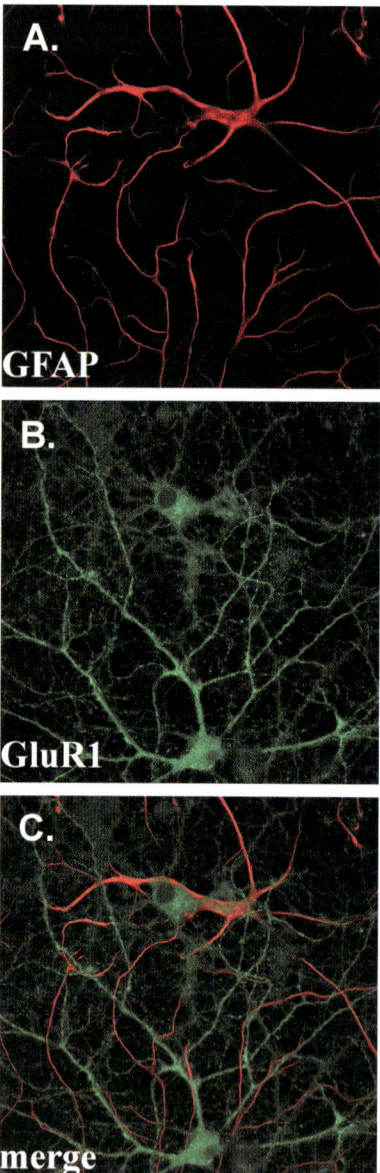

Fig. 2. Mixed rat hippocampal cultures stained for (A) astrocytes (glial fibrillary acidic protein [GFAP] stained, red) and (B) AMPAR subunits (GluR1, green), and (C) both together (merge). Panels show the two main cellular components of the hippocampal culture preparation at 18–21 days in vitro, namely hippocampal pyramidal neurons and astrocytes. In vivo, these cell types are intimately associated. In culture, after dissection disruption and recovery, they are still happy neighbors. In fact, neurons need this close association for healthy maintenance in culture.

TNF-ALPHA AND ABNORMAL AMPAR
TRAFFICKING DURING PATHOLOGIES

The trafficking of AMPARs in the normal state of neurons is a constitutive process regulated by activity. In neuronal disorders there must be an additional trigger that disrupts the trafficking process. Above, we described how cytokines released from glial cells, including the inflammatory cytokine TNF-α (Beattie et al. 2002a), are a major contributory factor to constitutive AMPAR trafficking. TNF-α is intimately involved in inflammation, immune activation, cell differentiation, and cell death, but its complex actions are increasingly implicated in diseases of the CNS (Perry et al. 1995; Allan and Rothwell 2001). TNF-α and other cytokines are rapidly induced in response to tissue injury or infection in the CNS (Perry et al. 1995; Allan and Rothwell 2001). TNF-α administered to cultured primary neurons causes a dose-dependent cytotoxicity (Zhao et al. 2001) as well as neuronal apoptosis (Reimann-Philipp et al. 2001). However, some in vitro studies have reported neuroprotective effects of TNF-α (Cheng et al. 1994; Bruce et al. 1996). Whether TNF-α is damaging or protective appears to depend on many factors. TNF-α during acute injury appears to be damaging, but its long-term presence can be protective (Wilde et al. 2000). The effect of TNF-α on distinct cell types is greatly influenced by the presence of specific receptors on target cells. TNF-α binds specifically to two distinct and co-expressed receptors, TNF-R1 and TNF-R2, which are both found on neurons (Vitkovic et al. 2000). The activation of TNF-R1 appears to be damaging to neurons, whereas activation of TNF-R2 is protective (Peschon et al. 1998; Fontaine et al. 2002; Yang et al. 2002). Furthermore, the presence or absence of compounds that modify TNF-α action also greatly influences possible neuroprotective or neurotoxic effects (Schubert et al. 1997; Carlson et al. 1998). There is a clear linkage between the actions of TNF-α released by glia and neuronal AMPAR trafficking events. TNF-α is involved in regulation of neuronal function and of AMPAR localization, but the complex actions and temporal profile of a neuron's response to this cytokine determines its ultimate effects on neuronal pathology.

HYPERALGESIA

Hyperalgesia is a condition of chronic heightened pain sensitivity that afflicts a large proportion of adults. Characterized by a shift in the perception of mild stimuli from nonpainful to painful, it is incompletely controlled by currently available drug regimens aimed at prostanoid reduction (nonsteroidal anti-inflammatory drugs) and opioid receptor activation (Curatolo and Bogduk 2001). Alternative pain pathways that may cause chronic hyperalgesia include the activity of pro-inflammatory cytokines, the release of glial factors, and the dependence on the availability of calcium-permeable AMPARs (Watkins and Maier 2003). In the preceding sections, we have discussed how TNF-α is a pro-inflammatory cytokine released by glia, which controls the neuronal surface expression of calcium-permeable AMPARs. We suggest that this process may be critical to understanding the induction of chronic hyperalgesia that develops centrally (e.g., in the spinal cord), and we propose that a more complete understanding of the functional relationship between TNF-α and AMPARs will provide insights into new avenues of pain treatment. A hypothetical model for the development of hyperalgesia with the novel mechanism of TNF-α-induced AMPAR surface expression is shown in Fig. 3.

A NEW MECHANISM IN THE MODEL FOR HYPERALGESIA BASED ON CENTRAL SENSITIZATION

The review of AMPAR trafficking above underscores the functional integration of neurons with glia. This area of study, together with current pain research, suggests that peripheral injury and inflammation leads to hyperactivity of spinal cord nociceptive neurons through a triad of components in the dorsal horn of the spinal cord (see Fig. 3). Here, incoming afferent pain fibers synapse with nociceptive neurons to form the first two components. This junction of pre- and postsynaptic connections is surrounded by a third functional component, namely astrocytes and microglia. We propose that an increased surface localization of postsynaptic AMPARs driven by glia-derived TNF-α is the missing mechanistic link between (1) the established activation of astrocytes and microglia by increased peripheral nociceptive input and (2) the overactivation of neighboring nociceptive neurons by afferent nociceptive pathways. Our observation that TNF-α increases surface localization of AMPARs over short (Beattie et al. 2002a; Leonoudakis et al. 2004; Stellwagen et al. 2005) or long time scales (Stellwagen and Malenka 2006) motivates us to suggest this activity as a key mechanism underlying hyperalgesia due to central sensitization.

HYPERALGESIA DUE TO CENTRAL SENSITIZATION

Peripheral injury activates nociceptive afferent pathways that carry input into the dorsal horn of the spinal cord; this type of persistent input can result in central sensitization and its behavioral consequence, hyperalgesia (Nozaki-Taguchi and Yaksh 1998; Sorkin et al. 1999, 2001; Guo et al. 2002; Wang et al. 2005). Here, chronic pain and hyperalgesia may be maintained in part by the close functional relationship between spinal glia and AMPAR-expressing dorsal horn nociceptive neurons. It is believed that central sensitization is activity dependent and acts upon either pre- or postsynaptic AMPA and NMDA-type glutamate receptors on dorsal horn neurons. Animal models of central sensitization can lead to behaviors that indicate spontaneous pain and/or mechanical hyperalgesia characterized by greater than normal levels of ambulation, escape responses, or startle reflexes (Zahn et al. 1998). Finally, central sensitization is the root cause of chronic pain that lasts past the time of injury and infection. This chronic pain is poorly controlled by currently available drugs that target

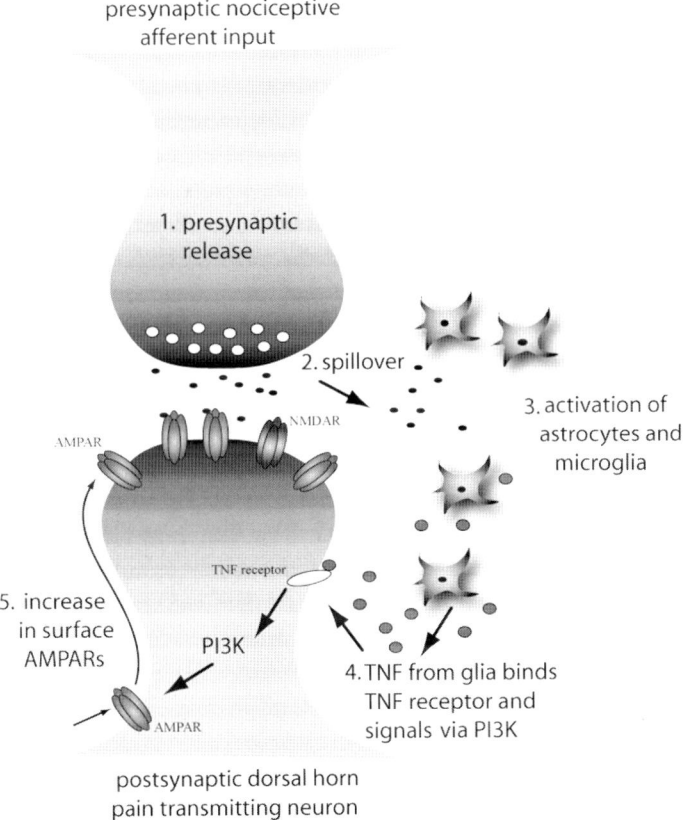

Fig. 3. A five-step hypothetical model for the development of hyperalgesia due to central sensitization. Depicted is a synapse located in the dorsal horn of the spinal cord. A presynaptic nociceptive neuron (1) carries pain messages from the periphery and releases neurotransmitters (e.g., glutamate, substance P) onto a postsynaptic nociceptive neuron (bottom). Activation of AMPA- and NMDA-type glutamate receptors and substance P-specific neurokinin-1 receptors transmits pain signals up the spinal cord and to the brain. Increased activity of this system caused by peripheral pain or nearby spinal cord injury causes spillover (2) of neurotransmitter or release of factors from either the pre- or postsynaptic neuron. These factors activate local astrocytes and microglia and induce the release of tumor necrosis factor alpha (TNF-α) (3). TNF-α binds to TNF-α receptors on the postsynaptic neuron and induces signaling through activated PI3 kinase (PI3K) (4). This process increases the surface localization of AMPARs (5) and leads to central sensitization of the postsynaptic neuron and hyperalgesia.

classical neurotransmission modalities (Curatolo and Bogduk 2001), but which importantly is reduced by AMPAR antagonists in animal models (Blackburn-Munro et al. 2004). Hyperalgesia stemming from dorsal horn neuronal sensitization can be activated by spinal cord injury and by the resultant neuroinflammation in nearby tissue (Christensen and Hulsebosch 1997; Bennett et al. 2000; Lindsey et al. 2000; Abraham et al. 2001). Whether spinal cord injury induces central sensitization in a manner akin to peripheral pain input is currently an area of strong interest (reviewed by Eaton 2006).

Recently, research examining hyperalgesia produced by central sensitization has focused on three main components in the superficial layers of the dorsal horn: (1) presynaptic terminals from peripheral nociceptive afferents, (2) postsynaptic terminals of nociceptive dorsal horn neurons, and (3) the glia that surround them (see Fig. 3). After increased activity from nociceptive afferents, a correlation of the following factors is observed: (1) an increase in molecules such as TNF-α, glutamate, substance P, prostaglandins, and nitric oxide and (2) an increase in activity in dorsal horn nociceptive neurons (reviewed by Watkins and Maier 2003). The key question is: What causes the long-lasting increase in activity in the postsynaptic dorsal horn neurons that underlies hyperalgesia? Here we discuss evidence that is consistent with the hypothesis that TNF-α derived from glia binds to TNF-α receptors on postsynaptic dorsal horn terminals and increases activity and calcium signaling via increased surface AMPARs.

EVIDENCE CONSISTENT WITH TNF-ALPHA AS AN ACTIVATOR OF HYPERALGESIA

Proinflammatory cytokines such as TNF-α, interleukin-1 (IL-1), and IL-6 are secreted by astrocytes and microglia in many CNS milieus (Allan and Rothwell 2001; Beattie et al. 2002a,b; Vezzani et al. 2002; Leonoudakis et al. 2004). Specifically, the pain-regulated secretion of TNF-α can be seen in astrocytes and glia of the spinal cord that surround the nociceptive neurons of the dorsal horn (Watkins et al. 1999; Hermann et al. 2001; Herzberg and Sagen 2001; Beattie et al. 2002b; Ohtori et al. 2004). Finally, both AMPARs and the receptors for TNF-α are known to be expressed by these nociceptive dorsal horn neurons that are postsynaptic to incoming nociceptive pathways (Ohtori et al. 2004; Wang et al. 2005; Tong and MacDermott 2006; Xu et al. 2006).

Microglia and astrocytes in the dorsal horn activated by afferent input or spinal cord injury can secrete many factors that may initiate many complex release cascades. What is the evidence that TNF-α alone has the potential to affect hypersensitivity of the nociceptive neurons in this area? In one study, thalidomide, an inhibitor of TNF-α production, was used to pretreat animals given subsequent spinal nerve ligation injury (Xu et al. 2006). Pretreated animals did not develop hyperalgesia, but in another group of animals, treatment with this compound did not block hyperalgesia 7 days after injury. This finding suggests that TNF-α is necessary for the development, but not the maintenance, of hyperalgesia.

In another study, TNF-α was applied to dorsal root ganglia in various concentrations in animals with or without spinal nerve ligation injury (Schäfers et al. 2003). TNF-α caused hyperalgesia and pain behaviors when applied alone to the ganglia, and subthreshold levels of TNF-α synergistically combined with nerve injury to cause more rapid onset of hyperalgesia and pain behaviors than did injury alone. Pretreatment with a soluble reagent that binds up and effectively removes TNF-α dramatically reduced hyperalgesia and pain behaviors after induced injury. Further, electrophysiological data obtained after in vitro perfusion of TNF-α to uninjured dorsal root ganglia resulted in a rapid and transient increase in neuronal activity, whereas subthreshold levels of TNF-α added to injured dorsal root ganglia caused higher and longer-lasting increases in neuronal activity (Schäfers et al. 2003).

THE INVOLVEMENT OF CALCIUM-PERMEABLE AMPARS IN THE DEVELOPMENT OF HYPERALGESIA

The results of Schäfers and colleagues are reminiscent of our studies showing rapid TNF-α-induced increases in synaptic activity in hippocampal cultures and in acute hippocampal slices (Beattie et al. 2002a; Stellwagen et al. 2005). More specifically, our studies showed that exogenous application of either purified TNF-α or TNF-α from astrocyte culture media dramatically increased surface delivery of AMPARs within 15 minutes of application (Beattie et al. 2002a). Interestingly, the immunohistochemical, biochemical, and electrophysiological data suggested that a large proportion of these rapidly delivered AMPARs were GluR2-lacking (i.e., calcium permeable) (Stellwagen et al. 2005). These rapid changes allow for more calcium influx, which, if confirmed in dorsal horn nociceptive neurons, could potentially contribute to the long-term changes in synaptic efficacy that underlie central sensitization.

These studies, together with current information regarding the expression of calcium-permeable AMPARs on nociceptive neurons in the dorsal horn and the importance of AMPARs to the development of hyperalgesia, complete the circuit of the proposed mechanism of hyperalgesia in our model. An early study that localized AMPARs to dorsal horn nociceptive neurons alerted the field to the potential involvement of a specific calcium-permeable subtype of AMPARs (GluR2-lacking) in the pain pathway (Engelman et al. 1999). Very recently, Tong and MacDermott (2006) detailed the amount of calcium-permeable AMPARs on neurons within the various lamina of the dorsal horn. They noted expression of these receptors in lamina I and especially high levels in laminae III/IV.

Other groups have come out with important studies supporting the necessity of GluR2-lacking AMPARs in the full expression of central hyperalgesia. A study by Hartmann et al. (2004) utilized GluR2-knockout transgenic mice and compared the development of central sensitization in vivo with and without calcium-permeable AMPARs on dorsal horn neurons. Here, in GluR2-lacking transgenic mice, the calcium current through AMPARs in dorsal horn neurons was increased and central sensitization was dramatically enhanced compared to wild-type mice. This study also showed that in GluR1-lacking mice, hyperalgesia was reduced, as was the number of calcium-permeable AMPARs. In other investigations, specific blockage of calcium-permeable AMPARs by Joro spider toxin prevented hyperalgesia when given intrathecally prior to nociceptive input to the spinal cord (Pogatzki et al. 2003; Jones and Sorkin 2004).

SUMMARY

We have reviewed the basic mechanisms of AMPAR trafficking in the context of chronic pain mechanisms in the spinal cord after peripheral or central injury and inflammation. We utilize a tripartite model of hyperalgesic pain development in which incoming nociceptive afferent input activates spinal astrocytes to release TNF-α onto nociceptive dorsal horn neurons. The mechanism we suggest here for the amplification of pain signals is based on our original observation that TNF-α increases calcium-permeable AMPAR surface expression in hippocampal neurons. Considering recent investigations into the development of pain that confirm a role for calcium-permeable AMPARs, the translation of this TNF-α-induced AMPAR trafficking mechanism to spinal cord dorsal horn neurons promises to provide new drug targets in the fight against chronic pain.

ACKNOWLEDGMENTS

The authors wish to acknowledge Dr. Dmitri Leonoudakis and Sarah McDowell for performing the experiments shown in Figs. 1 and 2 and for assistance in final manuscript preparation. Our laboratory is supported by grants from the National Institute of Mental Health, the California Pacific Medical Center Research Institute, and the Forbes/Norris Foundation.

REFERENCES

Abraham KE, McGinty JF, Brewer KL. The role of kainic acid/AMPA and metabotropic glutamate receptors in the regulation of opioid mRNA expression and the onset of pain-related behavior following excitotoxic spinal cord injury. *Neuroscience* 2001; 104:863–874.

Adesnik H, Nicoll RA, England PM. Photoinactivation of native AMPA receptors reveals their real-time trafficking. *Neuron* 2005; 48:977–985.

Allan SM, Rothwell NJ. Cytokines and acute neurodegeneration. *Nat Rev Neurosci* 2001; 2:734–744.

Aronica EM, Gorter JA, Paupard MC, et al. Status epilepticus-induced alterations in metabotropic glutamate receptor expression in young and adult rats. *J Neurosci* 1997; 17:8588–8595.

Ashby MC, Maier SR, Nishimune A, Henley JM. Lateral diffusion drives constitutive exchange of AMPA receptors at dendritic spines and is regulated by spine morphology. *J Neurosci* 2006; 26:7046–7055.

Beattie EC, Carroll RC, Yu X, et al. Regulation of AMPA receptor endocytosis by a signaling mechanism shared with LTD. *Nat Neurosci* 2000; 3:1291–1300.

Beattie EC, Stellwagen D, Morishita W, et al. Control of synaptic strength by glial TNF-alpha. *Science* 2002a; 295:2282–2285.

Beattie MS, Hermann GE, Rogers RC, Bresnahan JC. Cell death in models of spinal cord injury. *Prog Brain Res* 2002b;137:37–47.

Benke TA, Luthi A, Isaac JT, Collingridge GL. Modulation of AMPA receptor unitary conductance by synaptic activity. *Nature* 1998; 393:793–797.

Bennett AD, Everhart AW, Hulsebosch CE. Intrathecal administration of an NMDA or a non-NMDA receptor antagonist reduces mechanical but not thermal allodynia in a rodent model of chronic central pain after spinal cord injury. *Brain Res* 2000; 859:72–82.

Blackburn-Munro G, Bomholt SF, Erichsen HK. Behavioural effects of the novel AMPA/GluR5 selective receptor antagonist NS1209 after systemic administration in animal models of experimental pain. *Neuropharmacology* 2004; 47:351–362.

Bouschet T, Martin S, Henley JM. Receptor-activity-modifying proteins are required for forward trafficking of the calcium-sensing receptor to the plasma membrane. *J Cell Sci* 2005;118:4709–4720.

Braithwaite SP, Meyer G, Henley JM. Interactions between AMPA receptors and intracellular proteins. *Neuropharmacology* 2000; 39:919–930.

Bredt DS, Nicoll RA. AMPA receptor trafficking at excitatory synapses. *Neuron* 2003; 40:361–379.

Bruce AJ, Boling W, Kindy MS, et al. Altered neuronal and microglial responses to excitotoxic and ischemic brain injury in mice lacking TNF-α receptors. *Nat Med* 1996; 2:788–794.

Carlson NG, Bacchi A, Rogers SW, Gahring LC. Nicotine blocks TNF-alpha-mediated neuroprotection to NMDA by an alpha-bungarotoxin-sensitive pathway. *J Neurobiol* 1998; 35:29–36.

Carroll RC, Lissin DV, von Zastrow M, Nicoll RA, Malenka RC. Rapid redistribution of glutamate receptors contributes to long-term depression in hippocampal cultures. *Nat Neurosci* 1999a; 2:454–460.

Carroll RC, Beattie EC, Xia H, et al. Dynamin-dependent endocytosis of ionotropic glutamate receptors. *Proc Natl Acad Sci USA* 1999b; 96:14112–14117.

Carroll RC, Beattie EC, von Zastrow M, Malenka RC. Role of AMPA receptor endocytosis in synaptic plasticity. *Nat Rev Neurosci* 2001; 2:315–324.

Carroll RC, Zukin RS. NMDA-receptor trafficking and targeting: implications for synaptic transmission and plasticity. *Trends Neurosci* 2002; 25:571–577.

Chen L, Chetkovich DM, Petralia RS, et al. Stargazin regulates synaptic targeting of AMPA receptors by two distinct mechanisms. *Nature* 2000; 408:936–943.

Cheng B, Christakos S, Mattson MP. Tumor necrosis factors protect neurons against metabolic-excitotoxic insults and promote maintenance of calcium homeostasis. *Neuron* 1994; 12:139–153.

Chittajallu R, Braithwaite SP, Clarke VR, Henley JM. Kainate receptors: subunits, synaptic localization and function. *Trends Pharmacol Sci* 1999; 20:26–35.

Choi DW. Excitotoxic cell death. *J Neurobiol* 1992; 23:1261–1276.

Christensen MD, Hulsebosch CE. Chronic central pain after spinal cord injury. *J Neurotrauma* 1997; 14:517–537.

Clem RL, Barth A. Pathway-specific trafficking of native AMPARs by in vivo experience. *Neuron* 2006; 49:663–670.

Collingridge GL, Isaac JT, Wang YT. Receptor trafficking and synaptic plasticity. *Nat Rev Neurosci* 2004; 5:952–962.

Curatolo M, Bogduk N. Pharmacologic pain treatment of musculoskeletal disorders: current perspectives and future prospects. *Clin J Pain* 2001; 17:25–32.

Eaton MJ. Cell and molecular approaches to the attenuation of pain after spinal cord injury. *J Neurotrauma* 2006; 23:549–559.

Ehlers MD. Reinsertion or degradation of AMPA receptors determined by activity-dependent endocytic sorting. *Neuron* 2000; 28:511–525.

Ehrlich I, Malinow R. Postsynaptic density 95 controls AMPA receptor incorporation during long-term potentiation and experience-driven synaptic plasticity. *J Neurosci* 2004; 24:916–927.

Emch GS, Hermann GE, Rogers RC. TNF-α-alpha activates solitary nucleus neurons responsive to gastric distension. *Am J Physiol Gastrointest Liver Physiol* 2000; 279:G582–586.

Engelman HS, Allen TB, MacDermott AB. The distribution of neurons expressing calcium-permeable AMPA receptors in the superficial laminae of the spinal cord dorsal horn. *J Neurosci* 1999; 19:2081–2089.

Esteban JA, Shi SH, Wilson C, et al. PKA phosphorylation of AMPA receptor subunits controls synaptic trafficking underlying plasticity. *Nat Neurosci* 2003; 6:136–143.

Fontaine V, Mohand-Said S, Hanoteau N, et al. Neurodegenerative and neuroprotective effects of tumor Necrosis factor (TNF-α) in retinal ischemia: opposite roles of TNF-α receptor 1 and TNF-α receptor 2. *J Neurosci* 2002; 22:RC216.

Glazner GW, Mattson MP. Differential effects of BDNF, ADNF9, and TNF-α on levels of NMDA receptor subunits, calcium homeostasis, and neuronal vulnerability to excitotoxicity. *Exp Neurol* 2000; 161:442–452.

Grassi F, Mileo AM, Monaco L, et al. TNF-alpha increases the frequency of spontaneous miniature synaptic currents in cultured rat hippocampal neurons. *Brain Res* 1994; 659:226–230.

Guo W, Zou S, Guan Y, et al. Tyrosine phosphorylation of the NR2B subunit of the NMDA receptor in the spinal cord during the development and maintenance of inflammatory hyperalgesia. *J Neurosci* 2002; 22:6208–6217.

Hartmann B, Ahmadi S, Heppenstall PA, et al. The AMPA receptor subunits GluR-A and GluR-B reciprocally modulate spinal synaptic plasticity and inflammatory pain. *Neuron* 2004; 44:637–650.

Hayashi Y, Shi SH, Esteban JA, et al. Driving AMPA receptors into synapses by LTP and CaMKII: requirement for GluR1 and PDZ domain interaction. *Science* 2000; 287:2262–2267.

Hermann GE, Rogers RC, Bresnahan JC, Beattie MS. Tumor necrosis factor-alpha induces cFOS and strongly potentiates glutamate-mediated cell death in the rat spinal cord. *Neurobiol Dis* 2001; 8:590–599.

Herron CE, Lester RA, Coan EJ, Collingridge GL. Frequency-dependent involvement of NMDA receptors in the hippocampus: a novel synaptic mechanism. *Nature* 1986; 322:265–268.

Herzberg U, Sagen J. Peripheral nerve exposure to HIV viral envelope protein gp120 induces neuropathic pain and spinal gliosis. *J Neuroimmunol* 2001; 116:29–39.

Hirbec H, Francis JC, Lauri SE, et al. Rapid and differential regulation of AMPA and kainate receptors at hippocampal mossy fibre synapses by PICK1 and GRIP. *Neuron* 2003; 37:625–638.

Hollmann M, Heinemann S. Cloned glutamate receptors. *Annu Rev Neurosci* 1994; 17:31–108.

Isaac JT, Nicoll RA, Malenka RC. Evidence for silent synapses: implications for the expression of LTP. *Neuron* 1995; 15:427–434.

Jones TL, Sorkin LS. Calcium-permeable alpha-amino-3-hydroxy-5-methyl-4-isoxazolepropionic acid/kainate receptors mediate development, but not maintenance, of secondary allodynia evoked by first-degree burn in the rat. *J Pharmacol Exp Ther* 2004; 310:223–229.

Ju W, Morishita W, Tsui J, et al. Activity-dependent regulation of dendritic synthesis and trafficking of AMPA receptors. *Nat Neurosci* 2004; 7:244–253.

Kamenetz F, Tomita T, Hsieh H, et al. APP processing and synaptic function. *Neuron* 2003; 37:925–937.

Lee JM, Zipfel GJ, Choi DW. The changing landscape of ischaemic brain injury mechanisms. *Nature* 1999; 399:A7–14.

Lee HK, Barbarosie M, Kameyama K, Bear MF, Huganir RL. Regulation of distinct AMPA receptor phosphorylation sites during bidirectional synaptic plasticity. *Nature* 2000; 405:955–959.

Leonoudakis D, Braithwaite SP, Beattie MS, Beattie EC. TNF alpha-induced AMPA-receptor trafficking in CNS neurons; relevance to excitotoxicity? *Neuron Glia Biol* 2004; 1:263–273.

Liao D, Hessler NA, Malinow R. Activation of postsynaptically silent synapses during pairing-induced LTP in CA1 region of hippocampal slice. *Nature* 1995; 375:400–404.

Lin JW, Ju W, Foster K, et al. Distinct molecular mechanisms and divergent endocytotic pathways of AMPA receptor internalization. *Nat Neurosci* 2000; 3:1282–1290.

Lindsey AE, LoVerso RL, Tovar CA, et al. An analysis of changes in sensory thresholds to mild tactile and cold stimuli after experimental spinal cord injury in the rat. *Neurorehabil Neural Repair* 2000;14:287–300.

Lissin DV, Carroll RC, Nicoll RA, Malenka RC, von Zastrow M. Rapid, activation-induced redistribution of ionotropic glutamate receptors in cultured hippocampal neurons. *J Neurosci* 1999; 19:1263–1272.

Luscher C, Xia H, Beattie EC, et al. Role of AMPA receptor cycling in synaptic transmission and plasticity. *Neuron* 1999; 24:649–658.

Malenka RC, Nicoll RA. Long-term potentiation—a decade of progress? *Science* 1999; 285:1870–1874.

Malinow R, Malenka RC. AMPA receptor trafficking and synaptic plasticity. *Annu Rev Neurosci* 2002; 25:103–126.

Man HY, Lin JW, Ju WH, et al. Regulation of AMPA receptor-mediated synaptic transmission by clathrin-dependent receptor internalization. *Neuron* 2000; 25:649–662.

Man HY, Wang Q, Lu WY, et al. Activation of PI3-kinase is required for AMPA receptor insertion during LTP of mEPSCs in cultured hippocampal neurons. *Neuron* 2003; 38:611–624.

Mattson MP, Chan SL. Neuronal and glial calcium signaling in Alzheimer's disease. *Cell Calcium* 2003; 34:385–397.

Mattson MP, LaFerla FM, Chan SL, et al. Calcium signaling in the ER: its role in neuronal plasticity and neurodegenerative disorders. *Trends Neurosci* 2000; 23:222–229.

Miller BA, Sun F, Christensen RN, et al. A sublethal dose of TNF alpha potentiates kainate-induced excitotoxicity in optic nerve oligodendrocytes. *Neurochem Res* 2005; 30:867–875.

Mulkey RM, Malenka RC. Mechanisms underlying induction of homosynaptic long-term depression in area CA1 of the hippocampus. *Neuron* 1992; 9:967–975.

Nozaki-Taguchi N, Yaksh TL. A novel model of primary and secondary hyperalgesia after mild thermal injury in the rat. *Neurosci Lett* 1998; 254:25–28.

O'Brien RJ, Kamboj S, Ehlers MD, et al. Activity-dependent modulation of synaptic AMPA receptor accumulation. *Neuron* 1998; 21:1067–1078.

Ogoshi F, Weiss JH. Heterogeneity of Ca2+-permeable AMPA/kainate channel expression in hippocampal pyramidal neurons: fluorescence imaging and immunocytochemical assessment. *J Neurosci* 2003; 23:10521–10530.

Ogoshi F, Yin HZ, Kuppumbatti Y, et al. Tumor necrosis-factor-alpha (TNF-alpha) induces rapid insertion of Ca^{2+}-permeable alpha-amino-3-hydroxyl-5-methyl-4-isoxazole-propionate (AMPA)/kainate (Ca-A/K) channels in a subset of hippocampal pyramidal neurons. *Exp Neurol* 2005;193:384–393.

Ohtori S, Takahashi K, Moriya H, Myers RR. TNF-alpha and TNF-alpha receptor type 1 upregulation in glia and neurons after peripheral nerve injury: studies in murine DRG and spinal cord. *Spine* 2004; 29:1082–1088.

Passafaro M, Piech V, Sheng M. Subunit-specific temporal and spatial patterns of AMPA receptor exocytosis in hippocampal neurons. *Nat Neurosci* 2001; 4:917–926.

Pellegrini-Giampietro DE, Gorter JA, Bennett MV, Zukin RS. The GluR2 (GluR-B) hypothesis: Ca^{2+}-permeable AMPA receptors in neurological disorders. *Trends Neurosci* 1997; 20:464–470.

Perry VH, Bell MD, Brown HC, Matyszak MK. Inflammation in the nervous system. *Curr Opin Neurobiol* 1995; 5:636–641.

Peschon JJ, Torrance DS, Stocking KL, et al. TNF-α receptor-deficient mice reveal divergent roles for p55 and p75 in several models of inflammation. *J Immunol* 1998; 160:943–952.

Pogatzki EM, Niemeier JS, Sorkin LS, Brennan TJ. Spinal glutamate receptor antagonists differentiate primary and secondary mechanical hyperalgesia caused by incision. *Pain* 2003;105:97–107.

Reimann-Philipp U, Ovase R, Weigel PH, Grammas P. Mechanisms of cell death in primary cortical neurons and PC12 cells. *J Neurosci Res* 2001; 64:654–660.

Rumbaugh G, Sia GM, Garner CC, Huganir RL. Synapse-associated protein-97 isoform-specific regulation of surface AMPA receptors and synaptic function in cultured neurons. *J Neurosci* 2003; 23:4567–4576.

Schäfers M, Lee DH, Brors D, Yaksh TL, Sorkin LS. Increased sensitivity of injured and adjacent uninjured rat primary sensory neurons to exogenous tumor necrosis factor-alpha after spinal nerve ligation. *J Neurosci* 2003; 23:3028-3038.

Schubert P, Ogata T, Marchini C, Ferroni S, Rudolphi K. Protective mechanisms of adenosine in neurons and glial cells. *Ann NY Acad Sci* 1997; 825:1–10.

Shi SH, Hayashi Y, Petralia RS, et al. Rapid spine delivery and redistribution of AMPA receptors after synaptic NMDA receptor activation. *Science* 1999; 284:1811–1816.

Song I, Huganir RL. Regulation of AMPA receptors during synaptic plasticity. *Trends Neurosci* 2002; 25:578–588.

Sorkin LS, Yaksh TL, Doom CM. Mechanical allodynia in rats is blocked by a Ca^{2+} permeable AMPA receptor antagonist. *Neuroreport* 1999; 10:3523–3526.

Sorkin LS, Yaksh TL, Doom CM. Pain models display differential sensitivity to Ca^{2+}-permeable non-NMDA glutamate receptor antagonists. *Anesthesiology* 2001; 95:965–973.

Stein V, House DR, Bredt DS, Nicoll RA. Postsynaptic density-95 mimics and occludes hippocampal long-term potentiation and enhances long-term depression. *J Neurosci* 2003; 23:5503–5506.

Stellwagen D, Malenka RC. Synaptic scaling mediated by glial TNF-alpha. *Nature* 2006; 440:1054–1059.

Stellwagen D, Beattie EC, Seo JY, Malenka RC. Differential regulation of AMPA receptor and GABA receptor trafficking by tumor necrosis factor-alpha. *J Neurosci* 2005; 25:3219–3228.

Tanaka H, Grooms SY, Bennett MV, Zukin RS. The AMPAR subunit GluR2: still front and center-stage. *Brain Res* 2000; 886:190–207.

Tancredi V, D'Arcangelo G, Grassi F, et al. Tumor necrosis factor alters synaptic transmission in rat hippocampal slices. *Neurosci Lett* 1992; 146:176–178.

Tao YX, Rumbaugh G, Wang GD, et al. Impaired NMDA receptor-mediated postsynaptic function and blunted NMDA receptor-dependent persistent pain in mice lacking postsynaptic density-93 protein. *J Neurosci* 2003; 23:6703–6712.

Tomita S, Chen L, Kawasaki Y, et al. Functional studies and distribution define a family of transmembrane AMPA receptor regulatory proteins. *J Cell Biol* 2003; 161:805–816.

Tong CK, MacDermott AB. Both Ca^{2+} permeable and impermeable AMPA receptors contribute to primary synaptic drive onto rat dorsal horn neurons. *J Physiol* 2006; 575:133–144.

Tsai G, Coyle JT. Glutamatergic mechanisms in schizophrenia. *Annu Rev Pharmacol Toxicol* 2002; 42:165–179.

Turrigiano GG, Nelson SB. Homeostatic plasticity in the developing nervous system. *Nat Rev Neurosci* 2004; 5:97–107.

Tzschentke TM, Schmidt WJ. Glutamatergic mechanisms in addiction. *Mol Psychiatry* 2003; 8:373–382.

Vezzani A, Moneta D, Richichi C, et al. Functional role of inflammatory cytokines and antiinflammatory molecules in seizures and epileptogenesis. *Epilepsia* 2002; 43(Suppl 5):30–35.

Vitkovic L, Bockaert J, Jacque C. "Inflammatory" cytokines: neuromodulators in normal brain? *J Neurochem* 2000; 74:457–471.

Wang H, Kohno T, Amaya F, et al. Bradykinin produces pain hypersensitivity by potentiating spinal cord glutamatergic synaptic transmission. *J Neurosci* 2005; 25:7986–7992.

Watkins LR, Maier SF. Glia: a novel drug discovery target for clinical pain. *Nat Rev Drug Discov* 2003; 2:973–985.

Watkins LR, Nguyen KT, Lee JE, Maier SF. Dynamic regulation of proinflammatory cytokines. *Adv Exp Med Biol* 1999; 461:153–178.

Weiss JH, Sensi SL. Ca^{2+}-Zn^{2+} permeable AMPA or kainate receptors: possible key factors in selective neurodegeneration. *Trends Neurosci* 2000; 23:365–371.

Wierenga CJ, Ibata K, Turrigiano GG. Postsynaptic expression of homeostatic plasticity at neocortical synapses. *J Neurosci* 2005; 25:2895–2905.

Wilde GJ, Pringle AK, Sundstrom LE, Mann DA, Iannotti F. Attenuation and augmentation of ischaemia-related neuronal death by tumour necrosis factor-alpha in vitro. *Eur J Neurosci* 2000; 12:3863–3870.

Xia Y, Carroll RC, Nawy S. State-dependent AMPA receptor trafficking in the mammalian retina. *J Neurosci* 2006; 26:5028–5036.

Xu JT, Xin WJ, Zang Y, Wu CY, Liu XG. The role of tumor necrosis factor-alpha in the neuropathic pain induced by lumbar 5 ventral root transection in rat. *Pain* 2006; 123:306–321.

Yang L, Lindholm K, Konishi Y, Li R, Shen Y. Target depletion of distinct tumor necrosis factor receptor subtypes reveals hippocampal neuron death and survival through different signal transduction pathways. *J Neurosci* 2002; 22:3025–3032.

Yudowski GA, Puthenveedu MA, von Zastrow M. Distinct modes of regulated receptor insertion to the somatodendritic plasma membrane. *Nat Neurosci* 2006; 9:622–627.

Zahn PK, Umali E, Brennan TJ. Intrathecal non-NMDA excitatory amino acid receptor antagonists inhibit pain behaviors in a rat model of postoperative pain. *Pain* 1998; 74:213–223.

Zhao X, Bausano B, Pike BR, et al. TNF-alpha stimulates caspase-3 activation and apoptotic cell death in primary septo-hippocampal cultures. *J Neurosci Res* 2001; 64:121–131.

Correspondence to: Eric C. Beattie, PhD, Department of Neurosciences, California Pacific Medical Center Research Institute, 475 Brannan Street, Suite 220, San Francisco, CA 94107, USA; email: beattie@cpmcri.org.

Immune and Glial Regulation of Pain, edited by Joyce A. DeLeo, Linda S. Sorkin, and Linda R. Watkins, IASP Press, Seattle, © 2007.

13

Astrocyte Signaling Systems in Physiology and Pathology

Biljana Djukic, Todd A. Fiacco, and Ken D. McCarthy

Department of Pharmacology, University of North Carolina at Chapel Hill, Chapel Hill, North Carolina, USA

ASTROCYTES: UBIQUITOUS, MORPHOLOGICALLY COMPLEX, AND HIGHLY ADAPTABLE

Astrocytes are the most numerous cells in the mammalian brain and associate with all of its cellular elements. Most astrocytes can be classified as either protoplasmic or fibrous on the basis of their location and morphology. Protoplasmic astrocytes tend to reside in the gray matter and exhibit very fine processes radiating out from a central, small cell body. In contrast, fibrous astrocytes tend to reside in the white matter and extend a thicker network of processes. More specialized astrocytes exist in distinct brain regions including Bergmann glia in the cerebellum and Mueller glia in the retina. All of these cells express glial fibrillary acidic protein (GFAP), though the levels of this intermediate filament protein vary considerably as a function of brain region, stage of development, and injury. The morphological complexity of protoplasmic astrocytes is remarkable. These cells resemble a fine bush with processes that become progressively finer as they radiate out from the cell body. The general impression is that the processes of protoplasmic astrocytes fill the space not occupied by other cellular elements. As a consequence, they ensheathe most neuronal elements (synapses, axons, and dendrites) and vasculature within their morphological sphere. The extent to which an individual protoplasmic astrocyte associates with its local cellular environment is well illustrated in the hippocampus, where it is estimated that a single astrocyte envelops 80,000 synapses (Bushong et al. 2002). Less is known about the function of fibrous astrocytes residing within myelinated tracts. However, their association with myelinated axons and oligodendrocytes suggests that fibrous astrocytes may play a role in the development and maintenance of myelin.

The processes of individual astrocytes are highly connected through reflexive gap junctions, and gap junctions also interconnect adjacent astrocytes, thus forming a syncytium. The syncytial nature of protoplasmic astrocyte networks is readily demonstrated by intracellular injections of tracer dyes that can permeate the gap junction. Within the hippocampus, the injection of such dyes into a single astrocyte results in the filling of hundreds, if not thousands, of individual astrocytes (Konietzko and Muller 1994). The fact that gray matter astrocytes function as a syncytium has important functional consequences. First, signaling molecules smaller than 1 kDa (e.g., calcium, cyclic adenosine monophosphate [AMP], and inositol triphosphate [IP3]) readily diffuse between astrocyte processes. As a result, it is quite likely that astrocytes exhibit functional spheres, or microdomains, that function independently of other microdomains within the same astrocyte. Second, since the opening and closing of gap junctions is a highly regulated process, signals developing in one part of the astrocytic syncytium could propagate through a very specific morphological pathway to affect events distant from the initiation site. Third, an astrocytic syncytium provides a "sink" whereby molecules that might be detrimental if spatially restricted could dissipate to nontoxic levels. For example, elevated extracellular potassium creates a major problem by depolarizing cells, increasing their excitability. Protoplasmic astrocytes are thought to limit the build-up of extracellular potassium by K^+ uptake inwardly rectifying K^+ channels and by the dissipation of this ion within the astrocytic syncytium (Kofuji and Newman 2004).

Very little is known about how physiological changes in neural activity affect astrocytes. However, it is apparent that in the extreme case of central nervous system (CNS) injury (including chronic pain), astrocytes undergo extensive remodeling referred to as "gliosis" (Pekny and Nilsson 2005). In this situation, astrocytes enlarge and proliferate to form a dense tangle of astrocytic processes enriched in GFAP; such astrocytes are referred to as "reactive." Reactive astrocytes have been studied extensively because they appear to be detrimental to neuronal regeneration. It is clear that reactive astrocytes undergo significant changes in gene expression, which ultimately affects their function (Nakagawa et al. 2005). Less is known about how more subtle changes in neuronal activity affect astrocytes. One common observation among investigators studying astrocytic calcium responses in situ is that multiple applications of ligands can lead to increases in intrinsic calcium oscillations in these cells (Pasti et al. 1997). While the molecular basis of this plasticity remains unexplored, this observation suggests that, like neurons, astrocytic signaling responses will vary depending on their previous experiences.

GLIAL CELL SIGNALING: A HISTORICAL PERSPECTIVE

The first suggestion that glial cells might play a role in intercellular signaling can be traced back to 1907. In a remarkable paper based on the findings of early anatomists including Cajal and Del Rio-Hortega, Lugaro (1907) suggested that glial cells carry out a variety of supportive tasks necessary for neuronal activity (Somjen 1988). Among these tasks, Lugaro suggested that glia are well positioned to provide neurons with substances necessary for their function and to remove chemicals released from neuronal terminals during activity. Unfortunately, these visionary predictions remained untested for nearly 70 years. The prevailing concept during this period was that glial cells were primarily involved in insulating neurons from one another and that neurons alone were responsible for carrying out the many processes responsible for normal and abnormal brain function. The basis for this neurocentric view of brain function probably resided in the fact that most studies of brain cells during this period relied on electrophysiological recordings, and unlike neurons, glial cells are not electrically excitable.

Opinions began to change in the 1970s as neuroscientists began to use cell culture systems to study receptor-mediated changes in second messengers. Initially, most of these studies used transformed cell lines derived from neural tissue. A striking finding from these studies was that cell lines derived from glia responded to a variety of neuroligands with changes in second messengers (Clark and Perkins 1971; Gilman and Nirenberg 1971). At the time, it remained unclear whether the responses observed in glial cell lines reflected the signaling capacity of non-transformed glia or were induced by cell transformation. This issue was resolved in the late 1970s with a series of publications demonstrating that non-transformed astroglia derived from immature rodent brain exhibited similar responses to receptor activation (McCarthy and de Vellis 1978, 1980; Van Calker et al. 1978). During the 1980s a large number of investigators used primary cultures of astroglia to demonstrate that these cells express a large number of different receptor systems whose stimulation affects a wide variety of second messengers including cyclic AMP, cyclic guanosine monophosphate (GMP), calcium, nitric oxide, arachidonic acid, and prostaglandins (Hertz et al. 1984; Murphy and Pearce 1987). Further, it became apparent that astroglia exhibit transport systems that enable them to take up neurotransmitters (Roeder et al. 1988; Speciale et al. 1989; Levy et al. 1993; O'Connor et al. 1994). As glial biology entered the 1990s, a large amount of data supported Lugaro's early premise that glia, particularly astrocytes, play a critical role in neurophysiology. However, as the vast majority of work in this area relied on primary cultures of astroglia prepared from immature brain tissue, a question that remained unaddressed was whether mature astrocytes exhibited similar properties in vivo.

ASTROCYTES: LISTENING TO NEURONAL CONVERSATION

There is now overwhelming evidence that astrocytes in situ and in vivo express a large number of different neurotransmitter receptor signaling systems (Porter and McCarthy 1997). Methods used to demonstrate this finding include receptor immunocytochemistry (Aoki et al. 1987), receptor autoradiography (Salm and McCarthy 1989; Sutin and Shao 1992), electrophysiology (Seifert and Steinhauser 2001), and calcium imaging (Porter and McCarthy 1997; Volterra and Steinhauser 2004). Neurotransmitter receptor systems expressed by astrocytes include ionotropic and metabotropic glutamate receptors, type A gamma-aminobutyric acid (GABA$_A$) receptors, alpha- and beta-adrenergic receptors, adenosine receptors, adenosine triphosphate (ATP) receptors, serotonergic receptors, muscarinic cholinergic receptors, histaminergic receptors, substance P receptors, prostaglandin E$_1$ receptors, and opioid receptors (Porter and McCarthy 1997; Verkhratsky and Steinhauser 2000; Volterra and Steinhauser 2004). Importantly, the distribution of these astrocytic receptor systems varies throughout the brain and spinal cord and changes during development and under pathological conditions (Porter and McCarthy 1997; Binder and Steinhauser 2006). The fact that astrocytes in situ and in vivo express such a variety of neuroligand receptors strongly argues that these cells participate in intercellular signaling events in vivo.

The development of calcium indicator dyes that can be used to track temporal and spatial changes in intracellular calcium provided a critical tool in the study of astrocyte signaling in vitro, in situ, and more recently, in vivo (Porter and McCarthy 1997; Wang et al. 2006). Initially used in cultured astroglia, calcium imaging experiments demonstrated that astrocytes were remarkably heterogeneous in their ability to respond to different neuroligands and that their responsiveness changed as a function of time in culture (Shao and McCarthy 1991). Similar studies carried out in situ also demonstrated that astrocytes are heterogeneous with respect to their ability to respond to neuroligands with an increase in calcium (McCarthy and Salm 1991). It is clear from a large number of studies that astrocytes in situ respond to neuronal activity with increases in second messengers. Neuron-dependent excitation of astrocytes has been reported in many brain circuits following nerve fiber stimulation and the subsequent release of various neurotransmitters and factors including glutamate, GABA, acetylcholine, norepinephrine, dopamine, ATP, nitric oxide, and brain-derived neurotrophic factor (Haydon 2001). Interestingly, astrocytes appear to be able to discriminate and integrate neuronal inputs from different origins (Perea and Araque 2005b). Hippocampal astrocytes in the stratum oriens respond with elevated concentrations of intracellular Ca^{2+} to stimulation of either Schaffer collaterals (which are glutamatergic) or nerve fibers in the stratum oriens (which are mainly cholinergic). However, when both nerve fibers are stimulated simultaneously, astrocyte responses do not simply correspond to the sum of intracellular Ca^{2+} transients elicited by the separate stimulations. Instead, they are either smaller or larger, displaying either positive or negative cooperativity, depending on the frequency of the stimulation (Perea and Araque 2005b). The question is no longer whether or not astrocytic signaling systems are activated by the release of neurotransmitters from neurons, but rather, under what conditions are astrocytic receptors activated, what are the functional consequences of stimulating astrocytic receptors, and how does the neurotransmitter responsiveness of astrocytes change under pathological conditions?

ASTROCYTIC SIGNALING THROUGH CALCIUM WAVES AND INTRINSIC CALCIUM OSCILLATIONS

Studies from a large number of laboratories indicate that astroglia in culture and astrocytes in situ exhibit intracellular calcium waves that can propagate into adjacent astroglia to form a calcium wave moving through a syncytium of astrocytes (Scemes 2000; Perea and Araque 2005a). This observation led to the idea that astrocytes in vivo signal over long distances via calcium waves to affect a neuronal network. The concept that astrocytes, like neurons, signal over long distances was introduced by a series of remarkable calcium movies made in Stephen Smith's laboratory (Cornell-Bell et al. 1990). Smith and coworkers demonstrated that astrocytic calcium waves in hippocampal explant cultures propagated over long distances and are modulated both by neurotransmitters (e.g., glutamate) and by neuronal activity (Cornell-Bell et al. 1990). Studies using acutely isolated brain slices also demonstrated that astrocytes in situ exhibit intracellular calcium waves (Nett et al. 2002), although the distances traveled by such waves are generally much less than those observed in vitro. While the mechanisms underlying astrocytic calcium waves are still debated, it appears likely that such waves are dependent on the release of ATP from astrocytes and on the activation of purinergic receptors expressed by these cells (Guthrie et al. 1999; Gallagher and Salter 2003).

Intrinsic Ca^{2+} transients have been observed in astrocytes in acutely isolated brain slices (Parri et al. 2001; Aguado et al. 2002; Nett et al. 2002) and in vivo (Hirase et al. 2004; Nimmerjahn et al. 2004). They are generated by Ca^{2+} release from internal stores due to activation of inositol trisphosphate (IP3) receptors, with possible additional influx of extracellular Ca^{2+} through voltage-gated channels. Furthermore, they can either remain confined to distal processes that oscillate simultaneously or propagate to variable distances, intracellularly (Nett et al. 2002) or possibly even intercellularly (Parri et al. 2001; Nimmerjahn et al. 2004). Importantly, intrinsic calcium oscillations in astrocytes can result in the excitation of nearby neurons, suggesting that astrocytes and neurons may operate in coordinated networks (Parri and Crunelli 2001; Hirase et al. 2004; Nimmerjahn et al. 2004). Studies in our laboratory demonstrated that astrocytic calcium oscillations in acutely isolated hippocampal brain slices were unaffected by the presence of tetradotoxin (TTX), which blocks neuronal action potentials, or bafilomycin A, which blocks neurotransmitter release (Nett et al. 2002). These results are particularly interesting when coupled with the finding that increases in astrocytic calcium levels lead to the release of neurotransmitters (e.g., glutamate and ATP) from these cells (see below). These findings suggest that, independent of neuronal input, astrocytes may release neurotransmitters to modulate neuronal activity. There is little evidence to suggest that the release of neurotransmitters from astrocytes (subsequently referred to as "gliotransmitters") is sufficient to generate neuronal action potentials. Rather, astrocytes may release gliotransmitters to affect the excitability of neurons. For example, the release of glutamate from astrocytes could increase the ambient concentration of extracellular glutamate, leading to a small depolarization of neurons via the activation of ionotropic glutamate receptors; such neurons would have a greater tendency to fire action potentials. Alternatively, the release of ATP from astrocytes could lead to the activation of purinergic receptors, which can either increase (ATP) or decrease (adenosine) neuronal excitability. The role of intrinsic calcium oscillations or the mechanisms through which they are generated remain poorly understood. Nevertheless, as these have been observed in vitro, in situ, and in vivo, they are likely to represent an important mechanism in the astrocytic modulation of neuronal activity.

ASTROCYTES: TALKING TO NEURONS

The concept of astrocytes as non-excitable support cells has given way over the past 15 years due to the astonishing discovery that astrocytes are capable of talking to neuronal elements with chemical messages of their own. Today we view these multifunctional cells as the third essential element of the CNS signal-integration unit, the "tripartite synapse" (Araque et al. 1999). Even though they are not involved in fast electrical signaling, astrocytes are now thought of as excitable cells due to their ability to propagate chemical signals via intracellular Ca^{2+} mobilization. When activated by internal or external signals, astrocytes respond with intracellular Ca^{2+} transients and oscillations, leading to delivery of chemical messages to neighboring cells, an activity that has been termed "gliotransmission" (Bezzi et al. 2001).

An important response of astrocyte Ca^{2+}-mediated excitation, both by neuronal input and self-generated stimuli, is the release of gliotransmitters or chemicals that act on adjacent neurons, glial cells, and blood vessels. Over the years, the number of proposed gliotransmitters has increased, and some of their properties and actions have been revealed. They include, but are not limited to glutamate, ATP, adenosine, D-serine, eicosanoids, cytokines, proteins, and peptides, such as acetylcholine-binding protein and atrial natriuretic peptide (Volterra and Meldolesi 2005). In addition, several gliotransmitter release mechanisms have been identified, including the Ca^{2+}-dependent release via exocytosis of transmitter containing vesicles (Bezzi et al. 2004; Kreft et al. 2004; Montana et al. 2004; Chen et al. 2005), release through Na^+-dependent glutamate transporters operating in reverse mode (Rossi et al. 2000), release via activation of volume-regulated anion channels due to the cellular volume regulatory response (Kimelberg et al. 1990; Eggermont et al. 2001), release via functional hemichannels (Ye et al. 2003; Parpura et al. 2004b), and release via purinergic receptors forming permeable pores (Duan et al. 2003; Fellin et al. 2006). Properties of these release mechanisms in astrocytes, such as their specificity and regulation, are not yet clarified, but what is clear is the remarkable ability of gliotransmission to affect neuronal information processing.

Modulation of neuronal excitability and synaptic transmission by astrocytes was first shown to be mediated by glutamate (Parpura et al. 1994a; Volterra and Steinhauser 2004). Recently, modulatory effects mediated by ATP, adenosine, and D-serine have also emerged (Yang et al. 2003; Bowser and Khakh 2004). The experimental models that have been most intensely studied are the retinal and hippocampal circuits. Activation of retinal glia, astrocytes, and Müller cells has been shown to modulate the light-evoked spiking activity of ganglion cells that project to the brain, thereby affecting the processing of visual information (Newman and Zahs 1998). Two opposite effects have been identified so far. The first effect is inhibitory and is mediated by ATP released from Müller cells (Newman 2003), while the second is stimulatory and mediated by D-serine acting on N-methyl-D-aspartate (NMDA) receptors (Stevens et al. 2003). D-serine appears to be mainly synthesized and released by astrocytes and is proven to be an effective coagonist at the glycine-binding site of NMDA glutamate receptors (Miller 2004). In hippocampal slices, astrocyte-released glutamate can act on group I metabotropic glutamate receptors (mGluRs) to produce presynaptic facilitation, recorded as an increase in the frequency of spontaneous excitatory postsynaptic currents (EPSCs) in CA1 pyramidal neurons (Fiacco and McCarthy 2004). In contrast, astrocyte-released ATP mediates synaptic inhibition by suppressing glutamatergic synapses via presynaptic purinergic P2Y receptors (Zhang et al. 2003). Moreover, the observed heterosynaptic suppression of adjacent Schaffer collateral fibers during high-frequency activity is mediated by astrocytes, which sense the level of activity in the first fiber and tune the activity of the second by releasing ATP (Zhang et al. 2003). Astrocytes can also modulate inhibitory synaptic transmission. The best-characterized example of this modulatory activity is the potentiation of hippocampal synapses between the GABA-containing interneurons of the stratum radiatum and CA1 pyramidal neurons (Kang et al. 1998). This effect is not direct but depends on the activation of neighboring astrocytes by GABA. The feedback release of glutamate by astrocytes decreases GABA-mediated synaptic failures, possibly through the stimulation of GluR5-containing kainite receptors on the interneurons (Liu et al. 2004).

Furthermore, astrocytes appear to be involved in more global and longer-lasting changes of synaptic strength by direct stimulation of postsynaptic excitability, synchronization of neuronal networks, and modulation of synaptic plasticity mechanisms. In hippocampal slices under certain conditions, such as low extracellular Mg^{2+} concentration, CA1 pyramidal neurons show transient slow inward currents that are kinetically distinct and larger than synaptic currents. These currents, which are dependent on NMDA receptor activation and are unaffected by the blockade of synaptic transmitter release, depend on spontaneous intracellular Ca^{2+} oscillations of astrocytes and increase in frequency following astrocyte stimulation (Angulo et al. 2004; Fellin et al. 2004; Perea and Araque 2005b). Synchronized slow inward currents could be observed in clusters of neurons, suggesting that astrocytes may function as bridging units between circuits that are not directly connected to each other; however, the appearance of such currents needs to be verified in more physiologically relevant preparations. Several studies report astrocyte gliotransmission affecting synaptic strength and plasticity in the hippocampus. Astrocyte-released D-serine was shown to modulate NMDA-receptor-dependent long-term potentiation of CA1 pyramidal neurons (Yang et al. 2003). Astrocytes were also shown to control the strength of these synapses by increasing the surface expression of neuronal α-amino-3-hydroxy-5-methylisoxazole-4-propionic acid (AMPA) receptors through the release of tumor necrosis factor-α (Beattie et al. 2002). Pascual et al. (2005) have recently shown that impairment of astrocyte vesicular release machinery alters synaptic transmission and long-term potentiation in hippocampal slices by inhibiting ATP release. A glial-induced long-lasting depression of spontaneous synaptic currents of Purkinje neurons has also been shown in cerebellar slices (Brockhaus and Deitmer 2002).

These observations demonstrate that astrocyte release of gliotransmitters can influence synaptic transmission. By synchronizing neuronal activity and affecting long-term synaptic plasticity, astrocytes may modulate CNS information processing and memory formation under certain conditions. The new concept of synaptic physiology, the "tripartite synapse," in which astrocytes play an active role as dynamic regulatory elements of neurotransmission, is strongly supported. However, a considerable amount of work is still needed to fully understand the level of involvement of astrocyte-mediated synaptic modulation in physiological vs. pathological conditions, as well as the impact of this activity on brain function. Furthermore, the properties and mechanisms of astrocytic modulation of non-neuronal cellular activity are not well understood. For example, astrocytes coordinate spatial positioning of oligodendrocytes during development (Tsai et al. 2002), attract microglia and lymphocytes in response to inflammation or injury (Babcock et al. 2003; Marella and Chabry 2004), and might even bring reparative stem cells to lesion sites (Imitola et al. 2004). Astrocytes, therefore, appear to be the "all-capable" communication elements that have the capacity to regulate and coordinate different functional components of the CNS.

ASTROCYTES AND NEUROTRANSMITTER HOMEOSTASIS

Information processing within the CNS is based on intricately coordinated communication between excitatory and inhibitory synaptic units, composed of pre- and postsynaptic nerve endings enwrapped by astrocyte processes. The functional capacity of such synapses depends on the biosynthesis, release, receptor interaction, and inactivation of the neurotransmitter in question, and so each of these processes needs to be highly regulated and controlled. Even before synaptic transmission was understood, Lugaro (1907) suggested that glia might terminate the action of substances that transmit signals between neurons, based on his observations that glial processes surround "nervous articulations" (later identified as synapses; Somjen 1988). Since then it has become evident that astrocytes play a major role in neurotransmitter biosynthesis and in the uptake of neurotransmitters.

Glutamate is the main excitatory neurotransmitter in the CNS and a precursor for GABA, which is responsible for most of inhibitory neurotransmission. Both of these transmitters must be synthesized within the CNS, as they do not cross the blood-brain barrier. Since neurons lack pyruvate carboxylase, an essential enzyme for de novo synthesis of glutamate from glucose, much of the brain's glutamate is generated by astrocytes and supplied to neurons (Hertz and Zielke 2004). Astrocytes also control recycling of synaptically released glutamate. They accumulate glutamate from the synaptic cleft and convert it to glutamine by another astrocyte-specific enzyme, glutamine synthetase. Glutamine is then returned to neurons and reconverted to glutamate to power subsequent neurotransmission (Hallermayer et al. 1981; Loo et al. 1995). An almost instantaneous loss of normal vision upon inhibition of the astrocyte-specific metabolic pathways necessary for glutamate production clearly exemplifies the importance of astrocytes for normal function of glutamatergic neurons (Barnett et al. 2000).

Extensive research has also established that astrocyte glutamate transporters primarily accomplish glutamate uptake and termination of excitatory transmission in the CNS. As prolonged exposure of neurons to high levels of glutamate leads to excitotoxicity marked by neuronal degeneration and death, glutamate concentration in the interstitial space must be tightly controlled (Anderson and Swanson 2000). So far, five glutamate transporters have been cloned and named excitatory amino acid transporters 1–5 (EAAT1–5). EAAT1 (or GLAST) and EAAT2 (or GLT-1) account for the majority of the glutamate transport capacity in the CNS and are almost exclusively expressed in astrocytes (Gegelashvili and Schousboe 1997; Danbolt 2001). Glutamate transport in neurons is mainly accounted for by EAAT3 (or EAAC1; Kanai and Hediger 1992; Danbolt 2001). The two transporters, EAAT4 and EAAT5, are expressed in cerebellar Purkinje neurons and retinal Müller cells, respectively (Yamada et al. 1996; Arriza et al. 1997). Uptake of glutamate and H^+ is driven by the coupled transport of three sodium ions into the cell and one potassium ion out of the cell down their concentration gradients. This creates a net movement of positive charge into the cell, which can be monitored using electrophysiological techniques (Diamond et al. 1998). Excitatory synaptic activity has been shown to activate rapid glutamate transporter currents in astrocytes in the hippocampus (Mennerick and Zorumski 1994; Bergles and Jahr 1997; Kojima et al. 1999) and cerebellum (Bergles et al. 1997; Clark and Barbour 1997). Such transporter-associated currents cannot be detected in neurons (Bergles and Jahr 1998), perhaps due to localization of neuronal glutamate transporters away from the synaptic active zone (Furuta et al. 1997a,b; Pignataro et al. 2005). Furthermore, selective inhibition of astrocyte glutamate transporters has been reported to increase both the amplitude (Tong and Jahr 1994) and the duration (Barbour et al. 1994) of glutamate-induced EPSCs. Uptake inhibitors can also enhance the EPSC depression evoked by repetitive stimulation, suggesting a role for glutamate uptake in synaptic plasticity (Turecek and Trussell 2000). The crucial role of astrocyte transporters in vivo is supported by gene knockout and antisense studies. Antisense knockdown of GLAST and GLT-1, but not of the neuronal subtype EAAC1, produces elevated extracellular glutamate levels, excitotoxic neurodegeneration, and paralysis in rats (Rothstein et al. 1996). Mice lacking GLT-1 are prone to lethal spontaneous seizures and display increased susceptibility to loss of hippocampal neurons (Tanaka et al. 1997). Similarly, GLAST-deficient mice display motor discoordination and increased susceptibility to cerebellar injury (Watase et al. 1998). These studies have fostered increased interest in the role of astrocyte glutamate transport in disease states such as ischemia, epilepsy, and chronic pain.

ASTROCYTIC SIGNALING: ROLE IN
NEUROLOGICAL DISORDERS

Given the central role that astrocytes play in regulating neuronal communication, it is not surprising that astrocytic dysfunction appears to be involved in a number of clinical disorders. Disease states thought to involve astrocytic dysfunction include chronic pain (Wieseler-Frank et al. 2004; McMahon et al. 2005), epilepsy (Tian et al. 2005), multiple sclerosis (Lennon et al. 2005; Plant et al. 2005), Alzheimer's disease (Rossner 2004; Saez et al. 2004; Monnerie et al. 2005; Tzeng et al. 2005), amyotrophic lateral sclerosis (ALS) (Barbeito et al. 2004), Parkinson's disease (Teismann and Schulz 2004), and Alexander's disease (Brenner et al. 2001). Further, studies strongly suggest that activation of astrocytes leads to the release of cytokines that interfere with neuronal regeneration following spinal cord injury (Brambilla et al. 2005). Several recent studies suggest that a defect in the ability of astrocytes to buffer extracellular K^+, take up neuronally released glutamate, or limit their own glutamate release may underlie the development of chronic pain (Lee et al. 2005b), epilepsy (Tian et al. 2005), and certain neurodegenerative diseases including Alzheimer's and ALS (Miller 2005). Additionally, release of inflammatory cytokines, prostaglandins, and nitric oxide by reactive astrocytes appears to be an important factor in a number of neurodegenerative diseases including ALS and Alzheimer's (Barbeito et al. 2004; Schultz et al. 2004; Cartier et al. 2005; Deshpande et al. 2005). Two key properties of astrocytes are their ability to buffer extracellular K^+ and to control the concentration of extracellular glutamate via their uptake and release of glutamate. Changes in either of these parameters can lead to neuronal hyperexcitability. Optical measurements suggest that formalin-evoked nociceptor activation in skin decreases the ability of astrocytes to buffer extracellular K^+ and take up glutamate (Lee et al. 2005b). Interestingly, the primary gap junction protein associated with astrocytes, Cx43, is upregulated in reactive spinal cord astrocytes and remains so for at least 4 weeks after injury (Lee et al. 2005a). These findings suggest that reactive astrocytes may be able to propagate signaling molecules farther than nonreactive astrocytes, providing a potential explanation for the development of mirror-image pain (Spataro et al. 2004). It is also interesting that $mGluR_1$ and $mGluR_5$ glutamatergic receptors are upregulated in reactive astrocytes for at least 4 weeks after injury (Gwak and Hulsebosch 2005). Activation of these mGluR subtypes in astrocytes stimulates G_q-linked G-protein-coupled receptor signaling cascades, leading to an increase in cytoplasmic calcium and gliotransmitter release including glutamate, prostaglandin E_2 (PGE_2), and ATP (Haydon 2001; Pascual et al. 2005). All of these gliotransmitters are known to increase the activity of nociceptive neurons within the spinal cord.

There is little doubt that chronic pain initially arises from the hyperactivity of sensory neurons (Woolf and Salter 2000). However, the results from a number of studies suggest that it is the prolonged activation of spinal cord astrocytes that correlates best with persistent pain (Wieseler-Frank et al. 2004; Marchand et al. 2005; McMahon et al. 2005; Zhuang et al. 2005). Importantly, activated spinal cord astrocytes express molecules thought to be involved in the development and maintenance of chronic pain. For example, activated spinal cord astrocytes express proinflammatory cytokines such as interleukin-1β (IL-1β), IL-1β receptors, and cyclooxygenase-2 (COX-2, the enzyme responsible for the production of PGE_2) (Sweitzer et al. 1999; Okuno et al. 2004; Raghavendra et al. 2004; Wieseler-Frank et al. 2004; Zhang et al. 2005). Inhibition of either IL-1β receptors or COX-2 blocks the development and maintenance of certain types of chronic pain (Yaksh et al. 2001; Yeo et al. 2004; Ahn et al. 2005; Bingham et al. 2005). Further, intracellular signaling cascades thought to regulate the expression of IL-1β and COX-2 are stimulated in reactive astrocytes (Piao et al. 2003; Watkins et al. 2003; Tzeng et al. 2005). Reactive astrocytes also express nitric oxide and secrete nerve growth factor (Barbeito et al. 2004), molecules considered important in chronic pain (McMahon et al. 2005). In a recent report, Zhuang et al. (2006) reported that chronic neuropathic pain was associated with an increase in c-Jun N-terminal kinase 1 (JNK1) in spinal cord astrocytes. Selectively blocking the increase in astrocytic JNK1 not only blocked the development of chronic pain, but also reversed mechanical allodynia resulting from spinal nerve ligation (a model of neuropathic pain) (Zhuang et al. 2006). Importantly, one of the targets of JNK signaling is nuclear factor κB. This transcription factor is known to be important in cascades leading to the release of inflammatory cytokines that are thought to play a role in neuronal sensitization in chronic pain. Interestingly, studies demonstrate that blocking astrocyte function with a metabolic inhibitor abolishes chronic pain, whereas blocking microglial function inhibits the development, but not the maintenance, of chronic pain (Watkins and Maier 2003). These findings suggest that microglial cells are important in the development of chronic pain, perhaps by activating astrocytes, but it is the activated astrocytes that are responsible for the maintenance of the pain (Watkins and Maier 2003). Studies utilizing astrocyte-specific metabolic inhibitors as well as gap junction inhibitors suggest that astrocytes also play a role in mirror-image neuropathic pain via release of proinflammatory cytokines and prostaglandins (Milligan et al. 2003; Spataro et al. 2004). Overall, research in this area suggests that enhanced neuronal activity associated with painful stimuli leads to an "early phase" activation of microglial cells, which, in turn, induces a "late phase" activation of astrocytes and persistent sensitization of nociceptive neurons via astrocytic release of sensitizing molecules that include cytokines, prostaglandins, nerve growth factor, and nitric oxide.

SUMMARY

Findings obtained over the past several decades clearly demonstrate that astrocytes exhibit a wide variety of signaling systems capable of playing an important role in neurophysiology and disease. Further, it is likely that the expression and role of astrocytic signaling systems differs among brain regions and changes in disease states. While the study of these cells remains challenging, it is likely that unraveling the mysteries of processes ranging from learning and memory to the loss of cognition in Alzheimer's patients to chronic pain will require understanding of the role of astrocytic signaling systems in brain function.

ACKNOWLEDGMENTS

This work was supported by NIH grants R01 NS 033938-06 and R01 NS 020212-22.

REFERENCES

Aguado F, Espinosa-Parrilla JF, Carmona MA, Soriano E. Neuronal activity regulates correlated network properties of spontaneous calcium transients in astrocytes in situ. *J Neurosci* 2002; 22:9430–9444.

Ahn DK, Chae JM, Choi HS, et al. Central cyclooxygenase inhibitors reduced IL-1beta-induced hyperalgesia in temporomandibular joint of freely moving rats. *Pain* 2005; 117:204–213.

Anderson CM, Swanson RA. Astrocyte glutamate transport: review of properties, regulation, and physiological functions. *Glia* 2000; 32:1–14.

Angulo MC, Kozlov AS, Charpak S, Audinat E. Glutamate released from glial cells synchronizes neuronal activity in the hippocampus. *J Neurosci* 2004; 24:6920–6927.

Aoki C, Joh TH, Pickel VM. Ultrastructural localization of beta-adrenergic receptor-like immunoreactivity in the cortex and neostriatum of rat brain. *Brain Res* 1987; 437:264–282.

Araque A, Sanzgiri RP, Parpura V, Haydon PG. Astrocyte-induced modulation of synaptic transmission. *Can J Physiol Pharmacol* 1999; 77:699–706.

Arriza JL, Eliasof S, Kavanaugh MP, Amara SG. Excitatory amino acid transporter 5, a retinal glutamate transporter coupled to a chloride conductance. *Proc Natl Acad Sci USA* 1997; 94:4155–4160.

Babcock AA, Kuziel WA, Rivest S, Owens T. Chemokine expression by glial cells directs leukocytes to sites of axonal injury in the CNS. *J Neurosci* 2003; 23:7922–7930.

Barbeito LH, Pehar M, Cassina P, et al. A role for astrocytes in motor neuron loss in amyotrophic lateral sclerosis. *Brain Res Brain Res Rev* 2004; 47:263–274.

Barbour B, Keller BU, Llano I, Marty A. Prolonged presence of glutamate during excitatory synaptic transmission to cerebellar Purkinje cells. *Neuron* 1994; 12:1331–1343.

Barnett NL, Pow DV, Robinson SR. Inhibition of Muller cell glutamine synthetase rapidly impairs the retinal response to light. *Glia* 2000; 30:64–73.

Beattie EC, Stellwagen D, Morishita W, et al. Control of synaptic strength by glial TNFalpha. *Science* 2002; 295:2282–2285.

Bergles DE, Jahr CE. Synaptic activation of glutamate transporters in hippocampal astrocytes. *Neuron* 1997; 19:1297–1308.

Bergles DE, Jahr CE. Glial contribution to glutamate uptake at Schaffer collateral-commissural synapses in the hippocampus. *J Neurosci* 1998; 18:7709–7716.

Bergles DE, Dzubay JA, Jahr CE. Glutamate transporter currents in Bergmann glial cells follow the time course of extrasynaptic glutamate. *Proc Natl Acad Sci USA* 1997; 94:14821–14825.

Bezzi P, Domercq M, Vesce S, Volterra A. Neuron-astrocyte cross-talk during synaptic transmission: physiological and neuropathological implications. *Prog Brain Res* 2001; 132:255–265.

Bezzi P, Gundersen V, Galbete JL, et al. Astrocytes contain a vesicular compartment that is competent for regulated exocytosis of glutamate. *Nat Neurosci* 2004; 7:613–620.

Binder DK, Steinhauser C. Functional changes in astroglial cells in epilepsy. *Glia* 2006; 54:358–368.

Bingham S, Beswick PJ, Bountra C, et al. The cyclooxygenase-2 inhibitor GW406381X [2-(4-ethoxyphenyl)]-3-[4-(methylsulfonyl)phenyl]-pyrazolo[1,5-b]pyridazine] is effective in animal models of neuropathic pain and central sensitization. *J Pharmacol Exp Ther* 2005; 312:1161–1169.

Bowser DN, Khakh BS. ATP excites interneurons and astrocytes to increase synaptic inhibition in neuronal networks. *J Neurosci* 2004; 24:8606–8620.

Brambilla R, Bracchi-Ricard V, Hu WH, et al. Inhibition of astroglial nuclear factor kappaB reduces inflammation and improves functional recovery after spinal cord injury. *J Exp Med* 2005; 202:145–156.

Brenner M, Johnson AB, Boespflug-Tanguy O, et al. Mutations in GFAP, encoding glial fibrillary acidic protein, are associated with Alexander disease. *Nat Genet* 2001; 27:117–120.

Brockhaus J, Deitmer JW. Long-lasting modulation of synaptic input to Purkinje neurons by Bergmann glia stimulation in rat brain slices. *J Physiol* 2002; 545(Pt 2):581–593.

Bushong EA, Martone ME, Jones YZ, Ellisman MH. Protoplasmic astrocytes in CA1 stratum radiatum occupy separate anatomical domains. *J Neurosci* 2002; 22:183–192.

Cartier L, Hartley O, Dubois-Dauphin M, Krause KH. Chemokine receptors in the central nervous system: role in brain inflammation and neurodegenerative diseases. *Brain Res Brain Res Rev* 2005; 48:16–42.

Chen X, Wang L, Zhou Y, Zheng LH, Zhou Z. "Kiss-and-run" glutamate secretion in cultured and freshly isolated rat hippocampal astrocytes. *J Neurosci* 2005; 25:9236–9243.

Clark BA, Barbour B. Currents evoked in Bergmann glial cells by parallel fibre stimulation in rat cerebellar slices. *J Physiol(Lond)* 1997; 502:335–350.

Clark RB, Perkins JP. Regulation of adenosine 3':5'-cyclic monophosphate concentration in cultured human astrocytoma cells by catecholamines and histamine. *Proc Natl Acad Sci USA* 1971; 68:2757–2760.

Cornell-Bell AH, Finkbeiner SM, Cooper MS, Smith SJ. Glutamate induces calcium waves in cultured astrocytes: long-range glial signaling. *Science* 1990; 247:470–473.

Danbolt NC. Glutamate uptake. *Prog Neurobiol* 2001; 65:1–105.

Deshpande M, Zheng J, Borgmann K, et al. Role of activated astrocytes in neuronal damage: potential links to HIV-1-associated dementia. *Neurotox Res* 2005; 7:183–192.

Diamond JS, Bergles DE, Jahr CE. Glutamate release monitored with astrocyte transporter currents during LTP. *Neuron* 1998; 21:425–433.

Duan S, Anderson CM, Keung EC, Chen Y, Swanson RA. P2X7 receptor-mediated release of excitatory amino acids from astrocytes. *J Neurosci* 2003; 23:1320–1328.

Eggermont J, Trouet D, Carton I, Nilius B. Cellular function and control of volume-regulated anion channels. *Cell Biochem Biophys* 2001; 35:263–274.

Fellin T, Pascual O, Gobbo S, et al. Neuronal synchrony mediated by astrocytic glutamate through activation of extrasynaptic NMDA receptors. *Neuron* 2004; 43:729–743.

Fellin T, Pozzan T, Carmignoto G. Purinergic receptors mediate two distinct glutamate release pathways in hippocampal astrocytes. *J Biol Chem* 2006; 281:4274–4284.

Fiacco TA, McCarthy KD. Intracellular astrocyte calcium waves in situ increase the frequency of spontaneous AMPA receptor currents in CA1 pyramidal neurons. *J Neurosci* 2004; 24:722–732.

Furuta A, Martin LJ, Lin CLG, Dykes-Hoberg M, Rothstein JD. Cellular and synaptic localization of the neuronal glutamate transporters excitatory amino acid transporter 3 and 4. *Neuroscience* 1997a; 81:1031–1042.

Furuta A, Rothstein JD, Martin LJ. Glutamate transporter protein subtypes are expressed differentially during rat CNS development. *J Neurosci* 1997b; 17:8363–8375.

Gallagher CJ, Salter MW. Differential properties of astrocyte calcium waves mediated by P2Y1 and P2Y2 receptors. *J Neurosci* 2003; 23:6728–6739.

Gegelashvili G, Schousboe A. High affinity glutamate transporters: regulation of expression and activity. *Mol Pharmacol* 1997; 52:6–15.

Gilman AG, Nirenberg M. Regulation of adenosine 3',5'-cyclic monophosphate metabolism in cultured neuroblastoma cells. *Nature* 1971; 234:356–358.

Guthrie PB, Knappenberger J, Segal M, et al. ATP released from astrocytes mediates glial calcium waves. 1999; 19:520–528.

Gwak YS, Hulsebosch CE. Upregulation of Group I metabotropic glutamate receptors in neurons and astrocytes in the dorsal horn following spinal cord injury. *Exp Neurol* 2005; 195:236–243.

Hallermayer K, Harmening C, Hamprecht B. Cellular localization and regulation of glutamine synthetase in primary cultures of brain cells from newborn mice. *J Neurochem* 1981; 37:43–52.

Haydon PG. GLIA: listening and talking to the synapse. *Nat Rev Neurosci* 2001; 2:185–193.

Hertz L, Zielke HR. Astrocytic control of glutamatergic activity: astrocytes as stars of the show. *Trends Neurosci* 2004; 27:735–743.

Hertz L, Schousboe I, Schousboe A. Receptor expression in primary cultures of neurons or astrocytes. 1984; 8:521–527.

Hirase H, Qian L, Bartho P, Buzsaki G. Calcium dynamics of cortical astrocytic networks in vivo. *PLoS Biol* 2004; 2:E96.

Imitola J, Raddassi K, Park KI, et al. Directed migration of neural stem cells to sites of CNS injury by the stromal cell-derived factor 1alpha/CXC chemokine receptor 4 pathway. *Proc Natl Acad Sci USA* 2004; 101:18117–18122.

Kanai Y, Hediger MA. Primary structure and functional characterization of a high-affinity glutamate transporter. *Nature* 1992; 360:467–471.

Kang J, Jiang L, Goldman SA, Nedergaard M. Astrocyte-mediated potentiation of inhibitory synaptic transmission. *Nat Neurosci* 1998; 1:683–692.

Kimelberg HK, Goderie SK, Higman S, Pang S, Waniewski RA. Swelling-induced release of glutamate, aspartate, and taurine from astrocyte cultures. *J Neurosci* 1990; 10:1583–1591.

Kofuji P, Newman EA. Potassium buffering in the central nervous system. *Neuroscience* 2004; 129:1045–1056.

Kojima S, Nakamura T, Nidaira T, et al. Optical detection of synaptically induced glutamate transport in hippocampal slices. *J Neurosci* 1999; 19:2580–2588.

Konietzko U, Muller CM. Astrocytic dye coupling in rat hippocampus: topography, developmental onset, and modulation by protein kinase C. *Hippocampus* 1994; 4:297–306.

Kreft M, Stenovec M, Rupnik M, et al. Properties of Ca^{2+}-dependent exocytosis in cultured astrocytes. *Glia* 2004; 46:437–445.

Lee IH, Lindqvist E, Kiehn O, Widenfalk J, Olson L. Glial and neuronal connexin expression patterns in the rat spinal cord during development and following injury. *J Comp Neurol* 2005a; 489:1–10.

Lee J, Tommerdahl M, Favorov OV, Whitsel BL. Optically recorded response of the superficial dorsal horn: dissociation from neuronal activity, sensitivity to formalin-evoked skin nociceptor activation. *J Neurophysiol* 2005b; 94:852–864.

Lennon VA, Kryzer TJ, Pittock SJ, Verkman AS, Hinson SR. IgG marker of optic-spinal multiple sclerosis binds to the aquaporin-4 water channel. *J Exp Med* 2005; 202:473–477.

Levy LM, Lehre KP, Rolstad B, Danbolt NC. A monoclonal antibody raised against an [Na⁺⁺K⁺]coupled L-glutamate transporter purified from rat brain confirms glial cell localization. *FEBS Lett* 1993; 317:79–84.

Liu QS, Xu Q, Arcuino G, Kang J, Nedergaard M. Astrocyte-mediated activation of neuronal kainate receptors. *Proc Natl Acad Sci USA* 2004; 101:3172–3177.

Loo DT, Althoen MC, Cotman CW. Differentiation of serum-free mouse embryo cells into astrocytes is accompanied by induction of glutamine synthetase activity. *J Neurosci Res* 1995; 42:184–191.

Lugaro E. Sulle funzioni della nevroglia [On the functions of neuroglia]. *Riv Patol Nerv Ment* 1907; 12:225–233.

Marchand F, Perretti M, McMahon SB. Role of the immune system in chronic pain. *Nat Rev Neurosci* 2005; 6:521–532.

Marella M, Chabry J. Neurons and astrocytes respond to prion infection by inducing microglia recruitment. *J Neurosci* 2004; 24:620–627.

McCarthy KD, de Vellis J. Alpha-adrenergic receptor modulation of beta-adrenergic, adenosine and prostaglandin E1 increased adenosine 3':5'-cyclic monophosphate levels in primary cultures of glia. *J Cyclic Nucleotide Res* 1978; 4:15–26.

McCarthy KD, de Vellis J. Preparation of separate astroglial and oligodendroglial cell cultures from rat cerebral tissue. *J Cell Biol* 1980; 85:890–902.

McCarthy KD, Salm AK. Pharmacologically-distinct subsets of astroglia can be identified by their calcium response to neuroligands. *Neuroscience* 1991; 41:325–333.

McMahon SB, Cafferty WB, Marchand F. Immune and glial cell factors as pain mediators and modulators. *Exp Neurol* 2005; 192:444–462.

Mennerick S, Zorumski CF. Glial contributions to excitatory neurotransmission in cultured hippocampal cells. 1994; 368:59–62.

Miller G. Neuroscience. The dark side of glia. *Science* 2005; 308:778–781.

Miller RF. D-Serine as a glial modulator of nerve cells. *Glia* 2004; 47:275–283.

Milligan ED, Twining C, Chacur M, et al. Spinal glia and proinflammatory cytokines mediate mirror-image neuropathic pain in rats. *J Neurosci* 2003; 23:1026–1040.

Monnerie H, Esquenazi S, Shashidhara S, Le Roux PD. Beta-amyloid-induced reactive astrocytes display altered ability to support dendrite and axon growth from mouse cerebral cortical neurons in vitro. *Neurol Res* 2005; 27:525–532.

Montana V, Ni Y, Sunjara V, Hua X, Parpura V. Vesicular glutamate transporter-dependent glutamate release from astrocytes. *J Neurosci* 2004; 24:2633–2642.

Murphy S, Pearce B. Functional receptors for neurotransmitters on astroglial cells. 1987; 22:381–394.

Nakagawa T, Yabe T, Schwartz JP. Gene expression profiles of reactive astrocytes cultured from dopamine-depleted striatum. *Neurobiol Dis* 2005; 20:275–282.

Nett WJ, Oloff SH, McCarthy KD. Hippocampal astrocytes in situ exhibit calcium oscillations that occur independent of neuronal activity. *J Neurophysiol* 2002; 87:528–537.

Newman EA. Glial cell inhibition of neurons by release of ATP. *J Neurosci* 2003; 23:1659–1666.

Newman EA, Zahs KR. Modulation of neuronal activity by glial cells in the retina. *J Neurosci* 1998; 18:4022–4028.

Nimmerjahn A, Kirchhoff F, Kerr JN, Helmchen F. Sulforhodamine 101 as a specific marker of astroglia in the neocortex in vivo. *Nat Methods* 2004; 1:31–37.

O'Connor ER, Sontheimer H, Ransom BR. Rat hippocampal astrocytes exhibit electrogenic sodium-bicarbonate co-transport. *J Neurophysiol* 1994; 72:2580–2589.

Okuno T, Nakatsuji Y, Kumanogoh A, et al. Induction of cyclooxygenase-2 in reactive glial cells by the CD40 pathway: relevance to amyotrophic lateral sclerosis. *J Neurochem* 2004; 91:404–412.

Parpura V, Basarsky TA, Liu F, et al. Glutamate-mediated astrocyte-neuron signalling. *Nature* 1994a; 369:744–747.

Parpura V, Scemes E, Spray DC. Mechanisms of glutamate release from astrocytes: gap junction "hemichannels", puringeric receptors and exocytotic release. *Neurochem Int* 2004b; 45:259–264.

Parri HR, Crunelli V. Pacemaker calcium oscillations in thalamic astrocytes in situ. *Neuroreport* 2001; 12:3897–3900.

Parri HR, Gould TM, Crunelli V. Spontaneous astrocytic Ca^{2+} oscillations in situ drive NMDAR-mediated neuronal excitation. *Nat Neurosci* 2001; 4:803–812.

Pascual O, Casper KB, Kubera C, et al. Astrocytic purinergic signaling coordinates synaptic networks. *Science* 2005; 310:113–116.

Pasti L, Volterra A, Pozzan T, Carmignoto G. Intracellular calcium oscillations in astrocytes: a highly plastic, bidirectional form of communication between neurons and astrocytes in situ. *J Neurosci* 1997; 17:7817–7830.

Pekny M, Nilsson M. Astrocyte activation and reactive gliosis. *Glia* 2005; 50:427–434.

Perea G, Araque A. Glial calcium signaling and neuron-glia communication. *Cell Calcium* 2005a; 38:375–382.

Perea G, Araque A. Properties of synaptically evoked astrocyte calcium signal reveal synaptic information processing by astrocytes. *J Neurosci* 2005b; 25:2192–2203.

Piao CS, Yu YM, Han PL, Lee JK. Dynamic expression of p38beta MAPK in neurons and astrocytes after transient focal ischemia. *Brain Res* 2003; 976:120–124.

Pignataro L, Sitaramayya A, Finnemann SC, Sarthy VP. Nonsynaptic localization of the excitatory amino acid transporter 4 in photoreceptors. *Mol Cell Neurosci* 2005; 28:440–451.

Plant SR, Arnett HA, Ting JP. Astroglial-derived lymphotoxin-alpha exacerbates inflammation and demyelination, but not remyelination. *Glia* 2005; 49:1–14.

Porter JT, McCarthy KD. Astrocytic neurotransmitter receptors in situ and in vivo. *Prog Neurobiol* 1997; 51:439–455.

Raghavendra V, Tanga FY, DeLeo JA. Complete Freund's adjuvant-induced peripheral inflammation evokes glial activation and proinflammatory cytokine expression in the CNS. *Eur J Neurosci* 2004; 20:467–473.

Roeder LM, Hopkins IB, Kaiser JR, Hanukoglu L, Tildon JT. Thyroid hormone action on glucose transporter activity in astrocytes. *Biochem Biophys Res Commun* 1988; 156:275–281.

Rossi DJ, Oshima T, Attwell D. Glutamate release in severe brain ischaemia is mainly by reversed uptake. *Nature* 2000; 403:316–321.

Rossner S. New players in old amyloid precursor protein-processing pathways. *Int J Dev Neurosci* 2004; 22(7):467–474.

Rothstein JD, Dykes-Hoberg M, Pardo CA, et al. Knockout of glutamate transporters reveals a major role for astroglial transport in excitotoxicity and clearance of glutamate. 1996; 16:675–686.

Saez TE, Pehar M, Vargas M, Barbeito L, Maccioni RB. Astrocytic nitric oxide triggers tau hyperphosphorylation in hippocampal neurons. *In Vivo* 2004; 18:275–280.

Salm AK, McCarthy KD. Expression of beta-adrenergic receptors by astrocytes isolated from adult rat cortex. *Glia* 1989; 2:346–352.

Scemes E. Components of astrocytic intercellular calcium signaling. *Mol Neurobiol* 2000; 22:167–179.

Schultz J, Schwarz A, Neidhold S, et al. Role of interleukin-1 in prion disease-associated astrocyte activation. *Am J Pathol* 2004; 165:671–678.

Seifert G, Steinhauser C. Ionotropic glutamate receptors in astrocytes. *Prog Brain Res* 2001; 132:287–299.

Shao Y, McCarthy KD. Heterogeneity of receptor mediated responses within clones of type 1 astroglia. *Soc Neurosci Abstr* 1991; 17:56.

Somjen GG. Nervenkitt: notes on the history of the concept of neuroglia. *Glia* 1988; 1:2–9.

Spataro LE, Sloane EM, Milligan ED, et al. Spinal gap junctions: potential involvement in pain facilitation. *J Pain* 2004; 5:392–405.

Speciale C, Hares K, Schwarcz R, Brookes N. High-affinity uptake of L-kynurenine by a Na^+-independent transporter of neutral amino acids in astrocytes. *J Neurosci* 1989; 9:2066–2072.

Stevens ER, Esguerra M, Kim PM, et al. D-serine and serine racemase are present in the vertebrate retina and contribute to the physiological activation of NMDA receptors. *Proc Natl Acad Sci USA* 2003; 100:6789–6794.

Sutin J, Shao Y. Resting and reactive astrocytes express adrenergic receptors in the adult rat brain. *Brain Res Bull* 1992; 29:277–284.

Sweitzer SM, Colburn RW, Rutkowski M, DeLeo JA. Acute peripheral inflammation induces moderate glial activation and spinal IL-1beta expression that correlates with pain behavior in the rat. *Brain Res* 1999; 829:209–221.

Tanaka K, Watase K, Manabe T, et al. Epilepsy and exacerbation of brain injury in mice lacking the glutamate transporter GLT-1. *Science* 1997; 276:1699–1702.

Teismann P, Schulz JB. Cellular pathology of Parkinson's disease: astrocytes, microglia and inflammation. *Cell Tissue Res* 2004; 318:149–161.

Tian GF, Azmi H, Takano T, et al. An astrocytic basis of epilepsy. *Nat Med* 2005; 11:973–981.

Tong G, Jahr CE. Block of glutamate transporters potentiates postsynaptic excitation. *Neuron* 1994; 13:1195–1203.

Tsai HH, Frost E, To V, et al. The chemokine receptor CXCR2 controls positioning of oligodendrocyte precursors in developing spinal cord by arresting their migration. *Cell* 2002; 110:373–383.

Turecek R, Trussell LO. Control of synaptic depression by glutamate transporters. *J Neurosci* 2000; 20:2054–2063.

Tzeng SF, Hsiao HY, Mak OT. Prostaglandins and cyclooxygenases in glial cells during brain inflammation. *Curr Drug Targets Inflamm Allergy* 2005; 4:335–340.

Van Calker D, Muller M, Hamprecht B. Adrenergic alpha- and beta-receptors expressed by the same cell type in primary culture of perinatal mouse brain. *J Neurochem* 1978; 30:713–718.

Verkhratsky A, Steinhauser C. Ion channels in glial cells. *Brain Res Brain Res Rev* 2000; 32:380–412.

Volterra A, Meldolesi J. Astrocytes, from brain glue to communication elements: the revolution continues. *Nat Rev Neurosci* 2005; 6:626–640.

Volterra A, Steinhauser C. Glial modulation of synaptic transmission in the hippocampus. *Glia* 2004; 47:249–257.

Wang X, Lou N, Xu Q, et al. Astrocytic Ca^{2+} signaling evoked by sensory stimulation in vivo. *Nat Neurosci* 2006; 9:816–823.

Watase K, Hashimoto K, Kano M, et al. Motor discoordination and increased susceptibility to cerebellar injury in GLAST mutant mice. *Eur J Neurosci* 1998; 10:976–988.

Watkins LR, Maier SF. Glia: a novel drug discovery target for clinical pain. *Nat Rev Drug Discov* 2003; 2:973–985.

Watkins LR, Milligan ED, Maier SF. Glial proinflammatory cytokines mediate exaggerated pain states: implications for clinical pain. *Adv Exp Med Biol* 2003; 521:1–21.

Wieseler-Frank J, Maier SF, Watkins LR. Glial activation and pathological pain. *Neurochem Int* 2004; 45:389–395.

Woolf CJ, Salter MW. Neuronal plasticity: increasing the gain in pain. *Science* 2000; 288:1765–1769.

Yaksh TL, Dirig DM, Conway CM, et al. The acute antihyperalgesic action of nonsteroidal, anti-inflammatory drugs and release of spinal prostaglandin E$_2$ is mediated by the inhibition of constitutive spinal cyclooxygenase-2 (COX-2) but not COX-1. *J Neurosci* 2001; 21:5847–5853.

Yamada K, Watanabe M, Shibata T, et al. EAAT4 is a post-synaptic glutamate transporter at Purkinje cell synapses. *Neuroreport* 1996; 7:2013–2017.

Yang Y, Ge W, Chen Y, et al. Contribution of astrocytes to hippocampal long-term potentiation through release of D-serine. *Proc Natl Acad Sci USA* 2003; 100:15194–15199.

Ye ZC, Wyeth MS, Baltan-Tekkok S, Ransom BR. Functional hemichannels in astrocytes: a novel mechanism of glutamate release. *J Neurosci* 2003; 23:3588–3596.

Yeo JF, Ong WY, Ling SF, Farooqui AA. Intracerebroventricular injection of phospholipases A2 inhibitors modulates allodynia after facial carrageenan injection in mice. *Pain* 2004; 112:148–155.

Zhang JM, Wang HK, Ye CQ, et al. ATP released by astrocytes mediates glutamatergic activity-dependent heterosynaptic suppression. *Neuron* 2003; 40:971–982.

Zhang Z, Trautmann K, Schluesener HJ. Spinal cord glia activation following peripheral polyinosine-polycytidylic acid administration. *Neuroreport* 2005; 16:1495–1499.

Zhuang ZY, Gerner P, Woolf CJ, Ji RR. ERK is sequentially activated in neurons, microglia, and astrocytes by spinal nerve ligation and contributes to mechanical allodynia in this neuropathic pain model. *Pain* 2005; 114:149–159.

Zhuang ZY, Wen YR, Zhang DR, et al. A peptide c-Jun N-terminal kinase (JNK) inhibitor blocks mechanical allodynia after spinal nerve ligation: respective roles of JNK activation in primary sensory neurons and spinal astrocytes for neuropathic pain development and maintenance. *J Neurosci* 2006; 26:3551–3560.

Correspondence to: Ken D. McCarthy, PhD, Department of Pharmacology, University of North Carolina at Chapel Hill, Chapel Hill, NC 27599-7365, USA. Email: kdmc@med.unc.edu.

Part V

Glial-Pain Interactions: Spinal Cord and Brain

Immune and Glial Regulation of Pain, edited by Joyce
A. DeLeo, Linda S. Sorkin, and Linda R. Watkins,
IASP Press, Seattle, © 2007.

14

Steroid Hormone Regulation of Astrocyte Function: Implications for Central Nervous System Sensitization

Michael L. LaCroix-Fralish[a] and Joyce A. DeLeo[a,b]

[a]Department of Pharmacology and Toxicology, Dartmouth College, Hanover, New Hampshire, USA; [b]Departments of Anesthesiology and Pharmacology, Dartmouth-Hitchcock Medical Center, Lebanon, New Hampshire, USA

Steroid hormones are classically defined as a family of structurally related molecules produced by peripheral glands (testes, ovaries, and adrenals) that act through intracellular receptors to regulate specific gene expression in their target tissues. Recent studies of the central nervous system (CNS) have elucidated further complexities of this classical view. Steroids have been shown to have rapid effects on neuronal activity, consistent with a nongenomic, membrane-associated receptor-signaling mechanism (Schumacher 1990). Furthermore, the CNS is not only a key target tissue of steroids, but also an active site of steroid synthesis (Schlinger and Arnold 1991; Koenig et al. 1995) and steroid metabolism (Melcangi et al. 1999; Zwain and Yen 1999b). Indeed, mounting evidence suggests that the CNS itself may be an endocrine organ.

An interesting phenomenon in pain research has been the observation that significant differences exist between men and women in terms of pain sensitivity and incidence of chronic pain syndromes. Women typically have lower pain thresholds, resulting in higher pain ratings to constant stimuli, and have less tolerance to noxious stimuli than males (Berkley 1997). Furthermore, several chronic pain syndromes including fibromyalgia, rheumatoid arthritis, irritable bowel syndrome, and temporomandibular disorder have significant gender differences in clinical incidence, affecting primarily women (Yunus 2002). The symptoms can also be significantly different between men and women. Many studies have focused on the pivotal role of steroid hormones in the modulation of sensory systems and nociception in order to understand their role in mediating sex differences in pain (Fillingim and Ness 2000; Aloisi 2003; Blackburn-Munro and Blackburn-Munro 2003; LaCroix-Fralish et al. 2005, 2006a).

Our emerging understanding of the dynamic relationship between astrocytes and neurons at the level of the synapse suggests that steroid hormones acting on astrocytes may have important functional consequences for glial-neuronal communication and synaptic plasticity. Astrocytes express the entire repertoire of steroid hormone receptors (Kumar and deVillis 1988; Jung-Testas et al. 1992; Azcoitia et al. 1999; Finley and Kritzer 1999; Labombarda et al. 2000) and respond to a variety of steroid molecules in dynamic ways. For a diverse number of different processes in the CNS, it appears that astrocytes may be the direct targets of steroid hormones (Garcia-Ovejero et al. 2002). It follows that steroid hormones may regulate neurotransmission indirectly by acting on astrocytes to alter the expression of astrocyte-derived signaling molecules.

Steroid hormones encode the information of the hypothalamic-pituitary-gonadal (HPG) axis and the hypothalamic-pituitary-adrenal (HPA) axis controlling the reproductive and stress responses, respectively. Thus, steroids acting on the neurons and astrocytes that constitute the nociceptive axis may serve to integrate reproductive and stress-related information with nociceptive information, and this integration may give rise to the complex pain "experience" of the individual. This chapter provides an overview of the emerging evidence that suggests that steroid molecules may be important modulators of nociception by their myriad actions on astrocytes of the CNS.

EFFECTS OF GONADAL STEROIDS ON ASTROCYTES

The primary steroid hormone molecules produced by the ovaries and testes are broadly classified as the gonadal steroids. The ovarian hormones include the estrogens and progestins, while the testes principally produce the androgen steroids, testosterone and dihydrotestosterone. These gonadal steroids have been extensively studied for their role in modulating nociception in both humans and rodents (Riley et al. 1998; Fillingim and Ness 2000; Craft et al. 2004). The reported effects of gonadal hormones on nociceptive behaviors are robust, myriad, and seemingly contradictory. Whether gonadal hormones act as pro- or antinociceptive modulatory molecules appears to be highly dependent on the particular gonadal steroid in question, the dose or concentration, the duration and timing of exposure, the nociceptive stimuli applied, and the sex and genetic background of the animal. Despite these numerous nuances, several unifying concepts have emerged from the body of research examining the role of gonadal steroids in pain. First, gonadal steroids are generally neuroprotective and anti-inflammatory (Lee and McEwen 2001; Dhandapani and Brann 2002). Second, they modulate neurotransmission and synaptic plasticity in many different brain regions (Bicknell 1998). Third, gonadal steroids modulate nociceptive behavior in both rodents and humans, and these effects are sufficiently robust to be of consequence clinically (Aloisi and Bonifazi 2006).

An emerging topic that further complicates the issue of gonadal steroid action concerns the principal cell type in which these molecules exert their cellular action. It has only recently been appreciated that not only do glial cells (particularly astrocytes) possess gonadal steroid receptors, but steroid hormones can also have profound effects on cellular functions in these cells. The following are a few selected vignettes of how gonadal steroids acting on astrocytes can modulate pain-relevant processes.

GONADAL STEROID REGULATION OF GFAP EXPRESSION

It is hypothesized that astrocytes within the CNS are capable of maintaining a chronic pain state by becoming "activated" in response to peripheral or central injury or inflammation and that, in doing so, they alter neuronal excitability. This astrocytic activation includes a host of structural changes in these cells including hypertrophy, upregulation of intermediate filament proteins, and changes in morphology. Correspondingly, astrocytes also undergo significant alterations in cellular function and gene expression, including the upregulation of proinflammatory cytokines and growth factors and increased production of reactive oxygen species (Ridet et al. 1997). One particular intermediate filament protein, glial fibrillary acidic protein (GFAP), has long been recognized to be a selective marker of mature, differentiated astrocytes in the CNS (Eng 1985). Although not all astrocytes express GFAP, the vast majority of studies to date have focused on changes in GFAP immunoreactivity as an indicator of astrocytic activation.

The finding that gonadal steroids can alter the expression of GFAP in many different regions of the brain has led to the speculation that these steroids are capable of modulating astrocytic plasticity in significant ways. It has been observed that astrocyte morphology and function are modulated by fluctuations in gonadal steroid levels in the normal brain (Garcia-Segura et al. 1989; Chowen et al. 1995; Rasia-Filho et al. 2002; Conejo et al. 2005). Furthermore, it has been demonstrated that testosterone, progesterone, and 17β-estradiol treatment all decreased the number of hypertrophic, reactive GFAP-positive astrocytes adjacent to the site of injury following a cortical stab wound (Garcia-Estrada et al. 1993). Likewise, testosterone has been shown to attenuate the upregulation of GFAP mRNA and protein in the hamster facial motor nucleus following facial nerve transection (Jones et al. 1997; Coers et al. 2002). These findings suggest that gonadal hormones may decrease the morphological changes associated with astrocyte activation in response to nerve injury and that they may thus play an important regulatory role in modulating glially maintained chronic pain states.

GONADAL STEROID REGULATION OF GROWTH
FACTOR PRODUCTION IN ASTROCYTES

A growing body of evidence suggests that growth factors and neurotrophic factors in the CNS can act as algogenic mediators in chronic pain states. In particular, evidence is strong that the neurotrophins nerve growth factor (NGF) and brain-derived neurotrophic factor (BDNF) upregulate nociceptor gene expression in sensory neurons throughout the nociceptive axis (Pezet and McMahon 2006). Other growth factors that have been demonstrated to increase pain-related behaviors in various animal models of pain include acidic and basic fibroblast growth factor (aFGF and bFGF) (Ji et al. 1996), neuregulin-1-β1 (LaCroix-Fralish et al. 2007), and interleukin-6 (DeLeo et al. 1996). Conversely, exogenous administration of glial-cell-line-derived neurotrophic factor (GDNF) decreased pain-related behaviors in a neuropathic pain model (Boucher et al. 2000). Astrocytes appear to play a key role in the production and secretion of these growth factors and have been demonstrated to increase their expression of several of these factors after becoming activated in response to CNS injury (Ridet et al. 1997). The production of these factors by astrocytes appears to serve a dual purpose: to protect injured neurons from apoptosis by positively modulating the local trophic environment as well as to upregulate molecular components of nociceptive systems, leading to heightened responses to somatic stimuli. In this manner, increased local production of growth factors by astrocytes can simultaneously have a beneficial and detrimental function in chronic pain states.

The gonadal steroids are potent regulators of neurotrophins and associated neurotrophin receptor expression in the normal CNS. Several studies have demonstrated regulation of NGF and BDNF mRNA and protein expression in a number of different brain regions by 17β-estradiol and progesterone (Pan et al. 1999; Bimonte-Nelson et al. 2004) and in sensory neurons in the dorsal root ganglion (DRG) (Sohrabji et al. 1994). High-dose testosterone treatment in male rats also increased NGF protein expression in various regions of the brain (Tirassa et al. 1997).

It has also been demonstrated that these increases in neurotrophin expression by gonadal steroids are relevant for CNS disease. Progesterone increased the expression of BDNF mRNA and protein following spinal cord injury (Gonzalez et al. 2004; De Nicola et al. 2006). Similarly, spinal BDNF expression was enhanced by 17β-estradiol treatment, and this increase potentiated sensitivity to thermal stimuli after sciatic nerve chronic constriction injury (Zhao et al. 2003). Both 17β-estradiol and progesterone increased the expression of two neurotrophin receptors, tyrosine kinase A (trkA) and p75NTR, in DRG neurons (Lanlua et al. 2001). Following sciatic nerve axotomy, 17β-estradiol reversed injury-mediated decreases in trkA-receptor expression in DRG neurons. Likewise, progesterone treatment increased trkB-receptor immunoreactivity after spinal cord injury (De Nicola et al. 2006).

Similar effects of gonadal steroid regulation have been observed with other growth factors. First, 17β-estradiol increases GDNF expression in the brain (Ivanova et al. 2002), and this increase in GDNF expression has been shown to be neuroprotective and astrocyte-derived (Platania et al. 2005). It has also been shown that 17β-estradiol increases the expression and secretion of transforming growth factor-β in astrocytes and that this increase may be partially responsible for the neuroprotective effects of 17β-estradiol in the CNS (Dhandapani et al. 2005). Finally, it has been demonstrated that gonadal hormone status regulates the expression of astrocytic bFGF following 5-hydroxydopamine lesion in the brain (Moroz et al. 2003). These findings highlight the depth of gonadal steroid regulation on growth factor expression and demonstrate the possible ways in which astrocytic-derived growth factors can modulate CNS disease, including pathological pain.

PROGESTERONE-SPECIFIC REGULATION OF NEUREGULIN-1 IN ASTROCYTES

The neuregulin-1 family of growth factors has a variety of modulatory functions in the CNS (Buonanno and Fischbach 2001; Ozaki 2001; Murphy et al. 2002; Falls 2003). Neuregulin-1 protein is expressed and secreted by both neurons and astrocytes. Binding of neuregulin-1 ligand to the receptor tyrosine kinases ErbB3 and ErbB4 results in a signal transduction cascade that has numerous effects on CNS processes, including modulation of synaptic activity and synaptogenesis (Ozaki et al. 1997, 2000; Wolpowitz et al. 2000). Our laboratory has observed a sex difference in the expression of the neuregulin-1 gene and the high-affinity neuregulin-1 receptor, ErbB4, in the lumbar spinal cord of hormonally intact female rats following nerve root injury (LaCroix-Fralish et al. 2006b). Follow-up studies have demonstrated that an increase in neuregulin-1 mRNA and protein expression after nerve root injury is facilitated specifically by progesterone and not by 17β-estradiol. Furthermore, intrathecal injection of recombinant neuregulin-1 protein causes behavioral hypersensitivity in female rats (LaCroix-Fralish et al. 2007). Finally, we have observed that progesterone specifically increases the expression of neuregulin-1 in primary astrocytes, but not in neurons in vitro (see Fig. 1). These studies highlight an emerging role for progesterone-specific regulation of astrocyte-derived neuregulin-1 in modulating nociception in a sex-specific manner.

A.

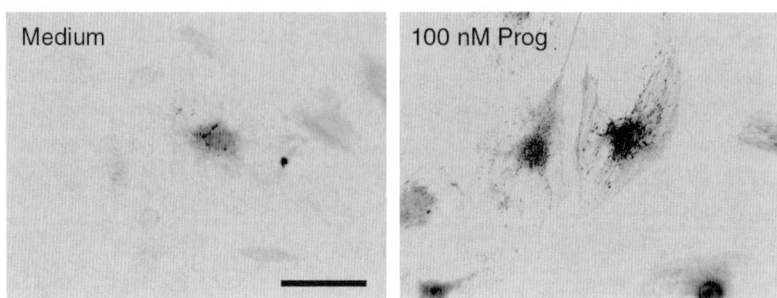

B.

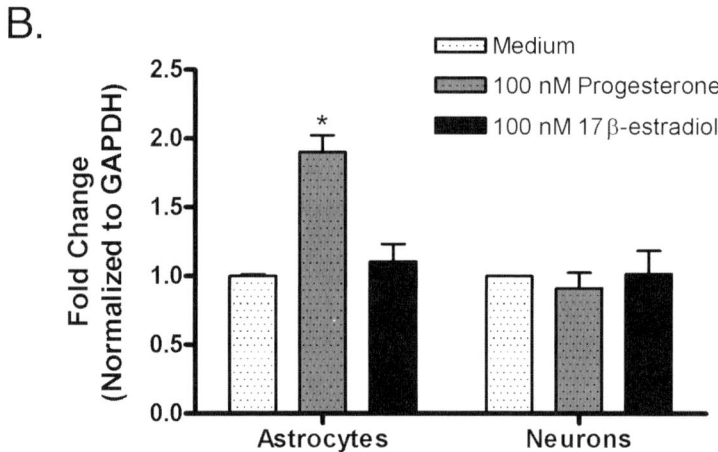

Fig. 1. (A) Immunocytochemical staining for intracellular neuregulin-1 protein expression in primary rat astrocytes treated with medium alone (Medium) or 100 nM of progesterone (100 nM Prog) for 6 hours. Scale bar = 30 μm. (B) Real-time RT-PCR analysis of neuregulin-1 mRNA expression in primary rat astrocytes and neurons treated with medium alone, 100 nM progesterone, or 100 nM 17β-estradiol for 6 hours. An asterisk (*) indicates a significant increase in neuregulin-1 expression ($P < 0.05$). GAPDH = glyceraldehyde 3-phosphate dehydrogenase.

GONADAL STEROID REGULATION
OF GLUTAMATE TRANSPORTERS

L-glutamate is the major excitatory neurotransmitter in the CNS and is absolutely critical for most functions in the CNS, including nociception. However, L-glutamate concentrations must also be tightly regulated in the CNS in order to prevent not only aberrant neurotransmission but also neurotoxic overstimulation of postsynaptic neurons, known as excitotoxicity. Astrocytes are responsible for the removal and metabolism of L-glutamate from the extrasynaptic space, predominantly through two high-affinity astrocyte glutamate transporters called GLT-1 and GLAST (Danbolt 2001). Mounting evidence indicates that potentiation of glutamatergic neurotransmission in chronic pain states may be mediated by decreases in astrocyte glutamate transporter activity or expression following nerve injury, resulting in a loss of the critical regulation of extrasynaptic L-glutamate concentrations (Sung et al. 2003; Binns et al. 2005; Weng et al. 2005).

Several studies have examined the role of gonadal steroids in regulating astrocytic glutamate transporter. For example, 17β-estradiol increased GLT-1 and GLAST expression in cultured astrocytes derived from brain tissue from Alzheimer's disease patients (Liang et al. 2002). Similarly, increases in GLT-1 and GLAST expression, along with subsequent increases in the uptake of extracellular L-glutamate, were demonstrated in cultured mouse astrocytes following treatment with nanomolar concentrations of 17β-estradiol (Pawlak et al. 2005). This effect was blocked by administration of a selective estrogen receptor antagonist, indicating a genomic action for the increased expression and activity of these glutamate transporters. Examination of L-glutamate transporter kinetics in cortical synaptosomes derived from female rats at various points of the estrous cycle demonstrated a significant effect of endogenous gonadal steroids in regulating glutamate transport in vivo (Mitrovic et al. 1999). Furthermore, L-glutamate transporter kinetics in females was significantly higher than L-glutamate transporter kinetics in male rats, depending on the stage of the estrous cycle in the female rats. These observations demonstrate that gonadal steroids are capable of regulating astrocytic glutamate transporter expression and activity and that this regulation may be relevant for modulation of nociception in chronic pain states.

NEUROSTEROID SYNTHESIS AND STEROID-CONVERTING ENZYMES IN ASTROCYTES

Steroids produced endogenously by the CNS or metabolized from circulating precursor steroids have been termed "neurosteroids" and are found in the CNS at concentrations considerable higher than (Baulieu and Robel 1990) and independent from those produced in the peripheral endocrine organs (Baulieu 1997). There is compelling evidence for de novo synthesis of the classical gonadal steroids (17β-estradiol, progesterone, and testosterone) by the conversion of cholesterol into pregnenolone precursor molecules by mitochondrial enzymes (Hu et al. 1987). Moreover, the brain can modify and metabolize many different steroid substrates through a host of enzyme systems. These enzymatic activities can drastically alter the effect of a given gonadal steroid. For example, testosterone can be aromatized to 17β-estradiol in a single step by the enzyme P450 aromatase, thus decreasing the activity of testosterone signaling. Conversely, testosterone can be modified to dihydrotestosterone by the enzyme 5α-reductase, which potently enhances the actions of testosterone (Melcangi et al. 1999). With this new understanding, we cannot view the actions of gonadal steroids on CNS function without investigating the possible involvement of secondary metabolites in mediating the observed effect of these steroids, particularly in vivo.

Glial cells, principally astrocytes, are a rich source of both gonadal steroid-converting enzymes and de novo neurosteroidogenesis (see Fig. 2). There is good evidence for the expression of all of the critical biosynthetic steroid-converting enzymes in astrocytes, including cholesterol side-chain cleavage cytochrome P450 (P450scc; Mellon and Deschepper 1993), P450c17 (Zwain and Yen 1999a), 5α-reductase (Melcangi et al. 1990), 3β- and 17β-hydroxysteroid dehydrogenase (Zwain and Yen 1999b), and P450 aromatase (Cesi et al. 1993). Furthermore, the functional activity of these enzymes has been demonstrated in cultured primary astrocytes treated with a variety of steroid molecule precursors (Zwain and Yen 1999b). Indeed, it appears that astrocytes are the most steroidogenic cells in the brain because they express more of the different steroidogenic enzymes than either neurons or oligodendrocytes in culture. The significance of all of these molecules, beyond being simply precursors to neurosteroids, is

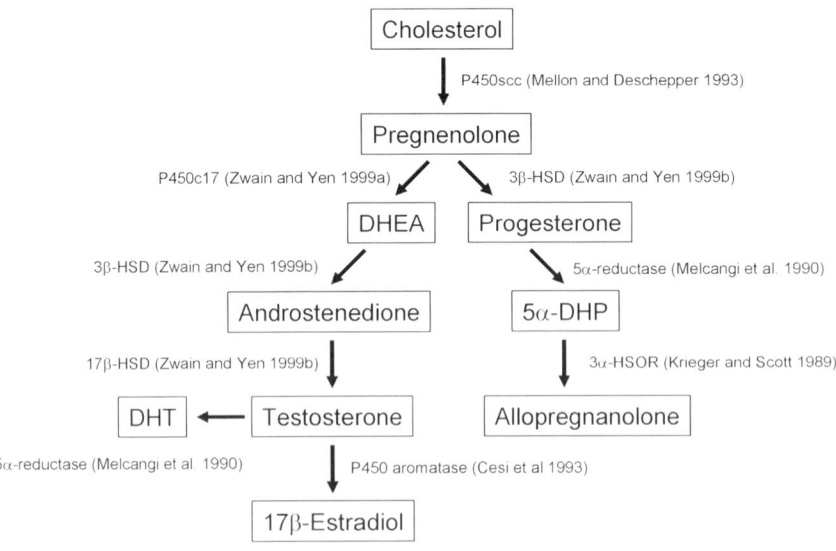

Fig. 2. Gonadal steroid synthesis pathways and key steroid-converting enzymes that are expressed in astrocytes. DHEA = dehydroepiandrosterone, 3β-HSD = 3β-hydroxysteroid dehydrogenase, 17β-HSD = 17β-hydroxysteroid dehydrogenase, 5α-DHP = 5α-dihydroprogesterone, 3α-HSOR = 3α-hydroxysteroid oxidoreductase, DHT = dihydrotestosterone.

still an area of much interest. Clearly, these lipophilic molecules are capable of passive membrane diffusion and thus may act as local glial-neuronal signaling molecules. In the presence of neurons, the activity of 5α-reductase is significantly increased in neighboring astrocytes (Melcangi et al. 1994). Several of these astrocyte-derived neurosteroids have also been demonstrated to be allosteric modulators of *N*-methyl-ᴅ-aspartate and gamma-aminobutyric acid A (GABA$_A$) receptors, resulting in modulation of excitatory and inhibitory neurotransmission, depending on the specific neurosteroid (Garcia-Ovejero et al. 2005; Schlichter et al. 2006).

A variety of neurosteroids have modulatory functions on nociceptive systems and play a modulatory role in a variety of pain models and experimental nociceptive stimuli. The key steroidogenic enzymes are localized to the superficial laminae of the dorsal horn in both astrocytes and neurons (Patte-Mensah et al. 2003). As previously discussed, the production and secretion of cytokines and growth factors have been implicated in the initiation and maintenance of chronic pain states. The neurosteroid dehydroepiandrosterone (DHEA) inhibited the expression of tumor necrosis factor-α and interleukin-6 in astrocytes following experimental autoimmune encephalomyelitis (Kipper-Galperin et al. 1999). A recent study has shown that the algogenic mediator, substance P, inhibits the conversion of progesterone to 5α-dihydroprogesterone (5α-DHP) (Patte-Mensah et al. 2005). Given that 5α-DHP has previously been shown to be a positive modulator of GABA$_A$-receptor activity, inactivation of its production could be involved in a shift in the inhibitory/excitatory balance in the spinal cord during chronic pain states. Inhibition of the P450 aromatase enzyme responsible for the conversion of testosterone to 17β-estradiol increased the withdrawal latency to a noxious thermal stimulus, implicating a role for endogenous, local production of spinal cord 17β-estradiol in the sensitization of sensory neurons in a rapid manner (Evrard and Balthazart 2004). Finally, a robust increase in the expression of P450scc was observed following sciatic nerve ligation, along with a corresponding increase in the production of pregnenolone and allopregnanolone, which are also potent positive modulators of GABA$_A$ receptor activity (Patte-Mensah et al. 2004). These series of studies have just begun to examine the role of neurosteroid production in modulating nociception in chronic neuropathic pain states. As we begin to understand the regulation of these different steroidogenic enzymes and the myriad neurosteroids produced by these enzymes, we will uncover a signaling network that may prove to be critically involved in the pathogenesis of chronic pain states and may represent novel therapeutic avenues for the treatment of painful diseases.

GLUCOCORTICOIDS

It is well known that chronic stress is a strong modulator of nociception. In rodents, exposure to a strong stressor increases behavioral responses to a variety of nociceptive stimuli (Gameiro et al. 2005; Boccalon et al. 2006; Imbe et al. 2006), and stress worsens pain perception in chronic pain patients (Schwartz et al. 1994; Ashkinazi and Vershinina 1999; Davis et al. 2001; Logan et al. 2001; Gil et al. 2003). These stress responses are largely mediated by circulating levels of corticosteroids, which are produced within the adrenal cortex and mediate a host of anti-inflammatory and immunosuppressive actions in the body. Corticosteroids exert their activities by binding to two distinct nuclear hormone receptors, the glucocorticoid receptor and the mineralocorticoid receptor. It has been demonstrated that glucocorticoid receptors are distributed throughout the peripheral and central nervous systems, and recent evidence has shown that glucocorticoid action in both of these compartments has significant modulatory activity on pain facilitation. Central glucocorticoid receptor activation results in plastic changes in neuronal activity related to nerve injury that is abolished by blocking glucocorticoid receptors (Cameron and Dutia 1999). Indeed, several studies found that central glucocorticoid receptor activation was partly responsible for mediating pain behaviors following peripheral nerve injury in rats (Wang et al. 2004, 2005).

Astrocytes express glucocorticoid receptors in a variety of CNS regions and appear to be major targets for glucocorticoid-mediated gene expression in the nervous system (Vielkind et al. 1990). Glucocorticoids regulate a significant number of important astrocyte genes discussed previously in this chapter, including GFAP (O'Callaghan et al. 1991; Maurel et al. 2000), NGF (Niu et al. 1997; Chang et al. 2005), and bFGF and glutamine synthase (Vardimon et al. 1999). Furthermore, a host of other unidentified mRNA transcripts were shown to be specifically regulated in astrocytes by glucocorticoids (O'Banion et al. 1994). These studies highlight the extensive regulation of gene expression in astrocytes by glucocorticoids and suggest that elevated levels of glucocorticoids, as occurs during stress, may regulate the homeostatic functions of astrocytes in a manner that could modulate nociception.

Several lines of evidence support a regulatory function of glucocorticoids in the expression of proteins involved in the initiation or maintenance of chronic pain syndromes. A recent study by Tanga et al. (2006) demonstrated that glial-derived S100β may be involved in mediating neuropathic pain states. Furthermore, glucocorticoids have been shown to regulate S100β expression in astrocytes in a biphasic manner (Niu et al. 1997), suggesting that they may regulate this algogenic mediator. Similarly, the chemokine CCL2 (also known as monocyte chemoattractant protein-1 [MCP-1]) is upregulated following

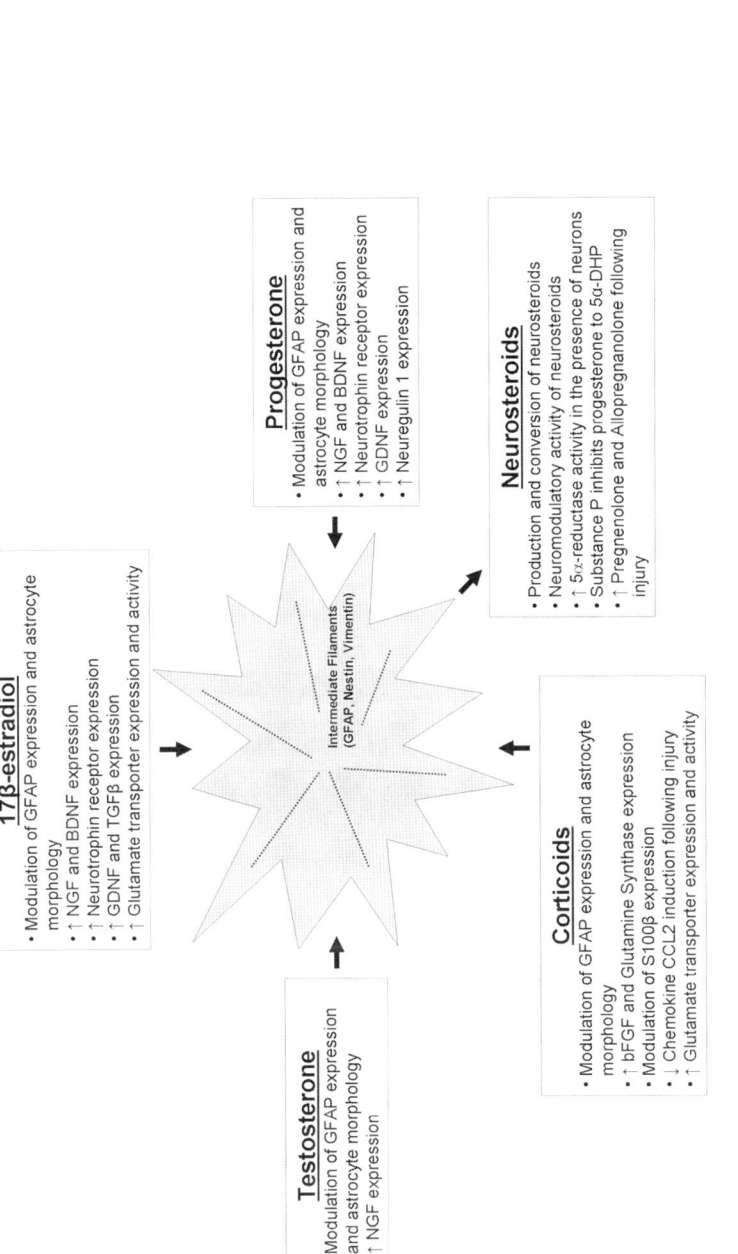

Fig. 3. Schematic diagram of the specific effects of steroid hormone signaling on nociception-relevant astrocyte functions discussed in this chapter. BDNF = brain-derived neurotrophic factor, bFGF = basic fibroblast growth factor, GFAP = glial fibrillary acidic protein, GDNF = glial-derived neurotrophic factor, NGF = nerve growth factor, TGF-β = transforming growth factor-β.

DRG injury (White et al. 2005), and the CCL2 receptor, CCR2, is significantly involved in pain processing (Abbadie et al. 2003; White et al. 2005). Glucocorticoid receptor signaling regulates CCL2 expression in peripheral monocytes and in the brain by maintaining a negative repression of CCL2 and CCR2 mRNA expression in response to injury (Little et al. 2006). Finally, the importance of astrocyte glutamate transporters in mediating L-glutamate homeostasis has been discussed previously in this chapter. The synthetic glucocorticoid, dexamethasone, has been shown to increase the expression of GLT-1, but not GLAST, in various brain regions while concomitantly increasing functional L-glutamate uptake (Zschocke et al. 2005). These studies provide mechanistic connections between stress responses and modulation of nociception in chronic and acute pain through the regulation of glucocorticoid receptor activation in astrocytes.

CONCLUSIONS

Increasing evidence of a key role for glial cells in modulating neuronal processes in the normal and diseased CNS has brought attention to the incredible diversity of function that these cells possess. In particular, it is clear that astrocytes are such active participants in synaptic transmission that the functional unit of neurotransmission must now be considered to include both neuronal and glial components (De Leo et al. 2006). This is particularly true in the case of chronic pain states, in which glial cells have been proven to be intimately involved.

Elucidation of endogenous modulators of glial function has provided and will continue to provide a mechanistic framework for understanding how astrocytes are able to dynamically modify CNS function in healthy and diseased tissue. We have discussed here the role of several of these endogenous astrocyte modulators, the steroid hormones. These steroid hormones are synthesized not only by the peripheral endocrine organs, but also by the astrocytes themselves. Furthermore, these steroid hormones signal through receptors expressed by the astrocytes and can significantly modify their gene expression patterns, morphology, homeostatic functions, and enzymatic activities (see Fig. 3). The studies summarized in this chapter represent the beginning of our understanding of how these steroid hormones can regulate nociceptive systems and, ultimately, pain perception, through their actions in modifying astrocyte function. Future studies designed to address how steroid hormones regulate astrocyte function will broaden our understanding of how astrocytes respond to CNS injury and will provide the basis for novel therapies for the treatment of chronic pain diseases.

ACKNOWLEDGMENTS

This work was supported by the National Institute of Arthritis and Musculo-skeletal and Skin Diseases grant AR44757 (J.A. DeLeo).

REFERENCES

Abbadie C, Lindia JA, Cumiskey AM, et al. Impaired neuropathic pain responses in mice lacking the chemokine receptor CCR2. *Proc Natl Acad Sci USA* 2003; 100:7947–7952.

Aloisi AM. Gonadal hormones and sex differences in pain reactivity. *Clin J Pain* 2003; 19:168–174.

Aloisi AM, Bonifazi M. Sex hormones, central nervous system and pain. *Horm Behav* 2006; 50:1–7.

Ashkinazi I, Vershinina EA. Pain sensitivity in chronic psychoemotional stress in humans. *Neurosci Behav Physiol* 1999; 29:333–337.

Azcoitia I, Sierra A, Garcia-Segura LM. Localization of estrogen receptor beta-immunoreactivity in astrocytes of the adult rat brain. *Glia* 1999; 26:260–267.

Baulieu EE. Neurosteroids: of the nervous system, by the nervous system, for the nervous system. *Recent Prog Horm Res* 1997; 52:1–32.

Baulieu EE, Robel P. Neurosteroids: a new brain function? *J Steroid Biochem Mol Biol* 1990; 37:395–403.

Berkley KJ. Sex differences in pain. *Behav Brain Sci* 1997; 20:371–380; discussion 435–513.

Bicknell RJ. Sex-steroid actions on neurotransmission. *Curr Opin Neurol* 1998; 11:667–671.

Bimonte-Nelson HA, Nelson ME, Granholm AC. Progesterone counteracts estrogen-induced increases in neurotrophins in the aged female rat brain. *Neuroreport* 2004; 15:2659–2663.

Binns BC, Huang Y, Goettl VM, Hackshaw KV, Stephens RL Jr. Glutamate uptake is attenuated in spinal deep dorsal and ventral horn in the rat spinal nerve ligation model. *Brain Res* 2005; 1041:38–47.

Blackburn-Munro G, Blackburn-Munro R. Pain in the brain: are hormones to blame? *Trends Endocrinol Metab* 2003; 14:20–27.

Boccalon S, Scaggiante B, Perissin L. Anxiety stress and nociceptive responses in mice. *Life Sci* 2006; 78:1225–1230.

Boucher TJ, Okuse K, Bennett DL, et al. Potent analgesic effects of GDNF in neuropathic pain states. *Science* 2000; 290:124–127.

Buonanno A, Fischbach GD. Neuregulin and ErbB receptor signaling pathways in the nervous system. *Curr Opin Neurobiol* 2001; 11:287–296.

Cameron SA, Dutia MB. Lesion-induced plasticity in rat vestibular nucleus neurones dependent on glucocorticoid receptor activation. *J Physiol* 1999; 518 (Pt 1):151–158.

Cesi PN, Melcangi RC, Celotti F, Martini L. Distribution of aromatase activity in cultured neurons and glia cells. *J Steroid Biochem Mol Biol* 1993; 44:637–639.

Chang CN, Yang JT, Lee TH, et al. Dexamethasone enhances upregulation of nerve growth factor mRNA expression in ischemic rat brain. *J Clin Neurosci* 2005; 12:680–684.

Chowen JA, Busiguina S, Garcia-Segura LM. Sexual dimorphism and sex steroid modulation of glial fibrillary acidic protein messenger RNA and immunoreactivity levels in the rat hypothalamus. *Neuroscience* 1995; 69:519–532.

Coers S, Tanzer L, Jones KJ. Testosterone treatment attenuates the effects of facial nerve transection on glial fibrillary acidic protein (GFAP) levels in the hamster facial motor nucleus. *Metab Brain Dis* 2002; 17:55–63.

Conejo NM, Gonzalez-Pardo H, Cimadevilla JM, et al. Influence of gonadal steroids on the glial fibrillary acidic protein-immunoreactive astrocyte population in young rat hippocampus. *J Neurosci Res* 2005; 79:488–494.

Craft RM, Mogil JS, Aloisi AM. Sex differences in pain and analgesia: the role of gonadal hormones. *Eur J Pain* 2004; 8:397–411.

Danbolt NC. Glutamate uptake. *Prog Neurobiol* 2001; 65:1–105.

Davis MC, Zautra AJ, Reich JW. Vulnerability to stress among women in chronic pain from fibromyalgia and osteoarthritis. *Ann Behav Med* 2001; 23:215–226.

DeLeo JA, Colburn RW, Nichols M, Malhotra A. Interleukin-6-mediated hyperalgesia/allodynia and increased spinal IL-6 expression in a rat mononeuropathy model. *J Interferon Cytokine Res* 1996; 16:695–700.

De Leo JA, Tawfik VL, LaCroix-Fralish ML. The tetrapartite synapse: path to CNS sensitization and chronic pain. *Pain* 2006; 122:17–21.

De Nicola AF, Gonzalez SL, Labombarda F, et al. Progesterone treatment of spinal cord injury: Effects on receptors, neurotrophins, and myelination. *J Mol Neurosci* 2006; 28:3–15.

Dhandapani KM, Brann DW. Protective effects of estrogen and selective estrogen receptor modulators in the brain. *Biol Reprod* 2002; 67:1379–1385.

Dhandapani KM, Wade FM, Mahesh VB, Brann DW. Astrocyte-derived transforming growth factor-β mediates the neuroprotective effects of 17β-estradiol: involvement of nonclassical genomic signaling pathways. *Endocrinology* 2005; 146:2749–2759.

Eng LF. Glial fibrillary acidic protein (GFAP): the major protein of glial intermediate filaments in differentiated astrocytes. *J Neuroimmunol* 1985; 8:203–214.

Evrard HC, Balthazart J. Rapid regulation of pain by estrogens synthesized in spinal dorsal horn neurons. *J Neurosci* 2004; 24:7225–7229.

Falls DL. Neuregulins: functions, forms, and signaling strategies. *Exp Cell Res* 2003; 284:14–30.

Fillingim RB, Ness TJ. Sex-related hormonal influences on pain and analgesic responses. *Neurosci Biobehav Rev* 2000; 24:485–501.

Finley SK, Kritzer MF. Immunoreactivity for intracellular androgen receptors in identified subpopulations of neurons, astrocytes and oligodendrocytes in primate prefrontal cortex. *J Neurobiol* 1999; 40:446–457.

Gameiro GH, Andrade Ada S, de Castro M, et al. The effects of restraint stress on nociceptive responses induced by formalin injected in rat's TMJ. *Pharmacol Biochem Behav* 2005; 82:338–344.

Garcia-Estrada J, Del Rio JA, Luquin S, Soriano E, Garcia-Segura LM. Gonadal hormones down-regulate reactive gliosis and astrocyte proliferation after a penetrating brain injury. *Brain Res* 1993; 628:271–278.

Garcia-Ovejero D, Veiga S, Garcia-Segura LM, Doncarlos LL. Glial expression of estrogen and androgen receptors after rat brain injury. *J Comp Neurol* 2002; 450:256–271.

Garcia-Ovejero D, Azcoitia I, Doncarlos LL, Melcangi RC, Garcia-Segura LM. Glia-neuron crosstalk in the neuroprotective mechanisms of sex steroid hormones. *Brain Res Brain Res Rev* 2005; 48:273–286.

Garcia-Segura LM, Torres-Aleman I, Naftolin F. Astrocytic shape and glial fibrillary acidic protein immunoreactivity are modified by estradiol in primary rat hypothalamic cultures. *Brain Res Dev Brain Res* 1989; 47:298–302.

Gil KM, Carson JW, Porter LS, et al. Daily stress and mood and their association with pain, health-care use, and school activity in adolescents with sickle cell disease. *J Pediatr Psychol* 2003; 28:363–373.

Gonzalez SL, Labombarda F, Gonzalez Deniselle MC, et al. Progesterone up-regulates neuronal brain-derived neurotrophic factor expression in the injured spinal cord. *Neuroscience* 2004; 125:605–614.

Hu ZY, Bourreau E, Jung-Testas I, Robel P, Baulieu EE. Neurosteroids: oligodendrocyte mitochondria convert cholesterol to pregnenolone. *Proc Natl Acad Sci USA* 1987; 84:8215–8219.

Imbe H, Iwai-Liao Y, Senba E. Stress-induced hyperalgesia: animal models and putative mechanisms. *Front Biosci* 2006; 11:2179–2192.

Ivanova T, Karolczak M, Beyer C. Estradiol stimulates GDNF expression in developing hypothalamic neurons. *Endocrinology* 2002; 143:3175–3178.

Ji RR, Zhang Q, Pettersson RF, Hokfelt T. aFGF, bFGF and NGF differentially regulate neuro-peptide expression in dorsal root ganglia after axotomy and induce autotomy. *Regul Pept* 1996; 66:179–189.

Jones KJ, Kinderman NB, Oblinger MM. Alterations in glial fibrillary acidic protein (GFAP) mRNA levels in the hamster facial motor nucleus: effects of axotomy and testosterone. *Neurochem Res* 1997; 22:1359–1366.

Jung-Testas I, Renoir M, Bugnard H, Greene GL, Baulieu EE. Demonstration of steroid hormone receptors and steroid action in primary cultures of rat glial cells. *J Steroid Biochem Mol Biol* 1992; 41:621–631.

Kipper-Galperin M, Galilly R, Danenberg HD, Brenner T. Dehydroepiandrosterone selectively inhibits production of tumor necrosis factor alpha and interleukin-6 in astrocytes. *Int J Dev Neurosci* 1999; 17:765–775.

Koenig HL, Schumacher M, Ferzaz B, et al. Progesterone synthesis and myelin formation by Schwann cells. *Science* 1995; 268:1500–1533.

Krieger NR, Scott RG. Nonneuronal localization for steroid converting enzyme: 3 alpha-hydroxy-steroid oxidoreductase in olfactory tubercle of rat brain. *J Neurochem* 1989; 52:1866-70.

Kumar S, deVillis J. Glucocorticoid-mediated functions in glial cells. In: Kimelberg HK (Ed). *Glial Cell Receptors.* New York: Raven Press, 1988, pp 243–264.

Labombarda F, Guennoun R, Gonzalez S, et al. Immunocytochemical evidence for a progesterone receptor in neurons and glial cells of the rat spinal cord. *Neurosci Lett* 2000; 288:29–32.

LaCroix-Fralish ML, Tawfik VL, DeLeo JA. The organizational and activational effects of sex hormones on tactile and thermal hypersensitivity following lumbar nerve root injury in male and female rats. *Pain* 2005; 114:71–80.

LaCroix-Fralish ML, Tawfik VL, Nutile-McMenemy N, Deleo JA. Progesterone mediates gonadal hormone differences in tactile and thermal hypersensitivity following l5 nerve root ligation in female rats. *Neuroscience* 2006a; 138:601–608.

LaCroix-Fralish ML, Tawfik VL, Spratt KF, DeLeo JA. Sex differences in lumbar spinal cord gene expression following experimental lumbar radiculopathy. *J Mol Neurosci* 2006b; 30:283–295.

LaCroix-Fralish ML, Tawfik VL, Nutile-McMenemy N, DeLeo JA. Neuregulin 1 is a pronocicep-tive cytokine that is regulated by progesterone in the spinal cord: Implications for sex specific pain modulation. *Euro J Pain* 2007; In press.

Lanlua P, Decorti F, Gangula PR, et al. Female steroid hormones modulate receptors for nerve growth factor in rat dorsal root ganglia. *Biol Reprod* 2001; 64:331–338.

Lee SJ, McEwen BS. Neurotrophic and neuroprotective actions of estrogens and their therapeutic implications. *Annu Rev Pharmacol Toxicol* 2001; 41:569–591.

Liang Z, Valla J, Sefidvash-Hockley S, Rogers J, Li R. Effects of estrogen treatment on glutamate uptake in cultured human astrocytes derived from cortex of Alzheimer's disease patients. *J Neurochem* 2002; 80:807–814.

Little AR, Sriram K, O'Callaghan JP. Corticosterone regulates expression of CCL2 in the intact and chemically injured hippocampus. *Neurosci Lett* 2006; 399:162–166.

Logan H, Lutgendorf S, Rainville P, et al. Effects of stress and relaxation on capsaicin-induced pain. *J Pain* 2001; 2:160–170.

Maurel D, Sage D, Mekaouche M, Bosler O. Glucocorticoids up-regulate the expression of glial fibrillary acidic protein in the rat suprachiasmatic nucleus. *Glia* 2000; 29:212–221.

Melcangi RC, Celotti F, Ballabio M, et al. 5 alpha-reductase activity in isolated and cultured neuronal and glial cells of the rat. *Brain Res* 1990; 516:229–236.

Melcangi RC, Celotti F, Martini L. Progesterone 5-alpha-reduction in neuronal and in different types of glial cell cultures: type 1 and 2 astrocytes and oligodendrocytes. *Brain Res* 1994; 639:202–206.

Melcangi RC, Magnaghi V, Martini L. Steroid metabolism and effects in central and peripheral glial cells. *J Neurobiol* 1999; 40:471–483.

Mellon SH, Deschepper CF. Neurosteroid biosynthesis: genes for adrenal steroidogenic enzymes are expressed in the brain. *Brain Res* 1993; 629:283–292.

Mitrovic AD, Maddison JE, Johnston GA. Influence of the oestrous cycle on L-glutamate and L-aspartate transport in rat brain synaptosomes. *Neurochem Int* 1999; 34:101–108.

Moroz IA, Rajabi H, Rodaros D, Stewart J. Effects of sex and hormonal status on astrocytic basic fibroblast growth factor-2 and tyrosine hydroxylase immunoreactivity after medial forebrain bundle 6-hydroxydopamine lesions of the midbrain dopamine neurons. *Neuroscience* 2003; 118:463–476.

Murphy S, Krainock R, Tham M. Neuregulin signaling via erbB receptor assemblies in the nervous system. *Mol Neurobiol* 2002; 25:67–77.

Niu H, Hinkle DA, Wise PM. Dexamethasone regulates basic fibroblast growth factor, nerve growth factor and S100beta expression in cultured hippocampal astrocytes. *Brain Res Mol Brain Res* 1997; 51:97–105.

O'Banion MK, Young DA, Bohn MC. Corticosterone-responsive mRNAs in primary rat astrocytes. *Brain Res Mol Brain Res* 1994; 22:57–68.

O'Callaghan JP, Brinton RE, McEwen BS. Glucocorticoids regulate the synthesis of glial fibrillary acidic protein in intact and adrenalectomized rats but do not affect its expression following brain injury. *J Neurochem* 1991; 57:860–869.

Ozaki M. Neuregulins and the shaping of synapses. *Neuroscientist* 2001; 7:146–154.

Ozaki M, Sasner M, Yano R, Lu HS, Buonanno A. Neuregulin-beta induces expression of an NMDA-receptor subunit. *Nature* 1997; 390:691–694.

Ozaki M, Tohyama K, Kishida H, et al. Roles of neuregulin in synaptogenesis between mossy fibers and cerebellar granule cells. *J Neurosci Res* 2000; 59:612–623.

Pan Y, Anthony M, Clarkson TB. Effect of estradiol and soy phytoestrogens on choline acetyl-transferase and nerve growth factor mRNAs in the frontal cortex and hippocampus of female rats. *Proc Soc Exp Biol Med* 1999; 221:118–125.

Patte-Mensah C, Kappes V, Freund-Mercier MJ, Tsutsui K, Mensah-Nyagan AG. Cellular distribution and bioactivity of the key steroidogenic enzyme, cytochrome P450side chain cleavage, in sensory neural pathways. *J Neurochem* 2003; 86:1233–1246.

Patte-Mensah C, Li S, Mensah-Nyagan AG. Impact of neuropathic pain on the gene expression and activity of cytochrome P450side-chain-cleavage in sensory neural networks. *Cell Mol Life Sci* 2004; 61:2274–2284.

Patte-Mensah C, Kibaly C, Mensah-Nyagan AG. Substance P inhibits progesterone conversion to neuroactive metabolites in spinal sensory circuit: a potential component of nociception. *Proc Natl Acad Sci USA* 2005; 102:9044–9049.

Pawlak J, Brito V, Kuppers E, Beyer C. Regulation of glutamate transporter GLAST and GLT-1 expression in astrocytes by estrogen. *Brain Res Mol Brain Res* 2005; 138:1–7.

Pezet S, McMahon SB. Neurotrophins: Mediators and Modulators of Pain. *Annu Rev Neurosci* 2006; 29:507–538.

Platania P, Seminara G, Aronica E, et al. 17beta-estradiol rescues spinal motoneurons from AMPA-induced toxicity: a role for glial cells. *Neurobiol Dis* 2005; 20:461–470.

Rasia-Filho AA, Xavier LL, dos Santos P, Gehlen G, Achaval M. Glial fibrillary acidic protein immunodetection and immunoreactivity in the anterior and posterior medial amygdala of male and female rats. *Brain Res Bull* 2002; 58:67–75.

Ridet JL, Malhotra SK, Privat A, Gage FH. Reactive astrocytes: cellular and molecular cues to biological function. *Trends Neurosci* 1997; 20:570–577.

Riley JL III, Robinson ME, Wise EA, Myers CD, Fillingim RB. Sex differences in the perception of noxious experimental stimuli: a meta-analysis. *Pain* 1998; 74:181–187.

Schlichter R, Keller AF, De Roo M, et al. Fast nongenomic effects of steroids on synaptic transmission and role of endogenous neurosteroids in spinal pain pathways. *J Mol Neurosci* 2006; 28:33–51.

Schlinger BA, Arnold AP. Brain is the major site of estrogen synthesis in a male songbird. *Proc Natl Acad Sci USA* 1991; 88:4191–4194.

Schumacher M. Rapid membrane effects of steroid hormones: an emerging concept in neuroendocrinology. *Trends Neurosci* 1990; 13:359–362.

Schwartz L, Slater MA, Birchler GR. Interpersonal stress and pain behaviors in patients with chronic pain. *J Consult Clin Psychol* 1994; 62:861–864.

Sohrabji F, Miranda RC, Toran-Allerand CD. Estrogen differentially regulates estrogen and nerve growth factor receptor mRNAs in adult sensory neurons. *J Neurosci* 1994; 14:459–471.

Sung B, Lim G, Mao J. Altered expression and uptake activity of spinal glutamate transporters after nerve injury contribute to the pathogenesis of neuropathic pain in rats. *J Neurosci* 2003; 23:2899–2910.

Tanga FY, Raghavendra V, Nutile-McMenemy N, Marks A, Deleo JA. Role of astrocytic S100beta in behavioral hypersensitivity in rodent models of neuropathic pain. *Neuroscience* 2006; 140:1003–1010.

Tirassa P, Thiblin I, Agren G, et al. High-dose anabolic androgenic steroids modulate concentrations of nerve growth factor and expression of its low affinity receptor (p75-NGFr) in male rat brain. *J Neurosci Res* 1997; 47:198–207.

Vardimon L, Ben-Dror I, Avisar N, Oren A, Shiftan L. Glucocorticoid control of glial gene expression. *J Neurobiol* 1999; 40:513–527.

Vielkind U, Walencewicz A, Levine JM, Bohn MC. Type II glucocorticoid receptors are expressed in oligodendrocytes and astrocytes. *J Neurosci Res* 1990; 27:360–373.

Wang S, Lim G, Zeng Q, et al. Expression of central glucocorticoid receptors after peripheral nerve injury contributes to neuropathic pain behaviors in rats. *J Neurosci* 2004; 24:8595–8605.

Wang S, Lim G, Zeng Q, et al. Central glucocorticoid receptors modulate the expression and function of spinal NMDA receptors after peripheral nerve injury. *J Neurosci* 2005; 25:488–495.

Weng HR, Aravindan N, Cata JP, et al. Spinal glial glutamate transporters downregulate in rats with Taxol-induced hyperalgesia. *Neurosci Lett* 2005; 386:18–22.

White FA, Sun J, Waters SM, et al. Excitatory monocyte chemoattractant protein-1 signaling is up-regulated in sensory neurons after chronic compression of the dorsal root ganglion. *Proc Natl Acad Sci USA* 2005; 102:14092–14097.

Wolpowitz D, Mason TB, Dietrich P, et al. Cysteine-rich domain isoforms of the neuregulin-1 gene are required for maintenance of peripheral synapses. *Neuron* 2000; 25:79–91.

Yunus MB. Gender differences in fibromyalgia and other related syndromes. *J Gend Specif Med* 2002; 5:42–47.

Zhao X, Liu J, Guan R, et al. Estrogen affects BDNF expression following chronic constriction nerve injury. *Neuroreport* 2003; 14:1627–1631.

Zschocke J, Bayatti N, Clement AM, et al. Differential promotion of glutamate transporter expression and function by glucocorticoids in astrocytes from various brain regions. *J Biol Chem* 2005; 280:34924–34932.

Zwain IH, Yen SS. Dehydroepiandrosterone: biosynthesis and metabolism in the brain. *Endocrinology* 1999a; 140:880–887.

Zwain IH, Yen SS. Neurosteroidogenesis in astrocytes, oligodendrocytes, and neurons of cerebral cortex of rat brain. *Endocrinology* 1999b; 140:3843–3852.

Correspondence to: Joyce A. De Leo, PhD, Department of Anesthesiology, HB 7125, One Medical Center Drive, Lebanon, NH 03756, USA. Tel: 1-603-650-6204; fax: 1-603-650-4928; email: joyce.a.deleo@dartmouth.edu.

Immune and Glial Regulation of Pain, edited by Joyce A. DeLeo, Linda S. Sorkin, and Linda R. Watkins, IASP Press, Seattle, © 2007.

15

The Role of ERK/MAPK in Spinal Glia for Neuropathic Pain: Signal Transduction in Spinal Microglia and Astrocytes after Nerve Injury

Ru-Rong Ji

Pain Research Center, Department of Anesthesiology, Brigham and Women's Hospital and Harvard Medical School, Boston, Massachusetts, USA

Mitogen-activated protein kinases (MAPKs) are a family of molecules that play a critical role in cell signaling. This family of proteins is evolutionarily well conserved, reflecting its indispensable role in signal transduction. The MAPK family includes three major members—extracellular signal-regulated kinase (ERK or p44/42 MAPK), p38, and c-Jun N-terminal kinase (JNK)—which represent three different signaling cascades. MAPKs transduce a broad range of extracellular stimuli into diverse intracellular responses by both transcriptional and nontranscriptional regulation. All the family members are activated by different upstream MAPK kinases (MKKs) via phosphorylation. The corresponding MKKs for ERK, p38, and JNK are MKK1/2 (also called MEK1/2), MKK3/6, and MKK4/7, respectively. MKKs are activated by MAPK kinase kinase (Ji et al. 1999; Widman et al. 1999).

Since MAPKs are activated by phosphorylation, phosphorylation-specific antibodies that only recognize the sites essential for kinase activation have been developed and extensively used to study the activation of MAPK pathways. These antibodies have greatly accelerated studies on the MAPK pathways. Studies on MAPKs have also greatly benefited from specific inhibitors that are available to explore the function of each pathway. Compared to other kinase inhibitors, MAPK inhibitors are relatively specific. Inhibitors of all three major MAPK pathways have been shown to attenuate pain hypersensitivity under different pain conditions, such as inflammatory pain and neuropathic pain. However, these inhibitors do not change basal pain sensitivity (Ji et al. 2007).

Extracellular signal-regulated kinase is the most studied member of the MAPK family. It was originally identified as a primary effector of growth factor receptor signaling, a cascade that involves sequential activation of RAS, RAF (a MAPK kinase kinase), MEK (MAPK/ERK kinase, a MAPK kinase), and finally ERK. Early studies indicated a critical role of ERK in regulating mitosis, proliferation, differentiation, and survival of mammalian cells during development. However, the activation of the ERK cascade is not restricted to growth factor signaling. ERK is activated in neurons of the peripheral and central nervous systems following neural activity. A growing body of evidence demonstrates an involvement of ERK in neuronal plasticity, such as learning and memory and pain hypersensitivity (Ji et al. 1999, 2003; Karim et al. 2001; Dai et al. 2002).

Although it was believed that pain hypersensitivity results exclusively from altered activity of neurons, mounting evidence indicates that spinal glia (e.g., microglia and astrocytes) play an essential role in pain facilitation. For example, peripheral nerve injury produces a profound activation of microglia and astrocytes in the spinal cord, and further, many drugs that modify glial actions can alter pain sensitivity (Garrison et al. 1991; Meller et al. 1994; Watkins et al. 1997, 2001; DeLeo and Yezierski 2001; Sweitzer et al. 2001a,b; Tsuda et al. 2003, 2005; Ji and Strichartz 2004; Tanga et al. 2005; Zhuang et al. 2006). It is of great interest that all three MAPK pathways are activated in spinal glial cells after nerve injury and play a crucial role in glial signal transduction and neuropathic pain sensitization (Ma and Quirion 2002; Jin et al. 2003; Tsuda et al. 2004; Zhuang et al. 2005, 2006). In particular, ERK is activated in spinal microglia (Fig. 1) and astrocytes (Fig. 2) at early and late stages of neuropathic pain development, respectively (Zhuang et al. 2005).

ERK ACTIVATION AND SIGNAL TRANSDUCTION
IN DORSAL HORN NEURONS

Under normal conditions, ERK activation in spinal dorsal horn neurons requires nociceptive activity (Ji et al. 1999). Injection of the C-fiber activator, capsaicin, into the hindpaw of rats induces marked ERK phosphorylation. Phosphorylated ERK (pERK) is rapidly induced (within 1 minute) in medial superficial dorsal horn neurons after C-fiber activation. pERK is induced by thermal noxious (heat and cold) and mechanical noxious stimuli or electrical stimulation at C-fiber intensity, but not by innocuous stimuli such as light touch or electrical stimulation at Aβ-fiber intensity (Ji et al. 1999). pERK is also induced in dorsal horn neurons in animal models of inflammatory pain and neuropathic pain (Ji et al. 2002; Ma and Quirion 2002; Adwanikar et al. 2004;

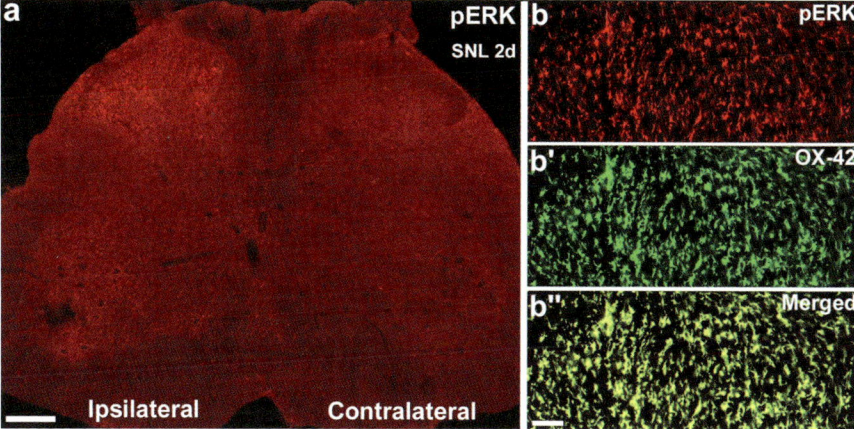

Fig. 1. (a) Immunofluorescence of phosphorylated extracellular signal-regulated kinase (pERK) demonstrates a marked activation of ERK in the ipsilateral spinal cord 2 days after spinal nerve ligation (SNL). Scale = 200 μm. (b-b") Double immunofluorescence of pERK (red) and OX-42 (antibody against CR3/CD11b) (green) reveals that pERK (b) colocalizes with OX-42 (b') in the medial superficial dorsal horn. Panel b" is merged from b and b'. Scale = 50 μm. Modified from Zhuang et al. (2005).

Zhuang et al. 2005). Whereas acute inflammation generated by intraplantar capsaicin or formalin produces only transient (<2-hour) ERK activation (Ji et al. 1999), chronic inflammation by intraplantar complete Freund's adjuvant induces more persistent (>24-hour) ERK activation in dorsal horn neurons (Ji et al. 2002; Adwanikar et al. 2004). In a model of neuropathic pain induced by spinal nerve ligation (SNL), pERK is induced in dorsal horn neurons within 10 minutes and declines after 6 hours. This transient activation is likely to be caused by the initial injury discharge elicited by ligation of the spinal nerve (Devor and Seltzer 1999).

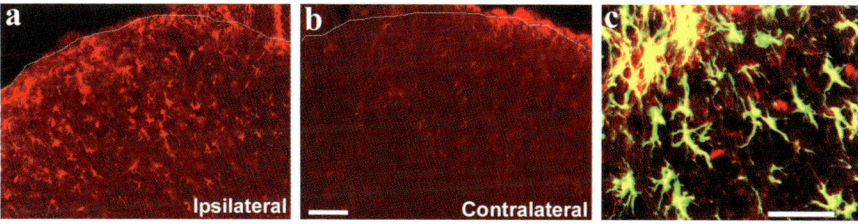

Fig. 2. (a, b) Immunofluorescence of phosphorylated extracellular signal-regulated kinase (pERK) indicates an increase in pERK-immunoreactive cells in the ipsilateral dorsal horn 21 days after spinal nerve ligation (SNL). Scale = 50 μm. (c) Double staining of pERK (red) and glial fibrillary acidic protein (GFAP) (green) reveals that pERK is largely colocalized with GFAP in laminae I–III 21 days after SNL. Scale = 50 μm. Modified from Zhuang et al. (2005), with permission.

While ERK activation in dorsal horn neurons requires high-threshold nociceptive input (e.g., C-fiber activation) under normal conditions, ERK can be activated in dorsal horn neurons by low-threshold stimulation (e.g., light touch or Aβ-fiber stimulation) after nerve injury or chronic inflammation (Wang et al. 2004; Cruz et al. 2005; Seino et al. 2006), indicating an important role of ERK in plastic changes of dorsal horn neurons. Taken together, these data indicate that pERK can serve as a marker for the activation of dorsal horn neurons following nociceptive activity. However, nociceptive activity appears to be insufficient to drive ERK activation in spinal glial cells, despite the fact that noxious stimulation can rapidly activate p38 MAPK in spinal microglia (Svensson et al. 2003; Sweitzer et al. 2004).

To define the signaling pathways involved in C-fiber activation of ERK, we have investigated ERK activation in isolated spinal slices (Kawasaki et al. 2004, 2006). We found that multiple neurotransmitter receptors, including N-methyl-D-aspartate (NMDA) receptors, α-amino-3-hydroxy-5-methylisoxazole-4-propionic acid (AMPA) receptors, and the metabotropic glutamate receptors neurokinin-1 (NK-1) and tyrosine kinase B (TrkB), all contribute to C-fiber-evoked ERK activation in spinal neurons (Kawasaki et al. 2004). Activation of these receptors results in a significant increase of intracellular Ca^{2+}, either through extracellular Ca^{2+} influx or through Ca^{2+} release from intracellular stores. Ca^{2+}-dependent activation of protein kinases A (PKA) and C (PKC) is both sufficient and necessary for ERK activation in spinal neurons (Ji et al. 1999; Hu et al. 2003; Lever et al. 2003; Kawasaki et al. 2004). The protein kinase Src is also implicated in ERK activation, possibly through the PKC pathway (Kawasaki et al. 2004).

Importantly, ERK activation in dorsal horn neurons contributes to both the induction and maintenance of central sensitization (Ji et al. 1999, 2002, 2003; Karim et al. 2001; Cruz et al. 2005). ERK activation induces central sensitization through the phosphorylation of the A-type voltage-gated potassium channel $K_V 4.2$, leading to increased membrane excitability (Hu et al. 2006), or through the trafficking of AMPA receptors from the cytoplasm to synapses (Ji et al. 2003). ERK also maintains inflammation-induced central sensitization through the transcriptional regulation of several genes, including, but almost certainly not limited to, genes of NK-1 and prodynorphin. The transcription factor cAMP (cyclic adenosine monophosphate) response element-binding protein (CREB) is activated by ERK and mediates gene expression in dorsal horn neurons (Ji et al. 2002, 2003; Kawasaki et al. 2004). However, ERK activation in dorsal horn neurons is transient after nerve injury, lasting only up to 6 hours, suggesting that this neuronal activation is more important for the early development of neuropathic pain.

ERK ACTIVATION AND SIGNAL TRANSDUCTION IN SPINAL MICROGLIA

Accumulating evidence suggests an important role of spinal microglia in the pathogenesis of pain, especially neuropathic pain (Tsuda et al. 2005). Microglia are regarded as resident macrophages in the central nervous system. They are ramified with thin branches at rest and become ameboid, with thick, short branches, once activated. Microglia show the quickest responses to nerve injury among all the glial cell types (Kreutzberg 1996). Nerve injury induces the expression of microglial markers such as macrophage-1 antigen (Mac-1/ CR3/CD11b), and CD14 within a few hours (DeLeo et al. 2004). Interestingly, several receptors, including the chemokine receptor CX3CR1, the adenosine triphosphate (ATP) receptor P2X4, and TLR-4, and enzymes such as cyclooxygenase-1 (COX-1) are specifically expressed or induced in spinal microglia; deleting or inhibiting these molecules can attenuate neuropathic pain (Tsuda et al. 2003; Zhu and Eisenach 2003; Verge et al. 2004; Tanga et al. 2005). A microglial inhibitor, minocycline, was able to prevent or delay neuropathic pain, but could not reverse it once established, suggesting a particular role of microglia in the early development of neuropathic pain (Raghavendra et al. 2003; Ledeboer et al. 2005).

We found that ERK is also activated in microglia of the spinal cord during the first few days of neuropathic pain development (Zhuang et al. 2005). Although pERK expression in dorsal horn neurons was transient after nerve injury, the overall level of pERK in the dorsal horn was persistently elevated for more than 3 weeks (Zhuang et al. 2005). On post-SNL day 2, there was a substantial increase in the number of pERK-immunoreactive cells in the ipsilateral spinal cord (Fig. 1a). We determined that pERK is induced in spinal microglia at this time point, because it is colocalized with the microglial marker OX-42 (CD11b, Fig 1b), but not with the neuronal marker NeuN or the astrocyte marker glial fibrillary acidic protein (GFAP) (Zhuang et al. 2005). Ten days after injury, pERK expression in microglia was substantially reduced. Blockade of ERK activation on day 2 with a MEK inhibitor attenuated SNL-induced mechanical allodynia, a major neuropathic pain symptom, indicating a role for microglia in the development of neuropathic pain (Zhuang et al. 2005).

It remains to be investigated how peripheral nerve injury activates ERK in spinal microglia. After nerve injury, spontaneous (ectopic) electrical activity produced in the axons and cell bodies of primary sensory neurons is believed to initiate neuropathic pain by inducing the release of neurotransmitters in the central terminals in the spinal cord (Devor and Seltzer 1999). However, it is unlikely that microglial activation of ERK is induced by nerve activity because persistent nerve activity in chronic inflammatory pain conditions does not activate ERK

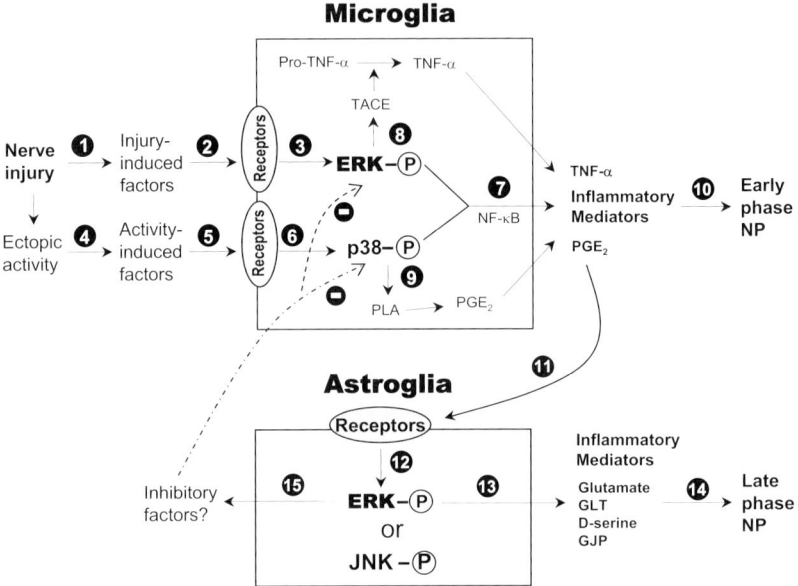

Fig. 3. Putative signaling in spinal microglia and astrocytes after nerve injury. Damage to the peripheral axons of primary sensory neurons will cause a change in central terminals of these neurons in the spinal cord. The affected terminals will release injury-induced factors (Step 1) that stimulate their receptors on microglia (Step 2), leading to activation (phosphorylation) of extracellular signal-regulated kinase (ERK) in spinal microglia (Step 3). Nerve injury will also produce spontaneous (ectopic) activity (discharge) in the axons and cell bodies of primary sensory neurons, and release activity-dependent factors (e.g., fractalkine and substance P) from central terminals (Step 4). These factors will activate their receptors (CX3CR1 and neurokinin-1 [NK-1], respectively) on microglia (Step 5), leading to the activation of p38 mitogen-activated protein kinase (MAPK) (Step 6). Upon activation, ERK or p38 activate the transcription factor nuclear factor (NF)-κB (Step 7), inducing the synthesis of multiple inflammatory mediators (e.g., interleukin [IL]-1β, IL-6, and tumor necrosis factor α [TNF-α]) and enzymes (e.g., inducible nitric oxide synthase [iNOS] and cyclooxygenase 1 and 2) for the production of the inflammatory mediators nitric oxide and prostaglandin E$_2$ (PGE$_2$). Furthermore, ERK activates TNF-α-converting enzyme (TACE, Step 8) that can cleave the extracellular domain of membrane-bound pro-TNF-α (26 kDa) to generate the mature TNF-α (18 kDa). p38 is known to activate phospholipase A (PLA, Step 9), leading to the production of PGE$_2$. All these mediators will increase dorsal horn neuron sensitivity and generate neuropathic pain (NP, Step 10). Inflammatory mediators released from microglia can further activate their receptors on astrocytes (Step 11), causing an activation of ERK or c-Jun N-terminal kinase (JNK) in spinal astrocytes (Step 12). ERK and JNK will increase the synthesis of multiple inflammatory mediators (Step 13). Activation of ERK or JNK may also regulate the expression of glutamate transporters (GLT) and gap junction proteins (GJP), as well as the release of glutamate or D-serine, contributing to the maintenance of neuropathic pain (Step 14). ERK or JNK may also produce inhibitory astroglial factors (Step 15), acting on microglial receptors to turn off the activation of ERK or p38 in microglia.

in spinal glia (Ji et al. 2002; Adwanikar et al. 2004). Rather, ERK activation in microglia requires axonal injury. In the spinal cord, some factors must be released from central nerve terminals of the damaged primary sensory neurons to activate ERK (Fig. 3).

Nerve injury (e.g., SNL) also activates p38 in spinal microglia, starting at 12 hours and peaking at 72 hours after injury (Jin et al. 2003). It remains unclear whether pERK and p-p38 are induced in the same population of microglia. However, studies indicate that the activation of ERK and p38 in spinal microglia is regulated by different mechanisms, because noxious stimulation activates p38 but not ERK in spinal microglia in conditions such as inflammatory pain (Ji et al. 2002; Svensson et al. 2003; Swetizer et al. 2004; see also Fig. 3), and because nerve conduction blockade prevents the activation of p38 but not ERK in spinal microglia following nerve injury (Wen et al. 2005). A recent study shows that Src family protein kinases are activated in spinal microglia after nerve injury, resulting in activation of ERK but not p38 in the spinal cord (Katsura et al. 2006).

Different types of receptors, such as the NK-1 receptor, NMDA receptor, chemokine CCR2 receptor, and tumor necrosis factor-α (TNF-α) receptor, have been implicated in p38 activation in spinal microglia (Abbadie et al. 2003; Svensson et al. 2003; 2005). In particular, inhibition of p38 has been implicated in minocycline's antinociceptive effects (Tikka et al. 2001; Hua et al. 2005; Hains and Waxman 2006). Whether these mechanisms are also involved in ERK activation remain to be tested.

How can activation of ERK in spinal microglia facilitate pain states? Microglia produce high levels of proinflammatory cytokines, such as interleukin (IL)-1β, IL-6, and TNF-α (Kreutzberg 1996; Hanisch 2002; Koistinaho and Koistinaho 2002). These cytokines are upregulated in the spinal cord after nerve injury and facilitate pain by enhancing synaptic transmission in dorsal horn neurons via pre- or postsynaptic mechanisms. ERK activation is likely to mediate the transcription of these cytokines in spinal microglia. Different transcription factors may be involved in ERK-mediated transcription in spinal neurons and microglia. While CREB is important for ERK-mediated transcription in spinal neurons, nuclear factor (NF)-κB appears to be induced in spinal microglia after nerve injury and seems to be essential for the transcription of the proinflammatory cytokines (Ji and Strichartz 2004). It is likely that the ERK and p38 pathways can act together to regulate neuropathic pain. For example, a combination of MEK and p38 inhibitors has been shown to suppress endotoxin-induced expression of iNOS and TNF-α in microglia with a much greater efficacy than each inhibitor alone (Bhat et al. 1998). In addition to slow transcriptional regulation, ERK also plays a role in fast post-translational regulation. ERK was shown to activate TNF-α-converting enzyme (TACE), a specific enzyme required to cleave the extracellular domain of membrane-bound pro-TNF-α (26 kDa) to generate the mature TNF-α (18 kDa) through a process known as ectodomain shedding (Watkins and Maier 2003; see also Fig. 3).

ERK ACTIVATION AND SIGNAL TRANSDUCTION IN SPINAL ASTROCYTES

Although astrocytes are five times more numerous than either neurons or microglia in the central nervous system, less is known about the role of spinal astrocytes in pain regulation compared to the role of microglia. Importantly, astrocytic processes form part of synapses (tripartite synapses; Araque et al. 1999). Glutamate released from presynaptic terminals not only acts on postsynaptic receptors, but also spills over to bind glutamate receptors on astrocytic processes. Activation of glutamate receptors on astrocytes leads to an increase in intracellular Ca^{2+} via release from Ca^{2+} stores. This increase induces glutamate release from astrocytic processes that are very close to synapses, altering synaptic transmission (Haydon 2001). Increasing evidence suggests a role of spinal astrocytes in pain hypersensitivity. First, an astroglial toxin can reverse neuropathic pain (Zhuang et al. 2006). Second, stem cells implanted into the spinal cord produce astrocytes and induce mechanical allodynia (Hofstetter et al. 2005). Third, astrocytes can form gap junctions with other astrocytes, allowing direct intercellular movements of ions, metabolites, and second messenger molecules, and contributing to local metabolic hemostats and synchronization of cellular activities. Gap junction blockade was shown to suppress the spread of pain (Spataro et al. 2004).

We also found that ERK is activated in astrocytes of the spinal cord in the later stages of neuropathic pain development (Zhuang et al. 2005). On post-SNL day 10, pERK is found in both spinal microglia and astrocytes. On post-SNL day 21, pERK is found predominantly in astrocytes (Fig. 2), as shown in another neuropathic pain model (Ma and Quirion 2002). Importantly, inhibition of this activation by the intrathecal MEK inhibitor PD98059 reverses mechanical allodynia. This finding supports a role for ERK in astrocytes in the maintenance of neuropathic pain (Zhuang et al. 2005).

What is the signal causing delayed ERK activation in spinal astrocytes? Given that microglia are not only activated before astrocytes, but also cause the activation of astrocytes (Aldskogius and Kozlova 1998; DeLeo et al. 2004), it is reasonable to postulate that ERK activation in astrocytes is initiated by factors released from microglia (Fig. 3). However, maintenance of ERK activation in spinal astrocytes may need additional signal molecules that are induced in astrocytes after nerve injury. For example, several growth factors, such as ciliary neurotrophic factor (CNTF) and basic fibroblast growth factor (bFGF), are induced in spinal astrocytes by nerve injury, maintaining the activation of astrocytes known as astrogliosis (Aldskogius and Kozlova 1998).

What signal turns off ERK activation in microglia at the later stages of nerve injury? The interaction between microglia and astrocytes has two aspects. First, microglia release factors such as inflammatory mediators to activate astrocytes (Ji and Wen 2006). Second, astrocytes may also release other factors such as TGF-β to suppress the activation of microglia at later stages (Fig. 3). These inhibitory factors from astrocytes may suppress ERK activation in spinal microglia, allowing microglia to have a protective, rather than destructive, role.

Recently, we also found that JNK/MAPK is activated in spinal astrocytes, a mechanism that is essential for the maintenance of neuropathic pain. Unlike ERK, nerve injury activates JNK in astrocytes at all time stages examined (Zhuang et al. 2006). Given that JNK is activated in only 30% of astrocytes, it would be interesting to determine whether JNK and ERK are activated in different astrocytes and to pinpoint their molecular targets. Very likely, these two pathways act together to control astroglial signaling, leading to increased pain sensitivity.

How does ERK activation in spinal astrocytes regulate pain sensitivity? And how do astrocytes regulate pain sensitivity? Like microglia, astrocytes could contribute to pain hypersensitivity by producing multiple inflammatory mediators and neuroactive substances, including proinflammatory cytokines, ATP, prostaglandin E_2, and growth factors such as brain-derived neurotrophic factor (BDNF), bFGF, and CNTF. These mediators in astrocytes could be more effective ways to enhance synaptic transmission due to the fact that astrocytes make closer contacts with synapses compared to microglia. ERK activation may also regulate the expression of the neuroactive mediators in astrocytes, although different transcription factors may be involved in different cell types.

Astrocytes may also enhance pain via other mechanisms. First, astrocytes express some glutamate transporters, such as Glu-transporter-1 (GLT-1) and Glu-Asp transporter (GLAST) (Tawfik et al. 2006). Nerve injury downregulates these transporters, leading to a decrease in glutamate uptake and a subsequent increase in excitatory synaptic transmission (Sung et al. 2003). Second, astrocytes produce a special type of amino acid, D-serine, which increases NMDA-receptor sensitivity in neurons by binding to the glycine site of the receptor. We have shown that a D-serine-degrading enzyme or a selective inhibitor of the glycine site of NMDA receptors attenuates pain-related negative affect (Ren et al. 2006). Finally, in the spinal cord, gap junctions are predominantly formed between astrocytes. Connexin 43, which is regarded as the main functional protein for gap junctions in astrocytes, is upregulated after injuries (Nagy et al. 2004). A gap junction inhibitor can suppress the spread of pain beyond the initial injury site (Spataro et al. 2004). ERK or JNK may participate in the mechanisms mentioned above by regulating the synthesis of GLT-1, GLAST, D-serine, or connexin (Fig. 3).

CONCLUDING REMARKS

The last few years have seen dramatically increasing interest in studying MAPK regulation of pain for the following reasons. First, activated (i.e., phosphorylated) MAPKs can be used as cellular markers to reflect the activation of different cells in nociceptive pathways under different pain conditions. Second, as a family of intracellular signaling molecules, MAPKs are important contributors to both neuronal mechanisms (such as peripheral and central sensitization) and glial mechanisms of pain. Third, MAPKs are potential targets for the treatment of clinical pain (Ji 2004; Ji et al. 2007).

We have demonstrated that different MAPKs exhibit different activation patterns in the spinal cord following nerve injury. Whereas JNK is persistently activated in spinal astrocytes, p38 appears to be transiently activated in spinal microglia, with peak activation in the first week after injury. In particular, ERK activation contributes to neuropathic pain through different mechanisms in different cell types at different times. ERK activation is dynamic after nerve injury: ERK is initially and transiently activated in dorsal horn neurons, then activated in spinal microglia in the first week, and then finally activated in spinal astrocytes (Zhuang et al. 2005; Figs. 1 and 2).

Neural-immune and neural-glial interactions are receiving more and more attention in recent years by investigators of pain mechanisms. However, it is still far from clear how neurons and glia interact to regulate pain sensitization. Microglia and astroglia can both be activated in the spinal cord after nerve injury and may release similar diffusible factors to affect neuronal sensitivity, thus exhibiting overlapping roles in neuropathic pain sensitization. However, the fact that astrocytes have very close contact with synapses and can be more persistently activated after nerve injury may support a more unique role of this subtype of glial cells in maintaining chronic pain. Recent studies have revealed an increasing list of proteins that are exclusively expressed in spinal microglia or astroglia. Current drugs that target neuronal mechanisms (e.g., opioids, gabapentin) have resulted in limited success in treating neuropathic pain, but identification of molecules expressed in glial cells will provide new targets for the management of such pain. Improved knowledge of the mechanisms underlying the activation and actions of MAPKs will greatly enhance our understanding of glial signaling and glial regulation of pain.

ACKNOWLEDGMENTS

The work was supported by NIH RO1 grants NS54932 and DE17794.

REFERENCES

Abbadie C, Lindia JA, Cumiskey AM, et al. Impaired neuropathic pain responses in mice lacking the chemokine receptor CCR2. *Proc Natl Acad Sci USA* 2003; 100:7947–7952.

Adwanikar H, Karim F, Gereau RW. Inflammation persistently enhances nocifensive behaviors mediated by spinal group I mGluRs through sustained ERK activation. *Pain* 2004; 111:125–135.

Aldskogius H, Kozlova EN. Central neuron-glial and glial-glial interactions following axon injury. *Prog Neurobiol* 1998; 55:1–26.

Araque A, Parpura V, Sanzgiri RP, Haydon PG. Tripartite synapses: glia, the unacknowledged partner. *Trends Neurosci* 1999; 22:208–215.

Bhat NR, Zhang P, Lee JC, Hogan EL. Extracellular signal-regulated kinase and p38 subgroups of mitogen-activated protein kinases regulate inducible nitric oxide synthase and tumor necrosis factor-alpha gene expression in endotoxin-stimulated primary glial cultures. *J Neurosci* 1998; 18:1633–1641.

Cruz CD, Neto FL, Castro-Lopes J, McMahon SB, Cruz F. Inhibition of ERK phosphorylation decreases nociceptive behaviour in monoarthritic rats. *Pain* 2005; 116:411–419.

Dai Y, Iwata K, Fukuoka T, et al. Phosphorylation of extracellular signal-regulated kinase in primary afferent neurons by noxious stimuli and its involvement in peripheral sensitization. *J Neurosci* 2002; 22:7737–7745.

DeLeo JA, Yezierski RP. The role of neuroinflammation and neuroimmune activation in persistent pain. *Pain* 2001; 90:1–6.

DeLeo JA, Tanga FY, Tawfik VL. Neuroimmune activation and neuroinflammation in chronic pain and opioid tolerance/hyperalgesia. *Neuroscientist* 2004; 10:40–52.

Devor M, Seltzer Z. Pathophysiology of damaged peripheral nerves in relation to chronic pain. In: Wall PD, Melzack R (Eds). *Textbook of Pain*. Edinburgh: Churchill Livingstone, 1999, pp 129–164.

Garrison CJ, Dougherty PM, Kajander KC, Carlton SM. Staining of glial fibrillary acidic protein (GFAP) in lumbar spinal cord increases following a sciatic nerve constriction injury. *Brain Res* 1991; 565:1–7.

Hains BC, Waxman SG. Activated microglia contribute to the maintenance of chronic pain after spinal cord injury. *J Neurosci* 2006; 26:4308–4317.

Hanisch UK. Microglia as a source and target of cytokines. *Glia* 2002; 40:140–155.

Haydon PG. GLIA: listening and talking to the synapse. *Nat Rev Neurosci* 2001; 2:185–193.

Hofstetter CP, Holmstrom NA, Lilja JA, et al. Allodynia limits the usefulness of intraspinal neural stem cell grafts; directed differentiation improves outcome. *Nat Neurosci* 2005; 8:346–353.

Hu HJ, Gereau RW. Integrates PKA and PKC signaling in superficial dorsal horn neurons II: modulation of neuronal excitability. *J Neurophysiol* 2003; 90:1680–1688.

Hu HJ, Carrasquillo Y, Karim F, et al. The $K_v4.2$ potassium channel subunit is required for pain plasticity. *Neuron* 2006; 50:89–100.

Hua XY, Svensson CI, Matsui T, et al. Intrathecal minocycline attenuates peripheral inflammation-induced hyperalgesia by inhibiting p38 MAPK in spinal microglia. *Eur J Neurosci* 2005; 22:2431–2440.

Ji RR. Mitogen-activated protein kinases as potential targets for pain killers. *Curr Opin Investig Drugs* 2004; 5:71–75.

Ji RR, Strichartz G. Cell signaling and the genesis of neuropathic pain. *Sci STKE* 2004:reE14.

Ji RR, Wen YR. Neural-glial interaction in the spinal cord for the development and maintenance of nerve injury-induced neuropathic pain. *Drug Dev Res* 2006; 67:331–338.

Ji RR, Baba H, Brenner JG, Woolf CJ. Nociceptive-specific activation of ERK in spinal neurons contributes to pain hypersensitivity. *Nat Neurosci* 1999; 2:1114–1119.

Ji RR, Befort K, Brenner GJ, Woolf CJ. ERK MAP kinase activation in superficial spinal cord neurons induces prodynorphin and NK-1 upregulation and contributes to persistent inflammatory pain hypersensitivity. *J Neurosci* 2002; 22:478–485.

Ji RR, Kohno T, Moore KA, Woolf CJ. Central sensitization and LTP: do pain and memory share similar mechanisms? *Trends Neurosci* 2003; 26:696–705.

Ji RR, Kawasaki Y, Zhuang ZY, Wen YR, Zhang YQ. Protein kinases as potential targets for the treatment of pathological pain. In: Stein C (Ed). *Handbook of Experimental Pharmacology,* Vol. 177. Berlin: Springer-Verlag, 2007, pp 359–389.

Jin SX, Zhuang ZY, Woolf CJ, Ji RR. p38 mitogen-activated protein kinase is activated after a spinal nerve ligation in spinal cord microglia and dorsal root ganglion neurons and contributes to the generation of neuropathic pain. *J Neurosci* 2003; 23:4017–4022.

Karim F, Wang CC, Gereau RW. Metabotropic glutamate receptor subtypes 1 and 5 are activators of extracellular signal-regulated kinase signaling required for inflammatory pain in mice. *J Neurosci* 2001; 21:3771–3779.

Katsura H, Obata K, Mizushima T, et al. Activation of Src-family kinases in spinal microglia contributes to mechanical hypersensitivity after nerve injury. *J Neurosci* 2006; 26:8680–8690.

Kawasaki Y, Kohno T, Zhuang ZY, et al. Ionotropic and metabotropic receptors, protein kinase A, protein kinase C, and Src contribute to C-fiber-induced ERK activation and cAMP response element-binding protein phosphorylation in dorsal horn neurons, leading to central sensitization. *J Neurosci* 2004; 24:8310–8321.

Kawasaki Y, Kohno T, Ji RR. Different effects of opioid and cannabinoid on C-fiber-induced ERK activation in dorsal horn neurons in normal and spinal nerve-ligated rats. *J Pharmacol Exp Ther* 2006; 316:601–607.

Koistinaho M, Koistinaho J. Role of p38 and p44/42 mitogen-activated protein kinases in microglia. *Glia* 2002; 40:175-83.

Kreutzberg GW. Microglia: a sensor for pathological events in the CNS. *Trends Neurosci* 1996; 19:312–318.

Ledeboer A, Sloane EM, Milligan ED, et al. Minocycline attenuates mechanical allodynia and proinflammatory cytokine expression in rat models of pain facilitation. *Pain* 2005; 115:71–83.

Lever IJ, Pezet S, McMahon SB, Malcangio M. The signaling components of sensory fiber transmission involved in the activation of ERK MAP kinase in the mouse dorsal horn. *Mol Cell Neurosci* 2003; 24:259–270.

Ma W, Quirion R. Partial sciatic nerve ligation induces increase in the phosphorylation of extracellular signal-regulated kinase (ERK) and c-Jun N-terminal kinase (JNK) in astrocytes in the lumbar spinal dorsal horn and the gracile nucleus. *Pain* 2002; 99:175–84.

Meller ST, Dykstra C, Grzybycki D, Murphy S, Gebhart GF. The possible role of glia in nociceptive processing and hyperalgesia in the spinal cord of the rat. *Neuropharmacology* 1994; 33:1471–1478.

Nagy JI, Dudek FE, Rash JE. Update on connexins and gap junctions in neurons and glia in the mammalian nervous system. *Brain Res Rev* 2004; 47:191–215.

Raghavendra V, Tanga F, DeLeo JA. Inhibition of microglial activation attenuates the development but not existing hypersensitivity in a rat model of neuropathy. *J Pharmacol Exp Ther* 2003; 306:624–30.

Ren WH, Guo JD, Cao H, et al. Is endogenous D-serine in the rostral anterior cingulate cortex necessary for pain-related negative affect? *J Neurochem* 2006; 96:1636–1647.

Seino D, Tokunaga A, Tachibana T, et al. The role of ERK signaling and the P2X receptor on mechanical pain evoked by movement of inflamed knee joint. *Pain* 2006; 123:193–203.

Spataro LE, Sloane EM, Milligan ED, et al. Spinal gap junctions: potential involvement in pain facilitation. *J Pain* 2004; 5:392–405.

Sung B, Lim G, Mao J. Altered expression and uptake activity of spinal glutamate transporters after nerve injury contribute to the pathogenesis of neuropathic pain in rats. *J Neurosci* 2003; 23:2899–2910.

Svensson CI, Marsala M, Westerlund A, et al. Activation of p38 mitogen-activated protein kinase in spinal microglia is a critical link in inflammation-induced spinal pain processing. *J Neurochem* 2003; 86:1534–44.

Svensson CI, Schafers M, Jones TL, Powell H, Sorkin LS. Spinal blockade of TNF blocks spinal nerve ligation-induced increases in spinal P-p38. *Neurosci Lett* 2005; 379:209–213.

Sweitzer S, Martin D, DeLeo JA. Intrathecal interleukin-1 receptor antagonist in combination with soluble tumor necrosis factor receptor exhibits an anti-allodynic action in a rat model of neuropathic pain. *Neuroscience* 2001a; 103:529–539.

Sweitzer SM, Schubert P, DeLeo JA. Propentofylline, a glial modulating agent, exhibits antiallodynic properties in a rat model of neuropathic pain. *J Pharmacol Exp Ther* 2001b; 297:1210–1217.

Sweitzer SM, Peters MC, Ma JY, et al. Peripheral and central p38 MAPK mediates capsaicin-induced hyperalgesia. *Pain* 2004; 111:278–285.

Tanga FY, Nutile-McMenemy N, DeLeo JA. The CNS role of Toll-like receptor 4 in innate neuroimmunity and painful neuropathy. *Proc Natl Acad Sci USA* 2005; 102:5856–5861.

Tawfik VL, Lacroix-Fralish ML, Bercury KK, et al. Induction of astrocyte differentiation by propentofylline increases glutamate transporter expression in vitro: Heterogeneity of the quiescent phenotype. *Glia* 2006; 54:193–203.

Tikka T, Fiebich BL, Goldsteins G, Keinanen R, Koistinaho J. Minocycline, a tetracycline derivative, is neuroprotective against excitotoxicity by inhibiting activation and proliferation of microglia. *J Neurosci* 2001; 21:2580–2588.

Tsuda M, Shigemoto-Mogami Y, Koizumi S, et al. P2X4 receptors induced in spinal microglia gate tactile allodynia after nerve injury. *Nature* 2003; 424:778–783.

Tsuda M, Mizokoshi A, Shigemoto-Mogami Y, Koizumi S, Inoue K. Activation of p38 mitogen-activated protein kinase in spinal hyperactive microglia contributes to pain hypersensitivity following peripheral nerve injury. *Glia* 2004; 45:89–95.

Tsuda M, Inoue K, Salter MW. Neuropathic pain and spinal microglia: a big problem from molecules in "small" glia. *Trends Neurosci* 2005; 28:101–107.

Verge GM, Milligan ED, Maier SF, et al. Watkins LR. Fractalkine (CX3CL1) and fractalkine receptor (CX3CR1) distribution in spinal cord and dorsal root ganglia under basal and neuropathic pain conditions. *Eur J Neurosci* 2004; 20:1150–1160.

Wang H, Dai Y, Fukuoka T, et al. Enhancement of stimulation-induced ERK activation in the spinal dorsal horn and gracile nucleus neurons in rats with peripheral nerve injury. *Eur J Neurosci* 2004; 19:884–890.

Watkins LR, Maier SF. Glia: a novel drug discovery target for clinical pain. *Nat Rev Drug Discov* 2003; 2:973–985.

Watkins LR, Martin D, Ulrich P, Tracey KJ, Maier SF. Evidence for the involvement of spinal cord glia in subcutaneous formalin induced hyperalgesia in the rat. *Pain* 1997; 71:225–235.

Watkins LR, Milligan ED, Maier SF. Glial activation: a driving force for pathological pain. *Trends Neurosci* 2001; 24:450–455.

Wen YR, Suter MR, Huang J, et al. Nerve conduction blockade prevents the activation of p38 MAPK in spinal microglia but not the activation of spinal microglia after spared nerve injury. *Soc Neurosci Abstr* 2005; 860.3.

Widmann C, Gibson S, Jarpe MB, Johnson GL. Mitogen-activated protein kinase: conservation of a three-kinase module from yeast to human. *Physiol Rev* 1999; 79:143–180.

Zhu X, Eisenach JC. Cyclooxygenase-1 in the spinal cord is altered after peripheral nerve injury. *Anesthesiology* 2003; 99:1175-1179.

Zhuang ZY, Gerner P, Woolf CJ, Ji RR. ERK is sequentially activated in neurons, microglia, and astrocytes by spinal nerve ligation and contributes to mechanical allodynia in this neuropathic pain model. *Pain* 2005; 114:149–159.

Zhuang ZY, Wen YR, Zhang DR, et al. A peptide JNK inhibitor blocks mechanical allodynia after spinal nerve ligation: respective roles of JNK activation in primary sensory neurons and spinal astrocytes for neuropathic pain development and maintenance. *J Neurosci* 2006; 26:3551–3560.

Correspondence to: Ru-Rong Ji, PhD Department of Anesthesiology, Brigham and Women's Hospital, 75 Francis Street, Medical Research Building, Room 604, Boston, MA 02115, USA. Tel: 1-617-732-8852; fax: 1-617-730-2801; email: rrji@ zeus.bwh.harvard.edu.

Immune and Glial Regulation of Pain, edited by Joyce
A. DeLeo, Linda S. Sorkin, and Linda R. Watkins,
IASP Press, Seattle, © 2007.

16

The Role of ATP and Microglia in Enhanced Pain States

Simon Beggs,[a,b,c] Tuan Trang,[b] and Michael W. Salter[a,b,c]

*[a]University of Toronto Centre for the Study of Pain; [b]Program in Neurosciences
& Mental Health, Hospital for Sick Children, Toronto; [c]Faculty of Dentistry,
University of Toronto, Toronto, Ontario, Canada*

Glial cells have historically been considered as having simply a supportive role in maintaining neuronal "health" within the central nervous system (CNS). Microglia, more specifically, have been implicated both in neuronal support and as a key component of the immune system. Recently, considerable evidence has accumulated to show that microglia have a critical role in the development and maintenance of neuropathic pain (Watkins et al. 2001; Watkins and Meier 2003; Salter 2005; Tsuda et al. 2005; Inoue and Tsuda 2006). Interestingly, there is no suggestion that microglia are involved in nonpathological nociception, such as acute pain. This seemingly restrictive role to pathological chronic neuropathic pain makes these cells of considerable interest as a target for future neuropathic pain therapies, a subject of keen pharmacological interest because many of these pain states remain refractory to conventional treatments.

It is well documented that microglia mount a response to peripheral nerve injury. Indeed, their functions as support cells for neurons and as phagocytes, and their ability to remove the debris of degenerating primary afferent central terminals, would suggest as much (Aldskogius 2001; Rotshenker 2003). However, to consider them as explicit effectors of neuropathic pain represents a conceptual change in microglial physiology (Jin et al. 2003; Tsuda et al. 2003; Coull et al. 2005). Damage to peripheral nerves resulting in neuropathic pain has long been considered a direct result of alterations in peripheral and central neuronal function. It is certainly true that nerve injury instigates a series of changes at the molecular and cellular level that directly affect neuronal plasticity, ultimately resulting in considerable physiological and anatomical alterations in pain pathways (Woolf and Salter 2000; Zimmermann 2001; Scholz and Woolf

2002; Woolf 2004). These effects are key to understanding the pathophysiology of neuropathic pain, but it is now apparent that a reductionist approach to understanding pain as restricted to neuronal function alone is an oversimplification. Clearly, a systems approach to central responses to peripheral nerve injury is required that takes into account all cell types within the CNS and the relative interplay between them. Neuronal-microglial communication is a bidirectional process, and a growing body of evidence indicates purinergic signaling as a key molecular component (Di Virgilio 2006). Neuronal release of adenosine triphosphate (ATP) directly modulates microglial functioning, and microglia are known to release a myriad array of cytokines, chemokines, and neurotrophic factors that in turn may have a profound effect on neuronal function (DeLeo and Yezierski 2001; Watkins et al. 2001; Tsuda et al. 2005; Inoue and Tsuda 2006).

SOURCE OF ATP IN CHRONIC PAIN STATES

ATP has been proposed to mediate both neuronal and injury-induced activation of microglia (Zimmerman 1994). ATP is released from damaged and/or inflamed tissue, from central terminals of nociceptive afferents within the spinal cord (Bardoni et al. 1997), and from astrocytes during calcium wave propagation. It is conceivable, therefore, that damage to a peripheral nerve will result in the release of ATP (among other molecules) from the nociceptive primary afferent terminals. This local release in itself will result in activation of microglia and in their recruitment to the source of ATP (Davalos et al. 2005). Whether continuous ATP release from peripherally damaged primary afferents is in itself sufficient to maintain chronic pain states is unlikely.

ATP-RECEPTOR EXPRESSION ON SPINAL MICROGLIA

ATP is an endogenous ligand for the P2 purinergic receptor family. Expressed on many cell types, the P2 family can be divided into two subgroups: the G-protein-coupled P2Y receptors and the ATP-gated cation channels of the P2X receptors. In neurons, ATP, acting through various P2 receptors, has been shown to be explicitly involved in both nonpathological pain transmission and pain hypersensitivity (Salter et al. 1993; Liu and Salter 2005; Burnstock 2006), specifically acute pain and inflammatory hyperalgesia (Liu and Salter 2005). There is a wide expression of P2Y receptors on microglia, including P2Y1, 2, 4, 6, and 12 receptors (Bouscein et al. 2003; Sasaki et al. 2003; Farber and Kettenmann 2005; Inoue and Tsuda 2006). No clear role for P2Y receptors in pain processing in the spinal cord has been described, their effects being related to chemotaxis and migration toward areas of damage. P2X receptor expression on microglia is restricted to P2X4 and P2X7 (Ferrari et al. 1996; Collo et al. 1997; Tsuda et al. 2003); the potential role of each of these receptor subtypes in mediating neuropathic pain is described below.

RESPONSE OF SPINAL MICROGLIA
TO PERIPHERAL NERVE INJURY

Conventionally regarded as macrophages, reactive microglia clearly have far more diverse roles within the CNS, responding to conditions such as trauma, ischemia, inflammation, and infection. Under normal homeostatic conditions, microglia appear to be dormant, with a small soma and long spindle-like processes radiating outwards. Although this state has long been described as a "resting" state, it is now clear that far from being inactive, microglia continuously monitor their local microenvironment and are able to mount responses to adverse stimuli within seconds (Nedergaard et al. 2003; Davalos et al. 2005). In experiments in which microglia have been imaged in vivo, local damage to the microenvironment elicits a rapid response whereby the microglia extend processes via an ATP-dependent mechanism that converge on the site of injury (Davalos et al. 2005). Longer-term changes occur in a process previously described as "activation" that includes changes in morphology, gene expression, migration, and proliferation (Kreutzberg 1996; Stoll and Jander 1999; Nakajima and Kohsaka 2001; Perry 2004). The process of activation remains a contentious issue. Although the term is often used to describe a single phenotype or event, "activation" is best described as a continuum of events that occur on a time scale of seconds to several days. A stereotypical "activation" response of spinal microglia has been reported in all experimental models of neuropathic pain involving peripheral nerve injury, such as ligation, compression, or transection (Liu et al. 1995; Tsuda et al. 2003; Zhang and De Koninck 2006). This response is typified by an increase in the number and density of microglia in the ipsilateral spinal cord; the degree to which this increase represents proliferation of resident spinal microglia versus infiltration of macrophages remains unclear, although evidence suggests that both occur. This response is accompanied by a distinct anatomical change in the morphology of the microglia, from the ramified, "resting" state to an ameboid, "activated" state.

This stage of activation of microglia is characterized by the production and secretion of proinflammatory cytokines that may contribute to the initiation and maintenance of pain hypersensitivity. Other proteins indicative of activation include members of the complement cascade: complement receptor 3 (CR3), Toll-like receptor 4 (TLR4), CD14, CD4, and major histocompatibility complex (MHC) class I and II. The upregulation of many of these markers in the spinal cord has long been correlated with peripheral nerve injury (Streit et al. 1988; Eriksson et al. 1993; Liu et al. 1995) and was later recognized to coincide with the onset of allodynia (Colburn et al. 1997, 1999; Coyle 1998), but it is only recently that a causal role of microglial activation in nerve-injury-induced pain behaviors has been established (Jin et al. 2003; Tsuda et al. 2003).

NEUROPATHIC PAIN IS MEDIATED BY MICROGLIAL P2X4-RECEPTOR ACTIVATION

The essential role of the P2X4 purinoceptor in mediating pain behaviors following peripheral nerve injury was first demonstrated by Tsuda et al. (2003). By pharmacological manipulation of the P2X receptor family, these investigators were able to determine the receptor subtypes active in central responses to peripheral nerve injury. Previous studies, focusing on the neuronal expression of P2X receptors, had suggested that P2X2 and P2X3 are abundantly expressed specifically on nociceptive neurons (Vulchanova et al. 1997; Novakovich et al. 1999). However, pharmacological blockade of these two receptors by intrathecal injection of a known antagonist, pyridoxal-phosphate-6-azophenyl-2',4'-disulfonate (PPADS), had no effect on the established allodynia, whereas treatment with an alternative P2X antagonist, the ATP analogue trinitrophenyl adenosine triphosphate (TNP-ATP), produced a rapid and transient reversal of the nerve-injury-induced pain behavior. The pharmacological profiles of these two antagonists suggested that P2X4 receptors were being selectively targeted. Subsequent experiments revealed an increase in P2X4 protein in the ipsilateral dorsal horn as soon as 1 day following peripheral nerve injury and that treatment with P2X4 antisense significantly attenuated the pain behavior. Further examination of the P2X4 protein upregulation revealed it to be restricted to microglia within the spinal dorsal horn. Together, this combination of pharmacological, molecular, and behavioral findings (Tsuda et al. 2003) indicated that ATP, acting through P2X4 receptors on spinal microglia, is necessary to induce the tactile allodynia associated with neuropathic pain.

The mechanism underlying P2X4-receptor upregulation in the spinal cord following injury to a peripheral nerve is not yet clear. As described above, the process of microglial "activation" involves a cascade or continuum of events. One facet of this process is a wide-ranging increase in transcription (Perry 1994; Wieseler-Frank et al. 2005), which may include the P2X4 receptor (Inoue and Tsuda 2006), although transcription factors and specific promoter regions involved in the regulation of the P2X4 gene remain unidentified. However, key intracellular signaling molecules with known transcriptional activity are modulated by peripheral nerve injury. Pharmacological inhibition of p38 and extracellular signal-regulated kinase (ERK)—two members of the family of mitogen-activated protein kinases—has been shown to both reverse and prevent the maintenance and induction of allodynia following experimental peripheral nerve lesions (Jin et al. 2003; Schafers et al. 2003; Tsuda et al. 2004; Zhuang et al. 2005). Indeed, peripheral nerve injury leads to a persistent, microglial-specific activation of p38. The maintenance of behavioral pain states is therefore dependent upon both P2X4-receptor and p38 protein expression. Whether the pathways influenced by P2X4-receptor activation and p38 phosphorylation are parallel or convergent is not known, but it is tempting to speculate a transcriptional role for p38 on P2X4 gene expression.

A recently proposed mechanism for P2X4-receptor upregulation following peripheral nerve injury involves the extracellular matrix molecule fibronectin (Nasu-Tada et al. 2006). Fibronectin is upregulated in the ipsilateral dorsal horn as a consequence of nerve injury and is consequently ideally placed to influence P2X4-receptor expression. Microglia grown in culture in the presence of fibronectin show a marked increase in P2X4-receptor expression and a consequent enhanced calcium response to ATP stimulation.

In neurons, P2X4 receptors are constitutively internalized and reinserted into the membrane (Bobanovic et al. 2002). Whether this is also the case for microglial P2X4 receptors is not known. Enhanced protein translation, such as through an interaction with fibronectin or augmented trafficking, could influence the potential of ATP to modulate the P2X4-expressing cell. Clearly, multiple potential pathways exist through which P2X4-receptor expression can be increased following damage to a peripheral nerve. Whichever mechanisms are elucidated as key in controlling receptor expression hold great therapeutic potential for future treatment of neuropathic disorders.

MODULATION OF NEURONAL EXCITABILITY AS A MECHANISM OF NEUROPATHIC PAIN: THE ROLE OF MICROGLIAL P2X4-RECEPTOR ACTIVATION

Traditionally, research into the mechanisms underlying pain states has concentrated on neuronal activity. It is now clear that this focus reflects a limited view of the complex cellular interactions that occur within the CNS. However, the perception of pain requires the involvement and active participation of higher CNS centers. Whatever the central changes at the spinal level following damage to a peripheral nerve, some form of altered communication to the brain is inevitable, and it is at this point that neuronal activity is key.

Pharmacological approaches to tackling pain have in general been restricted to manipulating ligand-receptor interactions, blocking neurotransmitter release, and modifying enzyme activity. That much of the suffering due to neuropathic pain still persists is testament to the inefficacy of such approaches. As stated above, the cellular environment of the spinal dorsal horn consists of a rich lattice of multiple cell types. Within the neuronal population there is considerable diversity, with excitation driven by primary afferent input and dampened by local and descending inhibitory circuitry. A large proportion of inhibitory control occurs via postsynaptic action on second-order dorsal horn neurons. Any imbalance in these competing systems will have profound effects on local excitability and subsequent ascending transmission.

Changes in dorsal horn neuronal excitability can be achieved by increasing the excitatory input, or by decreasing the inhibitory tone. This concept of disinhibition has been of considerable interest as a key mediator of the transmission of augmented sensory input to higher CNS regions in neuropathic pain states. Disinhibition permits polysynaptic low-threshold inputs to influence nociceptive pathways that are normally suppressed by local inhibitory activity. Furthermore, disinhibition can reverse the action of gamma-aminobutyric acid (GABA) to a net excitation, thereby mediating a direct excitatory effect on nociceptive pathways by low-threshold input.

Inhibitory transmission, be it GABAergic or glycinergic, is mediated by the net flow of chloride ions. For chloride to pass through open channels on the neuronal membrane, it must be driven by an electrical gradient. In normal inhibitory function, chloride ions pass from the extracellular space, an area of relatively high chloride concentration, into neurons where the chloride concentration is maintained at a low level by the actions of cation-chloride cotransporters. These cotransporters establish and maintain the reversal potential for GABAergic and glycinergic receptor channels and therefore directly control chloride ion flux.

The two classes of chloride cotransporters are the potassium-chloride cotransporters (KCCs) and the sodium-potassium cotransporters (NKCCs). In the dorsal horn, the latter are restricted to primary afferent terminals; the former are expressed by intrinsic neurons and comprise the focus of this section. One mechanism of increasing dorsal horn excitability following peripheral nerve injury that has recently been demonstrated in the spinal dorsal horn is a depolarizing shift in the chloride reversal potential (Coull et al. 2003). The shift was demonstrated in lamina I neurons, which constitute one of the main ascending nociceptive pathways, and was shown to be mediated by a marked decrease in KCC2 protein expression in those neurons.

Further experiments to elucidate the potential of altered KCC2 levels to influence neuronal excitability using antagonists or antisense targeted against the gene resulted in a much reduced nociceptive threshold, in effect mimicking the behavioral consequences of peripheral nerve injury. Disrupted anion homeostasis of lamina I neurons was sufficient to mediate the effect. Seemingly subtle changes in the balance of inhibition may have compounding effects as a consequence of disinhibition, resulting in net excitation, mediated through voltage-sensitive calcium channels and *N*-methyl D-aspartate (NMDA) receptors.

The role in neuropathic pain states of the dorsal horn neuron chloride reversal potential and of P2X4-receptor-expressing microglia in the spinal cord raised the question of whether one may influence the other. Microglia had not been considered a component in what was hitherto considered a neurocentric spinal neural network that processes and relays nociceptive input from the periphery. However, much is known of the responses of microglia to peripheral nerve injury, including the fact that their subsequent "activation" includes the release of many pro-inflammatory molecules. Is it possible that one of these molecules may have the potential to influence the chloride reversal potential of lamina I projection neurons and therefore directly influence nociceptive processing at the spinal level? This question was recently addressed by Coull et al. (2005). The microglial transfer experiments first demonstrated by Tsuda et al. (2003) showed that ATP acting through P2X4 receptors in microglia was necessary to maintain neuropathic pain states. In a further series of experiments by Coull et al. (2005), electrophysiological recordings were made from lamina I neurons in slices taken from rats that had behavioral allodynia induced by the intrathecal application of ATP-stimulated microglia. The results showed not only that the rats' behavior mimicked that of rats that had previously received a peripheral nerve injury, but that the chloride reversal potential also mimicked that found in the injured rats, with a significant depolarizing shift.

It is clear that microglia are capable of releasing a complex inflammatory "soup" of chemokines, cytokines, and other molecules, at least one of which must be capable of affecting neuronal chloride homeostasis. A series of experiments by Kaila and colleagues on hippocampal excitability had implicated brain-derived neurotrophic factor (BDNF) as a key modulator of anion gradients through a direct action on KCC2 expression (Rivera et al. 2002, 2004, 2005). BDNF has been implicated as a key mediator of central nociceptive processing for many years, although the main focus of research has been neuronally derived BDNF. Evidence suggests that inflammatory pain is indeed mediated by neuronally derived BDNF (Kerr et al. 1999; Mannion et al. 1999). Compelling evidence comes from the demonstration of a conditional knockout mouse where BDNF was selectively removed from nociceptive sensory neurons (Zhao et al. 2006). In these animals, pain-related behaviors were markedly reduced, both at basal levels and particularly in response to inflammation.

Intrathecal administration of BDNF induces an allodynic-like state in naive rats. Furthermore, subsequent electrophysiological studies on these rats show a depolarized anion reversal potential (Coull et al. 2005). The potential key role of BDNF as a mediator of neuropathic pain was strengthened by the demonstration that both function-blocking tropomyosin-related kinase B (trkB) antibodies and BDNF-sequestering TrkB-Fc fusion proteins reverse the behavioral consequences of peripheral nerve injury (Coull et al. 2005), indicating that BDNF-trkB signaling is a vital component of neuropathic pain.

The evidence that BDNF is microglially derived came from experiments in which cultured microglia were treated with siRNA targeted against BDNF before being stimulated with ATP and intrathecally injected into naive rats. This treatment resulted in a rapid onset of mechanical allodynia (within 5 hours) and a concomitant depolarizing shift in the chloride reversal potential of lamina I neurons recorded from slices taken from the same animals, again effectively mimicking the behavioral and physiological consequences of peripheral nerve injury. In vitro, ATP treatment of purified microglial cultures stimulated the secretion of BDNF, and this release was also preventable by TNP-ATP and prior siRNA transfection of the microglia. Taken together, this series of experiments clearly shows that P2X4-receptor activation is a key component of the signaling pathway, leading to a collapse of the transmembrane anion gradient of lamina I neurons, and that BDNF is a crucial component of that pathway (Fig. 1). Whether BDNF release from endogenous spinal microglia acts directly on lamina I neurons following peripheral nerve injury to set off the cascade of physiological and biophysical events that leads to a behavioral mechanical allodynia—a model of the neuropathic pain state—remains to be shown conclusively. Other sources of BDNF are conceivable and it is present in the central terminals of unmyelinated primary afferents in the superficial dorsal horn (Mannion et al. 1999; Thompson et al. 1999). However, mice engineered to remove all small sensory neuron-derived BDNF show deficits in inflammatory hyperalgesia, but no difference from wild-type mice in nerve-injury-induced allodynia (Zhao et al. 2006). This finding is consistent with a role for microglially derived BDNF in post-nerve-injury chronic pain states.

ROLE OF MICROGLIAL P2X7 RECEPTORS IN NEUROPATHIC PAIN

Functional P2X7 receptors are also expressed on microglia, and their activation has been implicated in microglial responses to CNS inflammation, resulting in hyperactive microglia and extensive cytokine release (Ferrari et al. 1997a,b; Brough et al. 2002; Chafke et al. 2002). Recent evidence has suggested an important role for P2X7 activation in controlling microglial proliferation (Bianco et al. 2006). Studies of P2X7 knockout mice revealed deficits in both inflammatory and neuropathic pain responses. However, P2X7-receptor expression is not limited to microglia, with receptors found on astrocytes and

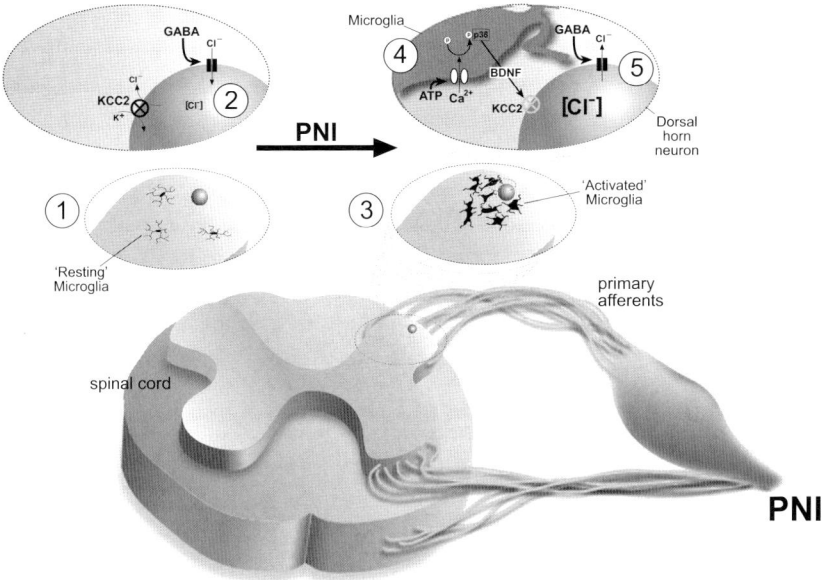

Fig. 1. Peripheral nerve injury elicits considerable functional changes in spinal microglia. Key to these changes are purinoceptors, which play a central role in the pathophysiology of neuropathic pain. The behavioral allodynia that accompanies post-nerve-injury pain states is mediated by activity of the P2X4 receptor and by the release of brain-derived neurotrophic factor (BDNF) from microglia. In turn, BDNF signals to second-order neurons within the spinal cord, resulting in enhanced excitability of spinal neuronal functioning. PNI = peripheral nerve injury.

presynaptic terminals of primary afferents (Deuchars et al. 2001; Chessell et al. 2005), although this evidence remains contentious (Sim et al. 2004).

CONCLUDING REMARKS

In the naive animal, microglia in the spinal dorsal horn exist in a lattice-like pattern, each contained within its own microenvironment, which it monitors with its fine spindle-like, ramified processes (Fig. 1-1). Neurons within the superficial laminae of the dorsal horn express the potassium-chloride cotransporter KCC2, responsible for extruding chloride and maintaining low intracellular levels (Fig. 1-2). GABA-receptor activation allows chloride to pass through the open receptor pore. In the normal state, the electrical gradient maintained by the constant extrusion of intracellular chloride drives the flow of chloride ions inward, resulting in a net hyperpolarization of the neuron and therefore the substrate for inhibition. Following peripheral nerve injury there is considerable "activation" of microglia (Fig. 1-3). Individual cells retract their long processes and become more ameboid in morphology. Cell proliferation and infiltration swell the numbers of cells within the dorsal horn. Considerable phenotypic changes occur as part of microglial activation, including a large increase in the expression of the P2X4 purinoceptor. Activation of this receptor initiates a cascade of signaling processes, including phosphorylation of p38, that results in increased synthesis and secretion of BDNF (Fig. 1-4). BDNF, via neuronal trkB signaling, causes a dramatic reduction in KCC2 expression, allowing chloride to accumulate intracellularly (Fig. 1-5). This process reverses the chloride gradient such that further GABA activity results in chloride ions leaving the neuron, the physiological consequence of which is net disinhibition and an overall increase in dorsal horn excitability.

Spinal microglia are a critical cellular component of the pathway mediating transsynaptic changes in neuronal excitability as a consequence of peripheral nerve injury. The identified molecular changes that underlie this effect are the upregulation of microglial P2X4 receptors and subsequent release of BDNF to effect the neuronal changes via KCC2 downregulation. These key events represent a framework of the signaling pathway underlying neuropathic pain. Further elucidation of the signaling cascade that triggers microglial activation, of the consequent increase in P2X4-receptor expression, and of how P2X4-receptor signaling causes release of BDNF may ultimately reveal new molecular targets for novel types of analgesics that are not conceivable at present.

REFERENCES

Aldskogius H. Microglia in neuroregeneration. *Microsc Res Tech* 2001; 54:40–46.

Bardoni R, Goldstein PA, Lee CJ, Gu JG, Macdermott AB. ATP P2X receptors mediate fast synaptic transmission in the dorsal horn of the rat spinal cord. *J Neurosci* 1997; 17:5297–5304.

Bianco F, Ceruti S, Colombo A, et al. A role for P2X in microglial proliferation. *J Neurochem* 2006; 99:745–758.

Bobanovic LK, Royle SJ, Murrell-Lagnado RD. P2X receptor trafficking in neurons is subunit specific. *J Neurosci* 2002; 22:4814–4824.

Boucsein, C, Zacharias R, Farber K, et al. Purinergic receptors on microglial cells: functional expression in acute brain slices and modulation of microglial activation in vitro. *Eur J Neurosci* 2003; 17:2267–2276.

Brough D, Le Feuvre RA, Iwakura Y, Rothwell NJ. Purinergic (P2X7) receptor activation of microglia induces cell death via an interleukin-1-independent mechanism. *Mol Cell Neurosci* 2002; 19:272–280.

Chakfe Y, Seguin R, Antel JP, et al. ADP and AMP induce interleukin-1beta release from microglial cells through activation of ATP-primed P2X7 receptor channels. *J Neurosci* 2002; 22:3061–3069.

Chessell IP, Hatcher JP, Bountra C, et al. Disruption of the P2X7 purinoceptor gene abolishes chronic inflammatory and neuropathic pain. *Pain* 2005; 114:386–396.

Colburn RW, DeLeo JA, Rickman AJ, et al. Dissociation of microglial activation and neuropathic pain behaviors following peripheral nerve injury in the rat. *J Neuroimmunol* 1997; 79:163–175.

Colburn RW, Rickman AJ, DeLeo JA. The effect of site and type of nerve injury on spinal glial activation and neuropathic pain behavior. *Exp Neurol* 1999; 157:289–304.

Coull JA, Beggs S, Boudreau D, et al. BDNF from microglia causes the shift in neuronal anion gradient underlying neuropathic pain. *Nature* 2005; 438:1017–1021.

Coyle DE. Partial peripheral nerve injury leads to activation of astroglia and microglia which parallels the development of allodynic behavior. *Glia* 1998; 23:75–83.

Davalos D, Grutzendler J, Yang G, et al. ATP mediates rapid microglial response to local brain injury in vivo. *Nat Neurosci* 2005; 8:752–758.

DeLeo JA, Yezierski RP. The role of neuroinflammation and neuroimmune activation in persistent pain. *Pain* 2001; 90:1–6.

Deuchars SA, Atkinson L, Brooke RE, et al. Neuronal P2X7 receptors are targeted to presynaptic terminals in the central and peripheral nervous systems. *J Neurosci* 2001; 21:7143–7152.

Di Virgilio F. Purinergic signalling between axons and microglia. *Novartis Found Symp* 2006 276:253–258.

Eriksson NP, Persson JK, Svensson M, et al. A quantitative analysis of the microglial cell reaction in central primary sensory projection territories following peripheral nerve injury in the adult rat. *Exp Brain Res* 1993; 96:19–27.

Farber K, Kettenmann H. Physiology of microglial cells. *Brain Res Brain Res Rev* 2005; 48:133–143.

Ferrari D, Chiozzi P, Falzoni S, et al. Extracellular ATP triggers IL-1 beta release by activating the purinergic P2Z receptor of human macrophages. *J Immunol* 1997a; 159:1451–1458.

Ferrari D, Chiozzi P, Falzoni S, Hanau S, Di Virgilio F. Purinergic modulation of interleukin-1 beta release from microglial cells stimulated with bacterial endotoxin. *J Exp Med* 1997b; 185:579–582.

Inoue K, Tsuda M. The role of microglia and ATP receptors in a mechanism of neuropathic pain. *Nippon Yakurigaku Zasshi* 2006; 127:14–17.

Jin SX, Zhuang ZY, Woolf CJ, Ji RR. p38 mitogen-activated protein kinase is activated after a spinal nerve ligation in spinal cord microglia and dorsal root ganglion neurons and contributes to the generation of neuropathic pain. *J Neurosci* 2003; 23:4017–4022.

Kerr BJ, Bradbury EJ, Bennett DL, et al. Brain-derived neurotrophic factor modulates nociceptive sensory inputs and NMDA-evoked responses in the rat spinal cord. *J Neurosci* 1999; 19:5138–5148.

Kreutzberg GW. Microglia: a sensor for pathological events in the CNS. *Trends Neurosci* 1996; 19:312–318.

Light AR, Wu Y, Hughen RW, Guthrie PB. Purinergic receptors activating rapid intracellular Ca increases in microglia. *Neuron Glia Biol* 2006; 2:125–138.

Liu L, Tornqvist E, Mattsson P, et al. Complement and clusterin in the spinal cord dorsal horn and gracile nucleus following sciatic nerve injury in the adult rat. *Neuroscience* 1995; 68:167–179.

Mannion RJ, Costigan M, Decosterd I, et al. Neurotrophins: peripherally and centrally acting modulators of tactile stimulus-induced inflammatory pain hypersensitivity. *Proc Natl Acad Sci* 1999; 96:9385–9390.

Nakajima K, Kohsaka S. Microglia: activation and their significance in the central nervous system. *J Biochem (Tokyo)* 2001; 130:169–175.

Nasu-Tada K, Koizumi S, Tsuda M, Kunifusa E, Inoue K. Possible involvement of increase in spinal fibronectin following peripheral nerve injury in upregulation of microglial P2X4, a key molecule for mechanical allodynia. *Glia* 2006; 53:769–775.

Nedergaard M, Ransom B, Goldman SA. New roles for astrocytes: redefining the functional architecture of the brain. *Trends Neurosci* 2003; 26:523–530.

Novakovic SD, Kassotakis LC, Oglesby IB, et al. Immunocytochemical localization of P2X3 purinoceptors in sensory neurons in naive rats and following neuropathic injury. *Pain* 1999; 80:273–282.

Perry VH. Modulation of microglia phenotype. *Neuropathol Appl Neurobiol* 1994; 20:177.

Rivera C, Li H, Thomas-Crusells J, et al. BDNF-induced TrkB activation down-regulates the K^+-Cl^- cotransporter KCC2 and impairs neuronal Cl^- extrusion. *J Cell Biol* 2002; 159:747–752.

Rivera C, Voipio J, Thomas-Crusells J. Mechanism of activity-dependent downregulation of the neuron-specific K-Cl cotransporter KCC2. *J Neurosci* 2004; 24:4683–4691.

Rivera C, Voipio J, Kaila K. Two developmental switches in GABAergic signalling: the $K+$-Cl^- cotransporter KCC2 and carbonic anhydrase CAVII. *J Physiol* 2005; 562:27–36.

Rotshenker S. Microglia and macrophage activation and the regulation of complement-receptor-3 (CR3/MAC-1)-mediated myelin phagocytosis in injury and disease. *J Mol Neurosci* 2003; 21:65–72.

Salter MW. Cellular signalling pathways of spinal pain neuroplasticity as targets for analgesic development. *Curr Top Med Chem* 2005; 5:557–567.

Sasaki Y, Hoshi M, Akazawa C, et al. Selective expression of Gi/o-coupled ATP receptor P2Y12 in microglia in rat brain. *Glia* 2003; 44:242–250.

Schafers M, Svensson CI, Sommer C, Sorkin LS. Tumor necrosis factor-alpha induces mechanical allodynia after spinal nerve ligation by activation of p38 MAPK in primary sensory neurons. *J Neurosci* 2003; 23:2517–2521.

Scholz J, Woolf CJ. Can we conquer pain? *Nat Neurosci* 2002; (5 Suppl):1062–1067.

Sim JA, Young MT, Sung HY, North RA, Surprenant A. Reanalysis of P2X7 receptor expression in rodent brain. *J Neurosci* 2004; 24:6307–6314.

Stoll G, Jander S. The role of microglia and macrophages in the pathophysiology of the CNS. *Prog Neurobiol* 1999; 58:233–247.

Streit WJ, Graeber MB, Kreutzberg GW. Functional plasticity of microglia: a review. *Glia* 1988; 1:301–307.

Suter MR, Papaloizos M, Berde CB, et al. Development of neuropathic pain in the rat spared nerve injury model is not prevented by a peripheral nerve block. *Anesthesiology.* 2003; 99:1402–1408.

Thompson SW, Bennett DL, Kerr BJ, Bradbury EJ, McMahon SB. Brain-derived neurotrophic factor is an endogenous modulator of nociceptive responses in the spinal cord. *Proc Natl Acad Sci USA* 1999; 96:7714–7718.

Tsuda M, Shigemoto-Mogami Y, Koizumi S, et al. P2X4 receptors induced in spinal microglia gate tactile allodynia after nerve injury. *Nature* 2003; 424:778–783.

Tsuda M, Mizokoshi A, Shigemoto-Mogami Y, Koizumi S, Inoue K. Activation of p38 mitogen-activated protein kinase in spinal hyperactive microglia contributes to pain hypersensitivity following peripheral nerve injury. *Glia* 2004; 45:89–95.

Tsuda M, Inoue K, Salter MW. Neuropathic pain and spinal microglia: a big problem from molecules in "small" glia. *Trends Neurosci* 2005; 28:101–107.

Vulchanova L, Riedl MS, Shuster SJ, et al. Immunohistochemical study of the P2X2 and P2X3 receptor subunits in rat and monkey sensory neurons and their central terminals. *Neuropharmacology* 1997; 36:1229–1242.

Watkins LR, Maier SF. Glia: a novel drug discovery target for clinical pain. *Nat Rev Drug Discov* 2003; 2:973–985.

Watkins LR, Milligan ED, Maier SF, Glial activation: a driving force for pathological pain. *Trends Neurosci* 2001; 24:450–455.

Wieseler-Frank J, Maier SF, Watkins LR. Central proinflammatory cytokines and pain enhancement. *Neurosignals* 2005; 14:166–174.

Woolf CJ. Dissecting out mechanisms responsible for peripheral neuropathic pain: implications for diagnosis and therapy. *Life Sci* 2004; 74:2605–2610.

Woolf CJ, Salter MW. Neuronal plasticity: increasing the gain in pain. *Science* 2000; 288:1765–1769.

Zhang J, De Koninck Y. Spatial and temporal relationship between monocyte chemoattractant protein-1 expression and spinal glial activation following peripheral nerve injury. *J Neurochem* 2006; 97:772–783.

Zhao J, Seereeram A, Nassar MA, et al. Nociceptor-derived brain-derived neurotrophic factor regulates acute and inflammatory but not neuropathic pain. *Mol Cell Neurosci* 2006; 31:539–548.

Zhuang ZY, Gerner P, Woolf CJ, Ji RR. ERK is sequentially activated in neurons, microglia, and astrocytes by spinal nerve ligation and contributes to mechanical allodynia in this neuropathic pain model. *Pain* 2005; 114:149–159.

Zimmermann H. Signaling via ATP in the nervous system. *Trends Neurosci* 1994; 17:420–426.

Zimmermann M. Pathobiology of neuropathic pain. *Eur J Pharmacol* 2001; 429:23–37.

Correspondence to: Michael W. Salter, MD, PhD, Hospital for Sick Children, 555 University Avenue, Toronto, ON, Canada M5G 1X8. Tel: 1-416-813-6272; fax: 1-416-813-7921; email: mike.salter@utoronto.ca.

Immune and Glial Regulation of Pain, edited by Joyce
A. DeLeo, Linda S. Sorkin, and Linda R. Watkins,
IASP Press, Seattle, © 2007.

17

The Role of p38 in Microglial Regulation of Spinal Pain Processing

Camilla I. Svensson, Tony L. Yaksh, and Linda S. Sorkin

Department of Anesthesiology, University of California, San Diego, La Jolla, California, USA

MICROGLIA

Tissue and nerve injury produces profound changes in behavior reflective of a facilitated pain state. As reviewed elsewhere, such injury leads to conditions in which otherwise nonaversive stimuli elicit signs of nociception. Recently, it has become evident that microglia may be an important component of these facilitated states (for review, see McMahon et al. 2005). Microglia are one of the principal types of immune cells in the central nervous system (CNS). Microglia are rapidly activated following brain and spinal cord injury such as lesion, stroke, neurodegenerative disorders, tumor invasion, and infection. Upon activation, microglia release factors that amplify inflammatory processes, coordinate host-defense responses, and facilitate tissue repair. At the extreme of activation, microglia transform into phagocytes to remove dead cells and other debris. The consequences of microglial activation, while necessary for certain beneficial activities, also contribute to a number of pathological conditions in the CNS, particularly those involving neuronal degeneration (for review, see Kreutzberg 1996; Aschner et al. 1999).

The literature predominantly describes the activation profile of these cells based on morphological changes classically associated with "activated" microglia. Thus, microglia under quiescent conditions have small cell bodies and highly ramified processes, while after stimulation, microglia are described as activated when they become enlarged with thickened, retracted processes. This change in appearance, occurring over hours to days, is a common feature seen in the dorsal horn after peripheral nerve injury, and it correlates with the development of functionally defined changes in pain behavior (allodynia) (for review, see Tsuda et al. 2005). Such morphological changes have become useful markers of microglial participation in neuraxial processes.

Although morphological changes of microglia occur after a variety of stress-related stimuli, it has become apparent that neural function is subject to ongoing modification by microglia in a manner that is not correlated with evident changes in morphology. Recent work suggests that microglia can play an ongoing role in neural function. Consider two sets of observations. First, imaging microglia in normal brain using 2-photon confocal microscopy has revealed that microglia in a normal environment display constant extension and retraction of their processes into the adjacent three-dimensional space (Davalos et al. 2005; Nimmerjahn et al. 2005). It is hypothesized that this activity represents a chemical surveillance of the parenchymal environment and that microglia participate in the regulation and maintenance of homeostatic CNS function in the absence of injury or infection (Davalos et al. 2005; Nimmerjahn et al. 2005). In support of this theory, microglia have been shown to respond within minutes to local increases in potassium, glutamate, and adenosine triphosphate (ATP) (Norenberg et al. 1994a,b; Lopez-Redondo et al. 2000; James and Butt 2002; Franchini et al. 2004; Davalos et al. 2005). Such sensitivity to products reflective of neuronal activation and transmitter overflow link microglia to changes in synaptic activity as well as to activity in non-neuronal cell systems (e.g., overflow of glutamate from astrocytes). Second, a temporal linkage of the microglial response to neuronal function is suggested by the observation that biochemical markers of microglial function can display rapid changes in response to stimulation. Thus, p38 mitogen-activated protein kinase (MAPK) is phosphorylated in microglia under certain circumstances within minutes of stimulation, clearly well in advance of any morphological signs of activation. As will be reviewed below, inhibition of microglial p38 at those early time points has a potent effect upon behavioral function. These observations suggest not only that microglia play an important role in conditions of severe pathology, but that they may also respond to and regulate ongoing neuronal and synaptic activity.

This chapter reviews the roles that microglia and the activation of microglial p38 signaling pathways play in pain processing. At one level, this association is important in our understanding of novel mechanisms of pain processing, while at another, these models provide important insights into the role of microglia in modulation of neuronal and synaptic function.

MORPHOLOGICAL CHANGES OF MICROGLIA IN ASSOCIATION WITH SPINAL SENSITIZATION

The characteristic morphology of quiescent or "resting" microglia shows a downregulated immunophenotype. For example, they do not express many of the surface antigens typical for macrophages such as CD45 and ED1. However, they constitutively express the complement type-3 receptor complex (known as CD11b or macrophage-1 antigen [Mac-1] and recognized by the antibody OX-42) (Akiyama and McGeer 1990), and ionized calcium binding adaptor molecule 1 (Iba-1) (Ito et al. 1998). Increased expression of these markers has been associated with Alzheimer's disease, Parkinson's disease, multiple sclerosis, amyotrophic lateral sclerosis, and AIDS-related dementia. The fact that these neurodegenerative disorders evoke a response of CNS immune cells may not be surprising. However, it is noteworthy that similar morphological alterations of microglia have been observed in the dorsal horn after induction of peripheral inflammation and nerve injury. Immunohistochemical staining of the rat spinal cord using OX-42 antibodies and measurement of CD11b mRNA showed microglial activation after subcutaneous injection of zymosan or formalin into the paw, as evidenced by increased cell surface marker expression and changes in morphology in the dorsal horn at intervals of 1–7 days. Microglial activation paralleled the development and/or maintenance of zymosan and formalin-induced mechanical allodynia, respectively (Colburn et al. 1997, 1999; Fu et al. 1999; Sweitzer et al. 1999; Zhang et al. 2003; Wu et al. 2004; Clark et al. 2006). It is unclear whether spinal microglia display these signs of activation following intraplantar injection of other commonly used inflammatory triggers, such as complete Freund's adjuvant (CFA). Using CD11b expression as an indicator, some studies have shown increases in this marker in spinal dorsal horn (Raghavendra et al. 2004; but see also Zhang et al. 2003; Clark et al. 2006). Despite contradictory data with regard to morphological changes of spinal microglia in models of peripheral inflammation, there is consensus that spinal microglia hypertrophy and show morphological signs of activation after injury to peripheral nerves (see Table I) and the spinal cord (Hains and Waxman 2006; Peng et al. 2006). Time of induction and duration of morphological changes vary among the models and the investigators, but generally these structural changes have been reported to occur from 1 day to 7 weeks after nerve injury.

MICROGLIAL INVOLVEMENT IN "ACUTE" PAIN PROCESSING

Proof of rapid microglial contributions to changes in nociceptive processing is provided by the anti-allodynic effects of agents that block microglial function at early time points in chronic pain models, as well as in pain models of short duration. The tetracycline derivatives, minocycline and doxycycline, represent an important class of agents that block activation of microglia in culture and in vivo. Intrathecal injection of minocycline (Hua et al. 2005) and doxycycline (X.Y. Hua, unpublished observations) attenuates hypersensitivity

Table I
Summary of nerve injury models leading to activation* of microglia

Model	Reference
Spinal nerve ligation (SNL)	Colburn et al. 1997
	Jin et al. 2003
	Zhang et al. 2003
	Narita et al. 2006
	Rahman et al. 2006
	Zhuang et al. 2006
SNL + transection	Colburn and DeLeo 1999
	Trang et al. 2003
	Tsuda et al. 2004
Partial SNL	Coyle 1998
	Clark et al. 2007
Spinal nerve cryoneurolysis	Colburn et al. 1997
	Colburn and DeLeo 1999
Chronic constriction injury	Colburn et al. 1997
	Stuesse et al. 2000
	Zhang et al. 2003
	Durrenberger et al. 2004, 2006
	Zhang and DeKoninck 2006
Spinal nerve transection	Arruda et al. 2000
	Raghavendra et al. 2003
Inferior alveolar and mental nerve transection	Piao et al. 2006
Sciatic inflammatory neuropathy	Ledeboer et al. 2005
Nerve root ligation	Hashizume et al. 2000
Cervical nerve root compression	Hubbard and Winkelstein 2005

* Activation is based on morphological changes and increased expression of microglial markers assessed by immunohistochemistry.

in short-term inflammation such as that which develops after intraplantar carrageenan, as well as in phase 2 of the formalin model; in these models there are no apparent changes in microglial morphology. In addition, hyperalgesia induced by intrathecal injection of *N*-methyl-D-aspartate (NMDA), which gives rise to a transient thermal hyperalgesia (lasting approximately 30 minutes), was prevented by spinal pretreatment with minocycline (Hua et al. 2005). These minocycline-sensitive pain behaviors occur within minutes rather than hours or days, suggesting that spinal microglia modulate synaptic transmission in an ongoing manner. This finding places in perspective the dichotomy noted above in which microglia in the absence of morphological changes (e.g., "activated") are in an active and contributing state.

ACTIVATION OF p38 MITOGEN-ACTIVATED PROTEIN KINASES IN SPINAL MICROGLIA

p38 is a stress-activated protein kinase that was originally isolated from lipopolysaccharide (LPS)-stimulated monocytes. This kinase mediates responses to environmental stress and constitutes a point of convergence for multiple upstream signaling processes. To date four isoforms of p38 have been identified: α, β, δ, and γ. The p38 isoforms differ in their distribution, substrate preference, activation modes, and response to inhibitors (Goedert et al. 1997; Vachon et al. 2002; Pramanik et al. 2003; Pratt et al. 2003; Kuma et al. 2004). Whereas p38δ and p38γ are found only in peripheral tissues (p38δ in the lung, kidney, testis, pancreas, and small intestine; p38γ in skeletal muscle), p38α and p38β are expressed ubiquitously in most tissues, including the brain and spinal cord (Smith et al. 2000; Shi and Gaestel 2002). Several of the pharmacological inhibitors (e.g., SB203580, Scio469, VX702, and AMG548) (Lee and Dominguez 2005; O'Neill 2006) potently block activity of both p38α and p38β, while having very low affinity for p38δ and p38γ. Little is known concerning the physiological role of p38δ and p38γ, but the other two isoforms are better characterized.

EVIDENCE FOR A ROLE OF SPINAL p38 IN EXPERIMENTAL MODELS OF PAIN

Peripheral inflammation and nerve injury are associated with sensitization of specialized sensory neurons that comprise the nociceptive pathway, leading to enhanced pain sensations in response to both noxious and non-noxious stimuli (termed "hyperalgesia" and "allodynia," respectively). Facilitation of nociceptive processing at the spinal level is a critical component in states of persistent pain. An increasing number of reports suggest that hypersensitivity following peripheral injury can be induced and maintained though activation of p38-mediated intracellular signaling. This involvement has been examined by assessment of the phosphorylated (activated) state of p38 (p-p38) in spinal cord tissue by Western blotting and by immunohistochemistry (see Table II), as well as by spinal delivery of agents that block p38 activation (see Table III). For details related to those experiments, see the references in Table II and Table III.

It is evident that peripheral injury and inflammation initiate increases in spinal p38 phosphorylation and that inhibition of spinal p38 significantly prevents the hyperalgesia otherwise observed. This observation leads to the question of where the p-p38 is to be found. Immunohistochemistry demonstrates that p38 is expressed in both neurons and microglia in the resting state (Svensson et al. 2005a). Of importance, in the studies where the cellular distribution of p-p38 was examined, it frequently colocalized with microglial markers (see Table II)

Table II
Summary of studies reporting p38 phosphorylation in the spinal cord of rodents
subjected to different experimental models of pain

Model	p-p38 Assessment Method	p-p38 Localization	p-p38 Time Frame and Change	Reference
IPLT carrageenan	WB, IHC	Microglia, neuron	1 h ⇑	Hua et al. 2005
IPLT CFA	WB, IHC	Microglia	6 h–7 d ⇔	Ji et al. 2002
IPLT formalin	WB		5–15 min ⇑	Svensson et al. 2003b, 2005a
Topical capsaicin	IHC		10–60 min ⇑	Sweitzer et al. 2004
i.t. IL-1β	WB		30–240 min ⇑	Sung et al. 2005
i.t. NMDA	IHC	Microglia, neuron	10 min ⇑	Svensson et al. 2003a
i.t. SP	WB, IHC	Microglia	5–30 min ⇑	Svensson et al. 2003b, 2005a
CCI	WB			Garry et al. 2005
PSNL	IHC		21 d ⇔	Ma and Quirion 2002
SNL	WB, IHC	Microglia	1–10 d ⇑	Jin et al. 2003
SNL	WB		5 h–3 d ⇑	Schäfers et al. 2003
SNL	WB		5 h–1 d ⇑	Svensson et al. 2005b
SNL	IHC	Microglia	3–21 d ⇑	Zhuang et al. 2006
SNL + transection	WB, IHC	Microglia	7–14 d ⇑	Tsuda et al. 2004
SNL + transection	WB		5 h–3 d ⇑	Svensson et al. 2006
SCI	WB		35 d ⇑	Crown et al. 2006
SCI	IHC	Microglia	33 d ⇑	Hains and Waxman 2006
SCI	IHC	Microglia	14 d ⇑	Peng et al. 2006

Abbreviations: CCI = chronic constriction injury, CFA = complete Freund's adjuvant, IHC = immunohistochemistry, IL-1β = interleukin-1β, IPLT = intraplantar, i.t. = intrathecal, PSNL = partial spinal nerve ligation, SCI = spinal cord injury, SNL = spinal nerve ligation, SP = substance P, WB = Western blot.

such as OX-42 (see Fig. 1). Activation of p38 in microglia is not restricted to a specific condition and appears to be an important signaling pathway in a number of experimental models of pain. Increased levels of p-p38 have been reported after peripheral inflammation, nerve injury, spinal cord injury, and intrathecal injection of neurotransmitters and cytokines (see Table II).

ROLE OF MICROGLIAL p38 IN PAIN EVOKED
BY PERIPHERAL INFLAMMATION

Peripheral inflammatory events evoke activation of p38 in spinal cord microglia (Kim et al. 2002; Svensson et al. 2003a, 2005a; Hua et al. 2005). This activation is transient and occurs in the early phase of the pain state. Importantly, morphology of microglia with activated p38 at early time points is not different from that of "resting microglia," indicating that these cells can be activated, and contribute to pain processing, in the absence of overt morphological changes.

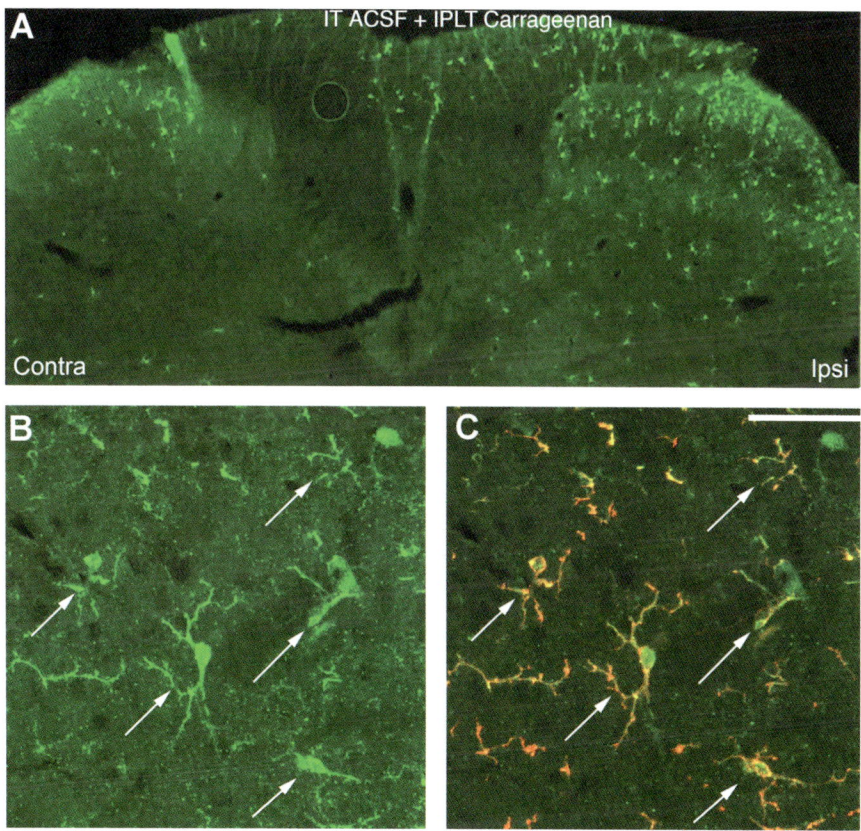

Fig. 1. (A) Image depicting phosphorylated p38 (p-p38) immunoreactivity in the lumbar dorsal horn of spinal cord from a rat 1 hour after unilateral intraplantar (IPLT) injection of carrageenan. Artificial cerebrospinal fluid (ACSF) was injected intrathecally 15 min prior to carrageenan injection. A profound increase in p-p38 immunoreactivity in the ipsilateral (Ipsi) dorsal horn (laminae I–V) was seen as compared to the contralateral side (Contra). (B) Close-up of p-p38 positive cells in the ipsilateral dorsal horn showing glia-like morphology colocalizing with the microglia marker OX-42 (red) (C), indicating that p38 is activated in microglia following peripheral inflammation. The scale bar represents 50 μm.

Table III
Summary of antinociceptive effects of intrathecal injection of p38 inhibitors
in different experimental models of pain

Model	Endpoint	Drug	Drug Effect	Reference
IPLT carrageenan	Thermal hyperalgesia	SB203580 (3–30 µg); SD-282 (30–60 µg)	Prevention of thermal hyper-algesia	Svensson et al. 2003b
IPLT capsaicin	Mechanical allodynia, thermal hyperalgesia	FR167653 (0.1–10 µg)	Prevention of thermal hyper-algesia, no effect on mechanical allodynia	Mizushima et al. 2005
IPLT CFA	Tactile allodynia	SB203580 (12 µg/d or 1 µg)	Prevention and reversal of allo-dynia	Ji et al. 2002
IPLT CFA	Cold and heat hyperalgesia	SB203580 (12 µg/d)	Prevention of heat, but not cold, hyperalgesia	Obata et al. 2005
IPLT formalin	Hindpaw flinching	SB203580 (3–30 µg); SD-282 (3–60 µg)	Prevention of 2nd phase flinching	Svensson et al. 2003b, 2005a
i.t. IL-1β	Thermal hyper-algesia	SB203580 (5 µg)	Prevention of thermal hyper-algesia	Sung et al. 2005
i.t. SP	Thermal hyper-algesia	SB203580 (3–30 µg); SD-282 (30–60 µg)	Prevention of thermal hyper-algesia	Svensson et al. 2003b, 2005a
CCI	Tactile allodynia and thermal hyperalgesia	SB203580 (12 µg/d)	Prevention of tactile and thermal hypersensitivity	Obata et al. 2004a
CCI	Tactile allodynia and thermal hyperalgesia	SB203580 (2 µg)	Reversal of tactile and thermal hypersensitivity	Garry et al. 2005
CCI	Tactile allodynia and thermal hyperalgesia	SB203580 (0.1–5 µg)	Reversal of tactile and thermal hypersensitivity	Zhang et al. 2005
SIN	Tactile allodynia	CNI-1493 (9 µg)	Prevention and reversal of allodynia	Milligan et al. 2003
SNL	Tactile allodynia	SB203580 (4 µg/d or 10 µg)	Prevention and reversal of allodynia	Jin et al. 2003

Table III (Continued)

SNL + transection	Tactile allodynia	SB203580 (11 µg/d)	Prevention of allodynia	Inoue et al. 2003
SNL + transection	Tactile allodynia	SB203580 (11 µg/d)	Prevention of allodynia	Tsuda et al. 2004
SNL + transection	Tactile allodynia and thermal hyperalgesia	SB203580 (12 µg/d)	Prevention of tactile and thermal hypersensitivity	Obata et al. 2004b

Abbreviations: CFA = complete Freund's adjuvant, IPLT = intraplantar, i.t. = intra-thecal, PSNL = partial spinal nerve ligation, SCI = spinal cord injury, SIN = sciatic inflammatory neuritis, SNL = spinal nerve ligation, SP = substance P.

Pretreatment with intrathecal injection of p38 inhibitors blocks hyperalgesia in these models (see Table III), indicating the importance of this signaling pathway in spinal sensitization induced by injection of formalin (Svensson et al. 2003b), carrageenan (Svensson et al. 2003b), or capsaicin (Sweitzer et al. 2004; Mizushima et al. 2005) to the paw. Activation of spinal p38 appears prominently only at early time points after induction of inflammation. For example, peripheral inflammation induced by carrageenan evokes a transient p38 activation peaking at 1 hour and absent at 4 and 15 hours (Svensson et al. 2005a; Beloeil et al. 2006), whereas the hyperalgesia in this model is robust for up to 24 hours. In another model in which peripheral inflammation was induced by intraplantar injection of CFA, no increase in spinal p-p38 was detected 6 hours or 7 days post-injection (Ji et al. 2002). It is possible that phosphorylation occurred at earlier time points, or that p38 does not become activated in the spinal cord in this model. However, CFA-induced activation of p38 was detected in dorsal root ganglia (DRG). It is important to note that p38 phosphorylation in the DRG was also observed in the models of nerve injury listed in Table II, indicating that p38 participates in regulation of nociceptive processing at the level of the primary afferent as well as at the spinal level.

ROLE OF MICROGLIAL p38 IN PAIN EVOKED BY NERVE INJURY

Peripheral nerve injury leads to multiple plastic alterations in spinal dorsal horn neurons and glia, and this neuroplasticity is thought to be an important component in the development of nerve-injury-evoked hyperalgesia and allodynia (for a recent review, see McMahon et al. 2005). One notable component in this scenario is activation of p38. It has been demonstrated that p38 is phosphorylated in the spinal dorsal horn after ligation of the L5 spinal nerve (SNL), modified SNL (in which L5 is ligated and then transected), chronic constriction injury (CCI), and axotomy of the sciatic nerve (see Table II). In addition, p38 is also activated in the medullary dorsal horn after inferior alveolar nerve and mental nerve transection (IAMNT) and spinal cord injury (SCI) (see Table II). Interestingly, even though p38 is expressed in spinal neurons (Svensson et al. 2005a), after nerve injury its activation seems to be restricted to microglia in the spinal cord (Jin et al. 2003). In the SNL model, p38 is activated in microglia within 1 day of nerve injury. In some studies, phosphorylation has been reported to decrease after 3 days, with a second peak of activity at 10 days post-surgery (Svensson et al. 2006), while other studies demonstrate persistent activity for up to 3 weeks (Zhuang et al. 2006). No time to onset is available for the other neuropathic pain models, but phosphorylated p38 has been reported in microglia 1 week after CCI and axotomy and 3 days after IAMNT. Pretreatment with the p38 inhibitor SB203580 attenuates allodynia both in the SNL (Inoue et al. 2003; Jin et al. 2003; Schäfers et al. 2003; Tsuda et al. 2004) and the CCI models (Zhang et al. 2005) of neuropathic pain, and intrathecal injection of the p38 inhibitor CNI-1493 prevents hyperalgesia in a model of peripheral nerve inflammation (Milligan et al. 2003) (see Table III), supporting a role for p38 in neuropathic pain processing. However, it is possible that intrathecal (i.t.) delivery of p38 inhibitors exerts additional effects at the level of the DRG. This possibility is important because it has been demonstrated that p38 is activated in DRG neurons in models of both inflammation and nerve-injury-evoked pain (Ji et al. 2002; Jin et al. 2003; Schäfers et al. 2003). Thus, it is possible that p38 contributes to hyperalgesia not only in microglia, but also in DRG neurons.

Interesting differences between laboratories have been observed with regards to the effect of postsurgical treatment with i.t. SB203580 in the SNL model. As stated above, there is agreement that pretreatment effectively blocks development of allodynia (Jin et al. 2003; Schäfers et al. 2003; Svensson et al. 2005b). In our laboratory, no antiallodynic effect was observed if treatment with p38 inhibitor was started 1 or 7 days after surgery. With regard to the time course of p38 phosphorylation in response to SNL, in our studies, p38 phosphorylation was increased in the spinal cord from 5 hours through 3 days after surgery, with a second peak at 10 days, but in DRG we observed increased p-p38 only from 5 hours to 1 day after surgery (Schäfers et al. 2003; Svensson et al. 2005b, 2006). However, lack of SB203580 post-treatment anti-allodynic effects and the brevity of the first peak of p38 phosphorylation have not been observed by others (Jin et al. 2003). These contentious findings led us to perform a series of studies to investigate the effects of age and modification of surgery (ligation alone vs. ligation and transection) on the time course of p38 phosphorylation. The outcome demonstrated that phosphorylation of p38 is sensitive to these variables (Svensson et al. 2006). Undoubtedly, these observations highlight the complexity of p38-mediated pain signaling, but an overall conclusion can be drawn: p38 is activated in response to nerve injury, and blocking that activation prevents allodynia. Clearly, standardization of experimental models of neuropathic pain is important.

ROLE OF MICROGLIAL p38 IN PAIN EVOKED BY SPINAL CORD INJURY

Spinal cord injury results not only in motor impairment, but also in chronic spontaneous and evoked pain. It is well documented that microglia display signs of activation (i.e., increased expression of Cd11b, de novo expression of ED-1 and MHC class II, and changes in morphology) in the spinal cord in models of contusion or hemisection SCI (Popovich et al. 1997; Carlson et al. 1998; Hains and Waxman 2006; Kigerl et al. 2006; Peng et al. 2006; Wang et al. 2006). Recently, it was demonstrated that phosphorylated p38 in microglia increases after SCI (Hains and Waxman 2006; Peng et al. 2006) and that reduction of p38 activity by i.t. infusion of minocycline (Hains and Waxman 2006) or by elimination of tumor necrosis factor-α (TNF-α) actions through herpes simplex virus-mediated gene transfer of the TNF soluble receptor (Peng et al. 2006) is associated with attenuation of SCI-evoked pain. It is noteworthy not only that TNF-α can drive p38 activation, but that p38 action also can lead to increased TNF-α release.

ROLE OF MICROGLIAL p38 IN PAIN EVOKED BY CENTRAL STIMULI

Human immunodeficiency virus-1 (HIV-1) envelope glycoprotein (gp120) binds to receptors on microglia and astrocytes and activates them. Intrathecal administration of gp120 evokes thermal hyperalgesia and tactile allodynia, and i.t. injection of minocycline and i.t. or systemic delivery of a p38 inhibitor (CNI-1493) (Milligan et al. 2000, 2001a,b; Ledeboer et al. 2005) blocks this hypersensitivity, indicating that microglial p38 signaling is important in this process. Minocycline also reduces spinal production and release of cytokines such as TNF and interleukin (IL)-1β, common products of p38 activation (Ledeboer et al. 2005).

Hyperalgesia is associated with persistent sensory afferent input-induced spinal sensitization. Substance P and glutamate, which are released from central terminals of afferent C fibers, contribute significantly to this facilitatory state in the spinal cord. Intrathecal injection of substance P or NMDA produces thermal hyperalgesia (Malmberg and Yaksh 1992) and leads to activation of p38 in microglia. Whether this is a direct or indirect effect on microglia is currently not known, although both NMDA and substance P activate p38 in primary microglial cultures, as stated below. Importantly, inhibition of spinal p38 using two different p38 inhibitors, SB203580 or SD-282, blocked this hyperalgesia (Svensson et al. 2003a,b).

ROLE OF MICROGLIAL p38 IN HYPERSENSITIVITY

p38 ISOFORMS

As reviewed above, two p38 isoforms are present within the CNS: p38α and p38β. It is important to note that most studies of spinal p38 in nociceptive processing have used inhibitors that block the activity of both p38α and p38β. In fact, there are no selective inhibitors for the p38 isoforms, hence the p38 inhibitors used in the studies referenced in Table I are all nonselective. Therefore, it has been difficult to determine which isoform is responsible and whether it is necessary to target both isoforms to block hypersensitivity. Immunohistochemistry indicates that p38α is expressed in neurons throughout the spinal parenchyma, whereas p38β is expressed in microglia in the dorsal horn and in microglia and large motor neurons in the ventral horn in the spinal cord of naive rats (Svensson et al. 2005a). The colocalization of activated p38 with microglial markers strongly suggests that if the role of p38 in microglia is critical to the hyperalgesic state, then the essential isoform will be p38β. Accordingly, we examined the effects of specifically downregulating the spinal expression of p38 isoforms through i.t. administration of p38-isoform-specific antisense oligonucleotides. In these studies, knock down of p38β, but not p38α, reversed the hyperalgesic states observed acutely after injection of formalin to the paw (Svensson et al. 2005a), after inflammation induced by injection of intraplantar carrageenan (X.Y. Hua and C.I. Svensson, unpublished observations), or after i.t. injection of substance P. These observations provide strong support for the thesis that it is the p38β isoform in microglia that is critical for the antihyperalgesic effect, and conversely, that the microglia are playing a critical role in the acute events that lead to hyperalgesia after peripheral inflammation and central receptor activation. Experiments with p38 knockout mice confirm that this isoform is necessary for facilitated pain behavior (Martin et al. 2005).

UPSTREAM AND DOWNSTREAM OF p38

The frequent reports that p38 is activated in spinal microglia in a variety of experimental models of pain point to an important role of this signaling pathway in pain processing. However, it is not well understood which factors are upstream and downstream of this kinase, and if those factors vary with different conditions. Below is a brief summary of mechanisms by which p38 is activated, both in neuronal and non-neuronal cells, as well as possible downstream targets by which p38 may contribute to spinal sensitization.

Activation of p38 has been observed in response to extracellular stimuli such as heat, osmotic shock, inflammatory cytokines, and growth factors. This broad range of activators conveys the complexity of the p38 pathway.

Furthermore, p38 activation depends not only on the stimulus, but also on cell type. In general, there are two distinct pathways that lead to activation of p38: (1) the mitogen-activated protein kinase kinase (MKK) pathway and (2) autophosphorylation of p38. Two principal MKKs are known to activate p38 in response to cytokines and other stressors: MKK3 and MKK6. In addition, MKK4 is reported to activate both p38 (Brancho et al. 2003) and c-Jun *N*-terminal kinase (JNK) (Derijard et al. 1995). The MKKs are activated by a variety of upstream MKK kinases. MKK6 is identified as an activator of p38α, β, and γ, while MKK3 activates only p38α and p38γ (Enslen et al. 1998), suggesting that the activation of p38 isoforms can be specifically controlled through different upstream mediators. Autophosphorylation of p38 is thought to occur through association with transforming growth factor-β-activated protein kinase 1 binding protein 1 (TAB1) (Ge et al. 2002). Interestingly, it was recently reported that neither phosphorylated MKK3, MKK4, nor MKK6 could be detected in spinal ventral horn microglia in a model of amyotrophic lateral sclerosis, despite the prominent increase of p-p38 (Veglianese et al. 2006) in these cells. This finding is in accordance with studies of dorsal horn microglia in our laboratory (L.S. Sorkin, unpublished observations) indicating that shortly after intraplantar formalin, p38 is phosphorylated in microglia, while phosphorylated MKK3 or MKK6 is confined to astrocytes.

From a mechanistic pain perspective, several factors that are released following increased neuronal activity in nociceptive afferent fibers can lead to activation of p38. However, the exact intracellular signaling pathways driving the p38 activation are not defined. Under in vitro conditions, neurotransmitters such as glutamate and substance P induce phosphorylation of p38 in primary cultures of microglia, neurons, astrocytes, and fibroblasts (Kawasaki et al. 1997; Fiebich et al. 2000; Rasley et al. 2002; Chen et al. 2003; Tokuda et al. 2005). In addition, other mediators of neuronal activity and/or CNS pathology, such as ATP, lysophosphatidic acid, TNF-α, and S100B cause activation of p38 in cultured glioma cells, microglia, macrophages, and fibroblasts (Hide et al. 2000; Adami et al. 2004; Chabaud-Riou and Firestein 2004; Malchinkhuu et al. 2005; Esposito et al. 2006). In vivo, blockade of spinal TNF-α prevents p38 phosphorylation following SNL (Svensson et al. 2005b).

Once activated, the p38 isoforms are able to phosphorylate a wide range of regulatory proteins in vitro and in vivo. p38 alters cellular activities by (1) activation of transcription factors, (2) activation of other protein kinases involved in transcription, (3) post-transcriptional regulation by mRNA stabilization, and (4) activation or enhancement of the activity of cytosolic enzymes other than kinases. Translocation of p38 to the nucleus induces transcription by phosphorylation of transcription factors such as activating transcription factor (ATF) subtypes 1, 2, and 6 and MAPK-activated protein kinase (MAPKAPK2).

MAPKAPK2 activates substrates such as lymphocyte-specific protein and cyclic adenosine monophosphate response element-binding protein (CREB). Microglia cultured ex vivo from MAPKAPK2-deficient mice have a reduced capacity to produce TNF-α in response to lipopolysaccharide (LPS) stimulation, which indicates that this signaling pathway is important for cytokine production (Culbert et al. 2006). Other substrates of p38 include mitogen and stress-activated protein kinase (MSK1), MAK kinase-interacting kinase (MNK1), and p38-regulated/activated kinase (PRAK) (for more extensive reviews, see Saklatvala 2004; Kaminska 2005; Zarubin and Han 2005).

Activated p38 can also affect protein synthesis at the post-transcriptional level. Messenger RNAs for inducible cytokines such as IL-1, IL-8, and TNF-α, as well as cyclooxygenase-2 contain an adenylate/uridylate (AU)-rich element in their 3' untranslated region that is responsible for their short half-lives. It is believed that under normal conditions, the AU-rich elements of these transcripts are occupied by AU-binding proteins and, as a result, are not translatable or are rapidly turned over. In response to stimuli such as LPS, these AU-binding proteins are phosphorylated in a p38-dependent manner, which results in stabilization and increased translation of these mRNAs (Winzen et al. 1999; Lasa et al. 2000; Ming et al. 2001; Neininger et al. 2002; Frevel et al. 2003).

A number of protein substrates are involved in cellular functions of p38 other than transcription. For example, p38 can activate calcium-dependent phospholipase A ($cPLA_2$) and 5-lipoxygenase (Kramer et al. 1996; Borsch-Haubold et al. 1997, 1999; You et al. 2005). Liberated from perinuclear cell membrane phospholipids by $cPLA_2$, arachidonic acid is converted to prostaglandins by cyclooxygenases and prostaglandin synthases. Inflammation evoked by formalin and carrageenan and intrathecal injection of agents that activate glutamate and neurokinin receptors (NMDA and substance P, respectively) evoke spinal release of PGE_2. Inhibition of spinal p38 by intrathecal injection of p38 inhibitors blocks this PGE_2 release (Svensson et al. 2003a,b), indicating a role for p38 in spinal prostaglandin-mediated sensitization.

Whereas many lines of evidence point to a role of microglia in spinal sensitization based on microglial morphology and the use of microglial modulators, less is known about the molecular mechanism by which microglia contribute to the development and maintenance of pain states. Research from other areas has shown that microglia, in common with other cells of monocyte–macrophage lineage, produce and secrete cytokines (Hanisch 2002) and chemokines (Ambrosini and Aloisi 2004). A number of reports indicate that these types of proinflammatory factors play an important role in spinal sensitization (for review, see Abbadie 2005; Wieseler-Frank et al. 2005). For example, peripheral and central inflammation and peripheral nerve injury lead to the central synthesis and release of cytokines involved in spinal pain processing such as TNF, IL-1, and

IL-6 (Milligan et al. 2001b; Samad et al. 2001; Beloeil et al. 2006), and p38 is known to be involved in regulating the synthesis of these molecules. However, although it is not fully understood which spinal cell type (at what time point) is responsible for the release of cytokines and chemokines, microglia clearly have the capacity to release them. For example, microglia release IL-1β, IL-6, TNF-α, CCL2 (monocyte chemoattractant protein-1, MCP-1), CCL3 (macrophage inflammatory protein-1α, MIP-1α), CCL4 (MIP-1β), CCL5 (RANTES), and CXCL8 (IL-8) (Hanisch 2002; Lee et al. 2002). Microglia also express receptors for cytokines and chemokines such as IL-1, IL-6, IL-8, TNF-α (Hanisch 2002; Lee et al. 2002; Ambrosini and Aloisi 2004), and fractalkine (Verge et al. 2004), indicating that microglia can respond to and be activated by these pro-inflammatory cytokines and thereby participate in spinal sensitization and development of hyperalgesia and allodynia.

SUMMARY

Microglia constantly sample their microenvironment. In response to short-term and long-term changes in their extracellular environment, microglia release factors that contribute to spinal sensitization and pain behavior. These processes are triggered by peripheral inflammation, by nerve and spinal cord injury, and by various pathological states, such as the presence of gp120 in the spinal cord. Activation of microglial p38 is a frequent feature of induction and maintenance of hypersensitivity. The time course of biochemical sequelae of microglial activation, e.g., signaling through the p38 pathway, and structural changes in microglia do not necessarily parallel each other, highlighting the fact that microglia may contribute to spinal sensitization in different ways depending on the particular conditions. Spinal inhibition of microglial p38 reduces allodynia and hyperalgesia in a number of inflammatory and neuropathic pain models, indicating the importance of this signaling pathway in spinal pain processing. Intriguingly, knockdown of p38β, the p38 isoform expressed in microglia, reduces hypersensitivity in models of inflammation, suggesting that this isoform plays a dominant role in inflammatory pain.

REFERENCES

Abbadie C. Chemokines, chemokine receptors and pain. *Trends Immunol* 2005; 26:529–534.
Adami C, Bianchi R, Pula G, Donato R. S100B-stimulated NO production by BV-2 microglia is independent of RAGE transducing activity but dependent on RAGE extracellular domain. *Biochim Biophys Acta* 2004; 1742:169–177.
Akiyama H, McGeer PL. Brain microglia constitutively express beta-2 integrins. *J Neuroimmunol* 1990; 30:81–93.

Ambrosini E, Aloisi F. Chemokines and glial cells: a complex network in the central nervous system. *Neurochem Res* 2004; 29:1017–1038.

Arruda JL, Sweitzer S, Rutkowski MD, DeLeo JA. Intrathecal anti-IL-6 antibody and IgG attenuates peripheral nerve injury-induced mechanical allodynia in the rat: possible immune modulation in neuropathic pain. *Brain Res* 2000; 879:216–225.

Aschner M, Allen JW, Kimelberg HK, et al. Glial cells in neurotoxicity development. *Annu Rev Pharmacol Toxicol* 1999; 39:151–173.

Beloeil H, Ji RR, Berde CB. Effects of bupivacaine and tetrodotoxin on carrageenan-induced hind paw inflammation in rats (Part 2): Cytokines and p38 mitogen-activated protein kinases in dorsal root ganglia and spinal cord. *Anesthesiology* 2006; 105:139–145.

Borsch-Haubold AG, Kramer RM, Watson SP. Phosphorylation and activation of cytosolic phospho-lipase A2 by 38-kDa mitogen-activated protein kinase in collagen-stimulated human platelets. *Eur J Biochem* 1997; 245:751–759.

Borsch-Haubold AG, Ghomashchi F, Pasquet S, et al. Phosphorylation of cytosolic phospholipase A2 in platelets is mediated by multiple stress-activated protein kinase pathways. *Eur J Biochem* 1999; 265:195–203.

Brancho D, Tanaka N, Jaeschke A, et al. Mechanism of p38 MAP kinase activation in vivo. *Genes Dev* 2003; 17:1969–1978.

Carlson SL, Parrish ME, Springer JE, Doty K, Dossett L. Acute inflammatory response in spinal cord following impact injury. *Exp Neurol* 1998; 151:77–88.

Chabaud-Riou M, Firestein GS. Expression and activation of mitogen-activated protein kinase kinases-3 and -6 in rheumatoid arthritis. *Am J Pathol* 2004; 164:177–184.

Chen RW, Qin ZH, Ren M, et al. Regulation of c-Jun N-terminal kinase, p38 kinase and AP-1 DNA binding in cultured brain neurons: roles in glutamate excitotoxicity and lithium neuroprotection. *J Neurochem* 2003; 84:566–575.

Clark AK, Gentry C, Bradbury EJ, McMahon SB, Malcangio M. Role of spinal microglia in rat models of peripheral nerve injury and inflammation. *Eur J Pain* 2007; 11:223–230.

Colburn RW, DeLeo JA. The effect of perineural colchicine on nerve injury-induced spinal glial activation and neuropathic pain behavior. *Brain Res Bull* 1999; 49:419–427.

Colburn RW, DeLeo JA, Rickman AJ, et al. Dissociation of microglial activation and neuro-pathic pain behaviors following peripheral nerve injury in the rat. *J Neuroimmunol* 1997; 79:163–175.

Colburn RW, Rickman AJ, DeLeo JA. The effect of site and type of nerve injury on spinal glial activation and neuropathic pain behavior. *Exp Neurol* 1999; 157:289–304.

Coyle DE. Partial peripheral nerve injury leads to activation of astroglia and microglia which parallels the development of allodynic behavior. *Glia* 1998; 23:75–83.

Crown ED, Ye Z, Johnson KM, et al. Increases in the activated forms of ERK 1/2, p38 MAPK, and CREB are correlated with the expression of at-level mechanical allodynia following spinal cord injury. *Exp Neurol* 2006; 199:397–407.

Culbert AA, Skaper SD, Howlett DR, et al. MAPK-activated protein kinase 2 deficiency in mi-croglia inhibits pro-inflammatory mediator release and resultant neurotoxicity. Relevance to neuroinflammation in a transgenic mouse model of Alzheimer disease. *J Biol Chem* 2006; 281:23658–23667.

Davalos D, Grutzendler J, Yang G, et al. ATP mediates rapid microglial response to local brain injury in vivo. *Nat Neurosci* 2005; 8:752–758.

Derijard B, Raingeaud J, Barrett T, et al. Independent human MAP-kinase signal transduction pathways defined by MEK and MKK isoforms. *Science* 1995; 267:682–685.

Durrenberger PF, Facer P, Gray RA, et al. Cyclooxygenase-2 (Cox-2) in injured human nerve and a rat model of nerve injury. *J Peripher Nerv Syst* 2004; 9:15–25.

Durrenberger PF, Facer P, Casula MA, et al. Prostanoid receptor EP1 and Cox-2 in injured human nerves and a rat model of nerve injury: a time-course study. *BMC Neurol* 2006; 6:1.

Enslen H, Raingeaud J, Davis RJ. Selective activation of p38 mitogen-activated protein (MAP) kinase isoforms by the MAP kinase kinases MKK3 and MKK6. *J Biol Chem* 1998; 273:1741–1748.

Esposito G, De Filippis D, Cirillo C, et al. The astroglial-derived S100beta protein stimulates the expression of nitric oxide synthase in rodent macrophages through p38 MAP kinase activation. *Life Sci* 2006; 78:2707–2715.

Fiebich BL, Schleicher S, Butcher RD, Craig A, Lieb K. The neuropeptide substance P activates p38 mitogen-activated protein kinase resulting in IL-6 expression independently from NF-kappa B. *J Immunol* 2000; 165:5606–5611.

Franchini L, Levi G, Visentin S. Inwardly rectifying K^+ channels influence Ca^{2+} entry due to nucleotide receptor activation in microglia. *Cell Calcium* 2004; 35:449–459.

Frevel MA, Bakheet T, Silva AM, et al. p38 Mitogen-activated protein kinase-dependent and -independent signaling of mRNA stability of AU-rich element-containing transcripts. *Mol Cell Biol* 2003; 23:425–436.

Fu KY, Light AR, Matsushima GK, Maixner W. Microglial reactions after subcutaneous formalin injection into the rat hind paw. *Brain Res* 1999; 825:59–67.

Garry EM, Delaney A, Blackburn-Munro G, et al. Activation of p38 and p42/44 MAP kinase in neuropathic pain: involvement of $VPAC_2$ and NK_2 receptors and mediation by spinal glia. *Mol Cell Neurosci* 2005; 30:523–537.

Ge B, Gram H, Di Padova F, et al. MAPKK-independent activation of p38alpha mediated by TAB1-dependent autophosphorylation of p38alpha. *Science* 2002; 295:1291–1294.

Goedert M, Cuenda A, Craxton M, Jakes R, Cohen P. Activation of the novel stress-activated protein kinase SAPK4 by cytokines and cellular stresses is mediated by SKK3 (MKK6); comparison of its substrate specificity with that of other SAP kinases. *Embo J* 1997; 16:3563–3571.

Hains BC, Waxman SG. Activated microglia contribute to the maintenance of chronic pain after spinal cord injury. *J Neurosci* 2006; 26:4308–4317.

Hanisch UK. Microglia as a source and target of cytokines. *Glia* 2002; 40:140–155.

Hashizume H, DeLeo JA, Colburn RW, Weinstein JN. Spinal glial activation and cytokine expression after lumbar root injury in the rat. *Spine* 2000; 25:1206–1217.

Hide I, Tanaka M, Inoue A, et al. Extracellular ATP triggers tumor necrosis factor-alpha release from rat microglia. *J Neurochem* 2000; 75:965–972.

Hua XY, Svensson CI, Matsui T, et al. Intrathecal minocycline attenuates peripheral inflammation-induced hyperalgesia by inhibiting p38 MAPK in spinal microglia. *Eur J Neurosci* 2005; 22:2431–2440.

Hubbard RD, Winkelstein BA. Transient cervical nerve root compression in the rat induces bilateral forepaw allodynia and spinal glial activation: mechanical factors in painful neck injuries. *Spine* 2005; 30:1924–1932.

Inoue K, Koizumi S, Tsuda M, Shigemoto-Mogami Y. Signaling of ATP receptors in glia-neuron interaction and pain. *Life Sci* 2003; 74:189–197.

Ito D, Imai Y, Ohsawa K, et al. Microglia-specific localisation of a novel calcium binding protein, Iba1. *Brain Res Mol Brain Res* 1998; 57:1–9.

James G, Butt AM. P2Y and P2X purinoceptor mediated Ca^{2+} signalling in glial cell pathology in the central nervous system. *Eur J Pharmacol* 2002; 447:247–260.

Ji RR, Samad TA, Jin SX, Schmoll R, Woolf CJ. p38 MAPK activation by NGF in primary sensory neurons after inflammation increases TRPV1 levels and maintains heat hyperalgesia. *Neuron* 2002; 36:57–68.

Jin SX, Zhuang ZY, Woolf CJ, Ji RR. p38 mitogen-activated protein kinase is activated after a spinal nerve ligation in spinal cord microglia and dorsal root ganglion neurons and contributes to the generation of neuropathic pain. *J Neurosci* 2003; 23:4017–4022.

Kaminska B. MAPK signalling pathways as molecular targets for anti-inflammatory therapy—from molecular mechanisms to therapeutic benefits. *Biochim Biophys Acta* 2005; 1754:253–262.

Kawasaki H, Morooka T, Shimohama S, et al. Activation and involvement of p38 mitogen-activated protein kinase in glutamate-induced apoptosis in rat cerebellar granule cells. *J Biol Chem* 1997; 272:18518–18521.

Kigerl KA, McGaughy VM, Popovich PG. Comparative analysis of lesion development and intraspinal inflammation in four strains of mice following spinal contusion injury. *J Comp Neurol* 2006; 494:578–594.

Kim SY, Bae JC, Kim JY, et al. Activation of p38 MAP kinase in the rat dorsal root ganglia and spinal cord following peripheral inflammation and nerve injury. *Neuroreport* 2002; 13:2483–2486.

Kramer RM, Roberts EF, Um SL, et al. p38 mitogen-activated protein kinase phosphorylates cytosolic phospholipase A2 (cPLA2) in thrombin-stimulated platelets. Evidence that proline-directed phosphorylation is not required for mobilization of arachidonic acid by cPLA2. *J Biol Chem* 1996; 271:27723–27729.

Kreutzberg GW. Microglia: a sensor for pathological events in the CNS. *Trends Neurosci* 1996; 19:312–318.

Kuma Y, Campbell DG, Cuenda A. Identification of glycogen synthase as a new substrate for stress-activated protein kinase 2b/p38beta. *Biochem J* 2004; 379:133–139.

Lasa M, Mahtani KR, Finch A, et al. Regulation of cyclooxygenase 2 mRNA stability by the mitogen-activated protein kinase p38 signaling cascade. *Mol Cell Biol* 2000; 20:4265–4274.

Ledeboer A, Sloane EM, Milligan ED, et al. Minocycline attenuates mechanical allodynia and pro-inflammatory cytokine expression in rat models of pain facilitation. *Pain* 2005; 115:71–83.

Lee MR, Dominguez C. MAP kinase p38 inhibitors: clinical results and an intimate look at their interactions with p38alpha protein. *Curr Med Chem* 2005; 12:2979–2994.

Lee YB, Nagai A, Kim SU. Cytokines, chemokines, and cytokine receptors in human microglia. *J Neurosci Res* 2002; 69:94–103.

Lopez-Redondo F, Nakajima K, Honda S, Kohsaka S. Glutamate transporter GLT-1 is highly expressed in activated microglia following facial nerve axotomy. *Brain Res Mol Brain Res* 2000; 76:429–435.

Ma W, Quirion R. Partial sciatic nerve ligation induces increase in the phosphorylation of extracellular signal-regulated kinase (ERK) and c-Jun N-terminal kinase (JNK) in astrocytes in the lumbar spinal dorsal horn and the gracile nucleus. *Pain* 2002; 99:175–184.

Malchinkhuu E, Sato K, Horiuchi Y, et al. Role of p38 mitogen-activated kinase and c-Jun terminal kinase in migration response to lysophosphatidic acid and sphingosine-1-phosphate in glioma cells. *Oncogene* 2005; 24:6676–6688.

Malmberg AB, Yaksh TL. Hyperalgesia mediated by spinal glutamate or substance P receptor blocked by spinal cyclooxygenase inhibition. *Science* 1992; 257:1276–1279.

Martin WM, Murphy BA, Parsons J, et al. p38b contributes to injury-induced nociceptive, but not inflammatory responses in mice. *Soc Neurosci Abstracts* 2005; 393.6.

McMahon SB, Cafferty WB, Marchand F. Immune and glial cell factors as pain mediators and modulators. *Exp Neurol* 2005; 192:444–462.

Milligan ED, Mehmert KK, Hinde JL, et al. Thermal hyperalgesia and mechanical allodynia produced by intrathecal administration of the human immunodeficiency virus-1 (HIV-1) envelope glycoprotein, gp120. *Brain Res* 2000; 861:105–116.

Milligan ED, O'Connor KA, Armstrong CB, et al. Systemic administration of CNI-1493, a p38 mitogen-activated protein kinase inhibitor, blocks intrathecal human immunodeficiency virus-1 gp120-induced enhanced pain states in rats. *J Pain* 2001a; 2:326–333.

Milligan ED, O'Connor KA, Nguyen KT, et al. Intrathecal HIV-1 envelope glycoprotein gp120 induces enhanced pain states mediated by spinal cord proinflammatory cytokines. *J Neurosci* 2001b; 21:2808–2819.

Milligan ED, Twining C, Chacur M, et al. Spinal glia and proinflammatory cytokines mediate mirror-image neuropathic pain in rats. *J Neurosci* 2003; 23:1026–1040.

Ming XF, Stoecklin G, Lu M, Looser R, Moroni C. Parallel and independent regulation of interleukin-3 mRNA turnover by phosphatidylinositol 3-kinase and p38 mitogen-activated protein kinase. *Mol Cell Biol* 2001; 21:5778–5789.

Mizushima T, Obata K, Yamanaka H, et al. Activation of p38 MAPK in primary afferent neurons by noxious stimulation and its involvement in the development of thermal hyperalgesia. *Pain* 2005; 113:51–60.

Narita M, Yoshida T, Nakajima M, et al. Direct evidence for spinal cord microglia in the development of a neuropathic pain-like state in mice. *J Neurochem* 2006; 97:1337–1348.

Neininger A, Kontoyiannis D, Kotlyarov A, et al. MK2 targets AU-rich elements and regulates biosynthesis of tumor necrosis factor and interleukin-6 independently at different post-transcriptional levels. *J Biol Chem* 2002; 277:3065–3068.

Nimmerjahn A, Kirchhoff F, Helmchen F. Resting microglial cells are highly dynamic surveillants of brain parenchyma in vivo. *Science* 2005; 308:1314–1318.

Norenberg W, Gebicke-Haerter PJ, Illes P. Voltage-dependent potassium channels in activated rat microglia. *J Physiol* 1994a; 475:15–32.

Norenberg W, Langosch JM, Gebicke-Haerter PJ, Illes P. Characterization and possible function of adenosine 5'-triphosphate receptors in activated rat microglia. *Br J Pharmacol* 1994b; 111:942–950.

Obata K, Yamanaka H, Dai Y, et al. Differential activation of MAPK in injured and uninjured DRG neurons following chronic constriction injury of the sciatic nerve in rats. *Eur J Neurosci* 2004a; 20:2881–2895.

Obata K, Yamanaka H, Kobayashi K, et al. Role of mitogen-activated protein kinase activation in injured and intact primary afferent neurons for mechanical and heat hypersensitivity after spinal nerve ligation. *J Neurosci* 2004b; 24:10211–10222.

Obata K, Katsura H, Mizushima T, et al. TRPA1 induced in sensory neurons contributes to cold hyperalgesia after inflammation and nerve injury. J Clin Invest (2005) 115:2393-2401.

O'Neill LA. Targeting signal transduction as a strategy to treat inflammatory diseases. *Nat Rev Drug Discov* 2006; 5:549–563.

Peng XM, Zhou ZG, Glorioso JC, Fink DJ, Mata M. Tumor necrosis factor-alpha contributes to below-level neuropathic pain after spinal cord injury. *Ann Neurol* 2006; 59:843–851.

Piao ZG, Cho IH, Park CK, et al. Activation of glia and microglial p38 MAPK in medullary dorsal horn contributes to tactile hypersensitivity following trigeminal sensory nerve injury. *Pain* 2006; 121:219–231.

Popovich PG, Wei P, Stokes BT. Cellular inflammatory response after spinal cord injury in Sprague-Dawley and Lewis rats. *J Comp Neurol* 1997; 377:443–464.

Pramanik R, Qi X, Borowicz S, et al. p38 isoforms have opposite effects on AP-1-dependent transcription through regulation of c-Jun. The determinant roles of the isoforms in the p38 MAPK signal specificity. *J Biol Chem* 2003; 278:4831–4839.

Pratt PF, Bokemeyer D, Foschi M, Sorokin A, Dunn MJ. Alterations in subcellular localization of p38 MAPK potentiates endothelin-stimulated COX-2 expression in glomerular mesangial cells. *J Biol Chem* 2003; 278:51928–51936.

Raghavendra V, Tanga F, DeLeo JA Inhibition of microglial activation attenuates the development but not existing hypersensitivity in a rat model of neuropathy. *J Pharmacol Exp Ther* 2003; 306:624–630.

Raghavendra V, Tanga FY, DeLeo JA. Complete Freund's adjuvant-induced peripheral inflammation evokes glial activation and proinflammatory cytokine expression in the CNS. *Eur J Neurosci* 2004; 20:467–473.

Rahman W, Suzuki R, Webber M, Hunt SP, Dickenson AH. Depletion of endogenous spinal 5-HT attenuates the behavioural hypersensitivity to mechanical and cooling stimuli induced by spinal nerve ligation. *Pain* 2006; 123:264-274.

Rasley A, Bost KL, Olson JK, Miller SD, Marriott I. Expression of functional NK-1 receptors in murine microglia. *Glia* 2002; 37:258–267.

Saklatvala J. The p38 MAP kinase pathway as a therapeutic target in inflammatory disease. *Curr Opin Pharmacol* 2004; 4:372–377.

Samad TA, Moore KA, Sapirstein A, et al. Interleukin-1beta-mediated induction of Cox-2 in the CNS contributes to inflammatory pain hypersensitivity. *Nature* 2001; 410:471–475.

Schäfers M, Svensson CI, Sommer C, Sorkin LS. Tumor necrosis factor-alpha induces mechanical allodynia after spinal nerve ligation by activation of p38 MAPK in primary sensory neurons. *J Neurosci* 2003; 23:2517–2521.

Shi Y, Gaestel M. In the cellular garden of forking paths: how p38 MAPKs signal for downstream assistance. *Biol Chem* 2002; 383:1519–1536.

Smith WL, DeWitt DL, Garavito RM. Cyclooxygenases: structural, cellular, and molecular biology. *Annual Rev Biochem* 2000; 69:145–182.

Stuesse SL, Cruce WL, Lovell JA, McBurney DL, Crisp T. Microglial proliferation in the spinal cord of aged rats with a sciatic nerve injury. *Neurosci Lett* 2000; 287:121–124.

Sung CS, Wen ZH, Chang WK, et al. Inhibition of p38 mitogen-activated protein kinase attenuates interleukin-1beta-induced thermal hyperalgesia and inducible nitric oxide synthase expression in the spinal cord. *J Neurochem* 2005; 94:742–752.

Svensson CI, Hua XY, Protter AA, Powell HC, Yaksh TL. Spinal p38 MAP kinase is necessary for NMDA-induced spinal PGE_2 release and thermal hyperalgesia. *Neuroreport* 2003a; 14:1153–1157.

Svensson CI, Marsala M, Westerlund A, et al. Activation of p38 mitogen-activated protein kinase in spinal microglia is a critical link in inflammation-induced spinal pain processing. *J Neurochem* 2003b; 86:1534–1544.

Svensson CI, Fitzsimmons B, Azizi S, et al. Spinal p38beta isoform mediates tissue injury-induced hyperalgesia and spinal sensitization. *J Neurochem* 2005a; 92:1508–1520.

Svensson CI, Schäfers M, Jones TL, Powell H, Sorkin LS. Spinal blockade of TNF blocks spinal nerve ligation-induced increases in spinal P-p38. *Neurosci Lett* 2005b; 379:209–213.

Svensson CI, Schäfers M, Jones TL, Yaksh TL, Sorkin LS. Covariance among age, spinal p38 MAP kinase activation and allodynia. *J Pain* 2006; 7:337–345.

Sweitzer SM, Colburn RW, Rutkowski M, DeLeo JA. Acute peripheral inflammation induces moderate glial activation and spinal IL-1beta expression that correlates with pain behavior in the rat. *Brain Res* 1999; 829:209–221.

Sweitzer SM, Peters MC, Ma JY, et al. Peripheral and central p38 MAPK mediates capsaicin-induced hyperalgesia. *Pain* 2004; 111:278–285.

Tokuda M, Miyamoto R, Sakuta T, Nagaoka S, Torii M. Substance P activates p38 mitogen-activated protein kinase to promote IL-6 induction in human dental pulp fibroblasts. *Connect Tissue Res* 2005; 46:153–158.

Trang T, Sutak M, Quirion R, Jhamandas K. Spinal administration of lipoxygenase inhibitors suppresses behavioural and neurochemical manifestations of naloxone-precipitated opioid withdrawal. *Br J Pharmacol* 2003; 140:295–304.

Tsuda M, Mizokoshi A, Shigemoto-Mogami Y, Koizumi S, Inoue K. Activation of p38 mitogen-activated protein kinase in spinal hyperactive microglia contributes to pain hypersensitivity following peripheral nerve injury. *Glia* 2004; 45:89–95.

Tsuda M, Inoue K, Salter MW. Neuropathic pain and spinal microglia: a big problem from molecules in "small" glia. *Trends Neurosci* 2005; 28:101–107.

Vachon PH, Harnois C, Grenier A, et al. Differentiation state-selective roles of p38 isoforms in human intestinal epithelial cell anoikis. *Gastroenterology* 2002; 123:1980–1991.

Veglianese P, Lo Coco D, Bao Cutrona M, et al. Activation of the p38MAPK cascade is associated with upregulation of TNF alpha receptors in the spinal motor neurons of mouse models of familial ALS. *Mol Cell Neurosci* 2006; 31:218–231.

Verge GM, Milligan ED, Maier SF, et al. Fractalkine (CX3CL1) and fractalkine receptor (CX3CR1) distribution in spinal cord and dorsal root ganglia under basal and neuropathic pain conditions. *Eur J Neurosci* 2004; 20:1150–1160.

Wang XF, Huang LD, Yu PP, et al. Upregulation of type I interleukin-1 receptor after traumatic spinal cord injury in adult rats. *Acta Neuropathol (Berl)* 2006; 111:220–228.

Wieseler-Frank J, Maier SF, Watkins LR. Central proinflammatory cytokines and pain enhancement. *Neurosignals* 2005; 14:166–174.

Winzen R, Kracht M, Ritter B, et al. The p38 MAP kinase pathway signals for cytokine-induced mRNA stabilization via MAP kinase-activated protein kinase 2 and an AU-rich region-targeted mechanism. *Embo J* 1999; 18:4969–4980.

Wu Y, Willcockson HH, Maixner W, Light AR. Suramin inhibits spinal cord microglia activation and long-term hyperalgesia induced by formalin injection. *J Pain* 2004; 5:48–55.

You HJ, Woo CH, Choi EY, et al. Roles of Rac and p38 kinase in the activation of cytosolic phospholipase A2 in response to PMA. *Biochem J* 2005; 388:527–535.

Zarubin T, Han J. Activation and signaling of the p38 MAP kinase pathway. *Cell Res* 2005; 15:11–18.

Zhang J, De Koninck Y. Spatial and temporal relationship between monocyte chemoattractant protein-1 expression and spinal glial activation following peripheral nerve injury. *J Neurochem* 2006; 97:772–783.

Zhang FE, Cao JL, Zhang LC, Zeng YM. Activation of p38 mitogen-activated protein kinase in spinal cord contributes to chronic constriction injury-induced neuropathic pain. *Sheng Li Xue Bao* 2005; 57:545–551.

Zhang J, Hoffert C, Vu HK, et al. Induction of CB2 receptor expression in the rat spinal cord of neuropathic but not inflammatory chronic pain models. *Eur J Neurosci* 2003; 17:2750–2754.

Zhuang ZY, Wen YR, Zhang DR, et al. A peptide c-Jun N-terminal kinase (JNK) inhibitor blocks mechanical allodynia after spinal nerve ligation: respective roles of JNK activation in primary sensory neurons and spinal astrocytes for neuropathic pain development and maintenance. *J Neurosci* 2006; 26:3551–3560.

Correspondence to: Camilla Svensson, PhD, Department of Anesthesiology, University of California, San Diego, 9500 Gilman Drive, La Jolla, CA 92093-0818, USA. Fax: 1-619-543-6070; email: csvensson@ucsd.edu.

Immune and Glial Regulation of Pain, edited by Joyce
A. DeLeo, Linda S. Sorkin, and Linda R. Watkins,
IASP Press, Seattle, © 2007.

18

Glially Driven Enhancement of Pain and Its Control by Anti-Inflammatory Cytokines

Erin D. Milligan, Annemarie Ledeboer,
Evan M. Sloane, Steven F. Maier, David A. Busha,
and Linda R. Watkins

*Department of Psychology and the Center for Neuroscience,
University of Colorado, Boulder, Colorado, USA*

Normally, pain occurs via clearly identifiable causes in the body, which can range from acute noxious stimulation to tissue injury and inflammation. When inflammation persists chronically, ongoing excitation occurs in primary sensory neurons that communicate to pain transmission neurons in the dorsal horn of the spinal cord. Injured or inflamed tissue in the central nervous system (CNS) can alter the activity of spinal or brain neurons as well, and if this process occurs in neurons relevant to the pain pathway, pain may ensue. Most often, treating the injury leads to a resolution of pain. However, a number of chronic pain conditions exist in which the underlying pathology cannot be treated, cannot be identified either in the peripheral or central nervous system, and leads to a sensitized, pain-facilitatory state in the dorsal horn of the spinal cord (central sensitization) due to the ongoing activity of primary sensory neurons or their central nerve terminals and/or dorsal horn pain transmission neurons (see Millan 1999 for a comprehensive review). Such pain conditions are often associated with trauma to and/or inflammation of peripheral nerves (i.e., peripheral neuropathy) or else are caused by chronic compression and inflammation of peripheral nerves such as occurs following disk herniation. Other neuropathies associated with trauma or inflammation are caused by spinal cord injury or inflammation or by cancer chemotherapeutics such as paclitaxel. Our understanding of the creation and maintenance of neuropathic pain has been based primarily on studies focused on neuronal mechanisms, an approach that currently mounting evidence suggests is too narrow. Indications that the true picture is far more complex may be one reason that drugs targeting neurons have not proven successful in treating chronic pain in many patients (Watkins and Maier 2003).

In the past 15 years, non-neuronal cells, namely astrocytes and microglia, in the CNS have been proposed to play a significant role in pain-facilitatory states, and glia are now recognized to modulate neuronal synaptic function and neuronal excitability by a variety of mechanisms (Haydon 2001; Fellin et al. 2006). Astrocytes and microglia are thought to have partly overlapping functions. While each have unique functions in the CNS (Benveniste 1997; Perry and Gordon 1997), both behave as immunocompetent cells and also release products that alter neuronal function (Benveniste 1997; Haydon 2001). Under conditions that lead to spinally mediated pain sensitization, such as after peripheral nerve injury or spinal cord inflammation or injury, glia respond to various neuronal factors that alter subsequent glial responsivity and ultimately affect glial-neuronal interactions (De Leo et al. 2006). This chapter reviews current evidence from rodent models for a major role of spinal cord glia in mediating pain facilitation created by diverse manipulations. Further, research that targets spinal cord glia using anti-inflammatory factors to control pain facilitation in these animal models is summarized with a focus on clinical implications for novel drug development.

ASTROCYTES ARE IDEALLY POSITIONED
TO MODULATE NEURONAL FUNCTION

Glial cells in the spinal cord consist of astrocytes, microglia, and oligodendrocytes and are the most abundant cell type in the CNS (Kettenmann and Ransom 2005). Astrocytes and oligodendrocytes are derived from neural tissue during development. Generally, astrocytes are best known for their regulation of water, ion clearance, and pH balance, as well as for providing energy and metabolic precursors to neurons, as these functions are critical for optimal neuronal function. Oligodendrocytes, which are cells responsible for myelin sheath formation that insulate axons for efficient neuronal signal transmission, will not be discussed further in this chapter because as yet, no direct evidence shows that they regulate pain. Microglia are mostly characterized as arising from hematopoietic cells, and they are traditionally considered to be the equivalent of macrophages in the CNS (Cuadros and Navascues 2001). However, both astrocytes and microglia are now known to exhibit a range of functions that reflects the repertoire of actions of these non-neuronal cells in their ability to respond to and modify neuronal synaptic activity (De Leo et al. 2006).

A more complete picture of the various functions performed by astrocytes has emerged over the past 15 years. Astrocytes are now known to play active, integrative roles during synaptic transmission (Castonguay et al. 2001). Thus, neurotransmitters released from presynaptic terminals during synaptic transmission activate receptors on nearby astrocytes, which in turn induce the release of astrocyte-derived transmitters. Astrocytes are closely associated with neuronal cell bodies, dendrites, and pre- and postsynaptic sites, as well as with other astrocytes and microglia. The close contact allows astrocytes to monitor neuronal synaptic activity. A variety of functional neurotransmitter receptors, initially characterized on neurons, are now known to be expressed by astrocytes. These include ionotropic non-N-methyl-D-aspartate (NMDA) and NMDA receptors (Porter and McCarthy 1997; Schipke et al. 2001; Seifert and Steinhauser 2001), group I and group II metabotropic glutamate receptors (Biber et al. 1999; Minoshima and Nakanishi 1999; Aronica 2003; Aronica et al. 2003, 2005), purinergic ionotropic (P2X) and metabotropic (P2Y) receptor families (Li and Perl 1995; Le et al. 1998), and substance P receptors (Porter and McCarthy 1997). Neurons releasing neuronal transmitters such as the extracellular purine, adenosine 5'-triphosphate (ATP), glutamate, and substance P are sources of stimuli for astrocytes. In turn, astrocytes release glutamate and/or ATP in response to substance P (Porter 1997), glutamate, and ATP (Fellin et al. 2006). However, astrocyte activation may not depend solely on neurotransmitter overflow from synaptic sites; recent data demonstrate their activation by direct synaptic innervation from neurons (Iino et al. 2001; Matsui and Jahr 2003, 2004). Whether direct synaptic contact onto astrocytes occurs in the spinal cord is as yet unknown. It is conceivable that, in addition to many of their maintenance functions, astrocytes can monitor and respond to neuronal synaptic activity via multiple mechanisms in the spinal cord.

The active and integrative functions that astrocytes perform during synaptic transmission are further demonstrated by the action of glutamate transporters, glutamate receptors, and purinoceptors on astrocytes. For example, astrocytes express glutamate excitatory amino acid transporters (GLT-1 and GLAST) that are believed to be the major mechanism for maintaining low extracellular glutamate (Danbolt 2001; Takano et al. 2005). In addition, during neuronal synaptic activity, both ATP and glutamate can induce astrocytes, via their respective receptors, to generate Ca^{2+} waves that provide both inhibitory (Newman 2003; Pascual et al. 2005) and excitatory effects on nearby neurons (Fellin et al. 2006). Taken together, the transmitters glutamate and ATP act via multiple pathways that may underlie the influence of astrocytes on neuronal synaptic activity.

Astrocyte function also extends to activities typically ascribed to cells of the immune system. That is, astrocytes are capable of phagocytosis (Iacono et al. 1991; Norenberg 1997) and are critical in mediating inflammatory processes, because they express receptors for and release a variety of chemical messages widely known to be associated with peripheral immune cells. These chemical mediators include a family of pro-inflammatory cytokines, namely interleukin-1 (IL-1), tumor necrosis factor-alpha (TNF-α), and interleukin-6 (IL-6) (Benveniste 1997). As discussed previously, a variety of signals activate astrocytes. However, in addition to releasing transmitter in response to glutamate, astrocytes also release IL-1, TNF-α, and IL-6 (Allan et al. 2005; Aronica et al. 2005), molecules that are able to act on nearby astrocytes, microglia, *and* neurons (Benveniste 1997; Perry and Gordon 1997). In turn, substances released by astrocytes such as TNF-α and IL-1 increase neuronal excitability and synaptic strength by increasing the conductivity of AMPA and NMDA receptors as well as by increasing the number of such receptors available on the surface of neurons (Beattie et al. 2002; Stellwagen and Malenka 2006). Thus, neurons respond to factors released by activated astrocytes. In sum, astrocytes not only support neuronal function, but also exert multifunctional roles, ranging from modulation of neuronal synaptic activity to phagocytosis, pathogen clearance, and participation in the inflammatory response.

MICROGLIA ARE IDEALLY POSITIONED TO MODULATE ASTROCYTE FUNCTION AND SYNAPTIC ACTIVITY

While it is clear that astrocytes have multifunctional roles in modulating neuronal communication, they are not alone in this regard because microglia are capable of a range of similar functions. Microglia, likely derived from hematopoietic cells during development, are most widely known to be the key resident immunocompetent cells of the CNS. Microglia, like astrocytes and neurons (Hanisch 2002), express receptors for and become activated by the same factors as hematopoietically-derived macrophages, namely IL-1, TNF-α, and IL-6 (Perry and Gordon 1997). Further, microglia express receptors for pathogens, such as viruses and bacteria, and phagocytose these foreign invaders, a process that induces the release of IL-1, TNF-α, and IL-6 from these activated microglia (Kreutzberg 1996).

As in the case of astrocytes, microglia are not limited to their traditionally classified functions. Microglial activation leads to the release of substances known to excite nearby astrocytes and neurons including nitric oxide (NO), leukotrienes, arachidonic acid, and prostaglandins, as well as proinflammatory cytokines (Kreutzberg 1996; Bezzi et al. 2001; Hanisch 2002; Marchand et al. 2005). Microglia are capable of responding to these substances as well as to the transmitters glutamate and ATP. Microglia express glutamate metabotropic group I–III receptors (Biber et al. 1999; Taylor et al. 2002, 2003) and respond to glutamate by releasing TNF-α (Taylor et al. 2005). In turn, TNF-α can exert excitatory actions on neighboring neurons, astrocytes, and microglia (Ohtori et al. 2004; Stellwagen and Malenka 2006). Interestingly, microglial cell cultures exposed to high levels of glutamate lead to decreased glutamate uptake by GLT-1 (Persson et al. 2006), thus increasing extracellular glutamate. Although glutamate uptake via GLAST and GLT-1 is predominantly characterized in astrocytes, both transporters have been found in microglia (Chretien et al. 2002; Vallat-Decouvelaere et al. 2003). Further, microglia express ionotropic and metabotropic purinoceptors (Tsuda et al. 2003; Bianco et al. 2005) and are activated in response to ATP (Suzuki et al. 2004). Coull and colleagues (2005) demonstrated that one effect of ATP is the induced release of brain-derived neurotrophic factor (BDNF) from microglia, which in turn converts gamma-aminobutyric acid (GABA) inhibition to GABA excitation in spinal lamina I neurons. Other reports have shown that the ionotropic P2X4 receptor, expressed solely on microglia, upregulates in response to peripheral neuropathy and that blocking this microglial P2X4 receptor blocks neuropathic pain (Tsuda et al. 2003). Activation of this microglial P2X4 receptor not only releases BDNF as noted above, but also induces the release of proinflammatory cytokines from microglia (Le Feuvre et al. 2002). Thus, activated microglia respond to and release transmitters and other substances that act to further stimulate themselves as well as nearby microglia, astrocytes, and neurons in an autocrine/paracrine fashion (Castonguay et al. 2001).

PAIN FACILITATION COINCIDES WITH SPINAL CORD GLIAL ACTIVATION

A large number of studies examining exaggerated pain states such as thermal hyperalgesia (exaggerated responses to noxious heat) and mechanical allodynia (exaggerated responses to normally non-noxious touch/pressure stimuli) document that spinal cord glia are activated coincidentally with the development of nociceptive facilitation resulting from peripheral nerve injury or inflammation (Watkins et al. 2001b). A direct correlation between pain facilitation produced by chronic constriction injury (CCI), a well-characterized model of partial nerve injury (Bennett and Xie 1988), and spinal cord astrocyte activation was first described by Garrison and colleagues (1991). These authors observed activated astrocytes in the spinal segments that receive input from nerve terminals of damaged sciatic nerves by examining upregulation of glial fibrillary acidic protein (GFAP) by immunohistochemistry. Indeed, intensity of spinal cord astrocyte activation observed in CCI-treated rats was directly correlated with the degree of hyperalgesia. The elevated GFAP expression demonstrated to be NMDA-dependent because MK-801, an NMDA antagonist, markedly reduced GFAP expression in CCI-treated rats (Garrison et al. 1994). This observation was important because it demonstrated that a drug known to block neuropathic pain (Davar et al. 1991; Mao et al. 1992) prevents glial activation as well.

Evidence for spinal glial activation, as reflected by increased GFAP expression in astrocytes and increased OX-42 labeling of complement type 3 receptors on microglia, has now accumulated for diverse models of inflammation and trauma. These include subcutaneous irritants, intraperitoneal inflammation, epineural immune activation, spinal inflammation, and spinal cord trauma (for review, see Watkins and Maier 2003). Often, glial activation occurs in parallel with exaggerated pain responses, which, in these studies, range from 45 minutes to as long as 30 days after a single inflammatory insult. Such glial activation is not limited to pain from purely inflammatory conditions but has also been demonstrated in studies of diverse nerve injury models that lead to pain facilitation. These manipulations include trauma to peripheral nerves, spinal nerves, and the spinal cord (for review, see Watkins and Maier 2003). A model of pain from bone cancer has also recently identified glial activation in the spinal cord (Schwei et al. 1999; Zhang et al. 2005). Early evidence of concurrent spinal cord glial activation with a variety of rodent models that produce exaggerated pain suggests that glia may prove to be important in clinical pain phenomena.

Evidence of glial activation based on immunohistochemical or mRNA analysis of so-called glial activation markers is informative as to which type of glial cell is activated, and for anatomical studies, their location in the spinal cord, but such data must be interpreted with caution. Activation markers simply indicate that glial activation has occurred at some point and cannot indicate which pain-relevant glial products are released and when, nor which events directly led to neuronal activation and pain enhancement. It is possible that products released from activated glia that alter neuronal function may be absent when glial activation markers become robustly expressed. That is, the activation of glia, as reflected by the release of glial products such as proinflammatory cytokines, can occur far sooner than the upregulation of glial activation markers. Indeed, increases in microglial and astrocytic activation markers have been observed by immunohistochemistry in the absence of pain, and the expression of microglial activation markers can be absent or blocked in the presence of pain (Colburn et al. 1997; DeLeo and Colburn 1999). Hence, examination of glial activation by anatomical markers alone is informative, but may not provide the temporal information about glial activation relative to the occurrence of pain facilitation.

SPINAL CORD GLIAL ACTIVATION IS NECESSARY
FOR PAIN FACILITATION

Measuring the increased production of the proinflammatory cytokines, IL-1, TNF-α, and IL-6 from glia has been a reliable method to assess glial activation (Benveniste 1997; Hanisch 2002). Studies blocking the action of IL-1, TNF-α, and/or IL-6 elucidated the critical role that proinflammatory cytokines play in a variety of enhanced pain states (Watkins et al. 2001a). For example, one approach to examining whether glia are involved in pain facilitation takes advantage of their capacity to act as immune-like cells, becoming activated and releasing substances that can act on nearby glia and neurons. Glia release pain-enhancing substances in response to pathogens such as lipopolysaccharide (LPS) (Nguyen et al. 2002). Both astrocytes and microglia express receptors for, and become activated by, LPS. It was first demonstrated by Meller and colleagues (1994) that activation of spinal cord glia with intrathecal LPS produces thermal and mechanical hyperalgesia. It was later demonstrated that spinal cord glia produce IL-1 fairly rapidly after a systemic injection of LPS at the same dose that produced thermal hyperalgesia (Watkins and Maier 1999).

Glia also express receptors for, and become activated by, the human immunodeficiency virus (HIV-1) surface glycoprotein, gp120 (Ma et al. 1994; Lazarini et al. 2000). We have used gp120 as a means to activate glia in the absence of peripheral inflammation or trauma so as to explore whether glial activation may be sufficient to enhance pain and, if so, how this enhancement may occur. Indeed, we have demonstrated that intrathecal gp120 induces robust thermal hyperalgesia and mechanical allodynia. In parallel, intrathecal gp120 activates both astrocytes and microglia, as reflected by upregulation of their activation markers by both immunohistochemistry (Milligan et al. 2001) and by real-time polymerase chain reaction (Ledeboer et al. 2005b). Importantly, pain enhancement by gp120 was due to glial activation because pain facilitation was blocked by either fluorocitrate (a glial metabolic inhibitor) or minocycline (a microglial activation inhibitor) (Ledeboer et al. 2005b). In exploring the underlying mechanisms, we have found that gp120 enhances pain via the activation of both p38 mitogen-activated protein kinase (Milligan et al. 2001b) and the cytokine regulatory transcription factor, nuclear factor (NF)-κB (Ledeboer et al. 2005a). In turn, these factors induced by intrathecal gp120 stimulate gene activation and the production and release of IL-1, TNF-α, and IL-6 from the dorsal spinal cord (Milligan et al. 2001; Holguin et al. 2004; Ledeboer et al. 2005b). Further, release of proinflammatory cytokines is sufficiently rapid to allow their accumulation in the surrounding cerebrospinal fluid (CSF) to detectable levels within as little as 20 minutes, mimicking the time course observed for thermal hyperalgesia and mechanical allodynia (Milligan et al. 2001). Importantly, spinal pretreatment with agents that neutralize the actions of proinflammatory cytokines, such as IL-1 receptor antagonist, TNF-soluble receptor-binding protein (sTNFbp), or IL-6-neutralizing antibody, blocks both thermal hyperalgesia and/or low-threshold mechanical allodynia. For example, intrathecal pretreatment with IL-1-receptor antagonist or sTNFbp blocked thermal hyperalgesia and mechanical allodynia produced by intrathecal gp120 (Milligan et al. 2001). These proinflammatory cytokines are most likely derived from glia because their production and release are prevented by blocking glial activation using either fluorocitrate (Milligan et al. 2000) or minocycline (Ledeboer et al. 2005b). Indeed, microglia rapidly isolated from the dorsal spinal cord following intrathecal gp120 administration exhibited elevated proinflammatory cytokine mRNAs, again supporting glia as a source of these neuroexcitatory products (Wieseler-Frank et al. 2005). The involvement of multiple proinflammatory cytokines is not surprising, as they are known to both synergize in their actions and to stimulate each other's production (Hanisch 2002).

However, activated glia, in response to viruses or bacteria, release factors in addition to proinflammatory cytokines that can further contribute to nearby glial activation and neuronal excitation. For example, gp120 induces the production and/or release of NO (Meller et al. 1994; Koka et al. 1995; Holguin et al. 2004; Ledeboer et al. 2005b), ATP (Murakami et al. 2003), prostaglandins (Benveniste 1997; Nguyen et al. 2002), and precursors to prostaglandins such as arachidonic acid or cyclooxygenase (Ushijima et al. 1995). In addition, glia inhibit excitatory amino acid (EAA) uptake as well as actively release glutamate (Dreyer and Lipton 1995; Tikka and Koistinaho 2001) in response to gp120. Proinflammatory cytokines from activated glia and substances such as NO may act together to produce allodynia and/or hyperalgesia. Indeed, we have reported that intrathecal gp120 rapidly induces NO from the dorsal spinal cord (Holguin et al. 2004; Ledeboer et al. 2005b) at a time that matches the development of allodynia. Spinal pretreatment with a NO synthase inhibitor (L-NAME, which inhibits neuronal and glial-derived NO) not only blocked allodynia in gp120-treated animals, but also blocked elevations in IL-1, TNF-α, and IL-6 mRNA and protein in the lumbar spinal cord (Holguin et al. 2004). These studies demonstrated that eliminating NO prevented the synthesis of glially derived components (IL-1, TNF-α, and IL-6) necessary for producing exaggerated pain. Thus, all of these substances can act on neurons in combination with proinflammatory cytokines to contribute to pain facilitation.

In addition to spinal glial activation by gp120, a number of models that lead to pain facilitation, such as intraplantar irritants, sciatic inflammatory neuropathy, spinal nerve trauma, and spinal cord injury, support the notion that glially derived proinflammatory cytokines are critical. As an example, sciatic inflammatory neuropathy is a model that creates neuropathic pain, not as a result of nerve trauma, but rather as a result of localized inflammation of one sciatic nerve at mid-thigh level (Chacur et al. 2001). Inflammation is induced by perisciatic microinjection of an immune activator (yeast cell walls; zymosan), which rapidly creates low-threshold mechanical allodynia and leads to microglial activation in the spinal cord dorsal horn (Ledeboer 2005). Allodynia created from this model was reversed, not only by disrupting glial activation (Milligan et al. 2003), but also by blocking the spinal action of IL-1, TNF-α, and IL-6 after intrathecal treatment with each respective proinflammatory cytokine antagonist (Milligan et al. 2003).

In other models, IL-1 expression was observed as early as 6 hours and at 1 week after subcutaneous hindpaw inflammation with zymosan (Sweitzer et al. 1999). In addition, spinal nerve transection resulted in increased spinal cord IL-1 levels 1 week after injury (Sweitzer et al. 2001). Importantly, spinal cord proinflammatory cytokines paralleled the development and maintenance of allodynia and glial activation (Sweitzer et al. 1999, 2001). In separate studies, spinal cord proinflammatory cytokine synthesis of IL-1, TNF-α, and/or IL-6 was increased in the spinal cord observed from 1 day to 1–3 weeks after nerve root injury in a rodent model of lumbar radiculopathy that produces mechanical allodynia and thermal hyperalgesia (Hashizume et al. 2000; Winkelstein et al. 2001). These studies were the first to demonstrate that proinflammatory cytokines are not simply expressed at the initiation of a variety of models for exaggerated pain, but rather continue to be produced for prolonged periods. Intrathecal administration of IL-1, TNF-α, and/or IL-6 antagonists prevented and/or reversed pain facilitation produced by intraplantar irritants (Watkins et al. 1997; Samad et al. 2001; Chacur et al. 2004a), as well as neuropathic pain produced by CCI (Milligan et al. 2005a), sciatic inflammation by phospholipase A2 (Chacur et al. 2004b) spinal nerve transection (Sweitzer et al. 2001), and systemic cancer chemotherapeutics (Milligan et al. 2005a; Ledeboer et al. 2006). Given that IL-1, TNF-α, and IL-6 lead to further increases of each of these proinflammatory cytokines (Chao et al. 1995; Gayle et al. 1998), the results of these studies suggest that multiple proinflammatory cytokines may be chronically released and demonstrate that acute or chronic pain is maintained by the actions of proinflammatory cytokines. What is notable from all of these studies using various models of pain facilitation is that blocking the actions of spinal cord IL-1, TNF-α, and/or IL-6 reverses or blocks neuropathic pain.

Importantly, most studies have demonstrated that proinflammatory cytokines are sufficient to cause pain facilitation. Are these spinal cord proinflammatory cytokines sufficient in and of themselves to produce this effect? A number of studies have demonstrated that proinflammatory cytokines administered in the CNS produce allodynia and/or hyperalgesia. In support of a direct action of proinflammatory cytokines on neurons (hence, a possible mechanism for pain facilitation), receptors for IL-1, TNF-α, and IL-6 are expressed on neurons in the brain and spinal cord (Dame and Juul 2000; Holmes et al. 2004; Ohtori et al. 2004). Indeed, IL-1, TNF-α, or IL-6 administered in the brain created thermal hyperalgesia (Oka and Hori 1999). However, cytokines such as IL-6 have also been shown to modulate neuropathic pain (Flatters et al. 2003, 2004). Indeed, IL-6 markedly suppressed electrically evoked C-fiber activity and dorsal horn neuronal hyperexcitability in neuropathic rats with spinal nerve ligation. Although the preponderance of data indicates that exogenous proinflammatory cytokines in the CNS are sufficient to produce exaggerated pain states, in some instances, such as in the case of IL-6, they may act to modulate neuropathic pain.

TARGETING ACTIVATED GLIA WITH ANTI-INFLAMMATORY CYTOKINES TO RESOLVE PAIN FACILITATION

As reviewed above, selective TNF-α, IL-1, and IL-6 antagonists have all successfully prevented or reversed various animal models of neuropathic pain upon acute administration. Indeed, proinflammatory cytokines appear to be the common spinal mediators of diverse pain states (see Watkins et al. 2006 for a comprehensive review). While acute disruption of proinflammatory cytokine action is sufficient to implicate these cytokines mechanistically in pain enhancement, prolonged disruption is required if clinical pain control is the goal.

In people, several chronic pain conditions have been reported to involve changes in proinflammatory *and* anti-inflammatory cytokine levels. Indeed, people with chronic widespread pain such as fibromyalgia show serum cytokine profiles that are significantly different from those of individuals without chronic pain (Üçeyler et al. 2006; see also Üçeyler and Sommer, this volume). This study demonstrated lower gene expression and protein levels of IL-10 and IL-4 in persons with chronic widespread pain. A separate study showed increased IL-1 and IL-6 in the CSF of patients with complex regional pain syndrome (Alexander et al. 2005), suggesting that spinal anti-inflammatory treatment may prove beneficial. In support of these observations, we know that the immune system has evolved the means to create negative feedback suppression of proinflammatory cytokine activity, most likely because these cytokines are powerful and potentially destructive. Inhibition is achieved by mechanisms that include the production of anti-inflammatory cytokines, such as interleukin-2 (IL-2), interleukin-4 (IL-4), transforming growth factor-beta (TGF-β) (Janeway et al. 2005), and IL-10 (Moore et al. 2001). If anti-inflammatory cytokines can be exploited as drug therapies, they may prove to be a novel and effective approach for clinical pain control.

One approach for achieving sustained suppression of proinflammatory cytokine action is via chronic overexpression of IL-4 by viral delivery of the IL-4 gene (Hao et al. 2006). This study characterized IL-4 gene expression in the dorsal root ganglion after subcutaneous injection into the plantar surface of the hindpaw of a replication-defective genomic herpes simplex virus (HSV) encoding IL-4 and demonstrated that this procedure attenuated mechanical allodynia and fully reversed thermal hyperalgesia in a rat model of neuropathic pain. This group further demonstrated that this IL-4 treatment greatly reduced touch-induced expression of dorsal horn c-Fos-like immunoreactivity, a gene product demonstrating neuronal activity. In addition, IL-1, microglial p38 activation, and prostaglandin expression were blocked in IL-4-treated neuropathic rats (Hao et al. 2006).

In a separate study, spinal cord overexpression of IL-2 after intrathecal adenovirus-mediated IL-2 gene delivery was almost perfectly correlated with pain blockade in neuropathic rats (Yao et al. 2003). Intrathecal injection of adenovirus-IL-2 gene led to mRNA expression of IL-2 in the spinal meninges and in the gray and white matter of the spinal cord as determined by in situ hybridization. This group had previously demonstrated that intrathecal IL-2 gene delivery using nonviral vectors was effective in blocking neuropathic pain produced by subcutaneous carrageenan (Yao et al. 2002b) or CCI (Yao et al. 2002a).

In addition to IL-4 and IL-2, a number of studies have examined the potential therapeutic benefit for controlling enhanced pain responses using IL-10. IL-10 has been documented to suppress the production and function of all proinflammatory cytokines (Moore et al. 2001). In addition, evidence to date suggests that spinal cord neurons do not express IL-10 receptors (Ledeboer et al. 2003), thus avoiding disruption of neuronal function by application of IL-10. Intrathecal IL-10 has been reported to block the onset of spinal IL-1-mediated mechanical allodynia induced by either intrathecal dynorphin (Laughlin et al. 2000) or perisciatic phospholipase A2 (Chacur et al. 2004b). IL-10 likewise blocks the development of pathological pain behaviors induced by spinal cord excitotoxic injury, a manipulation associated with increases in spinal cord glial activation and proinflammatory cytokines (Bethea et al. 1999; Brewer et al. 1999; Plunkett et al. 2001; Yu et al. 2003; Abraham et al. 2004). In all prior reports of spinal IL-10 effects on pain facilitation, IL-10 prevented the onset of such changes.

In support of these findings, our laboratory has been exploring the potential for intrathecal IL-10 gene therapy for prolonged control of neuropathic pain. We have shown that spinal cord overexpression of IL-10 with intrathecal administration of adenovirus or adeno-associated virus prevents pain facilitation produced by gp120-mediated spinal glial activation, sciatic inflammatory neuropathy, and CCI (Milligan et al. 2005a,b). Extraterritorial and mirror-image

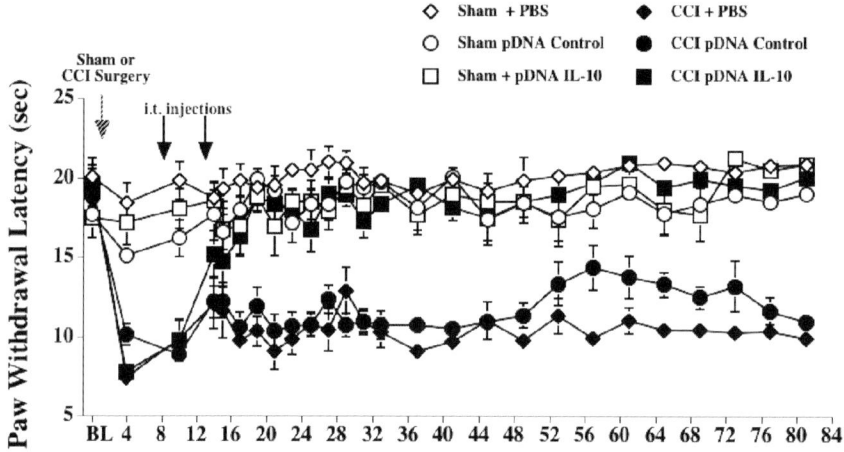

Fig. 1. Spinal cord IL-10 gene therapy reverses thermal hyperalgesia produced by chronic constriction injury (CCI) in rats. Rats received either sham or CCI surgery (indicated by the stippled arrow). Hindpaw withdrawal latency was assessed (in seconds) with the Hargreaves test (low radiant heat cut-off was set at 22 seconds to avoid tissue damage) at baseline (BL), prior to surgery, and 4 and 10 days after surgery. Rats received two intrathecal injections, spaced 3 days apart, of either plasmid DNA-IL-10 (pDNA IL-10; 100 and 25 μg, respectively) (indicated by the arrows), control plasmid DNA (pDNA without the IL-10 gene; 100 and 25 μg, respectively), or vehicle (phosphate-buffered saline [PBS]). Hindpaw thermal withdrawal responses were reassessed every 4 days after the first intrathecal injection, and up to 81 days after surgery. Based on data from Busha et al. (2006).

pain in addition to territorial pain produced by sciatic inflammatory neuropathy was reversed after intrathecal adenoviral delivery of the IL-10 gene. Presumably, IL-10 created this effect by blocking the actions of at least IL-1, because the increased protein expression of IL-1 from the CSF of IL-10-treated rats was suppressed. Although these single intrathecal viral vector injections infect cells in the meninges without expression in the spinal parenchyma (Iadarola et al. 1997; Mannes et al. 1998; Milligan et al. 2005a), the infection is short-lived, possibly due to recognition of the virus by the immune system (Jooss and Chirmule 2003; Liu and Muruve 2003). Thus, although this IL-10 viral gene therapy transiently reversed neuropathic pain, neither viral approach produced sufficiently sustained pain reversal to be clinically relevant.

More recently, our laboratory has been pursuing a nonviral gene therapy approach for intrathecal IL-10 gene transfer. This method involves nonsurgical delivery of the gene therapy, by means of percutaneous injections into the lumbosacral CSF space, similar to lumbar punctures in routine clinical use. In studies to date, intrathecal delivery of "naked" plasmid DNA encoding the IL-10 gene (pDNA-IL-10) leads to prolonged reversal (for 3 months) of neuropathic pain produced by CCI (Milligan et al. 2006; Sloane et al. 2006). Importantly, while intrathecal gene therapy to treat neuropathic pain is not unique (Wu et al. 2001a,b; Eaton et al. 2002; Yao et al. 2002a,b, 2003; Hao et al. 2006), IL-10 non-viral gene delivery shows excellent promise. Interestingly, repeated intrathecal injections were required to achieve long-lasting anti-allodynic effects of IL-10 gene therapy (Milligan et al. 2006). Results from our group demonstrate that two sequential injections of pDNA-IL-10 at intervals of 2–3 days reverses both CCI-induced mechanical allodynia (Ledeboer et al. 2006; Milligan et al. 2006) and thermal hyperalgesia (Fig. 1) (Busha et al. 2006). It is apparent that IL-10 is required for this prolonged therapeutic effect, because blocking the gene therapy-induced IL-10 actions with IL-10-neutralizing antibodies reinstates neuropathic pain (Sloane et al. 2006). Importantly, in models different from CCI, such as a well-established paclitaxel-induced allodynia, pain was also attenuated with this pDNA-IL-10 treatment for more than 35 days (Fig. 2) (Ledeboer et al. 2006). Thus, pathological pain states such as inflammatory, traumatic, and chemotherapy-induced neuropathies may be controlled by percutaneous injection of the gene encoding the anti-inflammatory cytokine IL-10.

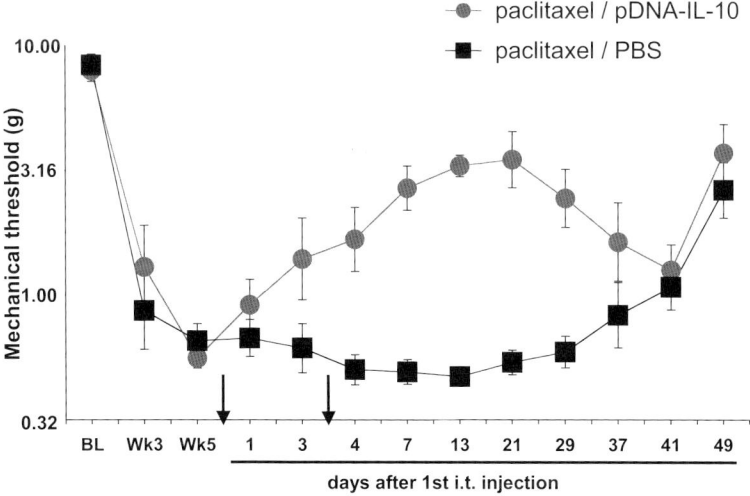

Fig. 2. Spinal cord IL-10 gene therapy attenuates mechanical allodynia produced by the chemotherapeutic agent paclitaxel (4 mg/kg) in rats. On alternate days, rats received four intraperitoneal injections of paclitaxel (1 mg/kg), which produced prolonged allodynia. Five weeks after the first paclitaxel injection, rats received two intrathecal injections of pDNA-IL-10 (100 and 25 μg, respectively) spaced 3 days apart (indicated by the arrows), or vehicle (phosphate-buffered saline [PBS]). Low-threshold mechanical sensitivity was assessed by the von Frey test, at baseline (BL), at 3 and 5 weeks after the first paclitaxel injection, and up to 49 days after the first intrathecal injection. From Ledeboer et al. (2006), with permission.

CONCLUSION

In conclusion, a number of chronic pain conditions are resistant to treatment with currently available therapeutics. Provocative evidence accumulating over the past 15 years demonstrates that astrocytes and microglia play a significant role in pain facilitation. Glia are now recognized to modulate neuronal synaptic function and neuronal excitability by a variety of mechanisms (Haydon 2001; Fellin et al. 2006). Under conditions that lead to spinally mediated pain sensitization, such as after peripheral nerve injury or spinal cord inflammation or injury, glia become activated in response to neuron-to-glia signals, leading to the release of pain-enhancing substances. Key among these substances are the proinflammatory cytokines. Suppressing the production or function of spinal cord proinflammatory cytokines will block pain facilitation induced by diverse manipulations, including various forms of neuropathy. The strength of these data shows that therapies targeting spinal cord glia and their proinflammatory cytokine products warrant exploration for clinical pain control.

REFERENCES

Abraham KE, McMillen D, Brewer KL. The effects of endogenous interleukin-10 on gray matter damage and pain behaviors following excitotoxic spinal cord injury in the mouse. *Neuroscience* 2004; 124:945–922.

Alexander GM, Rijn MA, van-Hilten JJ, Perreault MJ, Schwartzman RJ. Changes in cerebrospinal fluid levels of pro-inflammatory cytokines in CRPS. *Pain* 2005; 116:213–219.

Allan SM, Tyrrell PJ, Rothwell NJ. Interleukin-1 and neuronal injury. *Nat Rev* 2005; 5:629–640.

Aronica E. Expression and functional role of mGlu receptors in reactive astrocytes. *Glia* 2003; 43:S7.1.

Aronica E, Gorter JA, Ijlst-Keizers H, et al. Expression and functional role of mGluR3 and mGluR5 in human astrocytes and glioma cells: opposite regulation of glutamate transporter proteins. *Eur J Neurosci* 2003; 17:2106–2118.

Aronica E, Gorter JA, Rozemuller AJ, Yankaya B, Troost D. Activation of metabotropic glutamate receptor 3 enhances interleukin (IL)-1b-stimulated release of IL-6 in cultured human astrocytes. *Neuroscience* 2005; 130:927–933.

Beattie EC, Stellwagen D, Morishita W, et al. Control of synaptic strength by glial TNFalpha. *Science* 2002; 295:2282–2285.

Bennett GJ, Xie KY. A peripheral mononeuropathy in rat that produces disorders of pain sensation like those seen in man. *Pain* 1988; 33:87–107.

Benveniste EN. Cytokine expression in the nervous system. In: Keane RW, Hickey WF (Eds). *Immunology of the Nervous System.* New York: Oxford University Press, 1997, pp 419–459.

Bethea JR, Nagashima H, Acosta MC, et al. Systemically administered interleukin-10 reduces tumor necrosis factor-alpha production and significantly improves functional recovery following traumatic spinal cord injury in rats. *Neurotrauma* 1999; 16:851–863.

Bezzi P, Domercq M, Brambilla R, et al. CXCR4-activated astrocyte glutamate release via TNF-α: amplification by microglia triggers neurotoxicity. *Nat Neurosci* 2001; 4:702–710.

Bianco F, Fumagalli M, Pravettoni E, et al. Pathophysiological roles of extracellular nucleotides in glial cells: differential expression of purinergic receptors in resting and activated microglia. *Brain Res Rev* 2005; 48:144–156.

Biber K, Laurie DJ, Berthele A, et al. Expression and signalling of group I metabotropic glutamate receptors in astrocytes and microglia. *J Neurochem* 1999; 72:1671–1680.

Brewer KL, Bethea JR, Yezierski RP. Neuroprotective effects of interleukin-10 following spinal cord injury. *Exp Neurol* 1999; 159:484–493.

Busha D, Milligan ED, Murphy C, et al. Spinal cord gene transfer using naked plasmid DNA coding the anti-inflammatory gene, interleukin-10 (IL10) leads to long-term reversal of thermal hyperalgesia in chronic constriction injury (CCI) rats. Proceedings of the 25th Conference of the American Pain Society. *J Pain* 2006; 7(4) Suppl 2:S13.

Castonguay A, Levesque S, Robitaille R. Glial cells as active partners in synaptic functions. In: Castellano-Lopez B, Nieto-Sampedro M (Eds). *Glial Cell Function,* Progress in Brain Research, Vol. 132. Amsterdam: Elsevier, 2001, pp 227–240.

Chacur M, Milligan ED, Gazda, LS, et al. A new model of sciatic inflammatory neuritis (SIN): induction of unilateral and bilateral mechanical allodynia following acute unilateral peri-sciatic immune activation in rats. *Pain* 2001; 94:231–244.

Chacur M, Gutierrez JM, Milligan ED, et al. Snake venom components enhance pain upon subcutaneous injection: an initial examination of spinal cord mediators. *Pain* 2004a; 111:65–76.

Chacur M, Milligan ED, Sloane EM, et al. Snake venom phospholipase A2s (Asp49 and Lys49) induce mechanical allodynia upon peri-sciatic administration: involvement of spinal cord glia, proinflammatory cytokines and nitric oxide. *Pain* 2004b; 108:180–191.

Chao CC, Hu S, Ehrlich L, Peterson PK. Interleukin-1 and tumor necrosis factor-alpha synergistically mediate neurotoxicity: involvement of nitric oxide and *N*-methyl-D-aspartate receptors. *Brain Behav Immunol* 1995; 9:355–365.

Chretien F, Vallat-Decouvelaere AV, Boussuet C, et al. Expression of excitatory amino acid transporter-2 (EAAT-2) and glutamine synthesis (GS) in brain macrophages and microglia of SIVmac251-infected macaques. *Neuropathol Appl Neurobiol* 2002; 28:410–417.

Colburn RW, DeLeo JA, Rickman AJ, et al. Dissociation of microglial activation and neuropathic pain behaviors following peripheral nerve injury in the rat. *J Neuroimmunol* 1997; 79:163–175.

Coull JA, Beggs S, Boudreau D, et al. BDNF from microglia causes the shift in neuronal anion gradient underlying neuropathic pain. *Nature* 2005; 438:923–925.

Cuadros MA, Navascues J. Early origin and colonization of the developing central nervous system by microglial precursors. In: Castellano-Lopez B, Nieto-Sampedro M (Eds). *Glial Cell Function,* Progress in Brain Research, Vol. 132. Amsterdam: Elsevier, 2001, pp 51–59.

Dame JB, Juul SE. The distribution of receptors for the pro-inflammatory cytokine interleukin (IL)-6 and IL-8 in the developing human fetus. *Early Hum Dev* 2000; 58:25–39.

Danbolt NC. Glutamate uptake. *Prog Neurobiol* 2001; 65:1–105.

Davar G, Hama A, Deykin B, Vos B, Maciewicz R. MK-801 blocks the development of thermal hyperalgesia in a rat model of experimental painful neuropathy. *Brain Res* 1991; 553:327–330.

DeLeo JA, Tawfik VL, LaCroix-Fralish ML. The tetrapartite synapse: path to CNS sensitization and chronic pain. *Pain* 2006; 122:17–21.

DeLeo JA, Colburn RW. Proinflammatory cytokines and glial cells: their role in neuropathic pain. In: Watkins LR, Maier SF (Eds). *Cytokines and Pain.* Basel: Birkhauser, 1999, pp 159–182.

Dreyer EB, Lipton SA. The coat protein gp120 of HIV-1 inhibits astrocyte uptake of excitatory amino acids via macrophage arachidonic acid. *Eur J Neurosci* 1995; 7:2502–2507.

Eaton MJ, Blits B, Ruitenberg MJ, Verhaagen MJ, Oudega M. Amelioration of chronic neuropathic pain after partial nerve injury by adeno-associated viral (AAV) vector-mediated over-expression of BDNF in the rat spinal cord. *Gene Ther* 2002; 9:1387–1395.

Fellin T, Sul J-Y, D'Ascenzo, M, et al. Bidirectional astrocyte-neuron communication: the many roles of glutamate and ATP. *Novartis Found Symp* 2006; 276:208–217.

Flatters SJL, Fox AJ, Dickenson AH. Spinal interleukin-6 (IL-6) inhibits nociceptive transmission following neuropathy. *Brain Res* 2003; 984:54–62.

Flatters SJL, Fox AJ, Dickenson AH. Nerve injury alters the effects of interleukin-6 on nociceptive transmission in the peripheral. *Eur J Pharmacol* 2004; 484:183–191.

Garrison CJ, Dougherty PM, Kajander KC, Carlton SM. Staining of glial fibrillary acidic protein (GFAP) in lumbar spinal cord increases following a sciatic nerve constriction injury. *Brain Res* 1991; 565:1–7.

Garrison CJ, Dougherty PM, Carlton SM. GFAP expression in lumbar spinal cord of naive and neuropathic rats treated with MK-801. *Exp Neurol* 1994; 129:237–243.

Gayle D, Ilyin SE, Miele ME, Plata-Salaman CR. Modulation of TNF-alpha mRNA production in rat C6 glioma cells by TNFalpha, IL1beta, IL6 and IFNalpha: in vitro analysis of cytokine-cytokine interactions. *Brain Res Bull* 1998; 47:231–235.

Hanisch U-K. Microglia as a source and target of cytokines. *Glia* 2002; 40:140–155.

Hao S, Mata M, Glorioso JC, Fink DJ. HSV-mediated expression of interleukin-4 in dorsal root ganglion neurons reduces neuropathic pain. *Mol Pain* 2006; 2:6.

Hashizume H, DeLeo JA, Colburn RW, Weinstein JN. Spinal glial activation and cytokine expression after lumbar root injury in the rat. *Spine* 2000; 25:1206–1217.

Haydon PG. GLIA: Listening and talking to the synapse. *Nat Rev Neurosci* 2001; 2:185–193.

Holguin A, O'Connor KA, Biedenkapp J, et al. HIV-1 gp120 stimulates proinflammatory cytokine-mediated pain facilitation via activation of nitric oxide synthase-I (nNOS). *Pain* 2004; 110:517–530.

Holmes GM, Hebert SL, Rogers RC, Hermann GE. Immunohistochemical localization of the TNF type 1 and type 2 receptors in the rat spinal cord. *Brain Res* 2004; 1025:210–219.

Iacono RF, Berria MI, Lascano EF. A triple staining procedure to evaluate phagocytic role of differentiated astrocytes. *J Neurosci Methods* 1991; 39:225–230.

Iadarola MJ, Lee S, Mannes AJ. Gene transfer approaches to pain control. In: Borsook D (Ed). *Molecular Neurobiology of Pain,* Progress in Pain Research and Management, Vol. 9. Seattle: IASP Press, 1997, pp 337–360.

Iino M, Goto K, Kakegawa W, et al. Glia-synapse interaction through Ca^{2+}-permeable AMPA receptors in Bergmann glia. *Science* 2001; 292:926–929.

Janeway CA, Travers P, Walport M, Shlomchik MJ (Ed). *Immunobiology: The Immune System in Health and Disease*, 6th ed. New York: Garland Science, 2005.

Jooss K, Chirmule N. Immunity to adenovirus and adeno-associated viral vectors: implication for gene therapy. *Gene Ther* 2003; 10:995–963.

Kettenmann H, Ransom B (Ed). *Neuroglia*, 2nd ed. Oxford: Oxford University Press, 2005.

Koka P, He K, Zack JA, et al. Human immunodeficiency virus 1 envelope proteins induce interleukin 1, tumor necrosis factor alpha, and nitric oxide in glial cultures derived from fetal, neonatal and adult human brain. *J Exp Med* 1995; 182:941–951.

Kreutzberg GW. Microglia: a sensor for pathological events in the CNS. *Trends Neurosci* 1996; 19:312–318.

Laughlin TM, Bethea JR, Yezierski RP, Wilcox GL. Cytokine involvement in dynorphin-induced allodynia. *Pain* 2000; 84:159–167.

Lazarini F, Casanova P, Tham TN, et al. Differential signalling of the chemokine receptor CXCR4 by stromal cell-derived factor 1 and the HIV glycoprotein in rat neurons and astrocytes. *Eur J Neurosci* 2000; 12:117–125.

Le Feuvre R, Brough D, Rothwell N. Extracellular ATP and P2X7 receptors in neurodegeneration. *Eur J Pharmacol* 2002; 447:261–269.

Le KT, Villeneuve P, Ramjaun AR, et al. Sensory presynaptic and widespread somatodendritic immunolocalization of central ionotropic P2X ATP receptors. *Neuroscience* 1998; 83:177–190.

Ledeboer A, Wierinckx A, Bol JGJM, et al. Regional and temporal expression patterns of interleukin-10, interleukin-10 receptor and adhesion molecules in the rat spinal cord during chronic relapsing EAE. *J Neuroimmunol* 2003; 136:94–103.

Ledeboer A, Gamanos M, Lai W, et al. Involvement of spinal cord nuclear factor kappaB activation in rat models of proinflammatory cytokine-mediated pain facilitation. *Eur J Neurosci* 2005a; 22:1977–1986.

Ledeboer A, Sloane EM, Milligan ED, et al. Minocycline attenuates mechanical allodynia and proinflammatory cytokine expression in rat models of pain facilitation. *Pain* 2005b; 115:71–83.

Ledeboer A, Sloane EM, Milligan ED, et al. Paclitaxel-induced mechanical allodynia in rats is inhibited by spinal delivery of plasmid DNA encoding interleukin-10. In: Flor H, Kalso E, Dostrovsky JO (Eds). *Proceedings of the 11th World Congress on Pain.* Seattle: IASP Press, 2006, pp 187–194.

Li J, Perl ER. ATP modulation of synaptic transmission in the spinal substantia gelatinosa. *J Neurosci* 1995; 15:3357–3365.

Liu Q, Muruve DA. Molecular basis of the inflammatory response to adenovirus vectors. *Gene Ther* 2003; 10:935–940.

Ma M, Geiger JD, Nath A. Characterization of a novel binding site for the human immunodeficiency virus type 1 envelope protein gp120 on human fetal astrocytes. *J Virol* 1994; 68:6824–6928.

Mannes AJ, Caudle RM, O'Connell BC, Iadarola MJ. Adenoviral gene transfer to spinal cord neurons: intrathecal vs. intraparenchymal administration. *Brain Res* 1998; 793:1–6.

Mao J, Price DD, Mayer DJ, Lu J, Heyes RL. Intrathecal MK-801 and local nerve anesthesia synergistically reduce nociceptive behaviors in rats with experimental peripheral mononeuropathy. *Brain Res* 1992; 576:254–262.

Marchand F, Perretti M, McMahon SB. Role of the immune system in chronic pain. *Nat Rev* 2005; 6:521–530.

Matsui K, Jahr CE. Ectopic release of synaptic vesicles. *Neuron* 2003; 40:1173–1183.

Matsui K, Jahr CE. Differential control of synaptic and ectopic vesicular release of glutamate. *J Neurosci* 2004; 24:8932–8939.

Meller ST, Dykstra C, Grzybycki D, Murphy S, Gebhart GF. The possible role of glia in nociceptive processing and hyperalgesia in the spinal cord of the rat. *Neuropharmacology* 1994; 33:1471–1478.

Millan MJ. The induction of pain: an integrative review. *Prog Neurobiol* 1999; 57:1–164.

Milligan ED, Mehmert KK, Hinde JL, et al. Thermal hyperalgesia and mechanical allodynia produced by intrathecal administration of the human immunodeficiency virus-1 (HIV-1) envelope glycoprotein, gp120. *Brain Res* 2000; 861:105–116.

Milligan ED, O'Connor KA, Nguyen KT, et al. Intrathecal HIV-1 envelope glycoprotein gp120 enhanced pain states mediated by spinal cord proinflammatory cytokines. *J Neurosci* 2001a; 21:2808–2819.

Milligan ED, O'Connor KA, Armstrong CB, et al. Systemic administration of CNI-1493, a p38 mitogen-activated protein kinase inhibitor, blocks intrathecal human immunodeficiency virus-1 gp120-induced enhanced pain states in rats. *J Pain* 2001b; 2:326–333.

Milligan ED, Twining C, Chacur M, et al. Spinal glia and proinflammatory cytokines mediate mirror-image neuropathic pain in rats. *J Neuroscience* 2003; 23:1026–1040.

Milligan ED, Langer SJ, Sloane EM, et al. Controlling pathological pain by adenovirally driven spinal production of the anti-inflammatory cytokine, Interleukin-10. *Eur J Neurosci* 2005a; 21:2136–2148.

Milligan ED, Sloane EM, Langer SJ, et al. Controlling neuropathic pain by adeno-associated virus driven production of the anti-inflammatory cytokine, interleukin-10. *Mol Pain* 2005b; 1:9–22.

Milligan ED, Sloane EM, Langer SJ, et al. Repeated intrathecal injections of plasmid DNA encoding interleukin-10 produce prolonged reversal of neuropathic pain. *Pain* 2006; 126:294–308.

Minoshima T, Nakanishi S. Structural organization of the mouse metabotropic glutamate receptor type 3 gene and its regulation by growth factors in cultured cortical astrocytes. *J Biochem* 1999; 126:889–896.

Moore KW, de Waal Malefy, R, Coffman RL, O'Garra A. Interleukin-10 and the interleukin-10 receptor. *Annu Rev Immunol* 2001; 19:683–765.

Murakami K, Nakamura Y, Toneda Y. Potentiation by ATP of lipopolysaccharide-stimulated nitric oxide production in cultured astrocytes. *Neuroscience* 2003; 117:37–42.

Newman EA. Glial cell inhibition of neurons by release of ATP. *J Neurosci* 2003; 23:1659–1666.

Nguyen MD, Julien J-P, Rivest S. Innate immunity: the missing link in neuroprotection and neurodegeneration? *Nature Rev Neurosci* 2002; 3:216–227.

Norenberg MD. Astrocytes: Normal aspects and response to CNS injury. In: Keane RW, Hickey WF (Eds). *Immunology of the Nervous System.* New York: Oxford University Press, 1997, pp 173–199.

Ohtori S, Takahashi K, Moriya H, Myers RR. TNF-alpha and TNF-alpha receptor type 1 upregulation in glia and neurons after peripheral nerve injury: studies in murine DRG and spinal cord. *Spine* 2004; 29:1082–1088.

Oka T, Hori T. Brain cytokines and pain. In: Watkins LR, Maier SF (Eds). *Cytokines and Pain.* Basel: Birkhäuser Verlag, 1999, pp 183–204.

Pascual O, Casper KB, Kubera C, et al. Astrocytic puringeric signaling coordinates synaptic networks. *Science* 2005; 310:113–116.

Perry VH, Gordon S. Microglia and macrophages. In: Keane RW: Hickey WF (Eds). *Immunology of the Nervous System.* New York: Oxford University Press, 1997, pp 155–172.

Persson M, Sandberg M, Hansson E, Ronnback L. Microglial glutamate uptake is coupled to glutathione synthesis and glutamate release. *Eur J Neurosci* 2006; 24:1063–1070.

Plunkett JA, Yu C-G, Easton JM, Bethea JR, Yezierski RP. Effects of interleukin-10 (IL-10) on pain behavior and gene expression following excitotoxic spinal cord injury in the rat. *Exp Neurol* 2001; 168:144–154.

Porter JT, McCarthy KD. Astrocytic neurotransmitter receptors in situ and in vivo. *Prog Neurobiol* 1997; 51:439–455.

Samad TA, Moore KA, Sapirstein A, et al. Interleukin-1b-mediated induction of COX-2 in the CNS contributes to inflammatory pain hypersensitivity. *Nature* 2001; 410:471–475.

Schipke CG, Ohlemeyer C, Matyash M, et al. Astrocytes of the mouse neocortex express functional N-methyl-D-aspartate receptors. *FASEB J* 2001; 15:1270–1272.

Schwei MJ, Honore P, Rogers SD, et al. Neurochemical and cellular reorganization of the spinal cord in a murine model of bone cancer pain. *J Neurosci* 1999; 19:10886–10897.

Seifert G, Steinhauser C. Ionotropic glutamate receptors in astrocytes. In: Castellano-Lopez B, Nieto-Sampedro M (Eds). *Glial Cell Function,* Progress in Brain Research, Vol. 132. Amsterdam: Elsevier, 2001, pp 287–299.

Sloane EM, Langer SJ, Milligan ED, et al. A novel anti-inflammatory cytokine based non-viral gene therapy: controlling neuropathic pain and beyond. *Immunology 2006.* Boston, MA: American Association of Immunologists, 2006, S34.

Stellwagen D, Malenka RC. Synaptic scaling mediated by glial TNF-alpha. *Nature* 2006; 440:1054–1059.

Suzuki T, Hide I, Ido K, et al. Production and release of neuroprotective tumor necrosis factor by P2X7 receptor activated microglia. *J Neurosci* 2004; 24:1–7.

Sweitzer SM, Colburn RW, Rutkowski M, DeLeo JA. Acute peripheral inflammation induces moderate glial activation and spinal IL-1 beta expression that correlates with pain behavior in the rat. *Brain Res* 1999; 829:209–221.

Sweitzer SM, Martin D, DeLeo JA. Intrathecal interleukin-1 receptor antagonist in combination with soluble tumor necrosis factor receptor exhibits an anti-allodynia action in a rat model of neuropathic pain. *Neurosci* 2001; 103:529–539.

Takano H, Kang J, Jaiswal JK, et al. Receptor-mediated glutamate release from volume sensitive channels in astrocytes. *Proc Natl Acad Sci USA* 2005; 102:16466–16471.

Taylor DL, Diemel LT, Cuzner ML, Pocock JM. Activation of group II glutamate receptors underlies microglial reactivity and neurotoxicity following stimulation with peptides upregulated Alzheimer's disease. *J Neurochem* 2002; 82:1179–1191.

Taylor DL, Diemel LT, Pocock JM. Activation of microglial group III metabotropic glutamate receptors protects neurons against microglial neurotoxicity. *J Neurosci* 2003; 23:2150–2160.

Taylor DL, Jones F, Kubata ES, Pocock JM. Stimulation of microglial metabotropic glutamate receptor mGlu2 triggers tumor necrosis factor alpha–induced neurotoxicity in concert with microglial-derived Fas ligand. *J Neurosci* 2005; 25:2952–2964.

Tikka TM, Koistinaho JE. Minocycline provides neuroprotection against *N*-methyl-D-aspartate neurotoxicity by inhibiting microglia. *J Immunol* 2001; 166:7527–7533.

Tsuda M, Shigemoto-Mogami Y, Koizumi S, et al. P2X4 receptors induced in spinal microglia gate tactile allodynia after nerve injury. *Nature* 2003; 424:778–783.

Üçeyler N, Valenza R, Stock M, et al. Reduced levels of antiinflammatory cytokines in patients with chronic widespread pain. *Arthritis Rheum* 2006; 54:2656–2664.

Ushijima H, Nishio O, Klocking R, Perovic S, Muller WEG. Exposure to gp120 of HIV-1 induces an increased release of arachidonic acid in rat primary neuronal cell culture followed by NMDA receptor-mediated neurotoxicity. *Eur J Neurosci* 1995; 7:1353–1359.

Vallat-Decouvelaere AV, Chretien F, Gras G, et al. Expression of excitatory amino acid transporter-1 in brain macrophages and microglia of HIV-infected patients. A neuroprotective role for activated microglia? *J Neuropathol Exp Neurol* 2003; 62:475–485.

Watkins LR, Maier SF. Illness-induced hyperalgesia: Mediators, mechanisms and implications. In: Watkins LR, Maier SF (Eds). *Cytokines and Pain.* Switzerland: Birkhauser, 1999, pp 39–57.

Watkins LR, Maier SF. Glia: a novel drug discovery target for clinical pain. *Nat Rev Drug Discov* 2003; 2:973–985.

Watkins LR, Martin D, Ulrich P, Tracey KJ, Maier SF. Evidence for the involvement of spinal cord glia in subcutaneous formalin induced hyperalgesia in the rat. *Pain* 1997; 71:225–235.

Watkins LR, Milligan ED, Maier SF. Glial activation: a driving force for pathological pain. *Trends Neurosci* 2001a; 24:450–455.

Watkins LR, Milligan ED, Maier SF. Spinal cord glia: new players in pain. *Pain* 2001b; 93:201–205.

Watkins LR, Wieseler-Frank J, Milligan ED, Johnston I, Maier SF. Contribution of glia to pain processing in health and disease. In: Cervero F, Jensen TS (Eds). *Handbook of Clinical Neurology,* Vol. 81. Elsevier, 2006, pp 309–323.

Wieseler-Frank J, Maier SF, Watkins LR. Central proinflammatory cytokines and pain enhancement. *NeuroSignals* 2005; 14:166–174.

Winkelstein BA, Rutkowski MD, Sweitzer SM, Pahl JL, DeLeo JA. Nerve injury proximal or distal to the DRG induces similar spinal glial activation and selective cytokine expression but differential behavioral responses to pharmacologic treatment. *J Comp Neurol* 2001; 439:127–139.

Wu CL, Garry MG, Zollo RA, Yang J. Gene therapy for the management of pain: Part II: Molecular targets. *Anesthesiology* 2001a; 95:216–240.

Wu CL, Garry MG, Zollo RA, Yang J. Gene therapy for the management of pain: Part I: Methods and strategies. *Anesthesiology* 2001b; 94:1119–1132.

Yao MZ, Gu JF, Wang JH, et al. Interleukin-2 gene therapy of chronic neuropathic pain. *Neuroscience* 2002a; 112:409–416.

Yao MZ, Wang JH, Gu JF, et al. Interleukin-2 gene has superior antinociceptive effects when delivered intrathecally. *Clin Neurosci Neuropathol* 2002b; 13:791–794.

Yao MZ, Gu JF, Wang HJ, et al. Adenovirus-mediated interleukin-2 gene therapy of nociception. *Gene Ther* 2003; 10:1392–1399.

Yu C-G, Fairbanks CA, Wilcox GL, Yezierski RP. Effects of agmatine, interleukin-10 and cyclosporin on spontaneous pain behavior following excitotoxic spinal cord injury in rats. *J Pain* 2003; 4:129–140.

Zhang RX, Wang LB, Ren K, et al. Spinal glial activation in a new rat model of bone cancer pain produced by prostate cancer cell inoculation of the tibia. *Pain* 2005; 118:125–136.

Correspondence to: Erin D. Milligan, PhD, Department of Psychology and the Center for Neuroscience, Campus Box 345, University of Colorado at Boulder, Boulder, CO 80309-0345, USA. Tel: 1-303-735-2295; fax: 1-303-492-2967; email: erin.milligan@colorado.edu.

Part VI

Glial-Pain Interactions: Morphine Tolerance

Immune and Glial Regulation of Pain, edited by Joyce A. DeLeo, Linda S. Sorkin, and Linda R. Watkins, IASP Press, Seattle, © 2007.

19

Modulating Glial Activation in Opioid Tolerance and Neuropathic Pain: A Role for Glutamate Transporters

Vivianne L. Tawfik[a] and Joyce A. DeLeo[b,c]

[a]Department of Pharmacology, Dartmouth Medical School, Hanover, New Hampshire, USA; [b]Department of Anesthesiology, Dartmouth-Hitchcock Medical Center, Lebanon, New Hampshire, USA; [c]Neuroscience Center at Dartmouth, Lebanon, New Hampshire, USA

THE ROLE OF MICROGLIA AND ASTROCYTES IN NEUROPATHIC PAIN

Chronic neuropathic pain, characterized by both hyperalgesia (a heightened response to noxious stimuli) and allodynia (pain perceived following non-noxious stimuli), is a serious health concern, affecting patients with conditions as diverse as phantom limb pain and multiple sclerosis (Dworkin et al. 2003). The opioid family of drugs is only partially effective in treating neuropathic pain, and the high doses required cause a myriad of side effects. Dose escalation is often necessary due to the development of analgesic tolerance, a decreased efficacy of the opioid following repeated administration, rendering the initial dosing schedule inadequate (Cherny et al. 1994).

Over the years there has been a great deal of research into the mechanisms of chronic pain, with a strong focus on the development of central sensitization following nerve injury. Current theories suggest that a host of mediators including (but not limited to) adenosine triphosphate (ATP), gamma-aminobutyric acid (GABA), glutamate, nitric oxide, prostaglandins, and substance P produce alterations in the central nervous system (CNS) milieu that lead to permanent changes in synaptic processing. Our laboratory, among others, has proposed that central neuroimmune activation is a player in this complicated nociceptive signaling cascade. Specifically, we have postulated that spinal glial cell activation with subsequent cytokine and chemokine production may induce the expression of final common pain mediators such as glutamate and nitric oxide

(DeLeo and Yezierski 2001). Further knowledge of this interplay would help guide the development of novel therapeutic agents because events that induce hyperalgesia also activate immune cells, both centrally and in the periphery, suggesting that immune activation may mediate chronic pain (Watkins et al. 1995; DeLeo et al. 1996).

Microglia are the first non-neuronal cells to respond to a CNS perturbation such as nerve injury or chronic opioid administration (Raghavendra et al. 2002; Tanga et al. 2004). The exact mechanism of microglial cell activation may involve the release from injured or hyperactive neurons of algesic factors such as ATP, glutamate, and nitric oxide (Watkins et al. 2005). Recent work from our laboratory has indicated a role for the pattern recognition receptor Toll-like receptor 4 (TLR-4) in microglial activation that provides a link between central sensitization and innate immune responses (Tanga et al. 2005). Upon activation, microglia increase their expression of complement receptor 3/cluster of differentiation 11b (CR3/CD11b). Temporal and positional tracking of this molecule serves as a useful marker for experimental analysis of microglial activation. In fact, immunohistochemistry using OX-42, the antibody directed against CR3/CD11b, has demonstrated enhanced immunoreactivity in the spinal cord dorsal horn following various central and peripheral nerve injuries (Hashizume et al. 2000; Winkelstein et al. 2001). Microglia can release a host of factors to protect the CNS; however, when activated they can also produce free radicals and proinflammatory cytokines, including interleukin-1β (IL-1β), tumor necrosis factor-α (TNF-α), IL-6, and interferon-γ, in an aberrant fashion. Such factors are instrumental in the activation of astrocytes, induction of cell adhesion molecules, and T-leukocyte recruitment into the CNS following nerve injury (Sweitzer et al. 2002; Liu and Hong 2003; L. Cao and J.A. DeLeo, submitted manuscript).

Astrocytes, along with oligodendrocytes and ependymal cells, constitute the macroglia of the CNS. They are responsible for a plethora of tasks, including their well-known role in the formation of the blood-brain barrier, which limits the entry of circulating elements into the nervous system. In fact, the selective ablation of reactive astrocytes in the process of CNS restoration leads to failure of blood-brain barrier repair, an enhanced infiltration of leukocytes, and subsequent excitotoxic neuronal death (Bush et al. 1999). Such extreme consequences resulting from astrocytic loss underscore the crucial role of these glial cells in homeostasis and regeneration after injury. However, as discussed below, proper regulation of such functions is key to maintaining synaptic integrity.

Astrocytes derive from the neuroectoderm and express a series of "marker antigens" during development such as the intermediate filament proteins vimentin and nestin (Eliasson et al. 1999). Once they reach their adult phenotype, astrocytes express other markers including glial fibrillary acidic protein (GFAP).

This intermediate filament protein is commonly considered to be astrocyte-specific, although it may also be found on reactive choroid plexus epithelium cells (Reichenbach and Wolburg 2005). GFAP functions as a structural protein and has been shown to increase in hypertrophic, activated astrocytes (Eng et al. 2000). While enhancement of GFAP remains the mainstay for demonstrating astrocytic reactivity, it is important to note that estimates suggest that only 15% of the total cell volume is labeled with this marker (Bushong et al. 2002). In addition, there exist populations of astrocytes that are not GFAP positive, and the physiological relevance of these distinct groups is not well understood (Kimelberg 2004). It is clear that astrocytes are well poised in the CNS to modulate synaptic communication. For example, it is estimated that 56% of rat cortical synapses are ensheathed by astrocyte domains (Chao et al. 2002), suggesting an integral role of these complex cells. Phylogenetically, an increased astrocyte-to-neuron ratio is observed in parallel with species brain complexity (Nedergaard et al. 2003). This finding implies a greater requirement for network integration in higher mammals that is likely to be reliant on the functional domains imparted by astrocytic processes.

In the context of neuropathic pain, astrocytes are activated in the spinal cord following several types of nerve injury that result in behavioral hypersensitivity, including chronic constriction injury (Garrison et al. 1991) and L5 nerve ligation and transection (Colburn et al. 1999). It has been postulated that this aberrant activation results in the loss of homeostatic mechanisms and the expression of algesic mediators such as cytokines and chemokines (DeLeo et al. 1997; Abbadie et al. 2003), which may sensitize neurons.

Glia contribute in a fundamental way to synaptic events because they are capable of releasing transmitters such as D-serine, ATP, and glutamate (Parpura et al. 1994; Snyder and Kim 2000; Inoue et al. 2003). The role of such "gliotransmitters" is slowly being elucidated in the spinal cord in which the plasticity that characterizes chronic neuropathic pain is most likely due to prolonged central sensitization. Recent evidence suggests that astrocyte-derived D-serine may sensitize neurons in pain states by decreasing the threshold for N-methyl-D-aspartate (NMDA)-receptor activation (Guo et al. 2006). Moreover, Tsuda et al. (2003) demonstrated that ATP-activated microglia injected into the spinal cord were sufficient to cause allodynia. Interestingly, while astrocytic glutamate transporters hold a clear function in pain states, it remains to be demonstrated whether astrocytic glutamate release contributes to the elevated levels of spinal excitatory amino acids observed after nerve injury. A key feature of astrocytes is their proclivity to function as part of a syncytium and utilize intercellular communication ports such as connexins to transfer information in the form of ATP and Ca^{2+} (Cotrina et al. 1998). Fig. 1 summarizes the key features of the "tetrapartite synapse"—an astrocyte and microglial cell in relation to the pre- and post-

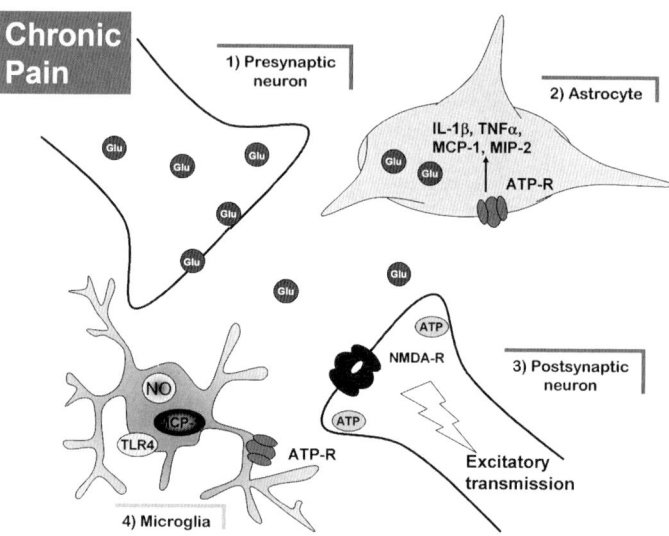

Fig. 1. The tetrapartite synapse in chronic neuropathic pain. The functional unit in the injured CNS consists of a presynaptic neuron (1), an astrocyte (2), a postsynaptic neuron (3), and a microglial cell (4). Under normal conditions, astrocytes orchestrate synaptic activity and microglia provide immune surveillance. After nerve injury, aberrant activation of these glial cells may lead to the release of sensitizing mediators, the upregulation of specific surface markers, and a loss of homeostatic mechanisms. Such alterations in the spinal cord result in excitatory effects on pre- and postsynaptic neurons, rendering them more responsive to incoming stimuli. ATP = adenosine triphosphate, ATP-R = ATP receptor, IL-1β = interleukin-1β, MCP-1 = monocyte chemoattractant protein-1, MIP-2 = macrophage inflammatory protein-2, NMDA-R = NMDA receptor, NO = nitric oxide, TLR4 = Toll-like receptor 4, TNF-α = tumor necrosis factor-α.

synaptic neuron after nerve injury. Prior work has highlighted a role for a tripartite synapse in long-term potentiation and other forms of spinal cord plasticity (Fellin et al. 2006). In the tripartite model, the microglial cell is excluded from the scheme. It is now clear, however, based on work from several laboratories (Raghavendra et al. 2003a; Svensson et al. 2003; Tsuda et al. 2004; Ledeboer et al. 2005), that microglia play a key role in central sensitization resulting from chronic pain. As such, we propose that our model of the tetrapartite synapse more accurately reflects the cell types that take part in spinal cord responses involved in neuropathic pain (De Leo et al. 2006).

GLIAL MODULATION THROUGH PROPENTOFYLLINE

Propentofylline is an atypical methylxanthine previously shown to attenuate astrocytic activation in a rodent model of ischemia (DeLeo et al. 1987).

As a result of this action, the drug has been used extensively to study the role of glial activation in behavioral sensitization after nerve injury. In an initial study, it was demonstrated that preemptive intrathecal or systemic treatment with propentofylline decreased mechanical allodynia after L5 spinal nerve transection (Sweitzer et al. 2001b). In concert with this antiallodynic effect, the expression of microglial and astrocytic activation markers (OX-42 and GFAP) was reduced. Further work established that propentofylline suppressed glial-activation-induced cytokine release and had an antihyperalgesic effect after peripheral nerve injury (Raghavendra et al. 2003b). In relation to a thera-peutically relevant action, we recently administered propentofylline 14 days after L5 spinal nerve transection to determine if it was capable of reversing existing chronic pain (Tawfik et al. 2007). We discovered that daily, systemic propentofylline reversed mechanical allodynia for the duration of dosing and furthermore, that this anti-allodynic effect was maintained for at least 14 days after the final dose, which suggests a disease-modifying effect. Microglial acti-vation was suppressed by propentofylline at this late time point, but a minimal contribution of GFAP-positive astrocytes was observed.

The exact mechanism of propentofylline's analgesic action remains un-known. However, propentofylline has been shown to inhibit adenosine transport and the cyclic-adenosine-5',3'-monophosphate (cAMP)-specific phosphodies-terase, leading to the induction of cAMP (Nagata et al. 1985; Parkinson and Fredholm 1991; Meskini et al. 1994). Furthermore, strengthening of cAMP-dependent signaling decreased microglial proliferation and activation in culture (Si et al. 1996), providing a possible mechanism of glial modulation via pro-pentofylline. Recent work from our laboratory has suggested a further function of propentofylline that may be crucial to its antiallodynic action: enhancement of astrocytic glutamate transporters, as described further below.

REGULATION OF GLUTAMATE BY ASTROCYTES

A crucial function ascribed to astrocytes is the control of extracellular glutamate homeostasis through sodium-dependent uptake via the excitatory amino acid transporters (EAATs) 1–5 (Danbolt 2001). Dysregulation of synap-tic glutamate has been implicated in many disease processes (Rothstein et al. 1996; Maragakis and Rothstein 2001), and therefore the exquisite regulation of glutamate by astrocytes is crucial to neuronal integrity. The glutamate-aspartate transporter (GLAST/EAAT1) and glutamate transporter-1 (GLT-1/EAAT2) are primarily localized in astrocytes, while the excitatory amino acid carrier (EAAC/EAAT3) is found in neurons (Kanai and Hediger 1992; Pines et al. 1992; Storck et al. 1992). The excitatory amino acid transporter 4 (EAAT4) is found in the cerebellum, and EAAT5 is the retinal glutamate transporter (Fairman et al. 1995; Arriza et al. 1997).

Injury to the central or peripheral nervous system increases GFAP immunoreactivity in astrocytes, suggesting that they have been "activated." Interestingly, in vitro studies have demonstrated that this activated phenotype includes reduced levels of the transporter GLT-1 (Schlag et al. 1998). Therefore, the potential exists for glutamate transporter downregulation in neuropathic pain states.

MODULATION OF GLUTAMATE TRANSPORTERS

Several studies in animal models have linked allodynia and hyperalgesia to excess levels of excitatory amino acids in the cerebral spinal fluid (Sluka and Westlund 1992; Malmberg and Yaksh 1995). It follows that after nerve injury, second-order neurons would be exposed to increased levels of glutamate in the synapse, which would lead to aberrant firing of action potentials. The role of glutamate transporters in this synaptic dysregulation has begun to be explored. Using the chronic constriction injury model of neuropathic pain, Sung et al. (2003) demonstrated that GLT-1, GLAST, and EAAC1 were all downregulated by day 7 post-nerve injury. In addition, after spinal nerve ligation, glutamate uptake in the lumbar spinal cord is attenuated (Binns et al. 2005). Interestingly, pharmacological inhibition of glutamate transporters has been shown to produce spontaneous nociceptive behaviors that could be attenuated by NMDA antagonists (Liaw et al. 2005). In our own studies, we have found that propentofylline is capable of reversing nerve-transection-induced reductions in GLT-1 and GLAST (Tawfik et al. 2006). Using primary astrocyte cultures, we showed that propentofylline shifted astrocytes from an activated, low-GLT-1-expressing state to a quiescent, high-GLT-1 phenotype that demonstrated enhanced glutamate clearance (Tawfik et al. 2006). In addition, we found that propentofylline was able to decrease lipopolysaccharide-induced chemokine release from these astrocytes, providing further evidence for a mechanism related to neuroimmune suppression. Taken together, this body of work highlights a role for deficient glutamate transport in pain behaviors and indicates the importance of returning astrocytes to a quiescent phenotype, competent of maintaining excitatory amino acid homeostasis, as depicted in Fig. 2.

Recently, a glial-restricted precursor cell line has been developed that overexpresses the glial glutamate transporter GLT-1. This cell line (called G3) has undergone preliminary testing in an organotypic spinal cord culture model of chronic glutamate neurotoxicity (Maragakis et al. 2005). It was demonstrated that the transplantation of G3s into the spinal slice protected against motor neuron death induced by excitotoxicity. Transplantation of similar cells into

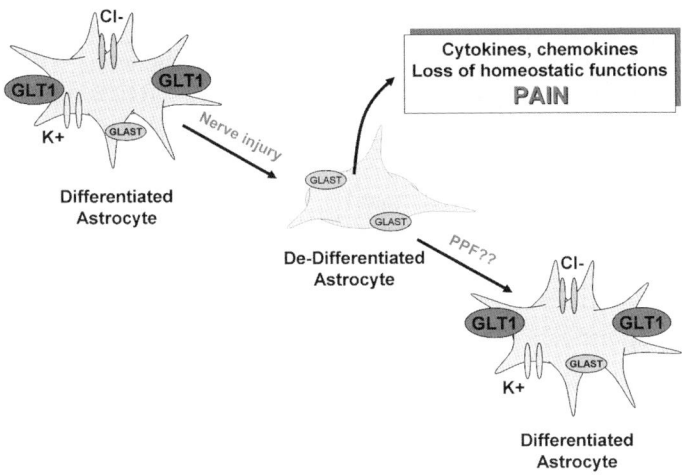

Fig. 2. Role of astrocytic glutamate transporters in neuropathic pain and modulation with propentofylline. In their differentiated, quiescent state, astrocytes express high levels of the glutamate transporter, GLT-1, as well as a normal complement of ion channels. Following nerve injury, the pathological activation of astrocytes leads to their de-differentiation, which comprises a phenotype shift and a dramatic decrease in the expression of GLT-1. In concert, activated astrocytes may release algesic mediators such as cytokines and chemokines that can sensitize the synaptic milieu and lead to the ectopic discharges characteristic of neuropathic pain. The glial-modulating agent propentofylline (PPF) reinstates the differentiated phenotype and enhances GLT-1 levels, allowing the astrocyte to resume its homeostatic functions in the central nervous system.

the adult rat spinal cord has been characterized, with results showing that differentiation occurs along astrocytic and oligodendrocytic lineages in response to endogenous proliferation signals (Han et al. 2004). Such a cell line offers an exciting and novel way to investigate neuroimmune activation-induced changes in glutamate transporter levels in neuropathic pain. Specifically, by introducing GLT-1 transporters via these glial-restricted precursor cells, it would be possible to confirm whether an enhancement of glutamate transport alone is sufficient to decrease injury-induced allodynia.

NEUROENERGETICS AND THE ASTROCYTE

Astrocytes are ideally located to couple synaptic activity to glucose utilization, which is known to be the major energy substrate for neurons. Recent evidence suggests that lactate may represent a further oxidative substrate in cases of enhanced activity because it reduces glutamate-induced neurotoxicity in vivo (Ros et al. 2001). In the context of the tetrapartite synapse, this lactate supply is thought to originate from astrocytes which, via end-feet on cerebral vasculature, may take up glucose through the glucose transporter 1 (GLUT1) and subsequently release lactate via specific monocarboxylate transporters (MCT1 and MCT4) (Pellerin et al. 2005). In contrast, neurons exhibit the higher-affinity transporter, MCT2, which is thought to lead to net uptake of lactate by neurons and export by astrocytes. This forms the hypothesized astrocyte-neuron lactate shuttle (Bonvento et al. 2005), seen in Fig. 3.

As outlined above, astrocytes express glutamate transporters, which are required for the exquisite control of glutamate levels in the synapse. Recent evidence suggests a further function of glutamate transporters in astrocytes: that of a neuronal metabolic sensor. The uptake process is electrogenic; three Na^+ ions and one proton are cotransported with glutamate, but only one K^+ ion is released. This shift in intracellular Na^+ is thought to trigger a signaling cascade of astrocytic glycolysis (Pellerin 2005). Concurrently, astrocytes release lactate, therefore supplying active synapses with increased metabolic substrates (Pellerin and Magistretti 1994). Interestingly, an elegant study by Voutsinos-Porche et al. (2003) demonstrated that GLT-1 and GLAST knockout mice display a dampened metabolic response to glutamate. Specifically, the study showed that

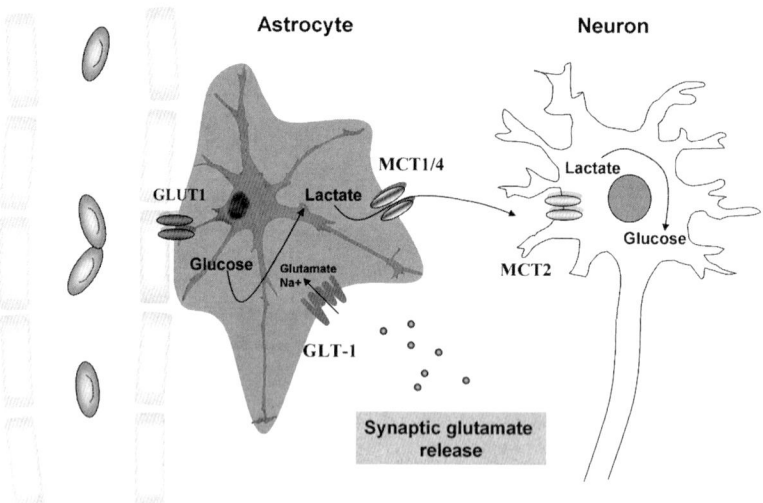

Fig. 3. The astrocyte-neuron lactate shuttle. Synaptic activity leads to glutamate release, which is "sensed" by astrocytes through glutamate transporters (such as GLT-1, depicted). Glucose is taken up via the glucose transporter (GLUT1) on astrocytic end-feet on the vasculature and converted to lactate when the intracellular Na^+ concentration is elevated by enhanced glutamate uptake. Lactate is then released through the monocarboxylate transporters, MCT1 or MCT4, and can then be taken up by the neuronal transporter, MCT2. Finally, lactate is converted back to glucose to satisfy neuronal energy requirements.

glucose utilization in the barrel cortex following whisker stimulation was re-duced in GLT and GLAST knockout mice. In addition, when cortical astrocytes from GLAST knockout mice were stimulated with glutamate, both glucose uptake and lactate release was suppressed—an effect that was correlated to the lack of an uptake-related increase in intracellular Na^+.

It is currently unknown how neuropathic pain affects neuronal energy balance and neuronal-astrocytic metabolic cross-talk. It is possible that fol-lowing nerve injury, activated astrocytes that exhibit lower levels of GLT-1 (Sung et al. 2003; also see White et al., this volume) could no longer sense the increased energy requirements of glutamatergic neurons, leading to the risk of excitotoxic damage. Specifically, as outlined in Fig. 4, the decreased ability of astrocytes to clear synaptic glutamate would hinder the conversion of glucose to lactate, therefore starving neurons of much-needed fuel. In combination with enhanced levels of synaptic glutamate, the corollary would be oxidative stress and aberrant neuronal firing, leading to sensitization. Our laboratory is currently investigating this hypothesis using astrocyte cultures and in vivo models of neuropathic pain.

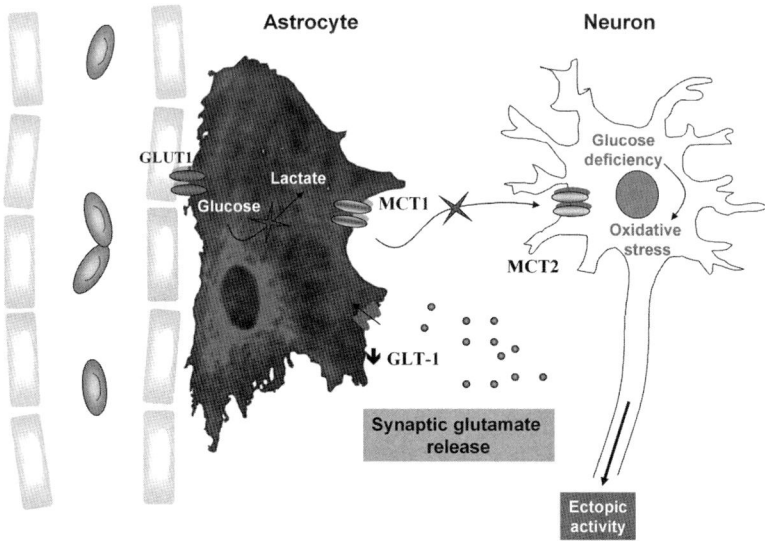

Fig. 4. Proposed disruption of glial-neuronal metabolic cross-talk in neuropathic pain. After an insult to the CNS, astrocytes may become activated and exhibit decreased numbers of glutamate transporters (such as GLT-1) on their surface. Without this "metabolic sensor," astrocytes can no longer respond to increased neuronal energy requirements by enhancing glucose uptake. The result is less lactate shuttled to neurons and oxidative stress ensues contributing further to ectopic neuronal activity.

THE GLIAL CONTRIBUTION TO OPIOID TOLERANCE

Opioids exert their analgesic effects through binding the opioid family of classic seven-transmembrane-spanning G-protein-coupled receptors, which include the mu, delta, and kappa opioid receptors (Martin et al. 1976; Mestek et al. 1995; Snyder and Pasternak 2003). These receptors are further linked to an inwardly rectifying potassium channel, and therefore, ligand binding leads to hyperpolarization of the cell (North et al. 1987). Subsequent signaling via the activated G protein initializes a range of intracellular cascades that have been hypothesized to mediate opioid tolerance. Although opioids decrease the probability of action potentials in pre- and postsynaptic cells of small nociceptive afferents and may prevent the release of pain neurotransmitters (Jessell and Iversen 1977), their exact mechanism of analgesic action is still unknown.

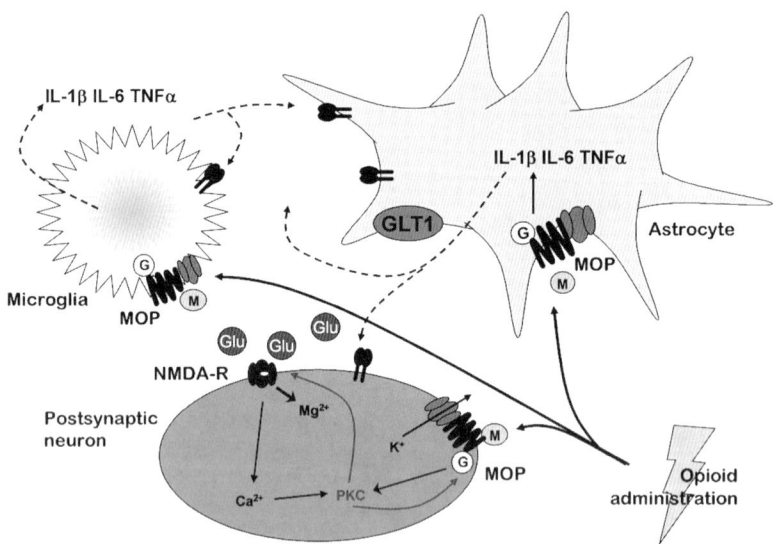

Fig. 5. Neuroimmune mediation of morphine tolerance/hyperalgesia. An administered opioid may act by several mechanisms including on the postsynaptic neuron via G-protein-coupled mu-opioid receptors (MOP) or on the glial cell network via G-protein-coupled mu-opioid receptors on microglia and astrocytes. Opioid binding to the neuronal mu-receptor activates G-protein-mediated protein kinase C (PKC) translocation and activation, promoting removal of the N-methyl-D-aspartate receptor (NMDA-R) Mg^{2+} plug. The ionotropic NMDA-R then responds to glutamate released from the presynaptic cell by allowing Ca^{2+} influx. This increase in intracellular Ca^{2+} leads to several downstream effects and causes further activation of PKC. With continual activation of these pathways by opioid receptor occupation, PKC may uncouple the G protein from the mu-opioid receptor, effectively short-circuiting the system and preventing any downstream signaling upon ligand binding. Glu = glutamate, G = G protein coupled to receptor, GLT1 = glutamate transporter-1, IL-1β = interleukin 1-β, IL-6 = interleukin 6, M = morphine, TNF-α = tumor necrosis factor-α.

At the cellular level, it has been demonstrated that opioids cause receptor phosphorylation that renders them unresponsive to further agonist stimulation, until rapid internalization by endocytosis allows for receptors to be recycled back to the membrane in an active form (see review by von Zastrow et al. 2003). Interestingly, opioid agonists differ in their ability to induce activation, desensitization, and endocytosis. Specifically, morphine fails to cause mu-opioid-receptor internalization in most (Keith et al. 1998; Finn and Whistler 2001), but not all, systems (Haberstock-Debic et al. 2005), whereas fentanyl or methadone stimulation always leads to rapid desensitization and endocytosis (Borgland et al. 2003; Bohn et al. 2004). This differential ability of various opioids to cause receptor recycling, the cellular hallmark of tolerance, may contribute to the discrepancy in the development of analgesic tolerance to various opioids (Paronis and Holtzman 1992; Duttaroy and Yoburn 1995).

An important addition to this scheme is the glial cell, which not only releases the mediators discussed above but also possesses opioid receptors and thus may directly respond to the presence of opioids (see Fig. 5). In addition, glutamate transporters on glia probably modulate the neuronal NMDA-receptor activation that ensues following chronic opioid administration. An integrated approach to the study of opioid tolerance would thus be beneficial, as it is now clear that these drugs are affecting both neurons and the crucial network of glial cells in the CNS.

As early as 1988, it was proposed that "astroglial cells" would play a role in morphine tolerance, given their strategic position and ability to contribute to synaptic events (Ronnback and Hansson 1988). It was Song and Zhao (2001), however, who provided the first evidence for a role for glial cells in the development of morphine tolerance. They reported increased GFAP in the spinal cord, posterior cingulate cortex, and hippocampus following chronic intraperitoneal treatment of rats with morphine sulfate. Furthermore, when the hypertrophy and hyperactivity of astrocytes was blocked using the glial metabolic inhibitor fluorocitrate, morphine analgesia was partially restored. Our laboratory has further shown that chronic, but not acute, morphine administration leads to glial activation and cytokine expression (Raghavendra et al. 2002). Specifically, we observed that daily morphine treatment alone led to increases in GFAP and OX-42 immunoreactivity as well as enhanced expression of IL-1β, IL-6, and TNF. These changes were further exacerbated when morphine was administered chronically to rats that had also received an L5 spinal nerve transection, suggesting a possible additive effect. In addition, we have shown that chronic subcutaneous and intrathecal morphine leads to analgesic tolerance within 6 and 3 days, respectively, which was associated with a robust activation of spinal glia (Tawfik et al. 2005). The key role of glial activation in morphine tolerance was demonstrated using the glial modulator propentofylline.

Suppression of glial activation with propentofylline was capable of restoring the acute analgesic activity of morphine in neuropathic rats (Raghavendra et al. 2003b) and of impeding the development of morphine tolerance (Raghavendra et al. 2004). A concurrent inhibition of chronic morphine-induced spinal glial activation and cytokine expression suggests a link between neuroimmune activation and morphine tolerance development. These findings indicate that inhibition of spinal glial action may be sufficient to re-establish the clinical utility of morphine (Watkins and Maier 2003), but further analysis is needed to determine the potential usefulness of this combination therapy in the treatment of neuropathic pain.

While no studies to date have focused specifically on the potential mechanism of morphine-induced glial activation and cytokine expression, Beitner-Johnson et al. (1993) demonstrated that naltrexone reversed the ability of chronic morphine to enhance GFAP levels in the rat ventral tegmental area. Astrocytes express functional mu, delta, and kappa opioid receptors in a region-specific manner (Eriksson et al. 1991; Ruzicka et al. 1995; Stiene-Martin et al. 1998), and morphine can modulate the astrocytic and microglial production of cytokines, chemokines, and their receptors in vitro in a mu-receptor-mediated fashion (Chao et al. 1994; Mahajan et al. 2002; El-Hage et al. 2005). In contrast, the non-opioid receptor antagonist D-naloxone blocked anti-analgesia produced by either morphine enantiomer, leading Wu et al. (2004, 2005) to propose that activation of a non-opioid receptor on glial cells is responsible for the decreased efficacy of morphine. In agreement, we have recently shown that neither chronic fentanyl nor methadone administration leads to spinal glial activation after continuous administration (V.L. Tawfik, unpublished manuscript). Given that fentanyl is a potent mu-receptor agonist, this finding lends further support to the hypothesis that morphine-induced glial activation occurs independently from this receptor. Further investigation of the differential ability of specific opioids to enhance astrocytic and microglial activation may therefore provide insight into the molecular mechanisms of tolerance-related neuroimmune activation.

Proinflammatory cytokines (IL-1β, IL-6, and TNF) have been shown to be elevated in nerve injury models (DeLeo et al. 1997) and to play a role in mediating other pain states (Watkins et al. 1995; Sweitzer et al. 2001a). Recent findings also suggest cytokine modulation of opioid analgesia and tolerance (Gul et al. 2000) as well as opioid control of cytokine action (Raghavendra and DeLeo 2006). Using a model of diabetes-induced neuropathy, Gul et al. (2000) showed that intracerebroventricularly injected IL-1β abolished the analgesic effects of morphine and also caused hyperalgesia in normal mice. For further information on the specific role of pro- and anti-inflammatory cytokines in the genesis of morphine tolerance, see the chapter by Shavit et al. in this book.

In addition to a proposed role for glutamate transporters in neuropathic pain, alterations in these important neurotransmitter modulators have also been linked to the development of morphine tolerance. Specifically, GLAST and EAAC mRNA and protein were downregulated during the development of morphine tolerance (Mao et al. 2002). Furthermore, the positive transporter regulator riluzole and the GLT-1 inhibitor L-trans-pyrrolidine-2,4-dicarboxylic acid (PDC) attenuated and potentiated the development of morphine tolerance, respectively (Ozawa et al. 2001; Mao et al. 2002). Dexamethasone has also been shown to attenuate morphine analgesic tolerance through an enhancement of astrocytic glutamate transporters and a subsequent reduction in excitatory amino acid levels (Wen et al. 2005). Alterations in glutamate transporters also play a role in morphine withdrawal. Xu et al. (2003) have demonstrated that cell surface GLT-1 expression increased during morphine withdrawal and that inhibition of glutamate transporters using the nonspecific inhibitor DL-threo-beta-benzyloxyaspartate led to an enhancement in naloxone-precipitated withdrawal symptoms (Sekiya et al. 2004). The relationship between glial modulators such as propentofylline or minocycline and glutamate transporter expression in morphine tolerance paradigms has yet to be explored and would be an interesting extension of the results obtained in neuropathy models.

RELATIONSHIP BETWEEN NEUROPATHIC PAIN AND MORPHINE TOLERANCE

While the sensation of pain is a direct result of enhanced neuronal firing, the overwhelming number of glial cells in the spinal cord necessitates further consideration. This chapter has focused not on the neuron, executor of CNS actions, but on the glial cell, orchestrator of CNS function. We have described research exploring the involvement of resident spinal glial cells in the generation of ectopic discharges that manifest as pain and the role of glia in the expression of morphine tolerance. We have framed this discussion using the tetrapartite synapse, consisting of an astrocyte, microglial cell, and pre- and postsynaptic neurons (DeLeo et al. 2006), as it relates to spinal mechanisms of central sensitization.

It has been proposed that nerve-injury-related pain and morphine tolerance share underlying molecular mechanisms (Mayer et al. 1999), which may explain the common clinical adage that neuropathic pain is opioid-resistant. This chapter has highlighted the role of glial activation, cytokine expression, and aberrant glutamate transporter function in both paradigms. The recruitment of these important mutual components may cause the injured CNS to react differently to exogenous morphine and possibly other opioids (Watkins et al. 2005).

In summary, discerning the role of spinal glia in modulating neuropathic pain and morphine tolerance remains key to improving our understanding of the CNS response to injury as a whole and may translate into improved pharmacological targets.

ACKNOWLEDGMENTS

The authors wish to thank Tracy Wynkoop for her editorial assistance.

REFERENCES

Abbadie C, Lindia JA, Cumiskey AM, et al. Impaired neuropathic pain responses in mice lacking the chemokine receptor CCR2. *Proc Natl Acad Sci USA* 2003; 100:7947–7952.

Arriza JL, Eliasof S, Kavanaugh MP, Amara SG. Excitatory amino acid transporter 5, a retinal glutamate transporter coupled to a chloride conductance. *Proc Natl Acad Sci USA* 1997; 94:4155–4160.

Beitner-Johnson D, Guitart X, Nestler EJ. Glial fibrillary acidic protein and the mesolimbic dopamine system: regulation by chronic morphine and Lewis-Fischer strain differences in the rat ventral tegmental area. *J Neurochem* 1993; 61:1766–1773.

Binns BC, Huang Y, Goettl VM, Hackshaw KV, Stephens RL Jr. Glutamate uptake is attenuated in spinal deep dorsal and ventral horn in the rat spinal nerve ligation model. *Brain Res* 2005; 1041:38–47.

Bohn LM, Dykstra LA, Lefkowitz RJ, Caron MG, Barak LS. Relative opioid efficacy is determined by the complements of the G protein-coupled receptor desensitization machinery. *Mol Pharmacol* 2004; 66:106–112.

Bonvento G, Herard AS, Voutsinos-Porche B. The astrocyte-neuron lactate shuttle: a debated but still valuable hypothesis for brain imaging. *J Cereb Blood Flow Metab* 2005; 25:1394–1399.

Borgland SL, Connor M, Osborne PB, Furness JB, Christie MJ. Opioid agonists have different efficacy profiles for G protein activation, rapid desensitization, and endocytosis of mu-opioid receptors. *J Biol Chem* 2003; 278:18776–18784.

Bush TG, Puvanachandra N, Horner CH, et al. Leukocyte infiltration, neuronal degeneration, and neurite outgrowth after ablation of scar-forming, reactive astrocytes in adult transgenic mice. *Neuron* 1999; 23:297–308.

Bushong EA, Martone ME, Jones YZ, Ellisman MH. Protoplasmic astrocytes in CA1 stratum radiatum occupy separate anatomical domains. *J Neurosci* 2002; 22:183–192.

Chao CC, Gekker G, Sheng WS, et al. Priming effect of morphine on the production of tumor necrosis factor-alpha by microglia: implications in respiratory burst activity and human immunodeficiency virus-1 expression. *J Pharmacol Exp Ther* 1994; 269:198–203.

Chao TI, Rickmann M, Wolff JR. The synapse-astrocyte boundary: an anatomical basis for an integrative role of glial in synaptic transmission. In: Volterra A, Magistretti P, Haydon P (Eds). *The Tripartite Synapse: Glia in Synaptic Transmission.* Oxford: Oxford University Press, 2002, pp 3–23.

Cherny NI, Thaler HT, Friedlander-Klar H, et al. Opioid responsiveness of cancer pain syndromes caused by neuropathic or nociceptive mechanisms: a combined analysis of controlled, single-dose studies. *Neurology* 1994; 44:857–861.

Colburn RW, Rickman AJ, DeLeo JA. The effect of site and type of nerve injury on spinal glial activation and neuropathic pain behavior. *Exp Neurol* 1999; 157:289–304.

Cotrina ML, Lin JH, Alves-Rodrigues A, et al. Connexins regulate calcium signaling by controlling ATP release. *Proc Natl Acad Sci USA* 1998; 95:15735–15740.

Danbolt NC. Glutamate uptake. *Prog Neurobiol* 2001; 65:1–105.

DeLeo JA, Yezierski RP. The role of neuroinflammation and neuroimmune activation in persistent pain. *Pain* 2001; 90:1–6.

DeLeo J, Toth L, Schubert P, Rudolphi K, Kreutzberg GW. Ischemia-induced neuronal cell death, calcium accumulation, and glial response in the hippocampus of the Mongolian gerbil and protection by propentofylline (HWA 285). *J Cereb Blood Flow Metab* 1987; 7:745–751.

DeLeo JA, Colburn RW, Nichols M, Malhotra A. Interleukin-6-mediated hyperalgesia/allodynia and increased spinal IL-6 expression in a rat mononeuropathy model. *J Interferon Cytokine Res* 1996; 16:695–700.

DeLeo JA, Colburn RW, Rickman AJ. Cytokine and growth factor immunohistochemical spinal profiles in two animal models of mononeuropathy. *Brain Res* 1997; 759:50–57.

DeLeo JA, Tawfik VL, LaCroix-Fralish ML. The tetrapartite synapse: path to CNS sensitization and chronic pain. *Pain* 2006; 122:17–21.

Duttaroy A, Yoburn BC. The effect of intrinsic efficacy on opioid tolerance. *Anesthesiology* 1995; 82:1226–1236.

Dworkin RH, Backonja M, Rowbotham MC, et al. Advances in neuropathic pain: diagnosis, mechanisms, and treatment recommendations. *Arch Neurol* 2003; 60:1524–1534.

El-Hage N, Gurwell JA, Singh IN, et al. Synergistic increases in intracellular Ca^{2+}, and the release of MCP-1, RANTES, and IL-6 by astrocytes treated with opiates and HIV-1 Tat. *Glia* 2005; 50:91–106.

Eliasson C, Sahlgren C, Berthold CH, et al. Intermediate filament protein partnership in astrocytes. *J Biol Chem* 1999; 274:23996–24006.

Eng LF, Ghirnikar RS, Lee YL. Glial fibrillary acidic protein: GFAP—thirty-one years (1969–2000). *Neurochem Res* 2000; 25:1439–1451.

Eriksson PS, Hansson E, Ronnback L. Mu and delta opiate receptors in neuronal and astroglial primary cultures from various regions of the brain-coupling with adenylate cyclase, localisation on the same neurones and association with dopamine (D1) receptor adenylate cyclase. *Neuropharmacology* 1991; 30:1233–1239.

Fairman WA, Vandenberg RJ, Arriza JL, Kavanaugh MP, Amara SG. An excitatory amino-acid transporter with properties of a ligand-gated chloride channel. *Nature* 1995; 375:599–603.

Fellin T, Pascual O, Haydon PG. Astrocytes coordinate synaptic networks: balanced excitation and inhibition. *Physiology (Bethesda)* 2006; 21:208–215.

Finn AK, Whistler JL. Endocytosis of the mu opioid receptor reduces tolerance and a cellular hallmark of opiate withdrawal. *Neuron* 2001; 32:829–839.

Garrison CJ, Dougherty PM, Kajander KC, Carlton SM. Staining of glial fibrillary acidic protein (GFAP) in lumbar spinal cord increases following a sciatic nerve constriction injury. *Brain Res* 1991; 565:1–7.

Gul H, Yildiz O, Dogrul A, Yesilyurt O, Isimer A. The interaction between IL-1beta and morphine: possible mechanism of the deficiency of morphine-induced analgesia in diabetic mice. *Pain* 2000; 89:39–45.

Guo JD, Wang H, Zhang YQ, Zhao ZQ. Distinct effects of D-serine on spinal nociceptive responses in normal and carrageenan-injected rats. *Biochem Biophys Res Commun* 2006; 343:401–406.

Haberstock-Debic H, Kim KA, Yu YJ, von Zastrow M. Morphine promotes rapid, arrestin-dependent endocytosis of mu-opioid receptors in striatal neurons. *J Neurosci* 2005; 25:7847–7857.

Han SS, Liu Y, Tyler-Polsz C, Rao MS, Fischer I. Transplantation of glial-restricted precursor cells into the adult spinal cord: survival, glial-specific differentiation, and preferential migration in white matter. *Glia* 2004; 45:1–16.

Hashizume H, DeLeo JA, Colburn RW, Weinstein JN. Spinal glial activation and cytokine expression after lumbar root injury in the rat. *Spine* 2000; 25:1206–1217.

Inoue K, Koizumi S, Tsuda M, Shigemoto-Mogami Y. Signaling of ATP receptors in glia-neuron interaction and pain. *Life Sci* 2003; 74:189–197.

Jessell TM, Iversen LL. Opiate analgesics inhibit substance P release from rat trigeminal nucleus. *Nature* 1977; 268:549–551.

Kanai Y, Hediger MA. Primary structure and functional characterization of a high-affinity glutamate transporter. *Nature* 1992; 360:467–471.

Keith DE, Anton B, Murray SR, et al. mu-Opioid receptor internalization: opiate drugs have differential effects on a conserved endocytic mechanism in vitro and in the mammalian brain. *Mol Pharmacol* 1998; 53:377–384.

Kimelberg HK. The problem of astrocyte identity. *Neurochem Int* 2004; 45:191–202.

Ledeboer A, Sloane EM, Milligan ED, et al. Minocycline attenuates mechanical allodynia and pro-inflammatory cytokine expression in rat models of pain facilitation. *Pain* 2005; 115:71–83.

Liaw WJ, Stephens RL Jr, Binns BC, et al. Spinal glutamate uptake is critical for maintaining normal sensory transmission in rat spinal cord. *Pain* 2005; 115:60–70.

Liu B, Hong JS. Role of microglia in inflammation-mediated neurodegenerative diseases: mechanisms and strategies for therapeutic intervention. *J Pharmacol Exp Ther* 2003; 304:1–7.

Mahajan SD, Schwartz SA, Shanahan TC, Chawda RP, Nair MP. Morphine regulates gene expression of alpha- and beta-chemokines and their receptors on astroglial cells via the opioid mu receptor. *J Immunol* 2002; 169:3589–3599.

Malmberg AB, Yaksh TL. Cyclooxygenase inhibition and the spinal release of prostaglandin E2 and amino acids evoked by paw formalin injection: a microdialysis study in unanesthetized rats. *J Neurosci* 1995; 15:2768–2776.

Mao J, Sung B, Ji RR, Lim G. Chronic morphine induces downregulation of spinal glutamate transporters: implications in morphine tolerance and abnormal pain sensitivity. *J Neurosci* 2002; 22:8312–8323.

Mao J, Sung B, Ji RR, Lim G. Neuronal apoptosis associated with morphine tolerance: evidence for an opioid-induced neurotoxic mechanism. *J Neurosci* 2002; 22:7650–7661.

Maragakis NJ, Rothstein JD. Glutamate transporters in neurologic disease. *Arch Neurol* 2001; 58:365–370.

Maragakis NJ, Rao MS, Llado J, et al. Glial restricted precursors protect against chronic glutamate neurotoxicity of motor neurons in vitro. *Glia* 2005; 50:145–159.

Martin WR, Eades CG, Thompson JA, Huppler RE, Gilbert PE. The effects of morphine- and nalorphine- like drugs in the nondependent and morphine-dependent chronic spinal dog. *J Pharmacol Exp Ther* 1976; 197:517–532.

Mayer DJ, Mao J, Holt J, Price DD. Cellular mechanisms of neuropathic pain, morphine tolerance, and their interactions. *Proc Natl Acad Sci USA* 1999; 96:7731–7736.

Meskini N, Nemoz G, Okyayuz-Baklouti I, Lagarde M, Prigent AF. Phosphodiesterase inhibitory profile of some related xanthine derivatives pharmacologically active on the peripheral microcirculation. *Biochem Pharmacol* 1994; 47:781–788.

Mestek A, Hurley JH, Bye LS, et al. The human mu opioid receptor: modulation of functional desensitization by calcium/calmodulin-dependent protein kinase and protein kinase C. *J Neurosci* 1995; 15:2396–2406.

Nagata K, Ogawa T, Omosu M, Fujimoto K, Hayashi S. In vitro and in vivo inhibitory effects of propentofylline on cyclic AMP phosphodiesterase activity. *Arzneimittelforschung* 1985; 35:1034–1036.

Nedergaard M, Ransom B, Goldman SA. New roles for astrocytes: redefining the functional architecture of the brain. *Trends Neurosci* 2003; 26:523–530.

North RA, Williams JT, Surprenant A, Christie MJ. Mu and delta receptors belong to a family of receptors that are coupled to potassium channels. *Proc Natl Acad Sci USA* 1987; 84:5487–5491.

Ozawa T, Nakagawa T, Shige K, Minami M, Satoh M. Changes in the expression of glial glutamate transporters in the rat brain accompanied with morphine dependence and naloxone-precipitated withdrawal. *Brain Res* 2001; 905:254–258.

Parkinson FE, Fredholm BB. Effects of propentofylline on adenosine A1 and A2 receptors and nitrobenzylthioinosine-sensitive nucleoside transporters: quantitative autoradiographic analysis. *Eur J Pharmacol* 1991; 202:361–366.

Paronis CA, Holtzman SG. Development of tolerance to the analgesic activity of mu agonists after continuous infusion of morphine, meperidine or fentanyl in rats. *J Pharmacol Exp Ther* 1992; 262:1–9.

Parpura V, Basarsky TA, Liu F, et al. Glutamate-mediated astrocyte-neuron signalling. *Nature* 1994; 369:744–747.

Pellerin L. How astrocytes feed hungry neurons. *Mol Neurobiol* 2005; 32:59–72.

Pellerin L, Magistretti PJ. Glutamate uptake into astrocytes stimulates aerobic glycolysis: a mechanism coupling neuronal activity to glucose utilization. *Proc Natl Acad Sci USA* 1994; 91:10625–10629.

Pellerin L, Bergersen LH, Halestrap AP, Pierre K. Cellular and subcellular distribution of mono-carboxylate transporters in cultured brain cells and in the adult brain. *J Neurosci Res* 2005; 79:55–64.

Pines G, Danbolt NC, Bjoras M, et al. Cloning and expression of a rat brain L-glutamate transporter. *Nature* 1992; 360:464–467.

Raghavendra V, DeLeo JA. Cytokine modulation of opioid action. In: Schmidt RF, Willis WD (Eds). *Encyclopedia of Pain.* New York: Springer, 2006, pp 227–235.

Raghavendra V, Rutkowski MD, DeLeo JA. The role of spinal neuroimmune activation in morphine tolerance/hyperalgesia in neuropathic and sham-operated rats. *J Neurosci* 2002; 22:9980–9989.

Raghavendra V, Tanga F, DeLeo JA. Inhibition of microglial activation attenuates the development but not existing hypersensitivity in a rat model of neuropathy. *J Pharmacol Exp Ther* 2003a; 306:624–630.

Raghavendra V, Tanga F, Rutkowski MD, DeLeo JA. Anti-hyperalgesic and morphine-sparing actions of propentofylline following peripheral nerve injury in rats: mechanistic implications of spinal glia and proinflammatory cytokines. *Pain* 2003b; 104:655–664.

Raghavendra V, Tanga FY, DeLeo JA. Attenuation of morphine tolerance, withdrawal-induced hyperalgesia, and associated spinal inflammatory immune responses by propentofylline in rats. *Neuropsychopharmacology* 2004; 29:327–334.

Reichenbach A, Wolburg H. Astrocytes and ependymal glia. In: Kettenmann H, Ransom BR (Eds). *Neuroglia,* 2nd ed. Oxford: Oxford University Press, 2005, pp 19–35.

Ronnback L, Hansson E. Are astroglial cells involved in morphine tolerance? *Neurochem Res* 1988; 13:87–103.

Ros J, Pecinska N, Alessandri B, Landolt H, Fillenz M. Lactate reduces glutamate-induced neurotoxicity in rat cortex. *J Neurosci Res* 2001; 66:790–794.

Rothstein JD, Dykes-Hoberg M, Pardo CA, et al. Knockout of glutamate transporters reveals a major role for astroglial transport in excitotoxicity and clearance of glutamate. *Neuron* 1996; 16:675–686.

Ruzicka BB, Fox CA, Thompson RC, et al. Primary astroglial cultures derived from several rat brain regions differentially express mu, delta and kappa opioid receptor mRNA. *Brain Res Mol Brain Res* 1995; 34:209–220.

Schlag BD, Vondrasek JR, Munir M, et al. Regulation of the glial Na^+-dependent glutamate transporters by cyclic AMP analogs and neurons. *Mol Pharmacol* 1998; 53:355–369.

Sekiya Y, Nakagawa T, Ozawa T, Minami M, Satoh M. Facilitation of morphine withdrawal symptoms and morphine-induced conditioned place preference by a glutamate transporter inhibitor DL-threo-beta-benzyloxyaspartate in rats. *Eur J Pharmacol* 2004; 485:201–210.

Si QS, Nakamura Y, Schubert P, Rudolphi K, Kataoka K. Adenosine and propentofylline inhibit the proliferation of cultured microglial cells. *Exp Neurol* 1996; 137:345–349.

Sluka KA, Westlund KN. An experimental arthritis in rats: dorsal horn aspartate and glutamate increases. *Neurosci Lett* 1992; 145:141–144.

Snyder SH, Kim PM. D-amino acids as putative neurotransmitters: focus on D-serine. *Neurochem Res* 2000; 25:553–560.

Snyder SH, Pasternak GW. Historical review: opioid receptors. *Trends Pharmacol Sci* 2003; 24:198–205.

Song P, Zhao ZQ. The involvement of glial cells in the development of morphine tolerance. *Neurosci Res* 2001; 39:281–286.

Stiene-Martin A, Zhou R, Hauser KF. Regional, developmental, and cell cycle-dependent differences in mu, delta, and kappa-opioid receptor expression among cultured mouse astrocytes. *Glia* 1998; 22:249–259.

Storck T, Schulte S, Hofmann K, Stoffel W. Structure, expression, and functional analysis of a Na⁺-dependent glutamate/aspartate transporter from rat brain. *Proc Natl Acad Sci USA* 1992; 89:10955–10959.

Sung B, Lim G, Mao J. Altered expression and uptake activity of spinal glutamate transporters after nerve injury contribute to the pathogenesis of neuropathic pain in rats. *J Neurosci* 2003; 23:2899–2910.

Svensson CI, Marsala M, Westerlund A, et al. Activation of p38 mitogen-activated protein kinase in spinal microglia is a critical link in inflammation-induced spinal pain processing. *J Neurochem* 2003; 86:1534–1544.

Sweitzer SM, Martin D, DeLeo JA. Intrathecal interleukin-1 receptor antagonist in combination with soluble tumor necrosis factor receptor exhibits an anti-allodynic action in a rat model of neuropathic pain. *Neuroscience* 2001a; 103:529–539.

Sweitzer SM, Schubert P, DeLeo JA. Propentofylline, a glial modulating agent, exhibits antiallodynic properties in a rat model of neuropathic pain. *J Pharmacol Exp Ther* 2001b; 297:1210–1217.

Sweitzer SM, Hickey WF, Rutkowski MD, Pahl JL, DeLeo JA. Focal peripheral nerve injury induces leukocyte trafficking into the central nervous system: potential relationship to neuropathic pain. *Pain* 2002; 100:163–170.

Tanga FY, Raghavendra V, DeLeo JA. Quantitative real-time RT-PCR assessment of spinal microglial and astrocytic activation markers in a rat model of neuropathic pain. *Neurochem Int* 2004; 45:397–407.

Tanga FY, Nutile-McMenemy N, DeLeo JA. The CNS role of Toll-like receptor 4 in innate neuroimmunity and painful neuropathy. *Proc Natl Acad Sci USA* 2005; 102:5856–5861.

Tawfik VL, Lacroix-Fralish ML, Nutile-McMenemy N, DeLeo JA. Transcriptional and translational regulation of glial activation by morphine in a rodent model of neuropathic pain. *J Pharmacol Exp Ther* 2005; 313:1239–1247.

Tawfik VL, Lacroix-Fralish ML, Bercury KK, et al. Induction of astrocyte differentiation by propentofylline increases glutamate transporter expression in vitro: heterogeneity of the quiescent phenotype. *Glia* 2006; 54:193–203.

Tawfik VL, Nutile-McMenemy N, LaCroix-Fralish ML, DeLeo JA. Efficacy of propentofylline, a glial modulating agent, on existing mechanical allodynia following peripheral nerve injury. *Brain Behav Immun* 2007; 21:238–246.

Tsuda M, Shigemoto-Mogami Y, Koizumi S, et al. P2X4 receptors induced in spinal microglia gate tactile allodynia after nerve injury. *Nature* 2003; 424:778–783.

Tsuda M, Mizokoshi A, Shigemoto-Mogami Y, Koizumi S, Inoue K. Activation of p38 mitogen-activated protein kinase in spinal hyperactive microglia contributes to pain hypersensitivity following peripheral nerve injury. *Glia* 2004; 45:89–95.

von Zastrow M, Svingos A, Haberstock-Debic H, Evans C. Regulated endocytosis of opioid receptors: cellular mechanisms and proposed roles in physiological adaptation to opiate drugs. *Curr Opin Neurobiol* 2003; 13:348–353.

Voutsinos-Porche B, Bonvento G, Tanaka K, et al. Glial glutamate transporters mediate a functional metabolic crosstalk between neurons and astrocytes in the mouse developing cortex. *Neuron* 2003; 37:275–286.

Watkins LR, Maier SF. Glia: a novel drug discovery target for clinical pain. *Nat Rev Drug Discov* 2003; 2:973–985.

Watkins LR, Maier SF, Goehler LE. Immune activation: the role of pro-inflammatory cytokines in inflammation, illness responses and pathological pain states. *Pain* 1995; 63:289–302.

Watkins LR, Hutchinson MR, Johnston IN, Maier SF. Glia: novel counter-regulators of opioid analgesia. *Trends Neurosci* 2005; 28:661–669.

Wen ZH, Wu GJ, Chang YC, Wang JJ, Wong CS. Dexamethasone modulates the development of morphine tolerance and expression of glutamate transporters in rats. *Neuroscience* 2005; 133:807–817.

Winkelstein BA, Rutkowski MD, Sweitzer SM, Pahl JL, DeLeo JA. Nerve injury proximal or distal to the DRG induces similar spinal glial activation and selective cytokine expression but differential behavioral responses to pharmacologic treatment. *J Comp Neurol* 2001; 439:127–139.

Wu HE, Thompson J, Sun HS, et al. Nonopioidergic mechanism mediating morphine-induced antianalgesia in the mouse spinal cord. *J Pharmacol Exp Ther* 2004; 310:240–246.

Wu HE, Thompson J, Sun HS, Terashvili M, Tseng LF. Antianalgesia: stereoselective action of dextro-morphine over levo-morphine on glia in the mouse spinal cord. *J Pharmacol Exp Ther* 2005; 314:1101–1108.

Xu NJ, Bao L, Fan HP, et al. Morphine withdrawal increases glutamate uptake and surface expression of glutamate transporter GLT1 at hippocampal synapses. *J Neurosci* 2003; 23:4775–4784.

Correspondence to: Joyce A. De Leo, PhD, Dartmouth-Hitchcock Medical Center, 1 Medical Center Drive, HB 7125, Lebanon, NH 03756, USA. Tel: 1-603-650-6204; fax: 1-603-650-4928; email: joyce.a.deleo@dartmouth.edu.

Immune and Glial Regulation of Pain, edited by Joyce
A. DeLeo, Linda S. Sorkin, and Linda R. Watkins,
IASP Press, Seattle, © 2007.

20

Proinflammatory Cytokines Modulate Neuropathic Pain, Opioid Analgesia, and Opioid Tolerance

Yehuda Shavit,[a] Gilly Wolf,[a] Ian N. Johnston,[b]
R. Frederick Westbrook,[c] Linda R. Watkins,[d]
and Raz Yirmiya[a]

[a]Department of Psychology, The Hebrew University of Jerusalem, Mount Scopus, Jerusalem, Israel; [b]School of Psychology, University of Sydney, Sydney, New South Wales, Australia; [c]School of Psychology, University of New South Wales, Sydney, New South Wales, Australia; [d]Department of Psychology and the Center for Neuroscience, University of Colorado at Boulder, Boulder, Colorado, USA

The perception of pain is dynamically modulated by pain-inhibitory and pain-facilitatory systems, implying that the pain experienced by an individual is determined by a combination of these modulatory effects. In several areas of the central nervous system (CNS), particularly within the dorsal horn of the spinal cord, activation of these systems results in the secretion of modulatory compounds that produce either pain suppression (analgesia) or pain facilitation (hyperalgesia). The endogenous opioid system plays a pivotal role in pain suppression; this system can also be activated by the administration of exogenous opioid drugs. In fact, opioid analgesia is the most potent and useful method for alleviating severe pain in many medical conditions.

Pain facilitation is mediated by many substances, including cholecystokinin (CCK), prostaglandins, dynorphin, substance P, and sympathetic amines (Verri et al. 2006). Over the last decade, it became evident that spinal cord glial cells play a major role in pain facilitation (Watkins and Maier 2002). The effects of glia are mediated, at least in part, by the secretion of proinflammatory cytokines—small proteins produced by activated immune cells, which regulate the amplitude and duration of the immune response. Recent research on the neurobiology of cytokines has shown that these molecules are also produced by other cells, including nerve and glial cells, and that they can act as modulators and potential neurotransmitters in the CNS.

Considerable evidence from animal studies suggests that glial-derived proinflammatory cytokines underlie pain facilitation associated with several medical conditions. Furthermore, interactions between proinflammatory cytokines and opioids prove to be theoretically and, most likely, clinically important. This chapter focuses on the modulatory role of proinflammatory cytokines in opioid analgesia, in the development of analgesic tolerance and withdrawal-induced pain enhancement following repeated opioid administration, and in the development of neuropathic pain.

PROINFLAMMATORY CYTOKINES AND NEUROPATHIC PAIN

Neuropathic pain is a severe, chronic condition, caused by injury to the nervous system. This condition is characterized by spontaneous pain, an exaggerated pain response to painful stimuli (hyperalgesia), and pain responses to normally nonpainful stimuli (allodynia). Abnormal pain after peripheral nerve injury is dependent on the activation of spontaneous and persistent abnormal discharge from ectopic foci at the site of injury (Wall and Gutnick 1974) and/or in the dorsal root ganglia (DRG) (Devor et al. 1994; Liu et al. 2000). This increased afferent discharge correlates well with the development of neuropathic pain (Liu et al. 2000; Draganic et al. 2001). Peripheral nerve injury is associated with inflammatory responses at the site of the tissue damage and in the CNS and is accompanied by the release of proinflammatory cytokines at both sites. In recent years, evidence has emerged showing the involvement of cytokines, especially proinflammatory cytokines, in the generation of pathological pain states, at both peripheral and central nervous system sites (for reviews see Watkins and Maier 2002, 2003; Sommer 2003; DeLeo et al. 2004; Verri et al. 2006). Proinflammatory cytokines, especially tumor necrosis factor-α (TNF-α), interleukin (IL)-1, and IL-6, induce a long-term alteration of synaptic transmission in the CNS and play a critical role in the development and maintenance of neuropathic pain (DeLeo and Yezierski 2001). The injection of exogenous proinflammatory cytokines over the spinal cord enhances nociception (DeLeo et al. 1996; Tadano et al. 1999; Reeve et al. 2000; Falchi et al. 2001), and electrophysiological studies document rapid enhancement of neuronal excitability in response to painful stimuli following the injection of proinflammatory cytokines to the region (Oka et al. 1995; Reeve et al. 2000). Protein and mRNA levels of proinflammatory cytokines in the spinal cord are elevated in several models of neuropathic and inflammatory pain (Watkins and Maier 2003; DeLeo et al. 2004), concomitantly with the development of thermal hyperalgesia and mechanical allodynia (Chacur et al. 2001; Winkelstein et al. 2001; Shamash et al. 2002; Watkins and Maier 2002). In the spinal cord, proinflammatory cytokines have been implicated in pain facilitation, including hyperalgesia, allodynia, and neuropathic pain (Watkins et al. 2001; DeLeo et al. 2004). Nerve injury also induces activation of spinal cord glia, which appears to play a crucial role in the development of neuropathic pain (Colburn et al. 1999; Raghavendra et al. 2003a,b; DeLeo et al. 2004).

Among the proinflammatory cytokines, IL-1 is particularly known to modulate pain sensitivity. Peripheral or central administration of IL-1β usually produces hyperalgesia (Ferreira et al. 1988; Watkins et al. 1994; Oka et al. 1995). Spinal administration of IL-1 induced both mechanical allodynia and thermal hyperalgesia (Tadano et al. 1999; Reeve et al. 2000; Falchi et al. 2001), whereas its blockade at the spinal level prevented hyperalgesia induced by various immune challenges (Watkins et al. 1994, 1997; Milligan et al. 2001; Samad et al. 2001). IL-1 has also been implicated in the development of neuropathic pain. Elevated levels of IL-1 following peripheral nerve injury were detected both in the periphery (Rotshenker et al. 1992; Shamash et al. 2002) and in the spinal cord (DeLeo et al. 1997). Furthermore, peripheral administration of neutralizing antibodies to IL-1 receptor type I reduced the development of experimental neuropathic pain in mice (Sommer et al. 1999), whereas intrathecal administration of a low dose of IL-1β increased spinal wind-up activity in normal rats (Constandil et al. 2003). Mice with genetic impairment of IL-1 signaling (mouse models with deletion of IL-1 receptor type I, or transgenic overexpression of IL-1-receptor antagonist [IL-1ra] within the brain and spinal cord) do not develop neuropathic pain behavior. In fact, such mice display delayed onset and reduced severity of autotomy and exhibit markedly attenuated ectopic neuronal activity in the DRG, emphasizing the role of IL-1 in the development and maintenance of neuropathic pain (Wolf et al. 2006) (Fig. 1).

Evidence has accumulated showing that glia importantly contribute to the creation and maintenance of neuropathic pain. First, spinal glia are activated in response to trauma to, or inflammation of, peripheral nerves, resulting in neuropathic pain (Watkins et al. 2001). This is reflected by increased expression of activation markers, including glial fibrillary acidic protein (GFAP) by astrocytes and complement-type-3 receptors (CR3/CD11b) by microglia. Second, glial activation drives neuropathic pain, because blockade of glial activation prevents or reverses such pain. Third, nerve injury downregulates glial glutamate transporters in the spinal cord dorsal horn, which would increase excitability of pain-transmission neurons by increasing extracellular glutamate levels (Sung et al. 2003). Fourth, neuropathy causes spinal cord glia to enhance pain by releasing neuroexcitatory glial proinflammatory cytokines (Watkins et al. 2001). Fifth, pain-enhancing effects of neuropathy are mimicked by spinal

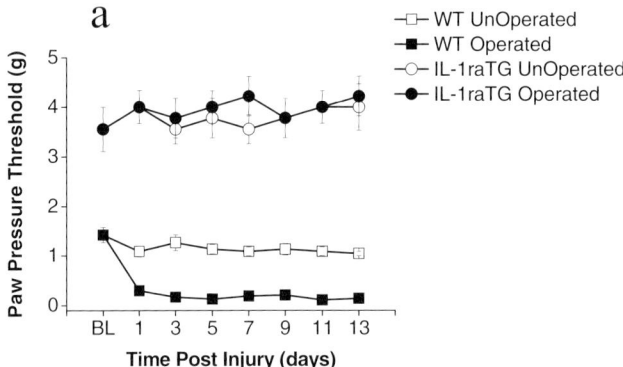

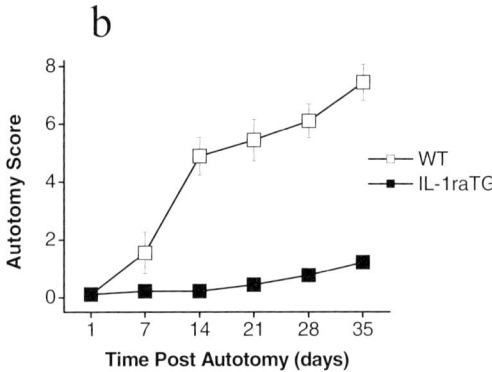

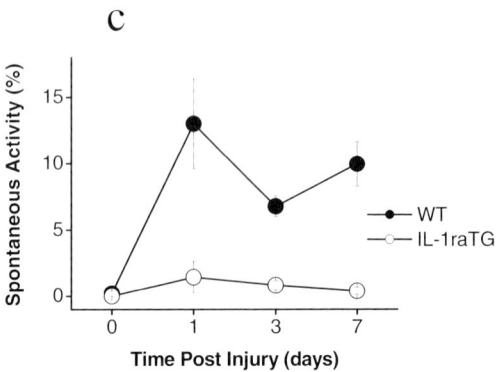

cord glial activation in the absence of peripheral nerve injury (Milligan et al. 2001) and by intrathecal administration of proinflammatory cytokines (DeLeo et al. 1996; Reeve et al. 2000). The last observation suggests that activation of glia, or elevation of proinflammatory cytokines, may be sufficient to drive enhanced pain states.

PROINFLAMMATORY CYTOKINES AND OPIOID TOLERANCE

Opioids remain the drug of choice for the alleviation of acute and chronic pain. However, the clinical efficacy of these drugs is reduced by the rapid development of analgesic tolerance with repeated administration of opioids, such as morphine, requiring increased dosage to maintain pain control. Dose increase is problematic because it is associated with increased side effects, such as nausea, respiratory depression, urinary retention, constipation, or miosis (Raith and Hochhaus 2004). Furthermore, tolerance often leads to pain amplification when opioid administration is discontinued (Mao 2002), which also presents a clinically relevant problem (Raith and Hochhaus 2004).

Many mechanisms have been proposed to account for opioid tolerance and withdrawal-induced pain enhancement. Some of these mechanisms involve adaptation within opioid- or opioid receptor-expressing neurons, rendering opioid actions at those neurons less effective. Such adaptations include decoupling, internalization, and/or downregulation of opioid receptors; upregulation of N-methyl-D-aspartate (NMDA) receptor function; downregulation of glutamate transporters; and production of nitric oxide (NO) (Raith and Hochhaus 2004). Other mechanisms activate pain facilitatory systems within the brain and spinal cord that actively oppose opioid analgesia. Such counter-regulatory adaptations include the release of CCK (Watkins et al. 1984) and dynorphin (Vanderah et al. 2000).

Despite decades of research, the study of mechanisms underlying morphine tolerance and withdrawal-induced pain enhancement remains incomplete (Raith and Hochhaus 2004). New evidence suggests that proinflammatory cytokines play a pivotal role in counter-regulating acute morphine analgesia, in morphine tolerance, and in withdrawal-induced pain enhancement. Furthermore,

---

← **Fig. 1.** The involvement of interleukin-1 (IL-1) signaling in neuropathic pain. (a) Mechanical pain sensitivity assessed by the von Frey filament test following transection of the left L5 spinal nerve in mice with impaired IL-1 signaling (transgenic overexpression of IL-1-receptor antagonist in the CNS; IL-1raTG) and their wild-type (WT) controls. IL-1raTG mice did not develop increased pain sensitivity in either hindpaw, whereas WT controls displayed lowered pain threshold in the hindpaw ipsilateral to the injury. (b) Autotomy scores following complete sciatic denervation. IL-1raTG mice displayed minimal autotomy behavior compared with the WT controls. (c) Ectopic neuronal activity measured from A-fiber axons ipsilateral to the nerve injury. In IL-1raTG mice, only a minimal proportion of axons were active, whereas in the WT controls a significant proportion was activated. Modified from Wolf et al. (2006).

the interactions between cytokines and opioids may be relevant to the basic mechanisms and pharmacological treatment of neuropathic pain.

Several lines of evidence implicate proinflammatory cytokines in opiate tolerance: (1) Proinflammatory cytokine transcription, translation, and protein release are elevated in the spinal cord in response to chronic morphine (Raghavendra et al. 2002; Johnston et al. 2004) (Fig. 2). (2) Mice with genetic impairment of IL-1 signaling (deletion of IL-1 receptor type I, deletion of IL-1-receptor accessory protein, or transgenic overexpression of IL-1ra) exhibit dramatically reduced morphine tolerance (Shavit et al. 2005). Similarly, morphine tolerance is markedly attenuated in control mice treated chronically with IL-1ra (Johnston et al. 2004; Shavit et al. 2005). (3) Morphine tolerance and withdrawal-induced pain facilitation after chronic morphine are attenuated by intrathecal injection of the anti-inflammatory cytokine IL-10 (Raghavendra et al. 2002; Johnston et al. 2004). (4) Furthermore, IL-1ra reinstates morphine analgesia in morphine-tolerant mice (Shavit et al. 2005), reduces opioid-withdrawal-induced hyperalgesia (Johnston et al. 2004), and attenuates further development of allodynia (Johnston et al. 2004) (Fig. 3).

The interactions between proinflammatory cytokines and opioids have important implications for neuropathic pain. Pain associated with neuropathy is difficult to treat; opioids, the most common and potent analgesics in clinical practice, are only partially effective in treating neuropathic symptoms, requiring high doses that are associated with a myriad of side effects (Cherny et al. 1994). Interestingly, neuropathy-induced hyperalgesia, which is thought to involve sensitization of primary afferent fibers, also leads to decreased analgesia and accelerated development of morphine tolerance (Mao et al. 1995b; Christensen and Kayser 2000; Raghavendra et al. 2002). Indeed, there are striking similarities between neuropathic pain and morphine tolerance (Mao et al. 1995a; Mayer et al. 1999). For example, in the spinal cord, both phenomena are associated with diminished morphine analgesia and pain facilitation (Mayer et al. 1999). Furthermore, both are mediated, in part, by excitatory amino acids, NO, and prostaglandins (Mayer et al. 1999) and can be blocked by NMDA-receptor antagonists (Ben-Eliyahu et al. 1992; Parsons 2001). Such findings led to the hypothesis that neuropathic pain shares cellular and molecular mechanisms of neural plasticity with opioid tolerance. Among those mechanisms, the release of proinflammatory cytokines and the activation of glia appear to play a pivotal role in both processes. Both neuropathic pain (Sung et al. 2003) and morphine tolerance (Ozawa et al. 2001) are associated with downregulation of glial glutamate transporters in the dorsal horn, where primary sensory neurons relay pain messages to spinal cord pain-transmitting secondary neurons. Both are also associated with the release of proinflammatory cytokines (Watkins et al. 2001; Johnston et al. 2004; Raghavendra et al. 2004).

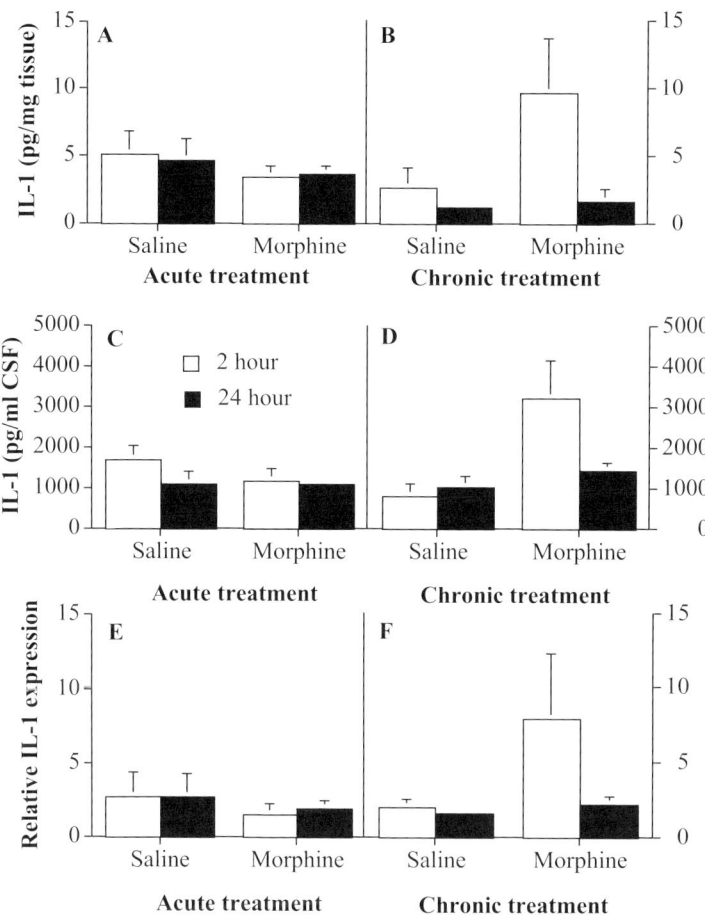

Fig. 2. Chronic, but not acute, intrathecal injections of morphine induce a rapid release of interleukin-1 (IL-1) protein from the lumbar spinal cord (as determined by ELISA) and tends to elevate IL-1 mRNA by reverse transcription polymerase chain reaction. (A–B) After five once-daily intrathecal injections of morphine (10 μg) or saline (Chronic treatment), there was an increase in IL-1 protein in lumbar dorsal spinal cord tissue 2 hours, but not 24 hours, after the last injection of morphine. There was no alteration in IL-1 levels in response to one morphine injection (Acute treatment). (C–D) After five once-daily (Chronic) intrathecal injections of morphine (10 μg) or saline, there was an increase in IL-1 protein in lumbar cerebrospinal fluid (CSF) 2 hours, but not 24 hours, after the last injection of morphine. There was no alteration in IL-1 levels in response to one morphine injection (Acute). (E–F) There was also a strong trend for the chronic morphine regimen described above to elevate IL-1 mRNA 2 hours, but not 24 hours, after morphine. Modified, with permission, from Johnston et al. (2004).

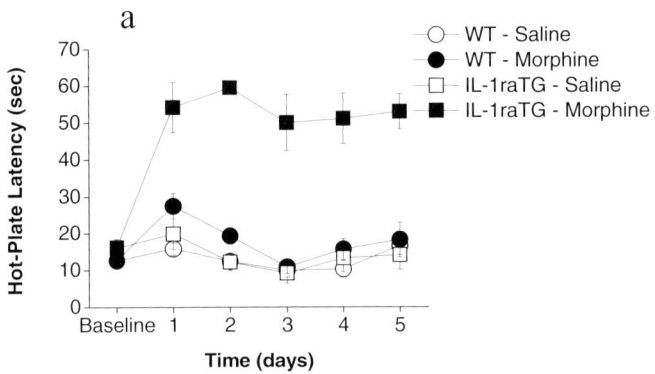

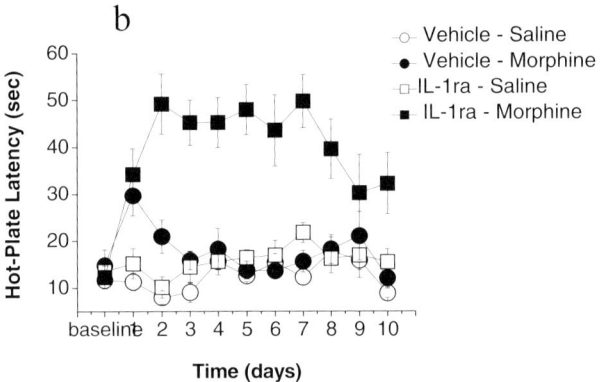

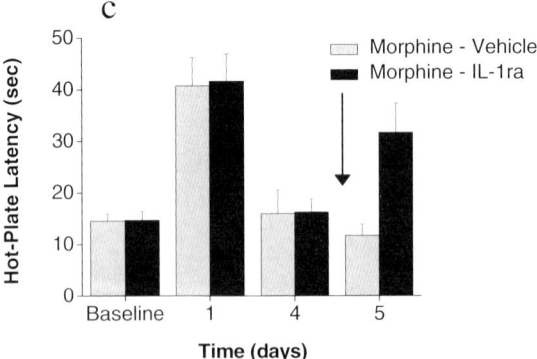

INTERACTIONS BETWEEN GLIAL-DERIVED CYTOKINES AND OPIOID SYSTEMS

Opioids can influence glial functioning by binding to opioid receptors. Glia express multiple opioid receptor subtypes, including μ-opioid receptors, which bind morphine (Chang et al. 1998). Morphine increases glial production of NO (Stefano 1998) and of proinflammatory cytokines (Peterson et al. 1998), which excite pain-responsive neurons. Morphine also primes microglia and macrophages to over-respond to subsequent stimuli, thereby increasing release of TNF, IL-1, and NO (Chao et al. 1994). Spinal glia become increasingly responsive to opioids upon repeated administration (Johnston et al. 2004), perhaps because glial exposure to morphine (Mahajan et al. 2002), or proinflammatory cytokines (Ruzicka and Akil 1997), enhances the constitutive expression of μ-opioid receptors on glia. Chronic morphine activates spinal cord glia, as indicated by upregulation of GFAP (Song and Zhao 2001; Raghavendra et al. 2002), and CR3 (Raghavendra et al. 2002) (Fig. 4). That glial activation causes morphine tolerance is supported by the fact that co-administration of morphine with a glial metabolic inhibitor (fluorocitrate) (Song and Zhao 2001), or with a glial modulator (propentofylline) associated with decreased glial activation (Raghavendra et al. 2004), greatly attenuated morphine tolerance.

Morphine might also indirectly affect glia via a neuron-to-glia signal mediated by the chemokine fractalkine (CX3CL1). Fractalkine is expressed by spinal cord neurons (Verge et al. 2004), and upon release, it forms a diffusible signal that activates nearby microglia to release proinflammatory cytokines (Johnston et al. 2004). Indeed, in the spinal cord, soluble fractalkine facilitates pain via proinflammatory cytokine release (Johnston et al. 2004; Milligan et al. 2004). Morphine appears to induce the release of fractalkine, because blockade of fractalkine receptors both potentiates the acute analgesic effects of morphine and blocks the development of morphine tolerance and withdrawal-associated pain enhancement (Johnston et al. 2004).

← **Fig. 3.** The involvement of interleukin-1-receptor antagonist (IL-1ra) in morphine tolerance. (a) Mice with genetic impairment of IL-1 signaling (IL-1raTG) were injected subcutaneously twice daily with morphine (10 mg/kg) or saline for 5 consecutive days. Hot-plate latency was assessed at baseline and 1 hour after each morning injection. IL-1raTG mice did not show morphine tolerance throughout the morphine injection days, whereas the wild-type (WT) controls developed tolerance within 3 days. (b) WT mice were implanted with osmotic micropumps secreting either IL-1ra or vehicle and were injected twice daily with morphine as described above. Mice chronically treated with IL-1ra did not develop morphine tolerance, whereas the vehicle-treated mice developed tolerance within 3 days. (c) WT mice were made tolerant to morphine (as described above). On day 5, half the mice received the morning injection of morphine in combination with IL-1ra (100 mg/kg, intraperitoneally); the other half received morphine with saline. Saline-treated mice continued to display complete tolerance, whereas in mice treated with IL-1ra morphine analgesia was reinstated. Modified, with permission, from Shavit et al. (2005).

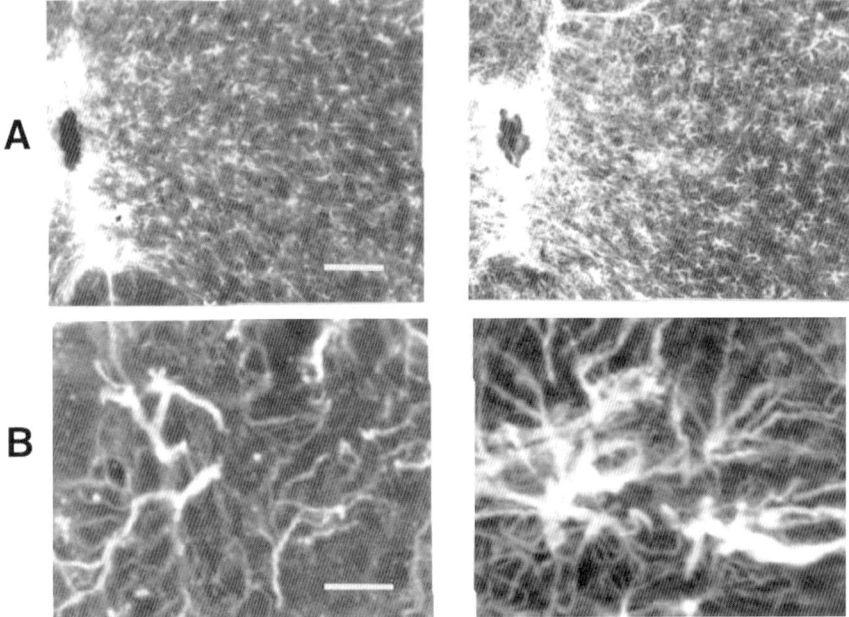

Fig. 4. Glial activation in response to morphine. One indication that morphine activates glia is the upregulation of cell-type-specific activation markers, which are detectable by immunohistochemistry. These photomicrographs show that morphine induces the upregulation of the astrocyte activation marker glial fibrillary acidic protein (GFAP) in the spinal cord. (A) Control rats are compared here with (B) rats after nine consecutive days of intraperitoneal morphine administration (50 mg/kg). Scale bars, 100 μm for the upper panels and 10 μm for the lower panels; section thickness = 30 μm. Modified, with permission, from Song and Zhao (2001).

Interesting relationships are emerging among glia, proinflammatory cytokines, and the endogenous neurotransmitters and neuromodulators that disrupt opioid responses. Mutual influences are becoming apparent in which proinflammatory cytokines affect glial cells, and vice versa, to produce hyperalgesia and counter-regulate morphine analgesia. As mentioned, opioids increase glial production of proinflammatory cytokines, whereby they may counter-regulate opioid analgesia either directly, by affecting opioid receptor activity, or indirectly, by inducing hyperalgesia. There are several potential mechanisms by which inflammatory molecules may rapidly and directly modulate opioid receptor function. For example, there is the potential for heterologous desensitization between opioid receptors and receptors for proinflammatory cytokines via shared G-protein-coupled systems (Szabo et al. 2002), or via other secondary messenger systems within neurons and glia, such as mitogen-activated protein (MAP) kinases, nuclear factor-κB, and calcium (Roy et al. 1998; Law et al.

2000; Haddad 2002). Alternatively, glia regulate glutaminergic NMDA-receptor-mediated neuroplastic changes known to contribute to opioid tolerance and hyperalgesia (Celerier et al. 1999; Ma and Zhao 2002). Chronic opioid treatment downregulates both neuronal and glial glutamate transporters (Mao 2002), increasing glutamate signaling accompanied by excessive NMDA-receptor activation. Glial glutamate transporters found in the spinal cord, GLAST and GLT-1, play a key role in maintaining homeostasis of extracellular glutamate concentrations (Danbolt 2001). Activated glia release other substances that contribute to analgesic tolerance, hyperalgesia, and allodynia, including NO, ATP, excitatory amino acids, prostaglandins, and dynorphin (Watkins and Maier 2003).

The mechanisms that underlie the anti-analgesic effects of IL-1 are not clear; they may involve either direct effects of IL-1 on opioid-receptor-associated mechanisms, or indirect effects, via the production of other anti-analgesic compounds, particularly CCK, prostaglandins, and dynorphin. Ample research has demonstrated that IL-1 evokes the release of neuronal CCK (Ohgo et al. 1992) and that CCK produces anti-analgesic effects. For example, administration of CCK or its receptor agonists diminishes the analgesic effects of morphine, whereas administration of CCK-receptor antagonists (particularly antagonists of the CCK-B receptor) potentiates the analgesic effects of morphine, inhibits the development of morphine tolerance, and restores morphine analgesia in morphine-tolerant animals (Faris et al. 1983, 1984; O'Neill et al. 1989; Idanpaan-Heikkila et al. 1997; McCleane 1998; Tortorici et al. 2003). Prostaglandins have also been demonstrated to produce anti-analgesic effects. Administration of prostaglandins (particularly PGE_2) reduces the analgesic effects of morphine, whereas blockade of prostaglandin production by cyclooxygenase (COX) inhibitors (particularly COX-2 inhibitors) potentiates the analgesic effects of morphine and delays the development of morphine tolerance (Rady et al. 2001; Deciga-Campos et al. 2003; Hernandez-Delgadillo et al. 2003). These reports, taken together with the findings that IL-1 induces the expression of COX-2 in spinal cord neurons (Samad et al. 2001) and causes the release of PGE_2 in both mixed glia cultures (Pinteaux et al. 2002) and the central nucleus of the amygdala (Beilin et al. 2006), suggest that prostaglandins are involved in IL-1-mediated anti-analgesia. Finally, dynorphin may also be involved in mediating the effects of IL-1. Chronic administration of morphine, like peripheral nerve injury, increases spinal levels of dynorphin (Rattan and Tejwani 1997; Gardell et al. 2002). Blocking dynorphin blocks nerve-injury-induced hyperalgesia, restores analgesia (Nichols et al. 1997), and prevents the development of opioid tolerance (Vanderah et al. 2000). Dynorphin exerts these effects via IL-1 release (Laughlin et al. 2000; Rady and Fujimoto 2001).

Another mechanism that may be involved in mediating the anti-analgesic effect of IL-1 is neural plasticity. Recent evidence indicates that IL-1 plays an important role in neural plasticity. For example, the induction of long-term potentiation (LTP) within the hippocampus is accompanied by the production of IL-1, and blockade of IL-1 receptors with IL-1ra abolished the maintenance of hippocampal LTP (Schneider et al. 1998). Genetic impairment of IL-1 signaling is associated with complete abolishment of hippocampal LTP induction, both in vivo and in vitro (Avital et al. 2003). Furthermore, genetic or pharmacological deficiency in IL-1 signaling is associated with a marked impairment in learning and memory functioning; correspondingly, administration of low levels of IL-1 can facilitate hippocampal-dependent memory consolidation (Yirmiya et al. 2002; Avital et al. 2003). Recent evidence indicates that LTP within the dorsal horn of the spinal cord may mediate the central sensitization underlying hyperalgesia (Ikeda et al. 2003; Ji et al. 2003), as well as the development of acute and chronic tolerance to opioids (Mayer et al. 1999). In fact, the molecular mechanisms involved in the generation and maintenance of central sensitization (underlying pain) and of hippocampal LTP (underlying memory) are strikingly similar (Ji et al. 2003). The findings that mice with genetic or pharmacological blockade of IL-1 signaling fail to exhibit hippocampal LTP or to develop morphine tolerance, suggest that IL-1-mediated neural plasticity is important for the development of opiate tolerance (Shavit et al. 2005).

INTERLEUKIN-1 MODULATES BASAL PAIN SENSITIVITY AND COUNTER-REGULATES ACUTE OPIOID ANALGESIA

Recent evidence indicates that IL-1 mediates pain sensitivity not only in inflammatory states, but also under normal, basal conditions. Mice with genetic impairment of IL-1 signaling exhibit lower basal thermal pain and mechanical sensitivity (Wolf et al. 2003). These findings have been confirmed in adult control mice chronically treated with IL-1ra, using continuous infusion by osmotic micropumps (Wolf et al. 2003), suggesting that IL-1 plays a hyperalgesic role in setting pain sensitivity in the normal state. However, we (Shavit et al. 2005), as well as others (e.g., Maier et al. 1993; Tadano et al. 1999), have found that peripheral or intrathecal acute administration of IL-1ra has no effect on basal pain sensitivity. These findings suggest that chronic disruption of IL-1 signaling may have a qualitatively different effect than acute blockade of IL-1 receptors. For example, IL-1ra may influence basal pain sensitivity by affecting IL-1-mediated adaptive changes that develop over time.

At least four lines of evidence indicate that IL-1 counter-regulates morphine analgesia, not only during chronic morphine administration, but also acutely. (1) IL-1, at a dose having no behavioral effects on its own, blocks the analgesic effects of systemic morphine (Gul et al. 2000; Shavit et al. 2005). Moreover, systemic or intrathecal administration of IL-1ra potentiates and prolongs the acute analgesic effect of morphine (Johnston et al. 2004; Shavit et al. 2005). Indeed, acute systemic administration of IL-1ra, at a time when the analgesic effect of acute morphine had subsided and pain sensitivity had returned to baseline, reinstated the analgesia; this reinstated analgesia was naloxone-sensitive (Shavit et al. 2005). These findings suggest that acute morphine analgesia is diminished soon after its peak due to elevated levels of endogenous IL-1, which counter-regulates the analgesic actions of morphine; thus, morphine analgesia can be unmasked by the blockade of IL-1 signaling (Shavit et al. 2005). (2) This suggestion is supported by the results of studies utilizing genetic approaches. Mice strains characterized by elevated levels of endogenous IL-1 (beige-J mutation and diabetic mice) display resistance to morphine analgesia (Raffa et al. 1993; Gul et al. 2000). Correspondingly, morphine analgesia is potentiated in magnitude and duration in mice with genetic impairment of IL-1 signaling (Shavit et al. 2005). (3) Intrathecal administration of drugs such as propentofylline and pentoxifylline that suppress production of IL-1 and other proinflammatory cytokines (Wordliczek et al. 2000; Raghavendra et al. 2003b), as well as administration of the anti-inflammatory cytokine IL-10 (Johnston et al. 2004), enhance morphine analgesia. (4) Finally, acute spinal tolerance after a single infusion of opioids can be attenuated by pretreatment with the anti-inflammatory cytokines IL-10 or IL-1ra (Fairbanks and Wilcox 2000) (Fig. 5).

Several studies have demonstrated that the analgesic effects of opioids are inhibited by the central administration of proinflammatory cytokines (Gul et al. 2000; Szabo et al. 2002), suggesting that at least some of the interactions between IL-1 signaling and opioids occur within the CNS. Moreover, the findings that morphine analgesia was potentiated in a mutant transgenic strain of mice, which overexpress IL-1ra only in astrocytes within the brain and spinal cord, and that IL-1 administration in this strain did not abolish morphine analgesia (Shavit et al. 2005), lend support to the notion that the anti-analgesic effect of IL-1 is mediated via receptors within the CNS.

Together, these findings suggest that morphine induces production and secretion of proinflammatory cytokines, which contribute to the activation of pain facilitatory systems and thus inhibit subsequent morphine analgesia. The mechanism by which acute morphine induces IL-1 release is not known, beyond the intermediary release of fractalkine (Johnston et al. 2004). As reviewed above, there is good evidence that chronic morphine activates spinal glia, which in turn release various pain modulatory agents. However, acute morphine does not appear to induce spinal glial activation as measured by glial activation markers or by elevations in proinflammatory cytokine mRNA or protein (Song and Zhao 2001; Raghavendra et al. 2002; Johnston et al. 2004). Nonetheless, systemic or intrathecal IL-1ra, as well as intrathecal IL-10, enhance acute

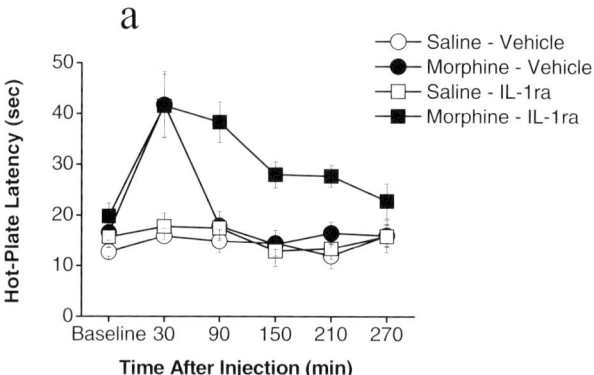

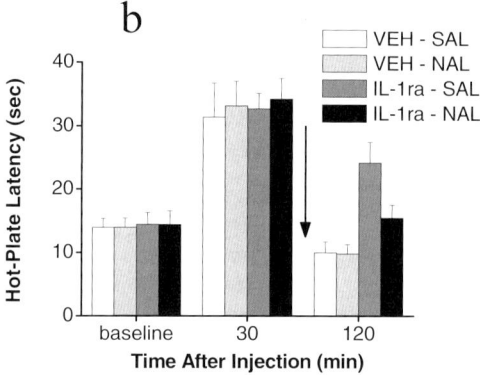

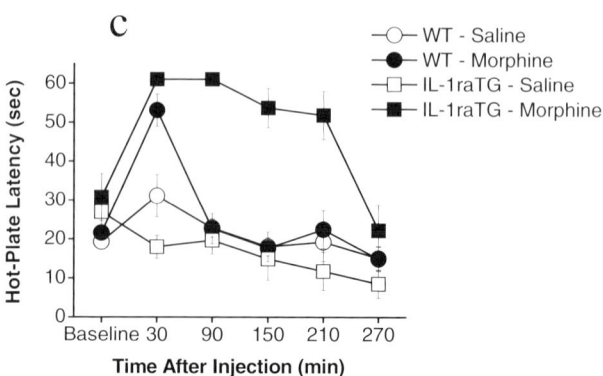

morphine analgesia (Johnston et al. 2004; Shavit et al. 2005). Based on these findings, Johnston et al. (2004) argued that acute morphine induces small local changes in IL-1, which are below detectable levels of the ELISA assay, but still sufficient to change opioid efficacy. It has recently been reported that the anti-analgesia induced by acute spinal opioids is mediated by the stimulation of a novel non-opioid receptor on glial cells (Wu et al. 2005). In any case, it is clear that either acute morphine or proinflammatory cytokines can induce hyperalgesia.

A growing body of evidence suggests that μ-opioid receptor agonists, such as morphine, activate both pain inhibitory and pain facilitatory systems. This paradoxical effect has been demonstrated in both clinical (Guignard et al. 2000; Angst et al. 2003) and laboratory studies (Laulin et al. 1998; Celerier et al. 1999, 2000). At analgesic doses, morphine induces analgesia that masks its hyperalgesic effect, but subsequently, when the opioid concentration has subsided and the analgesic effect has diminished, a delayed hyperalgesic phase is observed (Laulin et al. 1998; Celerier et al. 1999, 2000). Hyperalgesia is also observed in rodents immediately after systemic or central administration of low (subanalgesic) doses of morphine (Parvini et al. 1993; Crain and Shen 2001; Holtman and Wala 2005), or after spinally administered morphine at doses higher than those required for antinociception (Woolf 1981; Yaksh and Harty 1988). Although NMDA-receptor mechanisms are involved in both the immediate hyperalgesia produced by subanalgesic morphine and the delayed hyperalgesia observed after analgesic doses of μ-opioids (Holtman and Wala 2005; Galeotti et al. 2006), some notable differences have been described between the two hyperalgesic states (Holtman and Wala 2005). The hyperalgesia and allodynia induced by spinal high doses of morphine are not blocked by μ-opioid receptor antagonists, indicating mediation via non-opioid mechanisms (Sakurada et al. 2005). The exact mechanisms of morphine-induced nociception are unclear, but the findings described in this section suggest that IL-1, possibly released by glia cells, might be involved in certain forms of hyperalgesia observed following acute morphine administration.

⟵ **Fig. 5.** The involvement of interleukin-1 (IL-1) signaling in acute morphine analgesia. (a) Wild-type (WT) mice received a first intraperitoneal (i.p.) injection of either IL-1-receptor antagonist (IL-1ra, 100 mg/kg) or vehicle, and a second subcutaneous (s.c.) injection of morphine (4 mg/kg) or saline. IL-1ra significantly prolonged morphine analgesia compared with vehicle-treated controls. (b) WT mice were injected with morphine (4 mg/kg, s.c.) and tested for hot-plate latency. At 90 minutes, mice received two additional injections: either IL-1ra (100 mg/kg, i.p.) or vehicle (VEH), followed immediately by either naloxone (NAL; 4 mg/kg, i.p.) or saline (SAL). At 120 minutes, no analgesia was observed in the two vehicle-treated groups; however, analgesic response was re-instated in IL-1ra-treated mice, and this analgesia was significantly blocked by naloxone. (c) Mice were injected with morphine (4 mg/kg, s.c.) or saline. Hot-plate latency was assessed at baseline and at several time points post-injection. IL-1raTG mice displayed significantly prolonged morphine analgesia, compared with their WT controls. Modified, with permission, from Shavit et al. (2005).

CONCLUSIONS

The findings described in this chapter suggest that proinflammatory cytokines, particularly IL-1, are important pain modulatory molecules, playing an
ongoing pain facilitatory role and elevating basal pain sensitivity in the normal
state. Furthermore, these cytokines induce hyperalgesia and allodynia when
their concentration increases in response to peripheral or central inflammation
or infection, in response to peripheral neuropathy, and in response to drugs
such as morphine. In the spinal cord, proinflammatory cytokines are mainly
released by glia, which are activated by all the perturbations mentioned above,
and which appear to be crucial mediators of the pain facilitatory consequences
of these events.

These findings also suggest that among its many actions, morphine triggers the release of proinflammatory cytokines, and that these in turn exert an
anti-analgesic, homeostatic response, which not only limits the extent and
duration of acute morphine analgesia, but also underlies the development of
morphine tolerance following repeated administration. This opioid-induced glial
activation and cytokine release might be mediated by classical opioid receptors, as indicated by the report that naloxone blocked the reinstated analgesia
observed following blockade of IL-1 signaling in previously morphine-treated
mice (Shavit et al. 2005). However, involvement of nonclassical receptors
has also been demonstrated for opioid-mediated modulation of peripheral immune function (Hutchinson and Somogyi 2004), and for the hyperalgesia and
allodynia induced by spinal morphine (Sakurada et al. 2005). Investigations
of glial activation by analgesics have not yet extended beyond morphine, but
it is expected that other clinically relevant opioid analgesics might share this
property of morphine.

Finally, the findings reviewed here suggest that the analgesic efficacy of
opioids in broad clinical use is reduced by concomitant glial activation and
the release of proinflammatory cytokines, and thus may have major clinical
implications for the treatment of pain. Specifically, the administration of opioid
analgesics for the treatment of acute pain (e.g., surgical pain) could be accompanied by IL-1-blocking agents, which would potentiate and extend the analgesic
response. These blocking agents may also lower the effective dose of morphine
and thus reduce its side effects. Blocking glial activation and the subsequent
release of proinflammatory cytokines may minimize the development of opiate
tolerance, providing more effective treatment of chronic pain, which is currently
poorly controlled by opioid analgesics. Glial blockade and suppression of proinflammatory cytokine actions may be particularly advantageous for the treatment
of neuropathic pain, in which elevated levels of proinflammatory cytokines
play a critical role in pain facilitation and in opposing the analgesic effects of

opioids. Given that drugs modulating glial and cytokine functions are available—some already approved for human use, and others currently being evaluated for potential human pain control—therapies that could greatly increase the efficacy of clinically relevant analgesic drugs might be within reach.

ACKNOWLEDGMENTS

This work was partly supported by a grant from the Israel Science Foundation: The Charles H. Revson Foundation (grant no. 799/03) (R. Yirmaya and Y. Shavit), and by a grant from the Israel Foundations Trustees (G. Wolf); it was facilitated by the Leon and Clara Sznajderman Chair of Psychology (Y. Shavit). This work was also partly supported by NIH Grants DA015642, DA018156, and DA017670 (L.R. Watkins). We thank Prof. K. Iverfeldt for the IL-1raTG mice, and Amgen Inc., Thousand Oaks, CA, for the generous gift of IL-1ra.

REFERENCES

Angst MS, Koppert W, Pahl I, et al. Short-term infusion of the mu-opioid agonist remifentanil in humans causes hyperalgesia during withdrawal. *Pain* 2003; 106:49–57.

Avital A, Goshen I, Kamsler A, et al. Impaired interleukin-1 signaling is associated with deficits in hippocampal memory processes and neural plasticity. *Hippocampus* 2003; 13:826–834.

Beilin B, Shavit Y, Dekeyser F, et al. The involvement of glucocorticoids and interleukin-1 in the regulation of brain prostaglandin production in response to surgical stress. *Neuroimmunomodulation* 2006; 13:36–42.

Ben-Eliyahu S, Marek P, Vaccarino AL, et al. The NMDA receptor antagonist MK-801 prevents long-lasting non-associative morphine tolerance in the rat. *Brain Res* 1992; 575:304–308.

Celerier E, Laulin J, Larcher A, et al. Evidence for opiate-activated NMDA processes masking opiate analgesia in rats. *Brain Res* 1999; 847:18–25.

Celerier E, Rivat C, Jun Y, et al. Long-lasting hyperalgesia induced by fentanyl in rats: preventive effect of ketamine. *Anesthesiology* 2000; 92:465–472.

Chacur M, Milligan ED, Gazda LS, et al. A new model of sciatic inflammatory neuritis (SIN): induction of unilateral and bilateral mechanical allodynia following acute unilateral peri-sciatic immune activation in rats. *Pain* 2001; 94:231–244.

Chang SL, Sharp BM, Madden JJ. Cellular mechanisms involved in the modulation of the immune system by drugs of abuse. *Adv Exp Med Biol* 1998; 437:1–12.

Chao CC, Gekker G, Sheng WS, et al. Priming effect of morphine on the production of tumor necrosis factor-alpha by microglia: implications in respiratory burst activity and human immunodeficiency virus-1 expression. *J Pharmacol Exp Ther* 1994; 269:198–203.

Cherny NI, Thaler HT, Friedlander-Klar H, et al. Opioid responsiveness of cancer pain syndromes caused by neuropathic or nociceptive mechanisms: a combined analysis of controlled, single-dose studies. *Neurology* 1994; 44:857–861.

Christensen D, Kayser V. The development of pain-related behaviour and opioid tolerance after neuropathy-inducing surgery and sham surgery. *Pain* 2000; 88:231–238.

Colburn RW, Rickman AJ, DeLeo JA. The effect of site and type of nerve injury on spinal glial activation and neuropathic pain behavior. *Exp Neurol* 1999; 157:289–304.

Constandil L, Pelissier T, Soto-Moyano R, et al. Interleukin-1beta increases spinal cord wind-up activity in normal but not in monoarthritic rats. *Neurosci Lett* 2003; 342:139–142.

Crain SM, Shen KF. Acute thermal hyperalgesia elicited by low-dose morphine in normal mice is blocked by ultra-low-dose naltrexone, unmasking potent opioid analgesia. *Brain Res* 2001; 888:75–82.

Danbolt NC. Glutamate uptake. *Prog Neurobiol* 2001; 65:1–105.

Deciga-Campos M, Lopez UG, Reval MI, Lopez-Munoz FJ. Enhancement of antinociception by co-administration of an opioid drug (morphine) and a preferential cyclooxygenase-2 inhibitor (rofecoxib) in rats. *Eur J Pharmacol* 2003; 460:99–107.

DeLeo JA, Yezierski RP. The role of neuroinflammation and neuroimmune activation in persistent pain. *Pain* 2001; 90:1–6.

DeLeo JA, Colburn RW, Nichols M, Malhotra A. Interleukin-6-mediated hyperalgesia/allodynia and increased spinal IL-6 expression in a rat mononeuropathy model. *J Interferon Cytokine Res* 1996; 16:695–700.

DeLeo JA, Colburn RW, Rickman AJ. Cytokine and growth factor immunohistochemical spinal profiles in two animal models of mononeuropathy. *Brain Res* 1997; 759:50–57.

DeLeo JA, Tanga FY, Tawfik VL. Neuroimmune activation and neuroinflammation in chronic pain and opioid tolerance/hyperalgesia. *Neuroscientist* 2004; 10:40–52.

Devor M, Jänig W, Michaelis M. Modulation of activity in dorsal root ganglion neurons by sympathetic activation in nerve-injured rats. *J Neurophysiol* 1994; 71:38–47.

Draganic P, Miletic G, Miletic V. Changes in post-tetanic potentiation of A-fiber dorsal horn field potentials parallel the development and disappearance of neuropathic pain after sciatic nerve ligation in rats. *Neurosci Lett* 2001; 301:127–130.

Fairbanks CA, Wilcox GL. Spinal plasticity of acute opioid tolerance. *J Biomed Sci* 2000; 7:200–212.

Falchi M, Ferrara F, Gharib C, Dib B. Hyperalgesic effect of intrathecally administered interleukin-1 in rats. *Drugs Exp Clin Res* 2001; 27:97–101.

Faris PL, Komisaruk BR, Watkins LR, Mayer DJ. Evidence for the neuropeptide cholecystokinin as an antagonist of opiate analgesia. *Science* 1983; 219:310–312.

Faris PL, McLaughlin CL, Baile CA, et al. Morphine analgesia potentiated but tolerance not affected by active immunization against cholecystokinin. *Science* 1984; 226:1215–1217.

Ferreira SH, Lorenzetti BB, Bristow AF, Poole S. Interleukin-1 beta as a potent hyperalgesic agent antagonized by a tripeptide analogue. *Nature* 1988; 334:698–700.

Galeotti N, Stefano GB, Guarna M, et al. Signaling pathway of morphine induced acute thermal hyperalgesia in mice. *Pain* 2006; 123:294–305.

Gardell LR, Wang R, Burgess SE, et al. Sustained morphine exposure induces a spinal dynorphin-dependent enhancement of excitatory transmitter release from primary afferent fibers. *J Neurosci* 2002; 22:6747–6755.

Guignard B, Bossard AE, Coste C, et al. Acute opioid tolerance: intraoperative remifentanil increases postoperative pain and morphine requirement. *Anesthesiology* 2000; 93:409–417.

Gul H, Yildiz O, Dogrul A, et al. The interaction between IL-1beta and morphine: possible mechanism of the deficiency of morphine-induced analgesia in diabetic mice. *Pain* 2000; 89:39–45.

Haddad JJ. Cytokines and related receptor-mediated signaling pathways. *Biochem Biophys Res Commun* 2002; 297:700–713.

Hernandez-Delgadillo GP, Lopez-Munoz FJ, Salazar LA, Cruz SL. Morphine and dipyrone co-administration delays tolerance development and potentiates antinociception. *Eur J Pharmacol* 2003; 469:71–79.

Holtman JR Jr, Wala EP. Characterization of morphine-induced hyperalgesia in male and female rats. *Pain* 2005; 114:62–70.

Hutchinson MR, Somogyi AA. (S)-(+)-methadone is more immunosuppressive than the potent analgesic (R)-(–)-methadone. *Int Immunopharmacol* 2004; 4:1525–1530.

Idanpaan-Heikkila JJ, Guilbaud G, Kayser V. Prevention of tolerance to the antinociceptive effects of systemic morphine by a selective cholecystokinin-B receptor antagonist in a rat model of peripheral neuropathy. *J Pharmacol Exp Ther* 1997; 282:1366–1372.

Ikeda H, Heinke B, Ruscheweyh R, Sandkuhler J. Synaptic plasticity in spinal lamina I projection neurons that mediate hyperalgesia. *Science* 2003; 299:1237–1240.

Ji RR, Kohno T, Moore KA, Woolf CJ. Central sensitization and LTP: do pain and memory share similar mechanisms? *Trends Neurosci* 2003; 26:696–705.

Johnston IN, Milligan ED, Wieseler-Frank J, et al. A role for proinflammatory cytokines and fractalkine in analgesia, tolerance, and subsequent pain facilitation induced by chronic intrathecal morphine. *J Neurosci* 2004; 24:9353–9365.

Laughlin TM, Bethea JR, Yezierski RP, Wilcox GL. Cytokine involvement in dynorphin-induced allodynia. *Pain* 2000; 84:159–167.

Laulin JP, Larcher A, Celerier E, et al. Long-lasting increased pain sensitivity in rat following exposure to heroin for the first time. *Eur J Neurosci* 1998; 10:782–785.

Law PY, Wong YH, Loh HH. Molecular mechanisms and regulation of opioid receptor signaling. *Annu Rev Pharmacol Toxicol* 2000; 40:389–430.

Liu CN, Wall PD, Ben-Dor E, et al. Tactile allodynia in the absence of C-fiber activation: altered firing properties of DRG neurons following spinal nerve injury. *Pain* 2000; 85:503–521.

Ma JY, Zhao ZQ. The involvement of glia in long-term plasticity in the spinal dorsal horn of the rat. *Neuroreport* 2002; 13:1781–1784.

Mahajan SD, Schwartz SA, Shanahan TC, et al. Morphine regulates gene expression of alpha- and beta-chemokines and their receptors on astroglial cells via the opioid mu receptor. *J Immunol* 2002; 169:3589–3599.

Maier SF, Wiertelak EP, Martin D, Watkins LR. Interleukin-1 mediates the behavioral hyperalgesia produced by lithium chloride and endotoxin. *Brain Res* 1993; 623:321–324.

Mao J. Opioid-induced abnormal pain sensitivity: implications in clinical opioid therapy. *Pain* 2002; 100:213–217.

Mao J, Price DD, Mayer DJ. Experimental mononeuropathy reduces the antinociceptive effects of morphine: implications for common intracellular mechanisms involved in morphine tolerance and neuropathic pain. *Pain* 1995a; 61:353–364.

Mao J, Price DD, Mayer DJ. Mechanisms of hyperalgesia and morphine tolerance: a current view of their possible interactions. *Pain* 1995b; 62:259–274.

Mayer DJ, Mao J, Holt J, Price DD. Cellular mechanisms of neuropathic pain, morphine tolerance, and their interactions. *Proc Natl Acad Sci USA* 1999; 96:7731–7736.

McCleane GJ. The cholecystokinin antagonist proglumide enhances the analgesic efficacy of morphine in humans with chronic benign pain. *Anesth Analg* 1998; 87:1117–1120.

Milligan ED, O'Connor KA, Nguyen KT, et al. Intrathecal HIV-1 envelope glycoprotein gp120 induces enhanced pain states mediated by spinal cord proinflammatory cytokines. *J Neurosci* 2001; 21:2808–2819.

Milligan ED, Zapata V, Chacur M, et al. Evidence that exogenous and endogenous fractalkine can induce spinal nociceptive facilitation in rats. *Eur J Neurosci* 2004; 20:2294–2302.

Nichols ML, Lopez Y, Ossipov MH, et al. Enhancement of the antiallodynic and antinociceptive efficacy of spinal morphine by antisera to dynorphin A (1-13) or MK-801 in a nerve-ligation model of peripheral neuropathy. *Pain* 1997; 69:317–322.

O'Neill MF, Dourish CT, Iversen SD. Morphine-induced analgesia in the rat paw pressure test is blocked by CCK and enhanced by the CCK antagonist MK-329. *Neuropharmacology* 1989; 28:243–247.

Ohgo S, Nakatsuru K, Ishikawa E, Matsukura S. Stimulation of cholecystokinin (CCK) release from superfused rat hypothalamo-neurohypophyseal complexes by interleukin-1 (IL-1). *Brain Res* 1992; 593:25–31.

Oka T, Oka K, Hosoi M, et al. The opposing effects of interleukin -1 beta microinjected into the preoptic hypothalamus and the ventromedial hypothalamus on nociceptive behavior in rats. *Brain Res* 1995; 700:271–278.

Ozawa T, Nakagawa T, Shige K, et al. Changes in the expression of glial glutamate transporters in the rat brain accompanied with morphine dependence and naloxone-precipitated withdrawal. *Brain Res* 2001; 905:254–258.

Parsons CG. NMDA receptors as targets for drug action in neuropathic pain. *Eur J Pharmacol* 2001; 429:71–78.

Parvini S, Hamann SR, Martin WR. Pharmacologic characteristics of a medullary hyperalgesic center. *J Pharmacol Exp Ther* 1993; 265:286–293.

Peterson PK, Molitor TW, Chao CC. The opioid-cytokine connection. *J Neuroimmunol* 1998; 83:63–69.

Pinteaux E, Parker LC, Rothwell NJ, Luheshi GN. Expression of interleukin-1 receptors and their role in interleukin-1 actions in murine microglial cells. *J Neurochem* 2002; 83:754–763.

Rady JJ, Fujimoto JM. Confluence of antianalgesic action of diverse agents through brain interleukin(1beta) in mice. *J Pharmacol Exp Ther* 2001; 299:659–665.

Rady JJ, Campbell WB, Fujimoto JM. Antianalgesic action of nociceptin originating in the brain is mediated by spinal prostaglandin E_2 in mice. *J Pharmacol Exp Ther* 2001; 296:7–14.

Raffa RB, Mathiasen JR, Kimball ES, Vaught JL. The combined immunological and antinociceptive defects of beige-J mice: the possible existence of a 'mu-repressin'. *Life Sci* 1993; 52:1–8.

Raghavendra V, Rutkowski MD, DeLeo JA. The role of spinal neuroimmune activation in morphine tolerance/hyperalgesia in neuropathic and sham-operated rats. *J Neurosci* 2002; 22:9980–9989.

Raghavendra V, Tanga F, DeLeo JA. Inhibition of microglial activation attenuates the development but not existing hypersensitivity in a rat model of neuropathy. *J Pharmacol Exp Ther* 2003a; 306:624–630.

Raghavendra V, Tanga F, Rutkowski MD, DeLeo JA. Anti-hyperalgesic and morphine-sparing actions of propentofylline following peripheral nerve injury in rats: mechanistic implications of spinal glia and proinflammatory cytokines. *Pain* 2003b; 104:655–664.

Raghavendra V, Tanga FY, DeLeo JA. Attenuation of morphine tolerance, withdrawal-induced hyperalgesia, and associated spinal inflammatory immune responses by propentofylline in rats. *Neuropsychopharmacology* 2004; 29:327–334.

Raith K, Hochhaus G. Drugs used in the treatment of opioid tolerance and physical dependence: a review. *Int J Clin Pharmacol Ther* 2004; 42:191–203.

Rattan AK, Tejwani GA. Effect of chronic treatment with morphine, midazolam and both together on dynorphin (1-13) levels in the rat. *Brain Res* 1997; 754:239–244.

Reeve AJ, Patel S, Fox A, et al. Intrathecally administered endotoxin or cytokines produce allodynia, hyperalgesia and changes in spinal cord neuronal responses to nociceptive stimuli in the rat. *Eur J Pain* 2000; 4:247–257.

Rotshenker S, Aamar S, Barak V. Interleukin-1 activity in lesioned peripheral nerve. *J Neuroimmunol* 1992; 39:75–80.

Roy S, Cain KJ, Chapin RB, et al. Morphine modulates NF kappa B activation in macrophages. *Biochem Biophys Res Commun* 1998; 245:392–396.

Ruzicka BB, Akil H. The interleukin-1beta-mediated regulation of proenkephalin and opioid receptor messenger RNA in primary astrocyte-enriched cultures. *Neuroscience* 1997; 79:517–524.

Sakurada T, Komatsu T, Sakurada S. Mechanisms of nociception evoked by intrathecal high-dose morphine. *Neurotoxicology* 2005; 26:801–809.

Samad TA, Moore KA, Sapirstein A, et al. Interleukin-1beta-mediated induction of Cox-2 in the CNS contributes to inflammatory pain hypersensitivity. *Nature* 2001; 410:471–475.

Schneider H, Pitossi F, Balschun D, et al. A neuromodulatory role of interleukin-1beta in the hippocampus. *Proc Natl Acad Sci USA* 1998; 95:7778–7783.

Shamash S, Reichert F, Rotshenker S. The cytokine network of Wallerian degeneration: tumor necrosis factor-alpha, interleukin-1alpha, and interleukin-1beta. *J Neurosci* 2002; 22:3052–3060.

Shavit Y, Wolf G, Goshen I, et al. Interleukin-1 antagonizes morphine analgesia and underlies morphine tolerance. *Pain* 2005; 115:50–59.

Sommer C. Painful neuropathies. *Curr Opin Neurol* 2003; 16:623–628.

Sommer C, Petrausch S, Lindenlaub T, Toyka KV. Neutralizing antibodies to interleukin 1-receptor reduce pain associated behavior in mice with experimental neuropathy. *Neurosci Lett* 1999; 270:25–28.

Song P, Zhao ZQ. The involvement of glial cells in the development of morphine tolerance. *Neurosci Res* 2001; 39:281–286.

Stefano GB. Autoimmunovascular regulation: morphine and anandamide and ancondamide stimulated nitric oxide release. *J Neuroimmunol* 1998; 83:70–76.

Sung B, Lim G, Mao J. Altered expression and uptake activity of spinal glutamate transporters after nerve injury contribute to the pathogenesis of neuropathic pain in rats. *J Neurosci* 2003; 23:2899–2910.

Szabo I, Chen XH, Xin L, et al. Heterologous desensitization of opioid receptors by chemokines inhibits chemotaxis and enhances the perception of pain. *Proc Natl Acad Sci USA* 2002; 99:10276–10281.

Tadano T, Namioka M, Nakagawasai O, et al. Induction of nociceptive responses by intrathecal injection of interleukin-1 in mice. *Life Sci* 1999; 65:255–261.

Tortorici V, Nogueira L, Salas R, Vanegas H. Involvement of local cholecystokinin in the tolerance induced by morphine microinjections into the periaqueductal gray of rats. *Pain* 2003; 102:9–16.

Vanderah TW, Gardell LR, Burgess SE, et al. Dynorphin promotes abnormal pain and spinal opioid antinociceptive tolerance. *J Neurosci* 2000; 20:7074–7079.

Verge GM, Milligan ED, Maier SF, et al. Fractalkine (CX3CL1) and fractalkine receptor (CX3CR1) distribution in spinal cord and dorsal root ganglia under basal and neuropathic pain conditions. *Eur J Neurosci* 2004; 20:1150–1160.

Verri WA Jr, Cunha TM, Parada CA, et al. Hypernociceptive role of cytokines and chemokines: targets for analgesic drug development? *Pharmacol Ther* 2006; 112:116–138.

Wall PD, Gutnick M. Properties of afferent nerve impulses originating from a neuroma. *Nature* 1974; 248:740–743.

Watkins LR, Maier SF. Beyond neurons: evidence that immune and glial cells contribute to pathological pain states. *Physiol Rev* 2002; 82:981–1011.

Watkins LR, Maier SF. Glia: a novel drug discovery target for clinical pain. *Nat Rev Drug Discov* 2003; 2:973–985.

Watkins LR, Kinscheck IB, Mayer DJ. Potentiation of opiate analgesia and apparent reversal of morphine tolerance by proglumide. *Science* 1984; 224:395–396.

Watkins LR, Wiertelak EP, Goehler LE, et al. Characterization of cytokine-induced hyperalgesia. *Brain Res* 1994; 654:15–26.

Watkins LR, Martin D, Ulrich P, et al. Evidence for the involvement of spinal cord glia in subcutaneous formalin induced hyperalgesia in the rat. *Pain* 1997; 71:225–235.

Watkins LR, Milligan ED, Maier SF. Glial activation: a driving force for pathological pain. *Trends Neurosci* 2001; 24:450–455.

Winkelstein BA, Rutkowski MD, Sweitzer SM, et al. Nerve injury proximal or distal to the DRG induces similar spinal glial activation and selective cytokine expression but differential behavioral responses to pharmacologic treatment. *J Comp Neurol* 2001; 439:127–139.

Wolf G, Yirmiya R, Goshen I, et al. Impairment of interleukin-1 (IL-1) signaling reduces basal pain sensitivity in mice: genetic, pharmacological and developmental aspects. *Pain* 2003; 104:471–480.

Wolf G, Gabay E, Tal M, et al. Genetic impairment of interleukin-1 signaling attenuates neuropathic pain, autotomy, and spontaneous ectopic neuronal activity, following nerve injury in mice. *Pain* 2006; 120:315–324.

Woolf CJ. Intrathecal high dose morphine produces hyperalgesia in the rat. *Brain Res* 1981; 209:491–495.

Wordliczek J, Szczepanik AM, Banach M, et al. The effect of pentoxifylline on post-injury hyperalgesia in rats and postoperative pain in patients. *Life Sci* 2000; 66:1155–1164.

Wu HE, Thompson J, Sun HS, et al. Antianalgesia: stereoselective action of dextro-morphine over levo-morphine on glia in the mouse spinal cord. *J Pharmacol Exp Ther* 2005; 314:1101–1108.

Yaksh TL, Harty GJ. Pharmacology of the allodynia in rats evoked by high dose intrathecal morphine. *J Pharmacol Exp Ther* 1988; 244:501–507.

Yirmiya R, Winocur G, Goshen I. Brain interleukin-1 is involved in spatial memory and passive avoidance conditioning. *Neurobiol Learn Mem* 2002; 78:379–389.

Correspondence to: Yehuda Shavit, PhD, Department of Psychology, The Hebrew University of Jerusalem, Mount Scopus, Jerusalem 91905, Israel. Email: udi.shavit@huji.ac.il.

Part VII

Immune and Glial Interactions with Pain: Implications for Clinical Pain Control

Immune and Glial Regulation of Pain, edited by Joyce A. DeLeo, Linda S. Sorkin, and Linda R. Watkins, IASP Press, Seattle, © 2007.

21

New Perspectives on Sciatica

Jaro Karppinen

Department of Musculoskeletal Disorders, Finnish Institute of Occupational Health, Oulu, Finland

Sciatica, or lumbar radicular pain, is shooting pain radiating from the lower back to one or both legs, together with a band-like sensation. True radiculopathy is defined as radicular pain in the presence of a neurological deficit (Bogduk 1997). The prevalence of lumbar disk syndrome (herniated disk or typical sciatica) was studied as part of the Mini-Finland Health Survey (Heliövaara 1987). The syndrome was diagnosed in 5.1% of men and 3.7% of women aged 30 years and over. In a Finnish longitudinal birth cohort study, symptomatic lumbar disk disease appeared at approximately age 15, with the incidence rising more sharply after the age of 19 years (Zitting et al. 1998).

The long-term prognosis of lumbar radicular pain is thought to be good (Hakelius 1970), although in one study only one-third of patients with sciatica recovered fully within 1 year, whereas one-third underwent surgical treatment (Balague et al. 1999). This finding is in accordance with a systematic review on the long-term course of low back pain (Hestbaek et al. 2003). This study found that 62% of patients continued to experience low back pain at 12 months, 16% were sick-listed at 6 months, and 60% experienced relapses of pain within the first year. Vroomen et al. (2002) studied a cohort of primary care sciatica patients from the Netherlands. An unfavorable outcome was predicted by a disease duration of more than 30 days, increased pain on sitting, pain upon coughing, and restrictions in straight leg raising. This chapter reviews current views on the pathomechanism of sciatica, describes inflammatory mediators involved in nerve root pain, reviews the natural course of lumbar disk herniations, and outlines anticytokine treatments.

PATHOMECHANISM OF LUMBAR RADICULAR PAIN

The tissue origin of sciatic pain has been studied by means of surgical decompression performed under local anesthesia. In these studies, sciatic pain was produced only by applying pressure to the compressed, swollen nerve root, or on the dorsal root ganglion (DRG). Pressure on normal nerve roots or on other tissue did not produce sciatica (Smyth and Wright 1958; Kuslich et al. 1991). Mixter and Barr (1934) were the first to discover the connection between intervertebral disk herniations and symptoms of sciatica when they found that surgical removal of the herniated nucleus pulposus (HNP) relieved the symptoms.

LOCAL INFLAMMATION

Mechanical compression is not the sole mechanism behind sciatica symptoms. The nucleus pulposus of the intervertebral disk is chemically inflammatory and neurotoxic (McCarron et al. 1987) and can induce structural and functional changes in porcine nerve roots without any compression (Olmarker et al. 1993). It induces both macromolecular leakage and axonal spontaneous firing in vitro (Olmarker et al. 1995), and it attracts leukocytes, which play an essential role in radicular pain. In a rat model of mechanical hyperalgesia induced by nerve root exposure to nucleus pulposus, generation of hyperalgesia was inhibited by the depletion of leukocytes with nitrogen mustard (Kawakami et al. 2000). The cells first appearing in and around the HNP were polymorphonuclear leukocytes. Macrophages, originating from monocytes, became predominant a few days later and then remained in the affected region until the inflammation subsided (Kawakami et al. 2000). In an experimental animal herniation model, cells appeared three days after herniation consisting mainly of macrophages with some neutrophils. Macrophages are involved in pain-related behavior; enhancing their recruitment increases neuropathic pain behavior, whereas delaying their recruitment attenuates it (Clatworthy et al. 1995; Myers et al. 1996; Liu et al. 2000). Macrophages are thought to enhance Wallerian degeneration by secreting proteases and by upregulating the expression of adhesion molecules, which are needed to promote transendothelial migration of blood cells to the site of injury (Myers et al. 2006).

The involvement of T lymphocytes in lumbar radicular pain is controversial (Moalem et al. 2004; Yoshida et al. 2004; Kobayashi et al. 2005). A wound-healing reaction is suggested to take place instead of an autoimmune response. However, differentiation of T cells into T helper type 2 cells, an event that occurs in autoimmune reactions, was induced by porcine nucleus pulposus cells (Geiss et al. 2007). Thus, an autoimmune reaction may also be encountered among patients with sciatica, perhaps with greater frequency in chronic cases.

ISCHEMIA

Intraradicular blood flow, measured with a laser Doppler flow meter, has been studied in patients with disk herniation undergoing diskectomy (Kobayashi et al. 2003). A sharp 40–98% decrease in intraradicular blood flow in the L5 or S1 nerve roots was elicited by an intraoperative straight-leg-raising test at the angle that produced symptoms of sciatica. Blood flow normalized within 1 minute after the completion of the test. Surgery revealed that all nerve roots were adhered to herniations. After microdiskectomy, blood flow remained normal in the straight-leg-raising test (Kobayashi et al. 2003).This study highlights the importance of compression in the induction of ischemia. On the other hand, inflammation may also induce ischemia. Indeed, inflammation-induced capillary leakage increases endoneurial pressure and reduces blood flow, thereby causing a "compartment syndrome" in the DRG (Yabuki et al. 1998). The reduction of blood flow correlated with decreases in nerve conduction velocity in a canine model; blood flow reached its greatest decline within 1 week and returned to baseline within 1 month.

Schwann cells are extremely sensitive to ischemia (Wagner and Myers 1996a; Myers et al. 2006). The DRG are more vulnerable than nerve roots, as evidenced by the irreversible changes they undergo after direct application of nucleus pulposus (Otani et al. 1999). In contrast to nerve roots, intact DRG are very sensitive to compression, such that gentle pressure produces prolonged repetitive firing in single afferent fibers (Howe et al. 1977). According to the current view, leakage of nucleus pulposus tissue sensitizes nerve roots to produce pain when exposed to concurrent or subsequent mechanical deformation. These components, both chemical and mechanical irritation, initiate the pathophysiological events leading to pain and nerve dysfunction (Olmarker et al. 2004). This view is supported by experimental findings that the combination of these two factors produced more severe histological damage to the nerve roots than either factor alone (Olmarker and Myers 1998; Kawakami et al. 2003).

The molecular mechanism whereby ischemia/hypoxia induces cellular responses is very complex (Brines and Cerami 2005). Hypoxia-inducible factor (HIF), a transcription factor that responds to low oxygen concentrations, is a key molecule in these events. HIF, along with proinflammatory cytokines, triggers mitogen-activated protein kinase (MAPK) expression and erythropoietin synthesis (Brines and Cerami 2005; Risbud et al. 2005). It is difficult, however, to differentiate the mechanisms of action of mechanical compression because, in addition to hypoxia, compression induces the synthesis of inflammatory mediators such as proinflammatory cytokines, nitric oxide, and cyclooxygenase-2 (Kobayashi et al. 2005). Thus, inflammation and ischemia may be inextricable because both processes augment the immune defense against injuries or other insults.

CENTRAL NERVOUS SYSTEM ACTIVATION

Activation of the central nervous system (CNS) after peripheral nerve injury is discussed in more detail elsewhere in this book and has been extensively covered in two excellent reviews (Watkins and Maier 2002; Myers et al. 2006). DRG, which are composed of sensory neuron somas and their supporting glia-like satellite cells, are thought to be first-order sensory neurons that respond immediately and directly to axonal injuries. Exposure of DRG to low doses of interleukin (IL)-1β, tumor necrosis factor-α (TNF-α), and IL-6 resulted in increased mechanosensitivity of DRGs and sensitization of receptive fields (Ozaktay et al. 2006), in a manner similar to that previously observed with dorsal roots (Ozaktay et al. 2002). A key event in glial activation is the retrograde axonal transport of cytokines and neurotrophic factors (Myers et al. 2006). TNF-α tracer injected at the injury site is transported retrogradely to the DRG and then anterogradely to the spinal cord from the DRG (Shubayev and Myers 2001, 2002). Nerve injury activates p38 MAPK in both the DRG and the spinal cord (Kim et al. 2002; Igarashi et al. 2006). TNF-α is crucial in MAPK activation (Schäfers et al. 2003), which is significantly reduced, although not completely suppressed, in TNF-α knockout mice as compared to wild-type mice (Igarashi et al. 2006).

In the spinal cord, immune-like glial cells (astrocytes and microglia) are activated following nerve root injury. The activation and retrograde transport of TNF-α and its receptors from the injury site is thought to represent a mechanism for CNS activation and for upregulation of TNF-α and its receptors in the spinal cord (DeLeo et al. 2000; Ohtori et al. 2004; Myers et al. 2006). The glial cells are not only activated, but they may also create and maintain pathological pain states by locally releasing proinflammatory cytokines (Ruohonen et al. 2002; Watkins and Maier 2002). One of the clinically unwanted consequences of glial inflammatory activation is extraterritorial pain and mirror-image pain, as discussed by Milligan et al. (this volume). Mirror-image pain arises from the healthy body region contralateral to the actual site of trauma or inflammation. It can be reversed by intrathecal glial inhibitors, prevented by intrathecal p38 MAPK inhibitors, and reversed or prevented by intrathecal antagonists for IL-1, TNF-α, or IL-6 (Milligan et al. 2003).

INFLAMMATORY MEDIATORS IN RADICULAR PAIN

Symptomatic disk herniation tissue is known to contain many cytokines (Kang et al. 1996; Rand et al. 1997; Burke et al. 2002). Proinflammatory cytokines include IL-1, IL-6, granulocyte-macrophage colony-stimulating factor, and TNF-α. IL-10, the most important anti-inflammatory cytokine, has also been found in disks, and its expression increases after an inflammatory stimulus (Rand et al. 1997). The following subsections discuss the three most important pro-inflammatory cytokines found in disks in more detail. TNF-α is currently thought to be the crucial mediator in HNP-induced nerve root irritation (Myers et al. 2006). In addition to TNF-α, other inflammatory mediators may take part in the inflammatory component of radicular pain. These mediators could be either proximal or distal to TNF-α, i.e., they may increase its expression or be upregulated by it, respectively. Proinflammatory cytokines have synergistic activities and also stimulate their own production, as well as that of other proinflammatory cytokines. As a result, it is likely that all proinflammatory cytokines exert interrelated effects.

TUMOR NECROSIS FACTOR ALPHA

TNF-α is a cytokine produced mainly by activated macrophages and T cells in response to inflammation and by mast and Schwann cells in response to peripheral nerve injury (Bemelmans et al. 1996; Wagner and Myers 1996a). The initial increase of TNF-α release from Schwann cells serves to recruit macrophages to the injury site and activate them. Macrophage recruitment is achieved by activating adhesion molecules such as intercellular adhesion molecule-1 (ICAM-1) (Wagner and Myers 1996a; Lisak and Bealmear 1997; Schäfers et al. 2002). TNF-α activates the transcription factors nuclear factor (NF)-κB and activator protein 1 (AP-1) by binding to the p55 TNF-α-receptor-1 (TNFR1), thereby activating proinflammatory and immunomodulatory genes (Darnay and Aggarwal 1997; Myers et al. 2006). The intracellular signaling is mediated through activation of p38 MAPK and extracellular signal-regulated kinase (ERK) pathways (Myers et al. 2006; Takahashi et al. 2006). Interestingly, p38 is involved in stress-induced signaling, in addition to inflammatory responses (Martin-Blanco 2000).

Experiments have shown immunohistochemically and by reverse transcription polymerase chain reaction that TNF-α is expressed in the porcine nucleus pulposus (Olmarker and Larsson 1998; Ahn et al. 2002). TNF-α is also expressed in human intervertebral disks (from cadavers of persons with no known symptoms of sciatica), both in the nucleus pulposus and the annulus fibrosus, albeit at a lower level than in surgical disk tissue samples from sciatica patients (Weiler et al. 2005). In a rat model, the concentration of TNF-α was found to be approximately 0.5 ng per herniated disk (Igarashi et al. 2000). In disk cell cultures, no secreted TNF-α has been detected (Rand et al. 1997; Burke et al. 2002), which is probably explained by the transience of expression of this cytokine (Yoshida et al. 2004). In a disk herniation model, TNF-α is transiently expressed in disk tissue at day 1 after development of HNP

(Yoshida et al. 2004). The expression of TNF- α in human disks correlates with histological evaluation of disk degeneration (Weiler et al. 2004). This finding is in accordance with the ability of TNF-α to enhance the expression of matrix metalloproteinases and the catabolism of proteoglycans at low concentrations in bovine nucleus cells (Séguin et al. 2005).

Endoneurial TNF-α causes demyelination, axonal degeneration, and hyperalgesia (Redford et al. 1995; Wagner and Myers 1996b). Exogenous TNF-α applied to nerve roots produced neuropathological and behavioral changes, including Wallerian degeneration of nerve fibers, macrophage recruitment to phagocytose the debris, and splitting of the myelin sheath. These changes all mimicked those produced by nucleus pulposus (Igarashi et al. 2000). Application of TNF-α onto porcine nerve roots resulted in a reduction of nerve conduction velocity that was even more pronounced than with application of nucleus pulposus, whereas application of IL-1β and interferon (IFN)-γ resulted in slight, nonsignificant reductions of conduction velocity compared with fat (Aoki et al. 2002). In a sophisticated model, TNF-α-deficient mice were compared to wild-type animals with normal nucleus pulposus TNF-α expression. Application of normal (wild-type) nucleus pulposus to the sciatic nerve activated TNF-α receptors in DRG neurons and caused severe allodynia (Koshi et al. 2006). These responses were significantly attenuated when nucleus pulposus from TNF-α-deficient mice was applied to the nerve, indicating that TNF-α derived from the nucleus pulposus is the key player in sciatica.

INTERLEUKIN-1

IL-1 is involved in pain-related behavior indicating mechanical allodynia and thermal hyperalgesia in animal models. Increased spinal cord IL-1β expression is detected following chronic constriction injury (DeLeo et al. 1997), and the inflammatory consequences can be attenuated with monoclonal antibody against IL-1 receptor I (Sommer et al. 1999) or IL-1β (Perrin et al. 2005). Furthermore, genetic impairment of IL-1 signaling attenuates neuropathic pain in mice (Honore et al. 2006; Wolf et al. 2006). In a rat model of ischemia-reperfusion injury, mRNA of IL-1β peaked at 12 hours, whereas TNF-α gene expression peaked 24 hours after injury. The expression of both of these proinflammatory mediators correlated with severity of ischemia (Mitsui et al. 1999).

Both IL-1α and IL-1β are detectable in HNP homogenates (Takahashi et al. 1996). In murine nucleus pulposus-derived cells, no basal level secretion of IL-1 was observed. In contrast, after an inflammatory stimulus with lipopolysaccharide, IL-1 secretion increased sharply (Rand et al. 1997). In a peripheral nerve injury model, TNF-α and IL-1α were rapidly upregulated after the injury, whereas IL-1β was synthesized and secreted after a delay (Shamash et al. 2002).

Both TNF-α and IL-1 were transiently expressed in a disk herniation model at day 1 after the development of the herniation (Yoshida et al. 2004).

In rheumatoid arthritis, TNF-α is the dominant regulator of IL-1 (Feldmann et al. 1996). However, the exact role of these proinflammatory cytokines in HNP-induced radicular pain is unknown. Genetic studies have shown that IL-1 may modulate nociceptive responses in chronic pain conditions (Honore et al. 2006). An arthritis model showed that TNF-α and IL-1 may have separate activities (van den Berg et al. 1999). In fact, IL-1 is the primary inflammatory mediator in osteoarthritis, whereas TNF-α and IL-6 have lesser roles (Westacott and Sharif 1996). Furthermore, IL-1β may be the link between mechanical stress and pain. The responses in disk cells, especially in annulus fibrosus cells, increase exponentially with the combination of IL-1 and mechanical stress (Elfervig et al. 2001; Miyamoto et al. 2006).

INTERLEUKIN-6

IL-6 is involved in the cascade of events leading to the development and maintenance of neuropathic pain in animal models (DeLeo et al. 1996; Xu et al. 1997; Ramer et al. 1998). Increased levels of IL-6 have been observed in HNP culture media compared with control disks (Kang et al. 1996) and in disk extracts from patients undergoing spinal fusion for diskogenic pain (Burke et al. 2002). IL-1 is the major regulatory factor of the transcription factors needed for IL-6 gene expression in monocytes, although TNF-α and prostaglandin E_2 can also induce IL-6 upregulation in these cells (Shimizu et al. 1990; Matsusaka et al. 1993; Dendorfer et al. 1995). It has been demonstrated in vitro that IL-6 is produced mainly by macrophages and that upregulation of IL-6 requires an interaction between disk cells and macrophages (Takada et al. 2004). Moreover, IL-6 production follows TNF-α expression (Lee et al. 2004; Takada et al. 2006) and could be blocked with TNF-α-neutralizing antibody (Takada et al. 2006). Similarly, in a bacteremia model, blocking of TNF-α inhibited TNF-α-activated expression of IL-1 and IL-6 (Fong et al. 1989). The upregulation of IL-6 in invading macrophages seems to be mediated by prostaglandin E_2 receptor EP4, via autocrine or paracrine mechanisms (Ma and Quirion 2005).

IL-6 is particularly interesting in that it has a dual role in nerve injury, because its upregulation is required to promote regeneration within the CNS (Cafferty et al. 2004). IL-6 regulates, to a large extent, the hepatic acute phase and cachectic responses to an acute inflammatory stimulus (Oldenburg et al. 1993). It has been observed that patients with sciatica have an elevated acute phase response (Le Gars et al. 2000). Mean levels of C-reactive protein (CRP), an acute phase protein, were significantly higher in patients with sciatica compared to age- and sex-matched controls (1.68 vs. 0.74 mg/L; $P = 0.002$). However, normal concentrations of IL-6, IL-1β, IFN-γ, and TNF-α were detected in cerebrospinal fluid (CSF) and serum from patients with disk herniation and sciatica (Brisby et al. 2002). Only in patients with short symptom duration and a large herniation (extrusion or sequestration) could levels of IL-8, a chemokine, be detected in CSF. The normal levels of IL-6, IL-1β, and TNF-α are not surprising considering their temporally restricted expression (George et al. 1999).

NATURAL COURSE OF DISK HERNIATIONS

Clinicians should not forget the benign natural course of intervertebral disk herniation. Magnetic resonance imaging (MRI) follow-up examinations have shown that, in 66% of patients, HNP tends to regress over time, with partial to complete resolution within 6 months (Deyo and Weinstein 2001). We have recently evaluated MRIs of 21 patients with HNP-induced severe sciatica at 2 weeks, 3 months, and 6 months in an intervention trial. Significant resorption occurred as early as 3 months in most patients (Autio et al. 2006b). The resorption process appears to be associated with HNP-encircling rim enhancement (Komori et al. 1998), which is thought to represent a neovascularized zone with macrophage infiltration (Rothoerl et al. 1998). Neovascularization remains high in extrusions, as the disk has ruptured the posterior longitudinal ligament and entered the epidural space, allowing small vessels to penetrate the disk tissue more easily, whereas subligamentous herniations are immune-privileged (Ozaki et al. 1999). This finding is supported by the higher resorption rate for extrusion-type disk herniations (Ahn et al. 2000). It has also been demonstrated that the only significant determinants for resorption were the thickness of rim enhancement and the Komori classification, i.e., herniation extending above or below 67% of the adjacent vertebra (Komori et al. 1996; Autio et al. 2006a).

TNF-α has an important role in the resorption of disk herniations. Macrophages secrete matrix metalloproteinase (MMP)-7 (matrilysin), which releases soluble TNF-α from macrophage cell membranes. Soluble TNF-α induces secretion of MMP-3 (stromelysin), which is required for macrophage infiltration of the disk, from disk chondrocytes (Haro et al. 2000a,b). In addition to TNF-α, vascular endothelial growth factor (Haro et al. 2002) and monocyte chemoattractant protein-1 (Yoshida et al. 2004) are involved in the resorption process. Upregulation of TNF-α expression initiates the resorption process, followed by the upregulation of vascular endothelial growth factor, plasmin, and MMP-3 (Kato et al. 2004). Thus, anti-TNF-α treatment may inhibit resorption. However, a single infusion of infliximab did not interfere with the spontaneous resorption of disk herniations in an open-label trial (Korhonen et al. 2004). The observation of a nondeleterious effect of infliximab on herniation resorption was later confirmed in a randomized setting (Autio et al. 2006b).

TREATMENT OF SCIATICA

STEROIDS AND NERVE ROOT BLOCKS

Considering the inflammatory nature of sciatica, blocking the cytokine cascade by local or systemic corticosteroids appears to be a promising option. It is known from animal models that methylprednisolone injected within 2 days after application of the nucleus pulposus inhibits nucleus-induced vascular permeability and functional impairment of nerve conduction velocity (Olmarker et al. 1994). According to a systematic review on the treatment of lumbar radicular pain, intramuscular steroids were ineffective (Vroomen et al. 2000). A selective nerve root block is a precision method in which fluoroscopy or computed tomography is used to guide injections of steroid and local anesthetic in the area surrounding the irritated nerve root. In a randomized trial (Karppinen et al. 2001a), the effects of a single injection of methylprednisolone (80–120 mg) with bupivacaine (10–15 mg) ($n = 80$) were compared with placebo ($n = 80$) in patients with radicular pain extending below the knee who had not received surgical treatment. Eighty-two percent of all patients had a herniation confirmed by MRI. A short-term effect was observed in favor of the steroid injection, but the results from follow-up assessments showed that the treatments were of equal efficacy (Karppinen et al. 2001a). However, a recent systematic review found moderate evidence in support of selective root blocks in treating painful radicular symptoms (DePalma et al. 2005). Conclusive evidence in favor of root blocks is still lacking.

ANTICYTOKINE THERAPY FOR SCIATICA

Animal studies indicate that TNF-α plays a crucial role in the pathophysiology of radicular pain. TNF-α, or another molecule acting through the upregulation of TNF-α expression, causes hematogenously recruited leukocytes and macrophages to accumulate in the environment of the nerve root and DRG. This process leads to increased capillary permeability and endoneurial pressure, ultimately causing endoneurial ischemia. Thus, a strong theoretical rationale exists for the use of anti-TNF-α therapy in lumbar radicular pain. Other cytokines may also be involved (Burke et al. 2002), but to date the only anticytokine therapy used to treat radicular pain has been anti-TNF-α treatment.

In rheumatoid arthritis, a major result of TNF-α inhibition by infliximab is the inhibition of migration of blood cells into the joint (Feldmann and Maini 2001). A similar finding was obtained in a mouse model of Wallerian degeneration. In TNF-α-deficient mice, recruitment of macrophages from the periphery was impaired (Liefner et al. 2000). However, other mechanisms may be operational as well, because preemptive treatment with thalidomide, a selective blocker of TNF-α synthesis in activated macrophages, prevented allodynia and thermal hyperalgesia in the chronic constriction injury model (Sommer et al. 1998; George et al. 2000). Etanercept, a receptor for soluble TNF-α, reversed nucleus pulposus-induced nerve conduction block and nerve root edema in a porcine model (Olmarker and Rydevik 2001). In rats, soluble TNFR1 inhibited nociceptive spinal neuronal responses elicited by application of nucleus pulposus on L5 DRG (Cuellar et al. 2004). Neutralizing antibodies partially inhibited the nucleus pulposus-induced abnormal nociresponses in rat dorsal horn neurons (Onda et al. 2003). Finally, pentoxifylline, an anti-TNF-α drug, prevented the compartment syndrome in the DRG induced by the application of nucleus pulposus (Yabuki et al. 2001).

Currently, four commercial anticytokine preparations are available: chimeric, murine/human monoclonal antibody against TNF-α (infliximab) is infused intravenously over 2 hours; soluble TNF-α receptor (etanercept) is injected subcutaneously; humanized monoclonal antibody against TNF-α (adalimumab) can be delivered subcutaneously; and a recombinant IL-1-receptor antagonist (anakinra) is injected subcutaneously. The elimination half-life of infliximab is 10 days compared with 3–9 hours for anakinra, which therefore must be injected daily. Several new anti-TNF-α preparations, including one administered orally, will be commercially available shortly. The different preparations may vary in their safety profiles and in their efficacy in the treatment of lumbar radicular pain. Therefore, before large-scale clinical implementation of the various anticytokine preparations, both proof-of-concept trials and phase IV studies are needed to elucidate the clinical effectiveness and safety issues of these treatments.

CLINICAL EFFICACY OF ANTICYTOKINE THERAPY FOR SCIATICA

An open-label study indicated that a single infusion of infliximab at 3 mg/kg was efficacious for the treatment of HNP-induced acute sciatica. The benefit was seen within 3 hours after infusion and was sustained throughout the 3-month follow-up period (Karppinen et al. 2003). During a 1-year follow-up of this open-label study (Korhonen et al. 2004), the effect appeared to be sustained in all but one out of 10 patients, as evidenced by the outcomes reported both for leg pain and for disability, measured with the Oswestry scale. The nonresponder underwent surgical treatment shortly before the 1-year assessment (Korhonen et al. 2004). A dose of 1 mg/kg infliximab was administered to two patients, and one had rapid and complete relief of radicular pain, while the other reported no benefit from the treatment. In addition to infliximab, etanercept has also been used for the treatment of lumbar radicular pain in open-label trials. A single subcutaneous injection of 25 mg etanercept perispinally to the lower lumbar region appeared to produce rapid and sustained benefit in most patients (Tobinick and Britschgi-Davoodifar 2003; Tobinick and Davoodifar 2004). In a more recent study (Genevay et al. 2004), five patients with acute, severe sciatica received three injections of etanercept (25 mg every 3 days), and seven patients received three intravenous (i.v.) injections of methylprednisolone (250 mg every 3 days). At day 10, patients treated with etanercept reported significant improvement in both leg pain and disability. Further improvement was observed at week 6. In the methylprednisolone group, significant improvement was noted at day 10, but by week 6 symptoms had recurred.

The results of a 3-month follow-up of a randomized controlled trial by Korhonen et al. (2005) that examined the efficacy of infliximab (5 mg/kg) did not mirror the positive results of the open-label study by Karppinen et al. (2003). Patients in both treatment and placebo groups had a similar positive response, with approximately two-thirds responding well, with at least a 75% reduction in leg pain. The pronounced placebo effect was most pronounced in the straight-leg-raising test, with a 15-degree improvement 3 hours after the i.v. saline infusion. A one-year follow-up of the trial (Korhonen et al. 2006) found that 67% of patients in the infliximab group reported no leg pain at 52 weeks compared to 63% in the placebo group ($P = 0.72$). Similar event rates were observed between treatment groups for other outcomes. Eight patients in each group required surgery. Three non-serious adverse reactions (rhinitis, diarrhea, and otitis media with sinusitis maxillaris) were encountered in the infliximab group. Thus, current data do not support routine clinical use of infliximab for the treatment of sciatica.

An oral TNF-α inhibitor, REN-1654, was evaluated for treatment of lumbar radiculopathy in a randomized controlled setting (Carragee et al. 2006). REN-1654 belongs to a chemical class of compounds known as benzamides and acts as a functional TNF-α antagonist in vitro and in vivo. A total of 74 patients were randomized to REN-1654 ($n = 39$) or placebo ($n = 35$). The primary endpoint, improvement in daily spontaneous leg pain score at 3 weeks, was not reached. However, maximum daily leg pain at 1- and 2-week assessments revealed significant reduction in favor of REN-1654 (13% vs. 2.6% and 23% vs. 5.5%, respectively).

PROGNOSTIC FACTORS

There is so far no scientific evidence to justify any pharmaceutical intervention for the treatment of lumbar radicular pain. Nevertheless, uncontrolled studies suggest that a variety of interventions may be useful for radicular pain in clinical practice. One specific intervention is, however, unlikely to benefit all patients with radicular pain. Therefore, we need more information on prognostic factors, which may increase the treatment effect of different therapeutic interventions. Lumbar radicular pain may not be a homogenous entity as was previously thought.

Symptom duration is one prognostic factor that ought to be considered. In clinical practice, patients who have acute radicular pain (for less than 3 months) respond better to selective nerve root blocks than those with chronic radicular symptoms (for more than 1 year). In animal experiments, an injection of methylprednisolone within 2 days of the lesion reversed hyperalgesia after nucleus-pulposus-induced nerve root injury (Olmarker et al. 1994). Acute symptoms could be more susceptible to treatment, whereas it is less likely that local steroids or anticytokine therapy would be beneficial in the treatment of chronic neuropathic radicular pain. Severity of nerve root injury is another important prognostic factor because it influences spinal microglial activation (Winkelstein and DeLeo 2002). Other prognostic factors to be considered are the involvement of the DRG (Otani et al. 1999) and the type of symptomatic herniation (subligamentous vs. transligamentous) (Karppinen et al. 2001b). The role of disk level and genotype as prognostic factors is discussed in detail in the following subsections.

DISK LEVEL

A randomized trial studying the efficacy of selective nerve root blocks demonstrated that the combination of steroid and bupivacaine was more effective than placebo for the treatment of subligamentous HNP located at the L4–5 (or L3–4) level (Karppinen et al. 2001b). In the case of HNP at L5–S1, both treatments were of equal benefit, with a reasonably good chance of recovery. Another randomized controlled trial compared diskectomy with conservative treatment, and found no difference between the treatments, indicating that conservative treatment is justified in patients with sciatica (Österman et al. 2006). A subanalysis of this trial found evidence that surgery may be an effective treatment at the L4–5 level, whereas at L5–S1 both interventions were of equal benefit with a reasonable chance of recovery, similar to results observed in the selective nerve root block trial. Österman et al.'s analysis suggests that sciatica due to a herniation located at L4–5 may be less resistant to spontaneous improvement. The reason may be anatomical because there is more limited space at the L4–5 level compared to the L5–S1 level, so herniation may put the nerve roots and DRG at this lower level at risk of more extensive damage.

The importance of prognostic factors for predicting improvement was evaluated during the 1-year follow-up of the placebo-controlled infliximab trial (Korhonen et al. 2006). A significant improvement was defined as a reduction in leg pain score of at least 75% from baseline without any additional interventions, such as surgery. Interestingly, a better, although nonsignificant, response with infliximab was observed in patients with L4–5 (and L3–4) herniations or if a Modic change (vertebral endplate degeneration) was colocalized with the symptomatic herniation at any level. Modic changes are bone marrow lesions visible by MRI that are assumed to be associated with degenerative, symptomatic intervertebral disk disease (Modic et al. 1988; Kjaer et al. 2006; Kuisma et al. 2006, 2007).

GENOTYPE

Genotype can influence the development of radicular lumbar pain, inflammatory response to a disk herniation, or the response to a given treatment by either increasing or decreasing the effect of medication. Genetic factors influence the magnitude of pain in rodents (Mogil et al. 1999). Similarly, the magnitude of mechanical allodynia in a rodent model of lumbar radiculopathy is influenced by inheritance (LaCroix-Fralish et al. 2005). Recently, genotypes of patients with sciatica were compared with asymptomatic subjects, with regard to inflammatory genes. A genotype leading to increased production of IL-6 was present among patients with sciatica (Noponen-Hietala et al. 2005). IL-6, to a large extent, regulates the hepatic acute phase responses like CRP synthesis after an acute inflammatory stimulus (Oldenburg et al. 1993). Interestingly, in a German study, patients with sciatica who had higher CRP levels also had higher pain intensities (Sturmer et al. 2005), and in another study, patients with higher CRP levels had a lessened response to lumbar epidural steroid injection (Ackerman and Zhang 2006).

It is not likely that polymorphisms in a single gene could be responsible for complex traits such as nociceptive or inflammatory responses. Indeed, Solovieva and coworkers studied the IL-1 gene family, including IL-1α, IL-1β, and the IL-1 receptor antagonist, in 131 Finnish men, of whom 74% reported low back pain during the preceding year. The study identified mutations of C to T in the -889 position of *IL1A* and mutations of C to T in *IL1B* (+3954) that were associated with low back pain (Solovieva et al. 2004). Recently, similar results in an occupational cohort of middle-aged male workers indicated that one of the single polymorphisms of the inflammatory genes analyzed, C to T in the -889 position of *IL1A*, was associated with the intervertebral disk disease status (current and past symptoms). Moreover, whole-body vibration had an additive effect to this gene mutation (Virtanen et al. 2007). The observation correlates with the TT genotype (-889) in the *IL-1A* gene, which significantly increases the transcriptional activity of the *IL1A* gene (Dominici et al. 2002) and upregulates IL1-β expression (Hulkkonen et al. 2000). However, in patients with disk herniation and sciatica, CSF and serum concentrations of both IL-6 and IL-1β were normal (Brisby et al. 2002).

FUTURE PERSPECTIVES

In recent years the mechanisms of sciatica have been extensively studied. Nucleus-pulposus-derived TNF-α is the trigger of an inflammatory cascade in the nerve roots and DRG, although the effect of TNF-α may be augmented by IL-1 and some additional mediators. From animal models, it is known that TNF-α is produced at an early time point in the inflammatory cascade resulting in Wallerian degeneration and hyperalgesia (George et al. 1999). Anticytokine treatment is, however, not the only option. Inhibition of the phosphorylated p38 MAP kinase promotes neuronal regeneration through interaction with Schwann cell signaling and TNF-α activity (Myers et al. 2003). Intrathecal administration of p38 MAPK inhibitors is thought to block p38 phosphorylation in microglia (Myers et al. 2006). In a recent study, intrathecal p38 inhibitor decreased mechanical allodynia in an experimental disk herniation model; it also decreased TNF-α expression in the cauda equina and improved hypoalgesia (assessed with von Frey filaments) and walking distance in a spinal stenosis model. Also, phosphorylated p38 immunoreactivity was localized in spinal cord microglia but not in astrocytes or neurons (Ito et al. 2007).

Drugs that inhibit the activation of central glia in order to reduce neuropathic pain are currently under study (Watkins et al. 2003). Intrathecal administration of minocycline, an antimicrobial agent, attenuated mechanical allodynia and mRNA expression of proinflammatory cytokines such as IL-1β and TNF-α (Ledeboer et al. 2005). Furthermore, in patients with chronic widespread pain, levels of anti-inflammatory cytokines were reduced by minocycline (Uceyler et al. 2006). Therefore, one approach to attenuate neuropathic pain is to enhance endogenous anti-inflammatory mechanisms. Indeed, gene therapy aiming to augment the endogenous anti-inflammatory cytokine, IL-10, looks promising (Wieseler-Frank et al. 2005). Finally, erythropoietin, better known for its hematopoietic effects, is a neuroprotective agent for primary sensory neurons, spinal neurons, and their supporting glial cells (Myers et al. 2006). Systemically administered recombinant erythropoietin markedly downregulates TNF-α expression in Schwann cells after peripheral nerve injury (Campana et al. 2005; see the chapter by Campana in this volume). Carbamylated erythropoietin and peptide fragments of erythropoietin are devoid of the hematopoietic effects on the bone marrow and could be used for neuropathic pain (Leist et al. 2005).

The transient expression of cytokines may be one explanation for the disappointing efficacy of anti-TNF-α intervention in sciatica. The therapeutic window for beneficial pain-related effects seems to be narrow for all anti-TNF-α drugs (Sommer et al. 2001a; Schäfers et al. 2003), although etanercept may be effective at a later time point after the injury (Sommer et al. 2001b). Anticytokine therapy—possibly a combination of two different anticytokine drugs—may be beneficial for a subpopulation of patients with sciatica (Schäfers et al. 2001). However, to date, there is no evidence from randomized, controlled trials to justify the use of any of the available TNF-α-targeting drugs for the treatment of sciatica. Therefore, we strongly discourage off-label use of TNF-α inhibitors, despite some optimistic commentaries (Cooper and Freemont 2004), because of the potentially serious adverse effects associated with anticytokine therapies.

REFERENCES

Ackerman WE III, Zhang JM. Serum hs-CRP as a useful marker for predicting the efficacy of lumbar epidural steroid injections on pain relief in patients with lumbar disc herniations. *J Ky Med Assoc* 2006; 104:295–299.

Ahn SH, Ahn MW, Byun WM. Effect of the transligamentous extension of lumbar disc herniations on their regression and the clinical outcome of sciatica. *Spine* 2000; 25:475–480.

Ahn SH, Cho YW, Ahn MW, et al. mRNA expression of cytokines and chemokines in herniated lumbar intervertebral discs. *Spine* 2002; 27:911–917.

Aoki Y, Rydevik B, Kikuchi S, Olmarker K. Local application of disc-related cytokines on spinal nerve roots. *Spine* 2002; 27:1614–1617.

Autio R, Karppinen J, Niinimäki J, et al. Determinants of spontaneous resorption of intervertebral disc herniations. *Spine* 2006a; 31:1247–1252.

Autio RA, Karppinen J, Niinimäki J, et al. The effect of infliximab, a monoclonal antibody against TNF-α, on disc herniation resorption: a randomized controlled study. *Spine* 2006b; 31:2641–2645.

Balague F, Nordin M, Sheikhzadeh A, et al. Recovery of severe sciatica. *Spine* 1999; 24:2516–2524.

Bemelmans MH, van Tits LJ, Buurman WA. Tumor necrosis factor: function, release and clearance. *Crit Rev Immunol* 1996; 16:1–11.

Bogduk N (Ed). *Clinical Anatomy of the Lumbar Spine and Sacrum,* 3rd ed. New York: Churchill Livingstone, 1997.

Brines M, Cerami A. Emerging biological roles for erythropoietin in the nervous system. *Nat Rev Neurosci* 2005; 6:484–494.

Brisby H, Olmarker K, Larsson K, Nutu M, Rydevik B. Proinflammatory cytokines in cerebrospinal fluid and serum in patients with disc herniation and sciatica. *Eur Spine J* 2002; 11:62–66.

Burke JG, Watson RW, McCormack D, et al. Intervertebral discs which cause low back pain secrete high levels of proinflammatory mediators. *J Bone Joint Surg Br* 2002; 84:196–201.

Cafferty WB, Gardiner NJ, Das P, et al. Conditioning injury-induced spinal axon regeneration fails in interleukin-6 knock-out mice. *J Neurosci* 2004; 24:4432–4443.

Campana WM, Li X, Shubayev VI, et al. Erythropoietin reduces Schwann cell TNF-alpha, Wallerian degeneration and pain-related behaviors after peripheral nerve injury. *Eur J Neurosci* 2006; 23:617–626.

Carragee EJ, Klapper JA, Schaufele MK, et al. Oral REN-1654 in sciatica: a phase 2, randomized, double-blind, placebo-controlled, multi-center study in subjects with pain due to lumbosacral radiculopathy. Presented at: Annual Meeting of the International Society for the Study of the Lumbar Spine, Bergen, Norway June 13–17, 2006.

Clatworthy AL, Illich PA, Castro GA, Walters ET. Role of periaxonal inflammation in the development of thermal hyperalgesia and guarding behavior in a rat model of neuropathic pain. *Neurosci Lett* 1995; 184:5–8.

Cooper RG, Freemont AJ. TNF-alpha blockade for herniated intervertebral disc-induced sciatica: a way forward at last? *Rheumatology (Oxford)* 2004; 43:119–121.

Cuellar JM, Montesano PX, Carstens E. Role of TNF-alpha in sensitization of nociceptive dorsal horn neurons induced by application of nucleus pulposus to L5 dorsal root ganglion in rats. *Pain* 2004; 110:578–587.

Darnay BG, Aggarwal BB. Early events in TNF signaling: a story of associations and dissociations. *J Leukoc Biol* 1997; 61:559–566.

DeLeo JA, Colburn RW, Nichols M, Malhotra A. Interleukin-6-mediated hyperalgesia/allodynia and increased spinal IL-6 expression in a rat mononeuropathy model. *J Interferon Cytokine Res* 1996; 16:695–700.

DeLeo JA, Colburn RW, Rickman AJ. Cytokine and growth factor immunohistochemical spinal profiles in two animal models of mononeuropathy. *Brain Res* 1997; 759:50–57.

DeLeo JA, Rutkowski MD, Stalder AK, Campbell IL. Transgenic expression of TNF by astrocytes increases mechanical allodynia in a mouse neuropathy model. *Neuroreport* 2000; 11:599–602.

Dendorfer U, Oettgen P, Libermann TA. Interleukin-6 gene expression by prostaglandins and cyclic AMP mediated by multiple regulatory elements. *Am J Ther* 1995; 2:660–665.

DePalma MJ, Bhargava A, Slipman CW. A critical appraisal of the evidence for selective nerve root injection in the treatment of lumbosacral radiculopathy. *Arch Phys Med Rehabil* 2005; 86:1477–1483.

Deyo RA, Weinstein JN. Low back pain. *N Engl J Med* 2001; 344:363–370.

Dominici R, Cattaneo M, Malferrari G, et al. Cloning and functional analysis of the allelic polymorphism in the transcription regulatory region of interleukin-1 alpha. *Immunogenetics* 2002; 54:82–86.

Elfervig MK, Minchew JT, Francke E, Tsuzaki M, Banes AJ. IL-1beta sensitizes intervertebral disc annulus cells to fluid-induced shear stress. *J Cell Biochem* 2001; 82:290–298.

Feldmann M, Maini RN. Anti-TNF-α therapy of rheumatoid arthritis: what have we learned? *Annu Rev Immunol* 2001; 19:163–196.

Feldmann M, Brennan FM, Maini RN. Role of cytokines in rheumatoid arthritis. *Annu Rev Immunol* 1996; 14:397–440.

Fong Y, Tracey KJ, Moldawer LL, et al. Antibodies to cachectin/tumor necrosis factor reduce interleukin 1 beta and interleukin 6 appearance during lethal bacteremia. *J Exp Med* 1989; 170:1627–1633.

Geiss A, Larsson K, Rydevik B, Takahashi I, Olmarker K. Autoimmune properties of nucleus pulposus: an experimental study in pigs. *Spine* 2007; 32:168–173.

Genevay S, Stingelin S, Gabay C. Efficacy of etanercept in the treatment of acute and severe sciatica. A pilot study. *Ann Rheum Dis* 2004; 63:1120–1123.

George A, Schmidt C, Weishaupt A, Toyka KV, Sommer C. Serial determination of tumor necrosis factor-alpha content in rat sciatic nerve after chronic constriction injury. *Exp Neurol* 1999; 160:124–132.

George A, Marziniak M, Schäfers M, Toyka KV, Sommer C. Thalidomide treatment in chronic constrictive neuropathy decreases endoneurial tumor necrosis factor-alpha, increases interleukin-10 and has long-term effects on spinal cord dorsal horn met-enkephalin. *Pain* 2000; 88:267–275.

Hakelius A. Prognosis in sciatica. A clinical follow-up of surgical and non- surgical treatment. *Acta Orthop Scand* 1970; Suppl 129:1–76.1

Haro H, Crawford HC, Fingleton B, et al. Matrix metalloproteinase-3-dependent generation of a macrophage chemoattractant in a model of herniated disc resorption. *J Clin Invest* 2000a; 105:133–141.

Haro H, Crawford HC, Fingleton B, et al. Matrix metalloproteinase-7-dependent release of tumor necrosis factor-alpha in a model of herniated disc resorption. *J Clin Invest* 2000b; 105:143–150.

Haro H, Kato T, Komori H, Osada M, Shinomiya K. Vascular endothelial growth factor (VEGF)-induced angiogenesis in herniated disc resorption. *J Orthop Res* 2002; 20:409–415

Heliövaara M. Body height, obesity, and risk of herniated lumbar intervertebral disc. *Spine* 1987; 12:469–472.

Hestbaek L, Leboeuf-Yde C, Manniche C. Low back pain: what is the long-term course? A review of studies of general patient populations. *Eur Spine J* 2003; 12:149–165.

Honore P, Wade CL, Zhong C, et al. Interleukin-1alphabeta gene-deficient mice show reduced nociceptive sensitivity in models of inflammatory and neuropathic pain but not post-operative pain. *Behav Brain Res* 2006; 167:355–364.

Howe JF, Loeser JD, Calvin WH. Mechanosensitivity of dorsal root ganglia and injured axons: a physiological basis for the radicular pain of nerve root compression. *Pain* 1977; 3:25–41.

Hulkkonen J, Laippala P, Hurme M. A rare allele combination of the interleukin-1 gene complex is associated with high interleukin-1 beta plasma levels in healthy individuals. *Eur Cytokine Netw* 2000; 11:251–255.

Igarashi T, Kikuchi S, Shubayev V, Myers RR. Volvo Award winner in basic science studies: Exogenous tumor necrosis factor-alpha mimics nucleus pulposus-induced neuropathology. Molecular, histologic, and behavioral comparisons in rats. *Spine* 2000; 25:2975–2980.

Igarashi A, Campana WM, Shubayev VI, Kikuchi S, Myers RR. Immediate and delayed phosphorylation of p38 MAPK in nerve and DRG following crush injury: studies with TNF knockout mice. Presented at: Annual Meeting of the International Society for the Study of the Lumbar Spine, Bergen, Norway, June 13–17, 2006.

Ito T, Ohtori S, Inoue G, et al. Glial phosphorylated p38 MAP kinase mediates pain in a rat model of lumbar disc herniation and induces motor dysfunction in a rat model of lumbar spinal canal stenosis. *Spine* 2007; 32:159–167.

Kang JD, Georgescu HI, McIntyre-Larkin L, et al. Herniated lumbar intervertebral discs spontaneously produce matrix metalloproteinases, nitric oxide, interleukin-6, and prostaglandin E2. *Spine* 1996; 21:271–277.

Karppinen J, Malmivaara A, Kurunlahti M, et al. Periradicular infiltration for sciatica. A randomized controlled trial. *Spine* 2001a; 26:1059–1067.

Karppinen J, Ohinmaa A, Malmivaara A, et al. Cost effectiveness of periradicular infiltration for sciatica. Subgroup analysis of a randomized controlled trial. *Spine* 2001b; 26:2587–2595.

Karppinen J, Korhonen T, Malmivaara A, et al. Tumor necrosis factor-alpha monoclonal antibody, infliximab, used to manage severe sciatica. *Spine* 2003; 28:750–753.

Kato T, Haro H, Komori H, Shinomiya K. Sequential dynamics of inflammatory cytokine, angiogenesis inducing factor and matrix degrading enzymes during spontaneous resorption of the herniated disc. *J Orthop Res* 2004; 22:895–900.

Kawakami M, Tamaki T, Matsumoto T, et al. Role of leukocytes in radicular pain secondary to herniated nucleus pulposus. *Clin Orthop* 2000; 268–277.

Kawakami M, Hashizume H, Nishi H, et al. Comparison of neuropathic pain induced by the application of normal and mechanically compressed nucleus pulposus to lumbar nerve roots in the rat. *J Orthop Res* 2003; 21:535–539.

Kim SY, Bae JC, Kim JY, et al. Activation of p38 MAP kinase in the rat dorsal root ganglia and spinal cord following peripheral inflammation and nerve injury. *Neuroreport* 2002; 13:2483–2486.

Kjaer P, Korsholm L, Bendix T, Sorensen JS, Leboeuf-Yde C. Modic changes and their associations with clinical findings. *Eur Spine J* 2006; 15:1312–1319.

Kobayashi S, Shizu N, Suzuki Y, Asai T, Yoshizawa H. Changes in nerve root motion and intraradicular blood flow during an intraoperative straight-leg-raising test. *Spine* 2003; 28:1427-1434.

Kobayashi S, Baba H, Uchida K, et al. Effect of mechanical compression on the lumbar nerve root: localization and changes of intraradicular inflammatory cytokines, nitric oxide and cyclooxygenase. *Spine* 2005; 30:1699–1705.

Komori H, Shinomiya K, Nakai O, et al. The natural history of herniated nucleus pulposus with radiculopathy. *Spine* 1996; 21:225–229.

Komori H, Okawa A, Haro H, et al. Contrast-enhanced magnetic resonance imaging in conservative management of lumbar disc herniation. *Spine* 1998; 23:67–73.

Korhonen T, Karppinen J, Malmivaara A, et al. Efficacy of infliximab for disc herniation-induced sciatica: one-year follow-up. *Spine* 2004; 29:2115–2119.

Korhonen T, Karppinen J, Paimela L, et al. The treatment of disc herniation-induced sciatica with infliximab: results of a randomized, controlled, 3-month follow-up study. *Spine* 2005; 30:2724–2728.

Korhonen T, Karppinen J, Paimela L, et al. The treatment of disc herniation-induced sciatica with infliximab: one-year follow-up results of FIRST II, a randomized controlled trial. *Spine* 2006; 31:2759–2766.

Koshi T, Yamashita M, Ohtori S, et al. Role of tumor necrosis factor from the nucleus pulposus in regulation of the TNF receptors and radicular pain: a study using TNF-deficient mice. Presented at: Annual Meeting of the International Society for the Study of the Lumbar Spine, Bergen, Norway, June 13–17, 2006.

Kuisma M, Karppinen J, Niinimäki J, et al. A three-year follow-up of lumbar spine endplate (Modic) changes. *Spine* 2006; 31:1714–1718.

Kuisma M, Karppinen J, Niinimäki J, et al. Modic changes in endplates of lumbar vertebral bodies: prevalence and association with low-back and sciatic pain among middle-aged male workers. *Spine* 2007; 32:1116–1122.

Kuslich SD, Ulstrom CL, Michael CJ. The tissue origin of low back pain and sciatica: a report of pain response to tissue stimulation during operations on the lumbar spine using local anesthesia. *Orthop Clin N Am* 1991; 22:181–187.

LaCroix-Fralish ML, Rutkowski MD, et al. The magnitude of mechanical allodynia in a rodent model of lumbar radiculopathy is dependent on strain and sex. *Spine* 2005; 30:1821–1827.

Ledeboer A, Sloane EM, Milligan ED, et al. Minocycline attenuates mechanical allodynia and pro-inflammatory cytokine expression in rat models of pain facilitation. *Pain* 2005; 115:71–83.

Lee HL, Lee KM, Son SJ, Hwang SH, Cho HJ. Temporal expression of cytokines and their receptors mRNAs in a neuropathic pain model. *Neuroreport* 2004; 15:2807–2811.

Le Gars L, Borderie D, Kaplan G, Berenbaum F. Systemic inflammatory response with plasma C-reactive protein elevation in disk-related lumbosciatic syndrome. *Joint Bone Spine* 2000; 67:452–455.

Leist M, Ghezzi P, Grasso G, et al. Derivatives of erythropoietin that are tissue protective but not erythropoietic. *Science* 2004; 305:239–242.

Liefner M, Siebert H, Sachse T, et al. The role of TNF-alpha during Wallerian degeneration. *J Neuroimmunol* 2000; 108:147–152.

Lisak RP, Bealmear B. Upregulation of intercellular adhesion molecule-1 (ICAM-1) on rat Schwann cells in vitro: comparison of interferon-gamma, tumor necrosis factor-alpha and interleukin-1. *J Peripher Nerv Syst* 1997; 2:233–243.

Liu T, Vanrooijen N, Tracey DJ. Depletion of macrophages reduces axonal degeneration and hyperalgesia following nerve injury. *Pain* 2000; 86:25–32.

Ma W, Quirion R. Up-regulation of interleukin-6 induced by prostaglandin E from invading macrophages following nerve injury; an in vivo and in vitro study. *J Neurochem* 2005; 93:664–673.

Martin-Blanco E. p38 MAPK signaling cascades: ancient roles and new functions. *Bioessays* 2000; 22:637–645.

Matsusaka T, Fujikawa K, Nishio Y, et al. Transcription factors NF-IL6 and NF-kappa B synergistically activate transcription of the inflammatory cytokines, interleukin 6 and interleukin 8. *Proc Natl Acad Sci USA* 1993; 90:10193–10197.

McCarron RF, Wimpee MW, Hudkins PG, Laros GS. The inflammatory effect of nucleus pulposus. A possible element in the pathogenesis of low-back pain. *Spine* 1987; 12:760–764.

Milligan ED, Twining C, Chacur M, et al. Spinal glia and proinflammatory cytokines mediate mirror-image neuropathic pain in rats. *J Neurosci* 2003; 23:1026–1040.

Mitsui Y, Okamoto K, Martin DP, Schmelzer JD, Low PA. The expression of proinflammatory cytokine mRNA in the sciatic-tibial nerve of ischemia-reperfusion injury. *Brain Res* 1999; 844:192–195.

Mixter WJ, Barr JS. Rupture of the intervertebral disc with involvement of the spinal canal. *N Engl J Med* 1934; 211:210–215.

Miyamoto H, Doita M, Nishida K, et al. Effects of cyclic mechanical stress on the production of inflammatory agents by nucleus pulposus and annulus fibrosus derived cells in vitro. *Spine* 2006; 31:4–9.

Moalem G, Xu K, Yu L. T lymphocytes play a role in neuropathic pain following peripheral nerve injury in rats. *Neuroscience* 2004; 129:767–777.

Modic MT, Steinberg PM, Ross JS, Masaryk TJ, Carter JR. Degenerative disk disease: assessment of changes in vertebral body marrow with MR imaging. *Radiology* 1988; 166:193–199.

Mogil JS, Wilson SG, Bon K, et al. Heritability of nociception I: responses of 11 inbred mouse strains on 12 measures of nociception. *Pain* 1999; 80:67–82.

Myers RR, Heckman HM, Rodriguez M. Reduced hyperalgesia in nerve-injured WLD mice: relationship to nerve fiber phagocytosis, axonal degeneration and regeneration in normal mice. *Exp Neurol* 1996; 141:94–101.

Myers RR, Sekiguchi Y, Kikuchi S, et al. Inhibition of p38 MAP kinase activity enhances axonal regeneration. *Exp Neurol* 2003; 184:606–614.

Myers RR, Campana WM, Shubayev VI. The role of neuroinflammation in neuropathic pain: mechanisms and therapeutic targets. *Drug Discov Today* 2006; 11:8–20.

Noponen-Hietala N, Virtanen I, Karttunen R, et al. Genetic variations in IL6 associate with intervertebral disc disease characterized by sciatica. *Pain* 2005; 114:186–194.

Ohtori S, Takahashi K, Moriya H, Myers RR. TNF-α and TNF-α receptor type 1 upregulation in glia and neurons after peripheral nerve injury. Studies in murine DRG and spinal cord. *Spine* 2004; 29:1082–1088.

Oldenburg HS, Rogy MA, Lazarus DD, et al. Cachexia and the acute-phase protein response in inflammation are regulated by interleukin-6. *Eur J Immunol* 1993; 23:1889–1894.

Olmarker K, Larsson K. Tumor necrosis factor alpha and nucleus-pulposus-induced nerve root injury. *Spine* 1998; 23:2538–2544.

Olmarker K, Myers RR. Pathogenesis of sciatic pain: role of herniated nucleus pulposus and deformation of spinal nerve root and dorsal root ganglion. *Pain* 1998; 78:99–105.

Olmarker K, Rydevik B. Selective inhibition of tumor necrosis factor-alpha prevents nucleus pulposus-induced thrombus formation, intraneural edema, and reduction of nerve conduction velocity: possible implications for future pharmacologic treatment strategies of sciatica. *Spine* 2001; 26:863–869.

Olmarker K, Rydevik B, Nordborg C. Autologous nucleus pulposus induces neurophysiologic and histologic changes in porcine cauda equina nerve roots. *Spine* 1993; 18:1425–1432.

Olmarker K, Byrod G, Cornefjord M, Nordborg C, Rydevik B. Effects of methylprednisolone on nucleus pulposus-induced nerve root injury. *Spine* 1994; 19:1803–1808.

Olmarker K, Blomquist J, Stromberg J, et al. Inflammatogenic properties of nucleus pulposus. *Spine* 1995; 20:665–669.

Olmarker K, Myers R, Kikuchi S, Rydevik B. Pathophysiology of nerve root pain in disc herniation and spinal stenosis. In: Herkowits HN, Dvorak J, Bell G, Nordin M, Grob D (Eds). *The Lumbar Spine.* Philadelphia: Lippincott Williams & Wilkins, 2004, pp 11–30.

Onda A, Yabuki S, Kikuchi S. Effects of neutralizing antibodies to tumor necrosis factor-alpha on nucleus-pulposus-induced abnormal nociresponses in rat dorsal horn neurons. *Spine* 2003; 28:967–972.

Österman H, Seitsalo S, Karppinen J, Malmivaara A. Effectiveness of microdiscectomy for lumbar disc herniation. A randomised controlled trial with two years of follow-up. *Spine* 2006; 31:2409–1414.

Otani K, Arai I, Mao GP, Konno S, Olmarker K, Kikuchi S. Nucleus pulposus-induced nerve root injury: relationship between blood flow and motor nerve conduction velocity. *Neurosurgery* 1999; 45:614–619.

Ozaki S, Muro T, Ito S, Mizushima M. Neovascularization of the outermost area of herniated lumbar intervertebral discs. *J Orthop Sci* 1999; 4:286–292.

Ozaktay AC, Cavanaugh JM, Asik I, DeLeo JA, Weinstein JN. Dorsal root sensitivity to interleukin-1 beta, interleukin-6, and tumor necrosis factor in rats. *Eur Spine J* 2002; 11:467–475.

Ozaktay AC, Kallakuri S, Takebayashi T, et al. Effects of interleukin-1 beta, interleukin-6, and tumor necrosis factor on sensitivity of dorsal root ganglion and peripheral receptive fields in rats. *Eur Spine J* 2006; 15:1529–1537.

Perrin FE, Lacroix S, Aviles-Trigueros M, David S. Involvement of monocyte chemoattractant protein-1, macrophage inflammatory protein-1alpha and interleukin-1beta in Wallerian degeneration. *Brain* 2005; 128:854–866.

Ramer MS, Murphy PG, Richardson PM, Bisby MA. Spinal nerve lesion-induced mechanoallodynia and adrenergic sprouting in sensory ganglia are attenuated in interleukin-6 knockout mice. *Pain* 1998; 78:115–121.

Rand N, Reichert F, Floman Y, Rotshenker S. Murine nucleus pulposus-derived cells secrete interleukins-1-beta, -6, and -10 and granulocyte-macrophage colony-stimulating factor in cell culture. *Spine* 1997; 22:2598–2601.

Redford EJ, Hall SM, Smith KJ. Vascular changes and demyelination induced by the intraneural injection of tumour necrosis factor. *Brain* 1995; 118:869–878.

Risbud MV, Guttapalli A, Alber TJ, Shapiro IM. Hypoxia activates MAPK activity in rat nucleus pulposus cells. Regulation of integrin expression and cell survival. *Spine* 2005; 30:2503–2509.

Rothoerl RD, Woertgen C, Holzschuh M, Rueschoff J, Brawanski A. Is there a clinical correlate to the histologic evidence of inflammation in herniated lumbar disc tissue? *Spine* 1998; 23:1197–1200.

Ruohonen S, Jagodi M, Khademi M, et al. Contralateral non-operated nerve to transected rat sciatic nerve shows increased expression of IL-1beta, TGF-beta1, TNF-alpha, and IL-10. *J Neuroimmunol* 2002; 132:11–7.

Schäfers M, Brinkhoff J, Neukirchen S, Marziniak M, Sommer C. Combined epineurial therapy with neutralizing antibodies to tumor necrosis factor-alpha and interleukin-1 receptor has an additive effect in reducing neuropathic pain in mice. *Neurosci Lett* 2001; 310:113–116.

Schäfers M, Schmidt C, Vogel C, Toyka KV, Sommer C. Tumor necrosis factor-alpha (TNF) regulates the expression of ICAM-1 predominantly through TNF receptor 1 after chronic constriction injury of mouse sciatic nerve. *Acta Neuropathol (Berl)* 2002; 104:197–205.

Schäfers M, Svensson CI, Sommer C, Sorkin LS. Tumor necrosis factor-alpha induces mechanical allodynia after spinal nerve ligation by activation of p38 MAPK in primary sensory neurons. *J Neurosci* 2003; 23:2517–2521.

Séguin CA, Pilliar RM, Roughley PJ, Kandel RA. Tumor necrosis factor-α modulates matrix production and catabolism in nucleus pulposus tissue. *Spine* 2005; 30:1940–1948.

Shamash S, Reichert F, Rotshenker S. The cytokine network of Wallerian degeneration: tumor necrosis factor-alpha, interleukin-1alpha, and interleukin-1beta. *J Neurosci* 2002; 22:3052–3060.

Shimizu H, Mitomo K, Watanabe T, Okamoto S, Yamamoto K. Involvement of a NF-kappa B-like transcription factor in the activation of the interleukin-6 gene by inflammatory lymphokines. *Mol Cell Biol* 1990; 10:561–568.

Shubayev VI, Myers RR. Axonal transport of TNF-alpha in painful neuropathy: distribution of ligand tracer and TNF receptors. *J Neuroimmunol* 2001; 114:48–56.

Shubayev VI, Myers RR. Anterograde TNF alpha transport from rat dorsal root ganglion to spinal cord and injured sciatic nerve. *Neurosci Lett* 2002; 320:99–101.

Smyth MJ, Wright J. Sciatica and the intervertebral disk. An experimental study. *J Bone Joint Surg* 1958; 1401–1418.

Solovieva S, Leino-Arjas P, Saarela J, et al. Possible association of interleukin 1 gene locus polymorphisms with low back pain. *Pain* 2004; 109:8–19.

Sommer C, Marziniak M, Myers RR. The effect of thalidomide treatment on vascular pathology and hyperalgesia caused by chronic constriction injury of rat nerve. *Pain* 1998; 74:83–91.

Sommer C, Petrausch S, Lindenlaub T, Toyka KV. Neutralizing antibodies to interleukin 1-receptor reduce pain associated behavior in mice with experimental neuropathy. *Neurosci Lett* 1999; 270:25–28.

Sommer C, Lindenlaub T, Teuteberg P, et al. Anti-TNF-neutralizing antibodies reduce pain-related behavior in two different mouse models of painful mononeuropathy. *Brain Res* 2001a; 913:86–89.

Sommer C, Schäfers M, Marziniak M, Toyka KV. Etanercept reduces hyperalgesia in experimental painful neuropathy. *J Peripher Nerv Syst* 2001b; 6:67–72.

Sturmer T, Raum E, Buchner M, et al. Pain and high sensitivity C reactive protein in patients with chronic low back pain and acute sciatic pain. *Ann Rheum Dis* 2005; 64:921–925.

Takada T, Nishida K, Doita M, Miyamoto H, Kurosaka M. Interleukin-6 production is upregulated by interaction between disc tissue and macrophages. *Spine* 2004; 29:1089–1092.

Takada T, Nishida K, Doita M, et al. TNF-alpha is the trigger for IL-6 production in the interaction between intervertebral disc and macrophages. Presented at: Annual Meeting of the International Society for the Study of the Lumbar Spine, Bergen, Norway, June 13–17, 2006.

Takahashi H, Suguro T, Okazima Y, et al. Inflammatory cytokines in the herniated disc of the lumbar spine. *Spine* 1996; 21:218–224.

Takahashi N, Kikuchi S, Shubayev VI, Campana M, Myers RR. TNF-α and phosphorylation of ERK in DRG and spinal cord. Insights into mechanisms of sciatica. *Spine* 2006; 31:523–529.

Tobinick EL, Britschgi-Davoodifar S. Perispinal TNF-alpha inhibition for discogenic pain. *Swiss Med Wkly* 2003; 133:170–177.

Tobinick E, Davoodifar S. Efficacy of etanercept delivered by perispinal administration for chronic back and/or neck disc-related pain: a study of clinical observations in 143 patients. *Curr Med Res Opin* 2004; 20:1075–1085.

Uceyler N, Valenza R, Stock M, et al. Reduced levels of antiinflammatory cytokines in patients with chronic widespread pain. *Arthritis Rheum* 2006; 54:2656–2664

van den Berg WB, Joosten LA, Kollias G, van De Loo FA. Role of tumour necrosis factor alpha in experimental arthritis: separate activity of interleukin 1beta in chronicity and cartilage destruction. *Ann Rheum Dis* 1999; 58(Suppl 1):I40–I48.

Virtanen IM, Karppinen J, Taimela S, et al. Occupational and genetic risk factors associated with intervertebral disc disease. *Spine* 2007; 32:1129–1134.

Vroomen PC, de Krom MC, Slofstra PD, Knottnerus JA. Conservative treatment of sciatica: a systematic review. *J Spinal Disord* 2000; 13:463–469.

Vroomen PC, Wilmink JT, de Krom MC. Prognostic value of MRI findings in sciatica. *Neuroradiology* 2002; 44:59–63.

Wagner R, Myers RR. Schwann cells produce tumor necrosis factor alpha: expression in injured and non-injured nerves. *Neuroscience* 1996a; 73:625–629.

Wagner R, Myers RR. Endoneurial injection of TNF-alpha produces neuropathic pain behaviors. *Neuroreport* 1996b; 7:2897–1901.

Watkins LR, Maier SF. Beyond neurons: evidence that immune and glial cells contribute to pathological pain states. *Physiol Rev* 2002; 82:981–1011.

Watkins LR, Milligan ED, Maier SF. Glial proinflammatory cytokines mediate exaggerated pain states: implications for clinical pain. *Adv Exp Med Biol* 2003; 521:1–21.

Weiler C, Nerlich AG, Bachmeier BE, Boos N. Expression and distribution of tumor necrosis factor alpha in human lumbar intervertebral discs: a study in surgical specimen and autopsy controls. *Spine* 2005; 30:44–54.

Westacott CI, Sharif M. Cytokines in osteoarthritis: mediators or markers of joint destruction. *Semin Arthritis Rheum* 1996; 25:254–272.

Wieseler-Frank J, Maier SF, Watkins LR. Central proinflammatory cytokines and pain enhancement. *Neurosignals* 2005; 14:166–174.

Winkelstein BA, DeLeo JA. Nerve root injury severity differentially modulates spinal glial activation in a rat lumbar radiculopathy model: considerations for persistent pain. *Brain Res* 2002; 956:294–301.

Wolf G, Gabay E, Tal M, Yirmiya R, Shavit Y. Genetic impairment of interleukin-1 signaling attenuates neuropathic pain, autotomy, and spontaneous ectopic neuronal activity, following nerve injury in mice. *Pain* 2006; 120:315–324.

Xu XJ, Hao JX, Andell-Jonsson S, et al. Nociceptive responses in interleukin-6-deficient mice to peripheral inflammation and peripheral nerve section. *Cytokine* 1997; 9:1028–1033.

Yabuki S, Kikuchi S, Olmarker K, Myers RR. Acute effects of nucleus pulposus on blood flow and endoneurial fluid pressure in rat dorsal root ganglia. *Spine* 1998; 23:2517–2523.

Yabuki S, Onda A, Kikuchi S, Myers RR. Prevention of compartment syndrome in dorsal root ganglia caused by exposure to nucleus pulposus. *Spine* 2001; 26:870–875.

Yoshida M, Nakamura T, Sei A, et al. Intervertebral disc cells produce tumor necrosis factor α, interleukin-1β, and monocyte chemoattractant protein-1 immediately after herniation: an experimental study using a new hernia model. *Spine* 2004; 29:55–61.

Zitting P, Rantakallio P, Vanharanta H. Cumulative incidence of lumbar disc diseases leading to hospitalization up to the age of 28 years. *Spine* 1998; 23:2337–2343.

Correspondence to: Professor Jaro Karppinen, MD, MSc, PhD, Department of Musculoskeletal Disorders, Finnish Institute of Occupational Health, Aapistie 1, FIN-90220, Oulu, Finland. Email: jaro.karppinen@ttl.fi; jaro.karppinen@occuphealth.fi.

Immune and Glial Regulation of Pain, edited by Joyce A. DeLeo, Linda S. Sorkin, and Linda R. Watkins, IASP Press, Seattle, © 2007.

22

Immunomodulatory Therapies for Complex Regional Pain Syndrome: Thalidomide and Beyond

Donald C. Manning

Neurosciences Clinical Research and Development, Celgene Corporation, Summit, New Jersey, USA; Department of Anesthesiology and Pain Management, University of Virginia, Health Sciences Center, Charlottesville, Virginia, USA

Complex regional pain syndrome type I (CRPS-I) is a painful illness that can follow relatively minor trauma to a limb without overt nerve injury. It is characterized by spontaneous pain or hyperalgesia and is not limited to a defined nerve territory. Associated signs and symptoms in the affected limb include edema, cutaneous temperature changes, sweating, allodynia, ulcers, and decreased joint range of motion as well as trophic changes in the hair, skin, and nails (Veldman et al. 1993). Although it is self-limiting in many people, for some, the condition can become chronic, with spread of symptoms and a high degree of disability.

Treatment of CRPS is based on functional restoration and includes physical therapy accompanied by reduction in allodynia and pain. Treatment for pain has included regional anesthetic techniques such as blockade of peripheral nerves and sympathetic ganglia as well as systemic analgesic therapy with anti-inflammatory agents (nonsteroidal anti-inflammatory drugs [NSAIDs] and steroids), antiepileptics (sodium and calcium channel modifiers), opioids, and alpha-adrenergic receptor agonists and antagonists (Kingery 1997). In general the results have been disappointing for many patients, and the adverse events associated with pharmacotherapy have been burdensome. A reexamination of potential mechanisms and, by extension, new therapies are needed.

Paul Sudeck, a German surgeon, was the first to hypothesize in 1942 that a regional inflammatory response to injury might be the cause of "Sudeck's atrophy." A number of subsequent studies have suggested that the pathogenesis of CRPS is due, in part, to an exaggerated regional inflammatory response to injury (Oyen et al. 1993; Veldman et al. 1993). CRPS has features of both inflammatory and neuropathic pain states and is consistent with neurogenic inflammation associated with immune activation.

Although a complete understanding of the etiology of CRPS-I remains elusive, there is evidence that pro-inflammatory cytokines such as tumor necrosis factor alpha (TNF-α) and interleukins play an important pathological role in the signs and symptoms of neuropathic pain states (Watkins and Maier 2002). TNF-α is an inflammatory cytokine produced by macrophages or monocytes during acute inflammation; it is responsible for a diverse range of signaling events within cells (Lindenlaub and Sommer 2003). An increase in soluble TNF-α receptors has been noted in the serum of patients with allodynia, as compared with neuropathy patients who do not report allodynia (Empl et al. 2001). Expression of TNF-α in Schwann cells is increased in painful neuropathies (Wagner and Myers 1996). Given the clinical presentation of CRPS and the emerging appreciation of neuroimmune mechanisms in chronic pain, it would be logical to look for evidence of these mechanisms in patients with CRPS.

Increased cytokine levels were reported in the cerebrospinal fluid (CSF) of patients with CRPS compared to controls. CSF levels of the proinflammatory cytokines interleukin (IL)-6 and IL-1β were elevated, although the IL-1β measures were near the level of detection for the assay (Alexander et al. 2005). Furthermore, in animal models, IL-6 is elevated in the spinal cord in response to peripheral nerve injury (Arruda et al. 1998).

Schinkel et al. (2006) studied venous blood samples drawn from unaffected and affected arms in 25 patients with acute CRPS and compared them to 30 healthy volunteers. No differences were noted for white blood cell count or for levels of C-reactive protein, IL-6, neuropeptide Y, or calcitonin gene-related peptide. Significant elevations were noted for IL-8, soluble TNF receptors I and II, and substance P in CRPS patients vs. normal subjects, but no difference was found between the unaffected and CRPS-affected arms within the patient group. In other patients with chronic CRPS-I, systemic plasma levels of IL-1β, IL-6, L-8, IL-10, and TNF-α remained unchanged compared to those in healthy controls (Van de Beek et al. 2001).

Systemic activation of cytokines, however, may not occur in a regional condition such as CRPS, which may involve local upregulation of cytokine production. The localized inflammation of a CRPS-affected limb could involve a wide range of immunocompetent cells including activated T lymphocytes, monocytes, and macrophages, as well as skin-resident cells such as keratinocytes, fibroblasts, endothelial cells, and mast cells (Ansel et al. 1990; Kupper 1990; Huygen et al. 2002).

Regional differences of interstitial fluid cytokines between involved and uninvolved extremities have been demonstrated in patients with chronic CRPS (Huygen et al. 2002). Interstitial fluid produced in suction blisters induced in individuals with CRPS was analyzed for cytokines. Increased levels of IL-6 and TNF-α were found in the involved extremity compared to the uninvolved extremity (Huygen 2002). In a limited study of two patients, these investigators were able to show that infliximab (a TNF-α inhibitor) not only reduced cytokine levels but also reduced pain and improved joint mobility (Huygen et al. 2004). Interestingly, the levels of cytokines found in the blister fluids were in the same range as those found in psoriasis patients, where levels of cytokines correlate with disease severity (Bonifati et al. 1994a,b). In patients with psoriasis, steroid therapy such as betamethasone can reduce cytokine levels in the blister fluid, accompanied by disease improvement (Ameglio et al. 1994).

Given the regional elevation of proinflammatory cytokines in CRPS, therapies directed at cytokine modulation would seem to hold promise. One such drug is thalidomide.

THALIDOMIDE AS AN IMMUNOMODULATOR

Thalidomide was developed as a sedative and antinausea drug, but its teratogenic effects and propensity to cause peripheral neuropathy with prolonged use have limited its utility. It is orally active, readily crosses the blood-brain barrier, and is now appreciated to function as an immunomodulator by inhibiting the production of a broad range of proinflammatory mediators including TNF-α, IL-1β, IL-6, and IL-8 and by increasing levels of IL-10, IL-2, and interferon (IFN)-γ (Corral et al. 1999). It is also a potent costimulator of T-cell function and can mediate a shift to a T-helper-2 type of immune profile (Haslett et al. 1998). Thalidomide inhibits the activation of nuclear factor (NF)-κB in response to certain stimuli, such as TNF-α and hydrogen peroxide, but not in response to other stimuli including ceramide, lipopolysaccharide, or phorbol ester (Lokensgard et al. 2000; Majumdar et al. 2002). These findings suggest that the effects of thalidomide on NF-κB are signal dependent and therefore indirect. TNF-α-induced activation of NF-κB is inhibited by thalidomide through the suppression of IκB kinase activity (Keifer et al. 2001). Thalidomide also inhibits the production of TNF-α from human microglial cells (Peterson et al. 1995). The direct effects of thalidomide on cytokines may be at the level of transcription or may be due to destabilization of the cytokine mRNA (Corral et al. 1996).

Thalidomide can dose-dependently reduce the hyperalgesia induced by carrageenan and inhibit irritant-induced writhing in mice (Ribeiro et al. 2000).

It also reduced the TNF-α mRNA levels in the peritoneal cells of mice injected with zymosan (Ribeiro et al. 2000). Thalidomide can reduce allodynia- and hyperalgesia-related behaviors when given at the time of sciatic nerve injury as well as reduce the vascular pathology associated with this injury in rats (Sommer et al. 1998). This effect was observed when thalidomide was administered preoperatively and every day after surgery, but not if its administration was delayed 6 days after surgery (Sommer et al. 1998). The drug's poor bioavailability in rats and uncertainty about systemic levels may have made the dose and duration of therapy insufficient to reverse allodynia or hyperalgesia. Since thalidomide is believed to act at the level of gene transcription and translation, it may require a longer period of exposure to reverse an established pain state. Thalidomide reduces endoneurial TNF-α and increases endoneurial IL-10 and dorsal horn levels of met-enkephalin, but it does not alter IL-1β or IL-6 levels (George et al. 2000). It can reduce the expression of cyclooxygenase (COX)-2 in endotoxin- and cytokine-stimulated peripheral blood monocytes in a partially IL-10-dependent manner (Payvandi et al. 2004). Thalidomide can attenuate the development of vincristine-induced mechanical hyperalgesia in rats (Cata et al. 2004). The effect of thalidomide on IL-10 and other cytokines is very dependent upon the animal or cell model studied (George et al. 2000; Celgene Corporation, data on file).

Sometimes the testing paradigm will influence the results produced by thalidomide, as in the study by Parada et al. (2003). These investigators induced hyperalgesia in rats with carrageenan but also observed a long-lasting primed state for at least 3 weeks in which subsequent inflammation could produce enhanced and prolonged hyperalgesia. This primed state can also be produced by direct administration of TNF-α. NSAIDs and β$_2$-adrenergic antagonists were only able to attenuate the acute hyperalgesia. Thalidomide or TNF-α antibodies injected before carrageenan administration both reduced the acute hyperalgesia and prevented the primed state for at least 5 days. Chronic pain states can evolve after resolved episodes of acute inflammation, as seen in post-traumatic and repetitive strain injury. Perhaps these chronic pain conditions are really a chronic state of increased susceptibility to hyperalgesic stimuli (Parada et al. 2003). This state is analogous to clinical CRPS, which can go into remission only to be activated by a minor trauma or state of inflammation.

It is interesting to note that NSAIDs did not prevent hyperalgesic priming in the animal model (Parada et al. 2003), despite use of such drugs in many chronic pain states. The fact that hyperalgesic priming appears to be prevented by thalidomide treatment in animals raises the question whether thalidomide can be given after an injury associated with hyperalgesic priming and inhibit the maintenance of the primed state. Clinical experience has suggested that thalidomide may have analgesic activity in humans for postoperative and cancer pain (Miller et al. 1960).

CLINICAL EXPERIENCE WITH THALIDOMIDE IN CRPS

Rajkumar et al. (2001) reported on a 43-year-old woman with a 3-year history of severe CRPS treated with thalidomide for newly diagnosed multiple myeloma. Her CRPS resulted from a traumatic injury to her left hand. At the time of the multiple myeloma diagnosis, the patient was nonambulatory and was confined to a bed or wheelchair due to left leg pain, swelling, and ulceration. She complained of severe attacks of neuropathic pain and on physical examination had atrophy of the muscles of the left hand with contractures of the digits and swelling involving the upper and lower extremities on the left side. The patient was enrolled in a multiple myeloma clinical trial of single-agent thalidomide at 200 mg/d, increased to 400 mg/d after 2 weeks. After 1 month of thalidomide therapy, the patient had a marked improvement, with near-resolution of CRPS symptoms. Her leg ulcerations and edema healed completely, allowing her to walk normally. In subsequent months, she regained function in her left hand as well. The authors stated that the benefit observed from thalidomide in this patient's CRPS may be related to the drug's anti-inflammatory effect, specifically an effect on afferent sensory nerves or efferent sympathetic nerves (Rajkumar et al. 2001).

Additional reports of treatment success with thalidomide have followed. In an open-label study, Prager et al. (2003) reported positive results in seven of nine CRPS patients treated with thalidomide, 50–300 mg once daily, for 1–3 months. Of the responders, two patients noted a significant reduction in concomitant pain medication use, and one patient, who was bedridden, became able to perform normal activities of daily living. In another open-label CRPS study (Schwartzman et al. 2003), 42 patients were treated for a total of 3 months at three institutions, receiving thalidomide at doses of 200–400 mg per day. Thirteen of the patients experienced at least moderate relief, with seven reporting "dramatic" responses, including a reduction of concurrent analgesic medications. Treatment responses, which appeared within 4–6 weeks of starting thalidomide, included improvements in deep joint pain, allodynia, and inflammatory skin changes. Also of note was the fact that these patients experienced no significant change in quantitative sensory detection thresholds. Prager et al. (2003) reported similar findings in that no patients experienced new or exacerbated peripheral neuropathy symptoms. Bengston et al. (2003) reported positive results in a 6-month phase II study that used thalidomide, 100–400 mg per day, in the treatment of CRPS. Of the 12 patients enrolled, six reported significant reductions in their levels of pain. Patients often had a "flare" of symptoms in the first few weeks before improvement. Adverse events included rash, somnolence, and constipation, which were mostly mild and transient and were often managed by thalidomide dose reduction. Importantly, a longer duration of CRPS symptoms did not prevent the beneficial effect of thalidomide. At this point it is not possible to predict which patients will respond to thalidomide treatment.

STUDIES OF NEW IMMUNOMODULATORY AGENTS AND CRPS

Given that thalidomide is a known teratogen and is associated with a number of dose-limiting adverse events, including a high incidence of peripheral neuropathy, an effort to develop a class of drugs with enhanced cytokine modulatory and TNF-α inhibitory activity with diminished or absent adverse effects has been underway (Corral et al. 1996). Lenalidomide is the leading compound of this new class. It has been approved in the United States for 2 indications: (1) for the treatment of patients with transfusion-dependent anemia due to low- or intermediate-risk myelodysplastic syndromes associated with a deletion 5q cytogenetic abnormality with or without additional cytogenetic abnormalities and (2) for the treatment of multiple myeloma in combination with dexamethasone in patients who have received at least one prior therapy.

Lenalidomide is minimally, if at all, able to penetrate the blood-brain barrier. It is approximately 1,000 times as potent as thalidomide in stimulating the proliferation of T cells following primary induction by T-cell-receptor (TCR) activation and 100 to 200 times as potent as thalidomide in augmenting the production of IL-2 and IFN-γ following TCR activation of peripheral blood mononuclear cells (Corral et al. 1999).

Lenalidomide suppressed edema and mechanical and thermal hyperalgesia in a model of inflammatory pain. The rat model of carrageenan-induced paw edema and hyperalgesia was used to assess the anti-inflammatory and analgesic properties of lenalidomide in vivo. Rats were treated with lenalidomide at a dose of 50 mg/kg intraperitoneally prior to carrageenan injection into the footpad. Three hours after carrageenan injection, the lenalidomide-treated animals experienced a significant ($P < 0.05$) reduction in paw edema of 36%, a reduction in mechanical hyperalgesia of 50%, and a reduction in thermal hyperalgesia of 44% (P. Schafer, personal communication; data on file at Celgene Corporation). This suppression of edema and hyperalgesia by lenalidomide is consistent with the ability to inhibit the proinflammatory mediators TNF-α, IL-1β, and IL-6 and COX-2-derived prostaglandin E_2.

CLINICAL EXPERIENCE WITH LENALIDOMIDE IN CRPS

On the basis of reports of dramatic response of CRPS to treatment with thalidomide and the known pharmacological properties of lenalidomide,

Celgene, along with several clinical investigators, conducted a pilot study to assess the safety and preliminary efficacy of lenalidomide in patients with unilateral CRPS-I. This study has previously appeared only in abstract form (Schwartzman et al. 2005).

This six-center, open-label study was conducted in men and women with chronic, unilateral type I CRPS, lasting at least 1 year, diagnosed according to the criteria published by the International Association for the Study of Pain (Bruehl et al. 1999; Harden et al. 1999). After qualifying for the study, subjects entered a baseline phase lasting up to 2 weeks, in which a pretreatment average pain rating was determined. If subjects qualified by meeting all inclusion criteria and no exclusion parameters, they were entered into the core treatment phase and treated with lenalidomide at an oral dose of 10 mg/day for 12 weeks. During the study, subjects were allowed to continue their usual medications for CRPS, provided the doses remained stable. Following completion of the core phase, the subjects had an option to participate in an open-ended extension phase.

Pain was assessed on a numerical rating scale of pain intensity (NRS-PI), on the Short-Form McGill Pain Questionnaire (SF-MPQ; Melzack et al. 1987), and on the pain-rating scales of the Brief Pain Inventory (BPI; Daut et al. 1983). Mechanical allodynia was determined by stroking the most painfully sensitive area of the skin three times over 5 seconds at a rate of 5 cm/s with a foam brush. The pain rating was recorded on an 11-point NRS. Safety assessments included physical examination, recording of adverse events (type, frequency, severity, and relationship to the study drug), hematology, serum chemistry and thyroid function laboratory tests, and electrocardiography.

Forty subjects with chronic CRPS for an average of 6 years, 75% women, who were at least partially refractory to conventional therapy and had high pain scores (7.1 ± 1.3) enrolled in the baseline phase, and 31 completed the core treatment phase. Twenty-eight subjects entered the extension phase; 18 of them were still receiving treatment after 52 weeks, and 15 subjects have completed over 104 weeks of therapy.

Lenalidomide provided significant reduction in pain intensity as assessed by NRS-PI (34% achieved >2-point reduction, mean decrease = 1.2 [± 2.1 SD], $P < 0.001$), SF-MPQ (total score $P < 0.01$, sensory score $P < 0.01$), and BPI pain scores ($P < 0.05$). Mechanical allodynia assessed by NRS decreased by 1.3 (± 2.5) units from a baseline of 6.1 units (± 3.3 SD, $P < 0.005$). Any improvements experienced by subjects were sustained with significant effects for at least 1 year. Reduced patient numbers make conclusions difficult beyond 1 year of therapy.

Adverse events were mild and time-limited. Rash, pruritis, dizziness, headache, nausea, increased sweating, and decreased thyroid-stimulating hormone were the most common. Seven serious adverse events (three thromboembolic events, three cytopenias, and one case of rectal bleeding) were suspected to be related to lenalidomide, and 10 adverse events were considered to be un-related.

These results suggest that lenalidomide may be a potentially meaningful therapy for CRPS-I, with improvements in pain that were sustained in some cases for over 2 years of treatment. To further define the therapeutic potential of lenalidomide in CRPS, a large multicenter, randomized, placebo-controlled study of lenalidomide in CRPS-I has been initiated and is currently near completion.

Thalidomide and lenalidomide are both immunomodulators with apparent beneficial effects on CRPS-I. The improvement in pain with lenalidomide is even more remarkable given that the drug does not seem to enter the central nervous system. These findings question the need for centrally active agents in this disease and suggest that peripherally generated inflammatory mediators may have a continuing influence on the signs and symptoms of a chronic pain-ful condition such as CRPS.

ACKNOWLEDGMENTS

Donald Manning is an employee of Celgene Corporation, which also supported the study by Schwartzman et al. (2005). The clinical results discussed in this chapter include off-label and investigational uses of marketed drugs.

REFERENCES

Alexander GM, van Rijn MA, van Hilton JJ, et al. Changes in cerebrospinal fluid levels of pro-inflammatory cytokines in CRPS. *Pain* 2005; 116:213–219.

Ansel J, Perry P, Brown J, et al. Cytokine modulation of keratinocyte cytokines. *J Invest Dermatol* 1990; 94:101S–107S.

Arruda JL, Colburn RW, Rickman AJ, Ruthowski MD, DeLeo JA. Increase of interleukin-6 mRNA in the spinal cord following peripheral nerve injury in the rat: potential role of IL-6 in neuro-pathic pain. *Mol Brain Res* 1998; 62:228–235.

Bartlett JB, Dredge K, Dalgleish AG. The evolution of thalidomide and its IMiD derivatives as anticancer agents. *Nat Rev Cancer* 2004; 4:4314–322.

Bengtson K, Rajkumar S, Brault J, et al. A phase II study of thalidomide in the treatment of chronic complex regional pain syndrome (CRPS). *J Pain* 2003; 4(Suppl 1):85.

Bonifati C, Ameglio F, Carducci M, et al. Interleukin-1-beta, interleukin-6 and interferon-gamma in suction blister fluids of involved and uninvolved skin and in sera of psoriatic patients. *Acta Derm Venereol* 1994a; 186(Suppl):23–24.

Bonifati C, Carducci M, Cordialifei P, et al. Correlated increases of tumor necrosis factor-alpha, interleukin-6 and granulocyte monocyte-colony stimulating factor levels in suction blister fluids and sera of psoriatic patients: relationships with disease severity. *Clin Exp Dermatol* 1994b; 19:383–387.

Bruehl S, Harden RN, Galer BS, et al. External validation of IASP diagnostic criteria for complex regional pain syndrome and proposed research criteria. *Pain* 1999; 81:147–154.

Buysse DJ. Reynolds CF III, Monk TH, et al. The Pittsburgh Sleep Quality Index: a new instrument for psychiatric practice and research *Psychiatry Res* 1989; 28:193–213.

Cata JP, Weng HR, Dougherty PM. Cyclooxygenase inhibitors and thalidomide ameliorate vincristine-induced hyperalgesia in rats. *Cancer Chemother Pharmacol* 2004; 54:391–397.

Corral LG, Muller GW, Moreira AL, et al. Selection of novel analogs of thalidomide with enhanced tumor necrosis factor alpha inhibitory activity. *Mol Med* 1996; 2:506–515.

Corral LG, Haslett PA, Muller GW, et al. Differential cytokine modulation and T-cell activation by two distinct classes of thalidomide analogues that are potent inhibitors of TNF-alpha. *J Immunol* 1999; 163:380–386.

Daut RL, Cleeland CS, Flanery RC. Development of the Wisconsin Brief Pain Questionnaire to assess pain in cancer and other diseases *Pain* 1983; 17:197–210.

Empl M, Renaud S, Erne B, et al. TNF-alpha expression in painful and nonpainful neuropathies. *Neurology* 2001; 56:1371–1377.

George A, Marziniak M, Schafers M, Toyka KV, Sommer C. Thalidomide treatment in chronic constrictive neuropathy decreases endoneurial tumor necrosis factor-a, increases interleukin-10 and has long-term effects on spinal cord dorsal horn met-enkephalin. *Pain* 2000; 88:267–275.

Grabow TS, Christo PJ, Raja SN. Complex regional pain syndrome: diagnostic controversies, psychological dysfunction and emerging concepts *Adv Psychosom Med* 2004; 25:89–101.

Harden RN, Duc TA, Williams TR, et al. Norepinephrine and epinephrine levels in affected versus unaffected limbs in sympathetically maintained pain. *Clin J Pain* 1994; 10:324–330.

Harden RN, Bruel S, Galer BS, et al. Complex regional pain syndrome: are the IASP diagnostic criteria valid and sufficiently comprehensive? *Pain* 1999; 83:211–219.

Haslett PAJ, Corral LG, Albert M, Kaplan G. Thalidomide costimulates primary human T lymphocytes, preferentially inducing proliferation, cytokine production and cytotoxic responses in the CD8+ subset. *J Exp Med* 1998; 187:1885–1892.

Huygen FJ, de Bruijn AG, Klein J, Zijlstra FJ. Neuroimmune alterations of the complex regional pain syndrome type 1. *Eur J Pharmacol* 2001; 429:101–113.

Huygen FJ, de Brujin AG, de Bruin MT, et al. Evidence for local inflammation in complex regional pain syndrome type 1. *Mediators Inflamm* 2002; 11:47–51.

Huygen FJ, Niehof S, Zijlstra FJ, et al. Successful treatment of CRPS-1 with anti TNF. *J Pain Symptom Manage* 2004; 27:101–103.

Huygen FJ, Ramdhani N, van Toorenenbergen A, et al. Mast cells are involved in inflammatory reactions during complex regional pain syndrome type 1. *Immunol Lett* 2004; 91:147–154.

Keifer JA, Guttridge DC, Ashburner BP, Baldwin J. Inhibition of NF-kappa-B activity by thalidomide through the suppression of I-kappa-B kinase activity *J Biol Chem* 2001; 276:22382–22387.

Kerns RD, Turk DC, Rudy TE. The West Haven–Yale Multidimensional Pain Inventory (WHYMPI). *Pain* 1985; 23:345–356.

Kingery WS. A critical review of controlled clinical trials for peripheral neuropathic pain and complex regional pain syndromes. *Pain* 1997; 73:123–129.

Kupper TS. The activated keratinocyte: a model for inducible cytokine production by non-bone marrow-derived cells in cutaneous inflammatory and immune responses. *J Invest Dermatol* 1990; 94:146S–150S.

Lindenlaub T, Sommer C. Cytokines in sural nerve biopsies from inflammatory and non-inflammatory neuropathies. *Acta Neuropathol* 2003; 105:593–602.

Lokensgard JR, Hu S, van Fenema EM, et al. Effect of thalidomide on chemokine production by human microglia *J Infect Dis* 2000; 182: 983–987.

Majumdar S, Lamothe B, Aggarwal BB. Thalidomide suppresses NF-κB activation induced by TNF and H_2O_2, but not that activated by ceramide, lipopolysaccharides, or phorbol ester. *J Immunol* 2002; 168:2644–2651

Melzack R. The Short-form McGill Pain Questionnaire. *Pain* 1987; 30:191–197.

Miller JM, Ginsberg M, McElfatrick GC, Shonberg IL. The anti-inflammatory effect and the analgesic property of contergan-268. *Antibiot Med Clin Ther* 1960; 7:743–746.

Oyen WJ, Arntz IE, Claessens RM, et al. Reflex Sympathetic Dystrophy of the hand: an excessive inflammatory response? *Pain* 1993; 55:151–157.

Parada CA, Yeh JJ, Joseph EK, Levine JD. Tumor necrosis factor receptor type-1 in sensory neurons contributes to induction of chronic enhancement of inflammatory hyperalgesia in rat. *Eur J Neurosci* 2003; 17:1847–1852.

Payvandi F, Wu L, Haley M, et al. Immunomodulatory drugs inhibit expression of cyclooxygenase-2 from TNF-a, IL-1b and LPS-stimulated human PBMC in a partially IL-10-dependent manner. *Cell Immunol* 2004; 230:81–88.

Peterson PK, Hu S, Sheng WS, et al. Thalidomide inhibits tumor necrosis factor-alpha production by lipopolysaccharide- and lipoarabinomannan-stimulated human microglial cells. *J Infect Dis* 1995; 172:1137–1140.

Prager J, Fleischman J, Lingua G. Open label clinical experience of thalidomide in the treatment of complex regional pain. *J .Pain* 2003; 4(Suppl 1):68.

Rajkumar SU, Fonseca R, Witzig TE. Complete resolution of reflex sympathetic dystrophy with thalidomide treatment. *Arch Intern Med* 2001; 161: 2502–2503

Ribeiro RA, Vale ML, Ferreira SH, Cunha FQ. Analgesic effect of thalidomide on inflammatory pain. *Eur J Pharmacol* 2000; 391:97–103.

Schinkel C, Gaertner A, Zaspel J, et al. Inflammatory mediators are altered in the acute phase of posttraumatic complex regional pain syndrome. *Clin J Pain* 2006; 22:235–239.

Schwartzman RJ, Chevlen E, Bengtson K. Thalidomide has activity in treating complex regional pain syndrome. *Arch Intern Med* 2003; 163:1487–1488.

Schwartzman R, O'Conner D, Grothusen J. Open label trial of thalidomide in the treatment of complex regional pain syndrome type I. *J Pain* 2003; 4(Suppl 1):76.

Schwartzman R, Irving G, Wallace M, et al. A multicenter, open-label, 12-week study with extension to evaluate the safety and efficacy of lenalidomide (CC-5013) in the treatment of complex regional pain syndrome type-1. *Abstracts: 11th World Congress on Pain.* Seattle: IASP Press, 2005, p 580.

Sommer C, Marziniak M, Myers RR. The effect of thalidomide treatment on vascular pathology and hyperalgesia caused by chronic constriction injury of rat nerve. *Pain* 1998; 74:83–91.

Van de Beek WJ, Remarque EJ, Westendorp RG, van Hilten JJ. Innate cytokine profile in patients with complex regional pain syndrome is normal. *Pain* 2001; 91:259–261.

Veldman PH, Reynen HM, Arntz IE, Goris RJ. Signs and symptoms of reflex sympathetic dystrophy: prospective study of 829 patients. *Lancet* 1993; 342:1012–1016.

Wagner R, Myers RR. Endoneurial injection of TNF-alpha produces neuropathic pain behaviors. *Neuroreport* 1996; 7:2897–2901.

Watkins LR, Maier SF. Beyond neurons: evidence that immune and glial cells contribute to pathological pain states. *Physiol Rev* 2002 82:981–1011.

Correspondence to: Donald C. Manning, MD, PhD, Celgene Corporation, 86 Morris Avenue, Summit, NJ 07901, USA. Tel: 1-908-673-9529; fax: 1-908-673-2778; email: dmanning@celgene.com.

Immune and Glial Regulation of Pain, edited by Joyce A. DeLeo, Linda S. Sorkin, and Linda R. Watkins, IASP Press, Seattle, © 2007.

23

Cytokine Profiles in Patients with Chronic Widespread Pain

Nurcan Üçeyler and Claudia Sommer

Department of Neurology, University of Würzburg, Würzburg, Germany

Chronic widespread pain (CWP) is a challenging disorder with a high incidence in the general population (Wolfe et al. 1995; Hunt et al. 1999; Neumann and Buskila 2003; Cieza et al. 2004). These patients have pain of unexplained origin for at least 3 months in all four body quadrants (Wolfe et al. 1990). In a subgroup of patients with CWP, fibromyalgia (FM) can be diagnosed according to the criteria of the American College of Rheumatology (ACR) (Wolfe et al. 1990). These criteria include those for CWP as well as tenderness upon digital palpation with 4 kg pressure on at least 11 out of 18 designated points. The prevalence of FM is estimated to be around 0.7% to 3.3% in the general population, with a preponderance in middle-aged women (Neumann and Buskila 2003).

Depending on their field of expertise, clinicians may regard FM as a rheumatological or as a psychosomatic disease or may not recognize it as an entity in itself (Rau and Russell 2000). Pain and hyperalgesia are often associated with additional symptoms including fatigue, poor sleep, depression, and autonomic dysfunction such as irritable bladder or bowel disease. Treatment of CWP and FM is symptomatic and often frustrating. The most frequently utilized drugs are tricyclic antidepressants, selective serotonin reuptake inhibitors, antiepileptics, sedatives, opioids, and muscle relaxants. The $\alpha_2\delta$-adrenergic ligand pregabalin and the dual-action antidepressant duloxetine have recently been shown to be effective in patients suffering from FM (Arnold et al. 2004b; Crofford et al. 2005).

PATHOPHYSIOLOGY OF CHRONIC WIDESPREAD PAIN AND FIBROMYALGIA

PEPTIDES, AMINES, HORMONES, AND GENES

The pathophysiology of CWP and FM is only partly understood, although numerous hypotheses have emerged through intensive research. The better-substantiated theories suggest the involvement of neuropeptides, in particular substance P, which is elevated in the cerebrospinal fluid of patients with FM (Russell et al. 1994). The biogenic amine serotonin is reduced in the serum of FM patients (Russell et al. 1992; Samborski et al. 1996; Wolfe et al. 1997; Ernberg et al. 2000), and this finding is regarded as an indication for diminished endogenous analgesia. Brain-derived neurotrophic factor (BDNF), which plays a role in the structural and functional plasticity of nociceptive pathways in the dorsal root ganglia and the spinal cord, is increased in the serum of FM patients (Laske et al. 2007). Changes in the endocrine system may also have implications in the pathogenesis of FM (Griep et al. 1993, 1998; Neeck and Riedel 1999). The hypothalamic-pituitary-adrenal axis is perturbed in patients with FM, with adrenal hyporesponsiveness in response to exogenous corticosteroid-releasing hormone (CRH) (Crofford et al. 1994, 1996). Different studies point to a possible central mechanism of hyperalgesia in FM (Mense 2000), and an abnormal pattern of wind-up (temporal summation of pain), indicating hyperresponsiveness to pain, was found in patients with FM compared to controls (Staud et al. 2004).

Familial aggregation of FM has been observed (Pellegrino et al. 1989; Buskila et al. 1996; Arnold et al. 2004a). Genetic factors that have been investigated include the association of FM with distinct HLA regions (Yunus et al. 1999) or with polymorphisms in serotonin transporter and receptor genes and their promoter regions (Bondy et al. 1999; Offenbaecher et al. 1999; Gürsoy et al. 2001; Cohen et al. 2002; Gürsoy 2002), but no firm correlation has been found so far. A recent study with pairs of twins showed a modest influence of genetic factors for the likelihood of developing CWP (Kato et al. 2006).

THE ROLE OF CYTOKINES

In recent years, the impact of cytokine-mediated neuroimmune interactions on pain has been studied extensively (Marchand et al. 2005). Most data were obtained from animal experiments, which have shown that peripheral nerve injury leads to early and sustained alterations in cytokine expression (Taskinen et al. 2000; Kleinschnitz et al. 2004). The intraneural application of proinflammatory cytokines elicits pain behavior (Zelenka et al. 2005), and hyperalgesia can be effectively reduced by blocking distinct proinflammatory cytokines or their receptors (for review see Sommer 2006).

Wallace and colleagues (1988) were the first to assume a connection between the pathogenesis of FM and cytokines. They observed that patients with malignancies who were treated with interleukin 2 (IL-2) developed FM-like symptoms, comprising fatigue, poor sleep, and pain. Further studies of a possible involvement of cytokines in the pathophysiology of CWP and FM have led to sometimes conflicting results, probably due to the variety of body fluids analyzed and methods used.

Several groups have reported an upregulation of proinflammatory cytokines in patients with CWP or FM. In a study with 113 FM patients and 32 controls, serum IL-8 and IL-2-receptor protein levels were elevated in the patient group, and IL-8 levels were related to pain intensity (Gürsoy 2002). A time-dependent upregulation of IL-8 and IL-1-receptor antagonist was found in the serum and peripheral blood mononuclear cells (PBMCs) of 56 patients compared to healthy controls, while IL-1β, IL-2, IL-10, IL-2-receptor, interferon-gamma (IFN-γ), and tumor necrosis factor-alpha (TNF-α) were not altered (Wallace et al. 2001). The analysis of local cytokine levels in patients with FM revealed that IL-1β, IL-6, and TNF-α were detectable in skin samples of patients, whereas none of these cytokines were found in skin from control subjects (Salemi et al. 2003).

In contrast, no difference was seen in the production of IL-1α, IL-6, TNF-α, and the anti-inflammatory cytokine IL-10 in PBMCs of patients with FM compared to healthy controls in another study (Amel Kashipaz et al. 2003). Hader et al. (1991) showed in cell culture experiments that T cells of patients with FM needed higher amounts of mitogen for the induction of IL-2 secretion, with a delayed peak level. A recent study investigated the secretion rate of stimulated PBMCs of patients with Sjögren's syndrome with and without accompanying myalgia. IL-1β and IL-6 secretion was reduced in PBMCs from patients with myalgia (Eriksson et al. 2004).

CYTOKINE PROFILES IN A COHORT OF PATIENTS WITH CHRONIC WIDESPREAD PAIN

Assuming alterations in the cytokine expression profile of patients with CWP compared to controls, we collected blood samples from 55 patients and 40 age- and gender-matched healthy volunteers for determination of mRNA expression and protein levels of a panel of cytokines. The relative blood mRNA expression and serum protein levels of the proinflammatory cytokines IL-2, IL-8, and TNF-α and of the anti-inflammatory cytokines IL-4, IL-10, and transforming growth factor-β1 (TGF-β1) were investigated by real-time polymerase chain reaction (PCR) and enzyme-linked immunosorbent assay (ELISA) (Üçeyler et al. 2006).

The CWP group comprised 40 patients ("patients I"), who received human pooled intravenous immunoglobulin (IVIG) at a dose of 10 g on three consecutive days as a novel treatment for otherwise therapy-refractory pain (Goebel et al. 2002). Twenty-six patients in this group fulfilled the ACR criteria for FM. Since IVIG can reduce the levels of IL-1, TNF-α, and IFN-γ (Aukrust et al. 1999; Gonzalez et al. 2004), to exclude possible confounding effects we recruited another 15 patients with CWP who did not receive IVIG treatment ("patients II").

After screening for several exclusion criteria that might influence systemic cytokine levels, such as strenuous physical activity (Pedersen et al. 1998) or alcohol consumption (Kovacs and Messingham 2002), we obtained venous blood for routine blood analysis, real-time PCR, and ELISA studies. Routine blood analysis was performed primarily to avoid the inclusion of patients with acute or chronic inflammatory diseases, which can also alter blood cytokine levels. For real-time PCR, mRNA was extracted from frozen blood samples according to a previously described protocol, with slight modifications (Kruse et al. 1997). After reverse transcription of mRNA to cDNA, the relative mRNA expression of the proinflammatory cytokines IL-2, IL-8, and TNF-α and of the anti-inflammatory cytokines IL-4, IL-10, and TGF-β1 were measured. The values were normalized to the endogenous control 18s-RNA.

REDUCED EXPRESSION OF IL-4 AND IL-10 mRNA

Blood mRNA expression of the proinflammatory cytokines IL-2, IL-8, and TNF-α did not differ between patients in group I and controls (Fig. 1A, C, E). In contrast, the mRNA levels of the anti-inflammatory cytokines IL-4 and IL-10 were significantly lower in patients from group I, with reductions to 24% ($P < 0.0001$) and 52% ($P = 0.03$), respectively, of the levels in healthy controls (Fig. 1B, D). Blood TGF-β1 mRNA levels did not differ between groups (Fig. 1F).

Patients in group II also showed no alterations in mRNA expression of IL-2, IL-8, TNF-α, and TGF-β1 compared to controls, but they had significantly lower blood IL-4 mRNA levels ($P < 0.001$). Their IL-10 mRNA expression was lower compared to controls as well, but the difference was not statistically significant.

LOWERED IL-4 AND IL-10 PROTEIN EXPRESSION

Serum protein levels of the pro- and anti-inflammatory cytokines were measured with commercial ELISA kits following the manufacturer's instructions. The results paralleled the mRNA findings. In sera of patients from group I, protein levels of TNF-α and TGF-β1 did not differ from those of controls

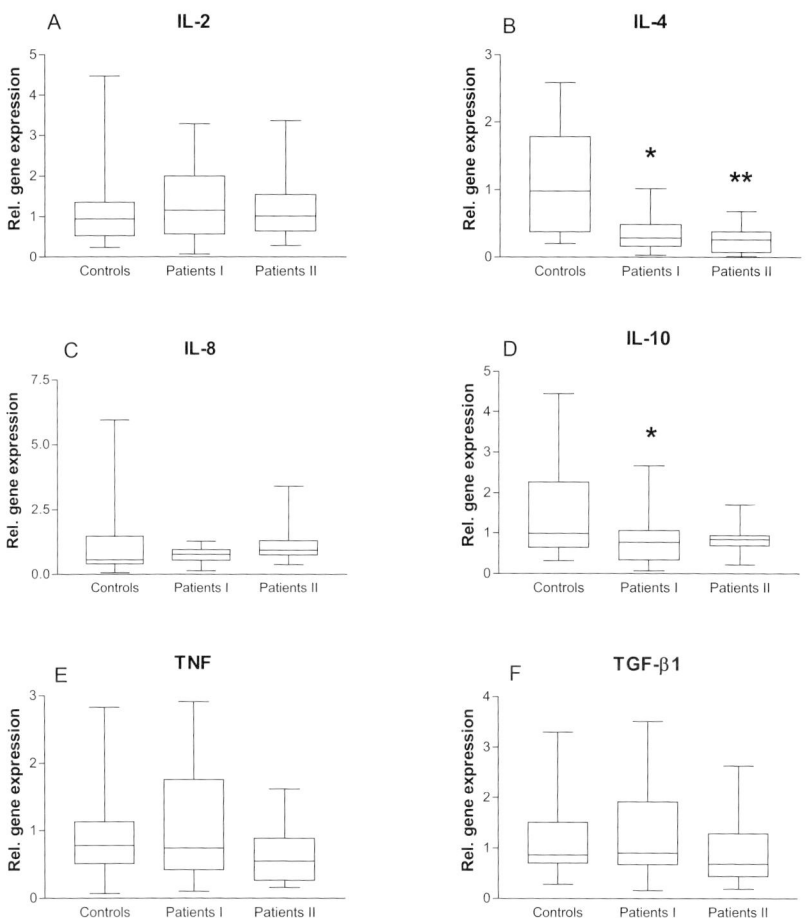

Fig. 1. Box plots showing the relative blood mRNA levels of the proinflammatory cytokines interleukin (IL)-2, IL-8, and tumor necrosis factor-α (TNF-α) (A, C, E) and the anti-inflammatory cytokines IL-4, IL-10, and transforming growth factor (TGF)-β1 (B, D, F) in two patient groups and in controls. Patients I: 40 patients with chronic widespread pain (CWP), who were enrolled in a treatment regimen with intravenous immunoglobulin (IVIG). Patients II: 15 patients with CWP, who did not receive IVIG. Relative IL-4 mRNA levels were significantly reduced in patients I and II compared to controls (patients I: * *P* < 0.0001; patients II: ** *P* < 0.001). IL-10 was also reduced in patients I (**P* = 0.03). No difference was found between patients and controls for IL-2, IL-8, TNF-α, and TGF-β1 relative mRNA levels. The box plots give the median (black horizontal line in the box), the upper 75th and lower 25th percentiles, and the outlier values. Data are from Üçeyler et al. (2006).

(Fig. 2C, D). However, for both the anti-inflammatory cytokines measured, IL-4 and IL-10, protein expression was significantly lower in the patients compared to controls (*P* < 0.0001 for IL-4 and *P* = 0.04 for IL-10) (Fig. 2A, B).

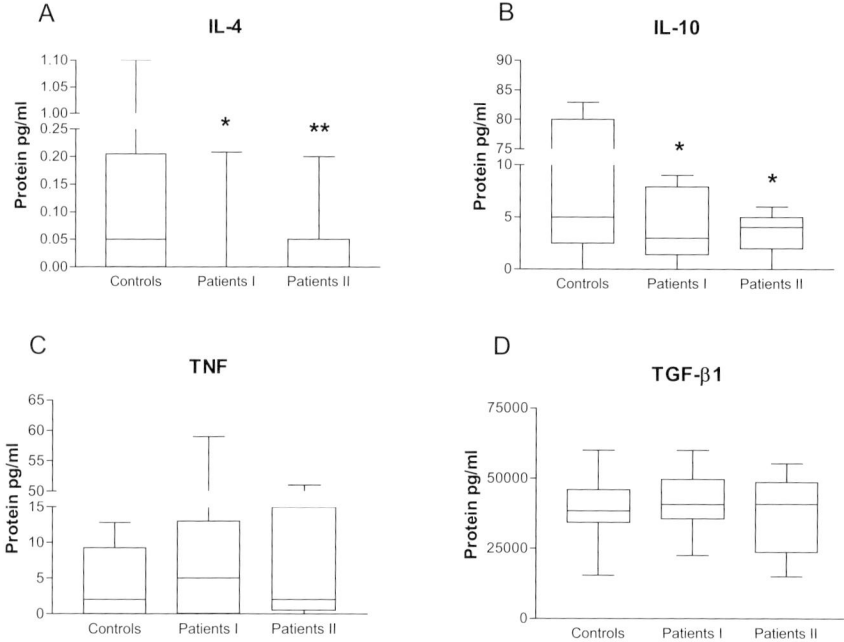

Fig. 2. Box plots showing the serum protein levels of (A) interleukin (IL)-4, (B) IL-10, (C) tumor necrosis factor-α (TNF-α), and (D) transforming growth factor (TGF)-β1 in two patient groups (as in Fig. 1) and in controls. TNF-α and TGF-β1 serum protein levels did not differ between groups. IL-4 and IL-10 protein levels were significantly lower in both patient groups compared to controls (IL-4: *$P < 0.0001$, **$P = 0.04$; IL-10: *$P = 0.04$). Data are from Üçeyler et al. (2006).

In sera of patients from group II, TNF-α and TGF-β1 protein levels again were similar to the control values (Fig. 2C, D). IL-4 and IL-10 protein levels were significantly lower in the patients than in the controls ($P = 0.04$ for both IL-4 and IL-10) (Fig. 2A, B).

ALTERATIONS IN CYTOKINE EXPRESSION

The reason for the observed reduction of IL-4 and IL-10 expression at the mRNA and protein level in patients with CWP is unknown. Besides the above-mentioned factors such as strenuous physical activity, IVIG treatment, alcohol consumption, or infectious diseases, several other conditions may have implications on systemic cytokine levels. For example, chronic pain is often accompanied by depression (Von Korff and Simon 1996). Cytokine expression may be influenced by depression and by antidepressant medication (Kubera et al. 2000; Gür et al. 2002; Miller and O'Callaghan 2005; Schiepers et al. 2005). However, no correlation was found between individual cytokine expression profiles and the assessment of items such as mood, sleep quality, fatigue, cognitive function, or pain (Üçeyler et al. 2006). Regulatory effects on DNA levels caused by polymorphisms in exons or promoter regions might be conceivable reasons for reduced cytokine levels, similar to other chronic diseases including schizophrenia or rheumatoid arthritis (Hobbs et al. 1998; Boin et al. 2001). However, no firm correlations between gene polymorphisms and pain have been shown for IL-4 or IL-10 to date.

ROLE OF ANTI-INFLAMMATORY CYTOKINES IN CHRONIC PAIN

While the impact of proinflammatory cytokines on pain perception is widely known and accepted, the importance of anti-inflammatory cytokines is less realized (Milligan et al. 2005; Hao et al. 2006). IL-4 and IL-10 are produced by a variety of different cells, and both are pleiotropic with several diverse actions. One major commonality, however, is their analgesic property (Kanaan et al. 1998; Vale et al. 2003; Milligan et al. 2005).

IL-10 is one of the main anti-inflammatory cytokines. The 18-kDa nonglycosylated human IL-10 polypeptide is encoded by a single-exon gene on chromosome 1q31-32. Several regulatory elements are known in the promoter region adjusting IL-10 production. The cells that produce IL-10 are T and B cells, macrophages, mast cells, and keratinocytes. The production of IL-10 is influenced by self-regulative circuits and by other cytokines such as IL-4, IL-13, and IFN-γ (Ding et al. 2003). In addition to its role in nociception, IL-10 is involved in many human disease states such as transplant rejection, autoimmunity, and angiogenesis (Ding 2003). In animal models of neuropathic pain, an increase of IL-10 mRNA levels is found, whereas IL-10 is reduced at the protein level (George et al. 2000, 2004; Kleinschnitz et al. 2004, 2005), and hyperalgesia is associated with low protein levels of IL-10. Thus, there is a discrepancy between the mRNA and protein levels. Low levels of the protein may reflect post-transcriptional or post-translational regulation of IL-10 synthesis. IL-10 protein exerts a negative feedback on its own production through IL-10 mRNA destabilization. The application of IL-10 protein directly or via gene transfer in turn reduces hyperalgesia (Kanaan et al. 1998; Vale et al. 2003; Milligan et al. 2005).

The human IL-4 gene is located on chromosome 5q23-31, close to the location of genes of related cytokines such as IL-13 or IL-3. The gene product is a 15-kDa glycoprotein. The human IL-4 gene has a number of binding sites for transcription factors, and its promoter displays several positive and negative regulatory sequences enhancing or silencing gene expression. Post-transcriptional regulation contains pathways of mRNA stabilization (via IL-7), and destabilization (via interferons). IL-4 acts on two receptor subtypes: the classical IL-4 receptor (consisting of the alpha and gamma chains) and the alternative IL-4 receptor (consisting of the alpha and alpha-1 chains). Because IL-13, another T-cell-derived cytokine, shares the alternative IL-4 receptor, both cytokines have overlapping effects. The main sources of IL-4 are activated CD4-positive T cells, mast cells, eosinophils, and basophils. IL-4 acts on T and B lymphocytes, natural killer cells, mast cells, synoviocytes, and endothelial cells and triggers the growth of B cells with consecutive antibody secretion. IL-4 is one of the major inducers of the Th2 immune pathway (Okada et al. 2003). IL-4 reduces the production of proinflammatory cytokines such as TNF-α, IL-1β, and IL-8 and enhances the production of IL-1-receptor antagonist. The analgesic effects of IL-4 are known from animal models in which pretreatment with IL-4 inhibited pain behavior after intraperitoneal application of acetic acid or zymosan (Vale et al. 2003). In a recent study, mechanical allodynia after L5 spinal nerve ligation in rats was attenuated by subcutaneous application of the viral vector S4IL-4 (Hao et al. 2006). In the context of the altered cytokine profiles in patients with CWP, it is thus conceivable that inflammation plays a role in the pathogenesis of the syndrome, in particular in FM. In fact, some clinicians would classify FM as a rheumatoid disorder.

Furthermore, a connection between the IL-4 and the opioid receptor system has been described. IL-4 induces and upregulates the transcription of μ- and δ-opioid receptors via a STAT6-binding site (Kraus et al. 2001; Börner et al. 2004). Lowered basal levels of IL-4 might entail a limited functional state of the endogenous opioid system due to reduced expression of opioid receptors. Diminished pain thresholds in patients with CWP and FM might be caused by reduced function of the endogenous opioid system. Additionally, reduced opioid receptor expression might result in the relative opioid resistance frequently seen in these patients.

In addition to the changes in cytokine profiles described above, further candidates from the large ligand families of pro- and anti-inflammatory cytokines may be involved in the pathophysiology of CWP. Different subgroups of chronic pain patients may even have distinct cytokine expression profiles. Characterizing these profiles and relating them to the clinical features may offer the chance to refine the differential diagnosis of chronic pain disorders. In addition, it is conceivable that restoring cytokine balance may be of therapeutic benefit in CWP and FM.

ACKNOWLEDGMENTS

This work was supported by research funds of the University of Würzburg.

REFERENCES

Amel Kashipaz MR, Swinden D, Todd I, Powell RJ. Normal production of inflammatory cytokines in chronic fatigue and fibromyalgia syndromes determined by intracellular cytokine staining in short-term cultured blood mononuclear cells. *Clin Exp Immunol* 2003; 132:360–365.

Arnold LM, Hudson JI, Hess EV, et al. Family study of fibromyalgia. *Arthritis Rheum* 2004a; 50:944–952.

Arnold LM, Lu Y, Crofford LJ, et al. A double-blind, multicenter trial comparing duloxetine with placebo in the treatment of fibromyalgia patients with or without major depressive disorder. *Arthritis Rheum* 2004b; 50:2974–2984.

Aukrust P, Muller F, Svenson M, et al. Administration of intravenous immunoglobulin (IVIG) in vivo—down-regulatory effects on the IL-1 system. *Clin Exp Immunol* 1999; 115:136–243.

Boin F, Zanardini R, Pioli R, et al. Association between –G308A tumor necrosis factor alpha gene polymorphism and schizophrenia. *Mol Psychiatry* 2001; 6:79–82.

Bondy B, Spaeth M, Offenbaecher M, et al. The T102C polymorphism of the 5-HT2A-receptor gene in fibromyalgia. *Neurobiol Dis* 1999; 6:433–439.

Börner C, Woltje M, Hollt V, Kraus J. STAT6 transcription factor binding sites with mismatches within the canonical 5'-TTC … GAA-3' motif involved in regulation of delta- and mu-opioid receptors. *J Neurochem* 2004; 91:1493–1500.

Buskila D, Neumann L, Hazanov I, Carmi R. Familial aggregation in the fibromyalgia syndrome. *Semin Arthritis Rheum* 1996; 26:605–611.

Cieza A, Stucki G, Weigl M, et al. ICF Core Sets for chronic widespread pain. *J Rehabil Med* 2004:63–68.

Cohen H, Buskila D, Neumann L, Ebstein RP. Confirmation of an association between fibromyalgia and serotonin transporter promoter region (5-HTTLPR) polymorphism, and relationship to anxiety-related personality traits. *Arthritis Rheum* 2002; 46:845–847.

Crofford LJ, Pillemer SR, Kalogeras KT, et al. Hypothalamic-pituitary-adrenal axis perturbations in patients with fibromyalgia. *Arthritis Rheum* 1994; 37:1583–1592.

Crofford LJ, Engleberg NC, Demitrack MA. Neurohormonal perturbations in fibromyalgia. *Baillieres Clin Rheumatol* 1996; 10:365–738.

Crofford LJ, Rowbotham MC, Mease PJ, et al. Pregabalin for the treatment of fibromyalgia syndrome: Results of a randomized, double-blind, placebo-controlled trial. *Arthritis Rheum* 2005; 52:1264–1273.

Ding YZ, Fu S, Zamarin D, Bromberg J. Interleukin 10. In: Thomson AW, Lotze MT (Eds). *The Cytokine Handbook,* 4th ed. London: Academic Press, 2003, pp 603–625.

Eriksson P, Andersson C, Ekerfelt C, Ernerudh J, Skogh T. Sjögren's syndrome with myalgia is associated with subnormal secretion of cytokines by peripheral blood mononuclear cells. *J Rheumatol* 2004; 31:729–735.

Ernberg M, Voog U, Alstergren P, Lundeberg T, Kopp S. Plasma and serum serotonin levels and their relationship to orofacial pain and anxiety in fibromyalgia. *J Orofac Pain* 2000; 14:37–46.

George A, Marziniak M, Schäfers M, Toyka KV, Sommer C. Thalidomide treatment in chronic constrictive neuropathy decreases endoneurial tumor necrosis factor-alpha, increases interleukin-10 and has long-term effects on spinal cord dorsal horn met-enkephalin. *Pain* 2000; 88:267–275.

George A, Buehl A, Sommer C. Wallerian degeneration after crush injury of rat sciatic nerve increases endo- and epineurial tumor necrosis factor-alpha protein. *Neurosci Lett* 2004; 372:215–219.

Goebel A, Netal S, Schedel R, Sprotte G. Human pooled immunoglobulin in the treatment of chronic pain syndromes. *Pain Med* 2002; 3:119–127.

Gonzalez H, Khademi M, Andersson M, et al. Prior poliomyelitis-IVIG treatment reduces proinflammatory cytokine production. *J Neuroimmunol* 2004; 150:139–144.

Griep EN, Boersma JW, de Kloet ER. Altered reactivity of the hypothalamic-pituitary-adrenal axis in the primary fibromyalgia syndrome. *J Rheumatol* 1993; 20:469–474.

Griep EN, Boersma JW, Lentjes EG, et al. Function of the hypothalamic-pituitary-adrenal axis in patients with fibromyalgia and low back pain. *J Rheumatol* 1998; 25:1374–1381.

Gür A, Karakoç M, Nas K, et al. Cytokines and depression in cases with fibromyalgia. *J Rheumatol* 2002; 29:358–361.

Gürsoy S. Absence of association of the serotonin transporter gene polymorphism with the mentally healthy subset of fibromyalgia patients. *Clin Rheumatol* 2002; 21:194–197.

Gürsoy S, Erdal E, Herken H, Madenci E, Alaşehirli B. Association of T102C polymorphism of the 5-HT2A receptor gene with psychiatric status in fibromyalgia syndrome. *Rheumatol Int* 2001; 21:58–61.

Hader N, Rimon D, Kinarty A, Lahat N. Altered interleukin-2 secretion in patients with primary fibromyalgia syndrome. *Arthritis Rheum* 1991; 34:866–872.

Hao S, Mata M, Glorioso JC, Fink DJ. HSV-mediated expression of interleukin-4 in dorsal root ganglion neurons reduces neuropathic pain. *Mol Pain* 2006; 2:6.

Hobbs K, Negri J, Klinnert M, Rosenwasser LJ, Borish L. Interleukin-10 and transforming growth factor-beta promoter polymorphisms in allergies and asthma. *Am J Respir Crit Care Med* 1998; 158:1958–1962.

Hunt IM, Silman AJ, Benjamin S, McBeth J, Macfarlane GJ. The prevalence and associated features of chronic widespread pain in the community using the 'Manchester' definition of chronic widespread pain. *Rheumatology (Oxford)* 1999; 38:275–279.

Kanaan SA, Poole S, Saade NE, Jabbur S, Safieh-Garabedian B. Interleukin-10 reduces the endo-toxin-induced hyperalgesia in mice. *J Neuroimmunol* 1998; 86:142–150.

Kato K, Sullivan PF, Evengard B, Pedersen NL. Importance of genetic influences on chronic widespread pain. *Arthritis Rheum* 2006; 54:1682–1686.

Kleinschnitz C, Brinkhoff J, Zelenka M, Sommer C, Stoll G. The extent of cytokine induction in peripheral nerve lesions depends on the mode of injury and NMDA receptor signaling. *J Neuroimmunol* 2004; 149:77–83.

Kleinschnitz C, Brinkhoff J, Sommer C, Stoll G. Contralateral cytokine gene induction after peripheral nerve lesions: dependence on the mode of injury and NMDA receptor signaling. *Brain Res Mol Brain Res* 2005; 136:23–28.

Kovacs EJ, Messingham KA. Influence of alcohol and gender on immune response. *Alcohol Res Health* 2002; 26:257–263.

Kraus J, Börner C, Giannini E, et al. Regulation of mu-opioid receptor gene transcription by interleukin-4 and influence of an allelic variation within a STAT6 transcription factor binding site. *J Biol Chem* 2001; 276:43901–43908.

Kruse N, Pette M, Toyka K, Rieckmann P. Quantification of cytokine mRNA expression by RT PCR in samples of previously frozen blood. *J Immunol Methods* 1997; 210:195–203.

Kubera M, Kenis G, Bosmans E, et al. Suppressive effect of TRH and imipramine on human inter-feron-gamma and interleukin-10 production in vitro. *Pol J Pharmacol* 2000; 52:481–486.

Laske C, Stransky E, Eschweiler GW, et al. Increased BDNF serum concentration in fibromyalgia with or without depression or antidepressants. *J Psychiatr Res* 2007; 41:600–605.

Marchand F, Perretti M, McMahon SB. Role of the immune system in chronic pain. *Nat Rev Neurosci* 2005; 6:521–532.

Mense S. Neurobiological concepts of fibromyalgia--the possible role of descending spinal tracts. *Scand J Rheumatol Suppl* 2000; 113:24–29.

Miller DB, O'Callaghan JP. Depression, cytokines, and glial function. *Metabolism* 2005; 54:33–38.

Milligan ED, Sloane EM, Langer SJ, et al. Controlling neuropathic pain by adeno-associated virus driven production of the anti-inflammatory cytokine, interleukin-10. *Mol Pain* 2005; 1:9.

Neeck G, Riedel W. Hormonal perturbations in fibromyalgia syndrome. *Ann N Y Acad Sci* 1999; 876:325–338.

Neumann L, Buskila D. Epidemiology of fibromyalgia. *Curr Pain Headache Rep* 2003; 7:362–368.

Offenbaecher M, Bondy B, de Jonge S, et al. Possible association of fibromyalgia with a polymorphism in the serotonin transporter gene regulatory region. *Arthritis Rheum* 1999; 42:2482–2488.

Okada H, Banchereau J, Lotze MT. Interleukin 4. In: Thomson AW, Lotze MT (Eds). *The Cytokine Handbook,* 4th ed. London: Academic Press, 2003, pp 227–262.

Pedersen BK, Ostrowski K, Rohde T, Bruunsgaard H. The cytokine response to strenuous exercise. *Can J Physiol Pharmacol* 1998; 76:505–511.

Pellegrino MJ, Waylonis GW, Sommer A. Familial occurrence of primary fibromyalgia. *Arch Phys Med Rehabil* 1989; 70:61–3.

Rau CL, Russell IJ. Is fibromyalgia a distinct clinical syndrome? *Curr Rev Pain* 2000; 4:287–294.

Russell IJ, Michalek JE, Vipraio GA, et al. Platelet 3H-imipramine uptake receptor density and serum serotonin levels in patients with fibromyalgia/fibrositis syndrome. *J Rheumatol* 1992; 19:104–109.

Russell IJ, Orr MD, Littman B, et al. Elevated cerebrospinal fluid levels of substance P in patients with the fibromyalgia syndrome. *Arthritis Rheum* 1994; 37:1593–1601.

Salemi S, Aeschlimann A, Gay RE, et al. Expression and localization of opioid receptors in muscle satellite cells: no difference between fibromyalgia patients and healthy subjects. *Arthritis Rheum* 2003; 48:3291–3293.

Samborski W, Stratz T, Schochat T, Mennet P, Müller W. Biochemische Veranderungen bei der Fibromyalgie [Biochemical changes in fibromyalgia]. *Z Rheumatol* 1996; 55:168–173.

Schiepers OJ, Wichers MC, Maes M. Cytokines and major depression. *Prog Neuropsychopharmacol Biol Psychiatry* 2005; 29:201–217.

Sommer C. Cytokines and pain. In: Aminoff MJ, Boller F, Swaab DF (Eds). *Handbook of Neurology.* Amsterdam: Elsevier, 2006, pp 231–248.

Staud R, Price DD, Robinson ME, Mauderli AP, Vierck CJ. Maintenance of windup of second pain requires less frequent stimulation in fibromyalgia patients compared to normal controls. *Pain* 2004; 110:689–696.

Taskinen HS, Olsson T, Bucht A, et al. Peripheral nerve injury induces endoneurial expression of IFN-gamma, IL-10 and TNF-alpha mRNA. *J Neuroimmunol* 2000; 102:17–25.

Üçeyler N, Valenza R, Stock M, et al. Reduced levels of antiinflammatory cytokines in patients with chronic widespread pain. *Arthritis Rheum* 2006; 54:2656–2664.

Vale ML, Marques JB, Moreira CA, et al. Antinociceptive effects of interleukin-4, -10, and -13 on the writhing response in mice and zymosan-induced knee joint incapacitation in rats. *J Pharmacol Exp Ther* 2003; 304:102–108.

Von Korff M, Simon G. The relationship between pain and depression. *Br J Psychiatry Suppl* 1996:101–108.

Wallace DJ, Margolin K, Waller P. Fibromyalgia and interleukin-2 therapy for malignancy. *Ann Intern Med* 1988; 108:909.

Wallace DJ, Linker-Israeli M, Hallegua D, et al. Cytokines play an aetiopathogenetic role in fibromyalgia: a hypothesis and pilot study. *Rheumatology (Oxford)* 2001; 40:743–749.

Wolfe F, Smythe HA, Yunus MB, et al. The American College of Rheumatology 1990 criteria for the classification of fibromyalgia. Report of the Multicenter Criteria Committee. *Arthritis Rheum* 1990; 33:160–172.

Wolfe F, Ross K, Anderson J, Russell IJ, Hebert L. The prevalence and characteristics of fibromyalgia in the general population. *Arthritis Rheum* 1995; 38:19–28.

Wolfe F, Russell IJ, Vipraio G, Ross K, Anderson J. Serotonin levels, pain threshold, and fibromyalgia symptoms in the general population. *J Rheumatol* 1997; 24:555–559.

Yunus MB, Khan MA, Rawlings KK, et al. Genetic linkage analysis of multicase families with fibromyalgia syndrome. *J Rheumatol* 1999; 26:408–412.

Zelenka M, Schäfers M, Sommer C. Intraneural injection of interleukin-1beta and tumor necrosis factor-alpha into rat sciatic nerve at physiological doses induces signs of neuropathic pain. *Pain* 2005; 116:257–263.

Correspondence to: Prof. Dr. Claudia Sommer, Department of Neurology, University of Würzburg, Josef-Schneider-Str. 11, 97080 Würzburg, Germany. Tel: 49-931-201-23763; fax: +49-931-201-23697; email: sommer@mail.uni-wuerzburg.de.

Index

Locators in italic refer to figures; locators followed by t refer to tables.

A

Aβ fibers, 158
Acetyl coenzyme A, 27
Action potentials, 90
Adalimumab, 74, 87, 394
Adenosine monophosphate, cyclic (cAMP), 67
Adenosine triphosphate (ATP)
  in chronic pain, 284
  inducing tactile allodynia in neuropathic pain, 286
  interactions with P2X4 receptor, 289
  microglial response to, 23
  receptor expression on spinal microglia, 284–285
Adhesion molecules, 179, 389
AIDS-related dementia, 299
Alexander's disease, 239
Allodynia
  ATP-stimulated microglia in, 23, 343
  definition, 68–69
  hyperalgesia vs., 69
  mechanical
    in experimental autoimmune neuropathy, 4
    microglial activation in, 299
    propentofylline for, 345
  p38 inhibition preventing, 306–307
  tactile
    ATP/P2X4-receptor induction of, 286
    chemokines causing, 132
    glycoprotein 120 causing, 307
    thalidomide preventing, 393–394
Alzheimer's disease, 47, 239, 299
Amines, sympathetic, 67
γ-aminobutyric acid (GABA), 237, 288
AMPA (α-amino-3-hydroxy-5-methyl-4-isoxazolepropionic acid), 25–26, 98
AMPA receptors (AMPARs)
  activity-dependent changes in trafficking, 210–211
  calcium-permeable, 221–222

excitatory postsynaptic function, 210–212
surface localization in neuronal dysfunction, 212–216
TNF-α and, 200–201, 213–215, 216
Amyotrophic lateral sclerosis, 47, 239, 299
Anakinra, 74, 190, 394
Analgesia, stress-induced, 113–114
Anti-TNF-α therapy
  for rheumatoid arthritis, 72
  for sciatica, 190, 393–395, 398–399
Arthritis. See also Rheumatoid arthritis
  collagen-induced, 76
  osteoarthritis, 391
Astrocyte-neuron lactate shuttle, 347–349, 348, 349
Astrocytes
  blood-brain barrier and, 47, 342
  in CNS glial cells, 46
  cytokine/chemokine secretion, 47–48
  in dorsal horn, 167
  as excitable cells, 234
  fibrous, 229
  function of, 25–33, 320–322
    in calcium ion homeostasis, 27–29, 30–31
    glutamatergic activity, 25–27, 26
    potassium ion homeostasis, 29, 31–33, 32
  glutamate regulation by, 345–346
  glutamate transporters and, 238, 277, 321, 348
  glycolysis, 348
  as immunocompetent cells, 320
  in inflammatory mediation, 321–322
  interleukin-6 activation of STAT-3 in, 49–50
  marker antigen expression, 342–343
  microglia interactions with, 24–25, 320
  morphology and ultrastructure, 21–22, 229–230
  neuroenergetics and, 347–349, 348, 349
  in neuronal function, 29, 33–34, 47–48, 320–322